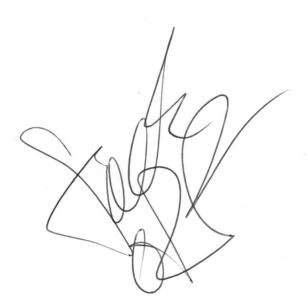

Handbook of
Methods in Gastrointestinal Pharmacology

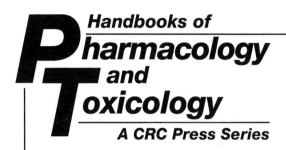

Handbooks of Pharmacology and Toxicology
A CRC Press Series

Mannfred A. Hollinger, Series Editor
University of California, Davis

Published Titles

Handbook of Pharmacokinetics/Pharmacodynamic Correlation
Hartmut Derendorf and Günther Hochhaus

Handbook of Methods in Gastrointestinal Pharmacology
Timothy S. Gaginella

Forthcoming Titles

Handbook of Mammalian Models in Biomedical Research
David B. Jack

Handbook of Pharmacology of Aging
Jay Roberts

Handbook of Theoretical Models in Biomedical Research
David B. Jack

Handbook of
Methods in Gastrointestinal Pharmacology

Edited by

Timothy S. Gaginella, Ph.D.
Adjunct Professor of Pharmacology
School of Pharmacy
University of Wisconsin
Madison, Wisconsin

CRC Press
Boca Raton   New York   London   Tokyo

Library of Congress Cataloging-in-Publication Data

Handbook of methods in gastrointestinal pharmacology / edited by
    Timothy S. Gaginella.
       p. cm. – (Handbook of pharmacology and toxicology)
    Includes bibliographical references and index.
    ISBN 0-8493-8304-8 (hardcover : alk. paper)
      1. Gastrointestinal agents–Research–Methodology.
    2. Gastroenterology–Research–Methodology. I. Gaginella, Timothy
    S. II. Series.
      [DNLM: 1. Gastrointestinal Diseases–drug therapy–handbooks.
    2. Gastrointestinal Agents–therapeutic use–handbooks. WI 39 M592
    1995]
    RM355.M48 1995
    615′.73—dc20
    DNLM/DLC
    for Library of Congress   95-15500
                                                                               CIP

PREFACE

Gastroenterology has advanced through the development and application of increasingly sophisticated methods to measure changes in gastrointestinal function. While methods for studying the effects of endogenous mediators and drugs on the gut exist, they are widely scattered throughout the scientific literature. This volume brings together, in one reference work (a handbook), details on the most commonly employed experimental approaches in investigative gastroenterology. *In vivo* techniques involving whole animals, isolated tissue methodology, the use of single cell systems, and molecular biology approaches are discussed.

Central and peripheral control of gastroduodenal secretion, intestinal transport, intestinal motility and sphincter function, enteric neural control mechanisms (including evaluation of visceral pain), and motion sickness are covered. Approaches to studying drug and electrolyte absorption and secretion by the intestine, smooth muscle contractility and central nervous system control of motility are included. Additional chapters deal with the intestine as a model of opiate dependence and methods for studying splanchnic blood flow and mucosal mast cells. The concluding chapter provides the reader with an overview of molecular pharmacology/cell biology techniques that have been or can be applied to study gastrointestinal pharmacology.

An especially important value of the book is the emphasis on advantages and disadvantages of each technique as approaches to answering specific research questions. The wide variety of topics included should make this book useful to established investigators, research fellows, and graduate students. It is anticipated that it will also be useful to reviewers of grants and manuscripts to clarify questions that arise regarding appropriate use of a technique in a particular research setting.

I wish to thank all of the authors for the conscientious and thorough preparation of their respective chapters, and for their patience in coping with the details necessary to bring this volume to completion. The thoughtful editorial assistance of Gerry Jaffe at CRC Press is greatly appreciated. Special thanks to BJ for untiring effort and support during all stages of the work on this book.

Timothy S. Gaginella, Ph.D.

EDITOR

Timothy S. Gaginella, Ph.D. is Adjunct Professor of Pharmacology in the School of Pharmacy, the University of Wisconsin and a consultant to the pharmaceutical industry. Dr. Gaginella earned a B.S. degree in Pharmacy in 1968, an M.S. in 1972, and a Ph.D. in Pharmacology in 1974, all from the University of Wisconsin. After a two year Research Fellowship in gastroenterology at the Mayo Clinic, Dr. Gaginella joined The Ohio State University College of Pharmacy as Assistant Professor of Pharmacology in 1976. Subsequently, he held positions of Associate Professor of Pharmacology at the College of Pharmacy and Associate Professor of Medicine and Physiology at the College of Medicine, The Ohio State University; Research Group Chief, Department of Pharmacology, Hoffmann LaRoche, Inc.; Director of Gastrointestinal Biology, Searle Research and Development; and Vice President, Aphton Corporation.

Dr. Gaginella is a member of The American Gastroenterological Association, American Physiological Society, and the American Society for Pharmacology and Experimental Therapeutics (ASPET). He is Chairman of the ASPET Section for Gastrointestinal Pharmacology and Chairman of the Gastrointestinal Pharmacology Section of The International Union of Pharmacology (IUPHAR).

Dr. Gaginella has been a Specific Field Editor for Gastrointestinal Pharmacology for the *Journal of Pharmacology and Experimental Therapeutics*, and he has been or is now a member of the Editorial Boards of the *American Journal of Physiology, Digestive Diseases and Sciences, Annals of Pharmacotherapy*, and the *Journal of Pharmacology and Experimental Therapeutics*.

Dr. Gaginella's research interests include the effect of drugs on gastrointestinal absorption and secretion, particularly the mechanism of action of laxatives, antidiarrheal drugs, and drugs used as therapy for inflammatory bowel disease. His research has been funded by the National Institutes of Health, the Crohn's and Colitis Foundation, and the pharmaceutical industry. Dr. Gaginella is the recipient of an NIH Research Career Development Award and has served on various NIH grant review committees. He is co-inventor on one patent, and his bibliography includes over 150 peer-reviewed research articles and reviews.

CONTRIBUTORS

Jose C. Barreto, Ph.D.
Department of Surgery
University of Texas Medical School
Houston, Texas

Paul Bass, Ph.D.
School of Pharmacy
University of Wisconsin
Madison, Wisconsin

A. Dean Befus, Ph.D.
Department of Medicine
University of Alberta
Edmonton, Alberta, Canada

Elyse Bissonnette, Ph.D.
Department of Medicine
University of Alberta
Edmonton, Alberta, Canada

David R. Brown, Ph.D.
Department of Veterinary Pathobiology
University of Minnesota
St. Paul, Minnesota

Lionel Bueno, Ph.D.
Department of Pharmacology
INRA
Toulouse, France

Thomas F. Burks, Ph.D.
Department of Research and Academic
  Affairs
University of Texas Health Science Center
Houston, Texas

Geoffrey Burnstock, D.Sc., F.A.A.
Department of Anatomy and Developmental
  Biology and Centre for Neuroscience
University College
London, United Kingdom

Beth Chin, M.Sc.
Department of Gastrointestinal Sciences
University of Calgary
Calgary, Alberta, Canada

Karen D. Crissinger, M.D., Ph.D.
Department of Physiology
Louisiana State University Medical Center
Shreveport, Louisiana

Kenneth R. DeVault, M.D.
Department of Medicine
Mayo Clinic Jacksonville
Jacksonville, Florida

Timothy S. Gaginella, Ph.D.
School of Pharmacy
University of Wisconsin
Madison, Wisconsin

James J. Galligan, Ph.D.
Department of Pharmacology and
  Toxicology
Michigan State University
East Lansing, Michigan

Gerald F. Gebhart, Ph.D.
Department of Pharmacology
University of Iowa
Iowa City, Iowa

D. Neil Granger, Ph.D.
Department of Physiology and Biophysics
Louisiana State University Medical Center
Shreveport, Louisiana

John R. Grider, Ph.D.
Department of Physiology
Medical College of Virginia
Richmond, Virginia

Charles H. V. Hoyle, Ph.D.
Department of Anatomy and Developmental
  Biology and Centre for Neuroscience
University College
London, United Kingdom

Vicente Martínez, Ph.D.
CURE/Gastroenteric Biology Center
VA Wadsworth Medical Center and
Department of Medicine and Brain
  Research Institute
University of California Los Angeles
Los Angeles, California

Laurence J. Miller, M.D.
Center for Basic Research in Digestive
  Diseases
Mayo Clinic and Foundation
Rochester, Minnesota

Thomas A. Miller, M.D.
Department of Surgery
University of Texas Medical School
Houston, Texas

K. S. Murthy, Ph.D.
Department of Physiology
Medical College of Virginia
Richmond, Virginia

Scott M. O'Grady, Ph.D.
Department of Physiology and Animal
  Science
University of Minnesota
St. Paul, Minnesota

William H. Percy, Ph.D.
Department of Physiology and
  Pharmacology
University of South Dakota Medical School
Vermillion, South Dakota

Satish Rattan, D.V.M.
Department of Medicine
Jefferson Medical College
Thomas Jefferson University
Philadelphia, Pennsylvania

Jyotirindra N. Sengupta, Ph.D.
Department of Pharmacology
College of Medicine
University of Iowa
Iowa City, Iowa

Terez Shea-Donohue, Ph.D.
Department of Medicine
Uniformed Services University of the
  Health Sciences
Bethesda, Maryland

Gregory S. Smith, Ph.D.
Department of Surgery
University of Texas Medical School
Houston, Texas

Philip L. Smith, Ph.D.
Department of Drug Delivery
SmithKline Beecham
King of Prussia, Pennsylvania

John J. Stewart, Ph.D.
Department of Pharmacology
Louisiana State University Medical School
Shreveport, Louisiana

Yvette Taché, Ph.D.
CURE/Gastroenteric Biology Center
VA Wadworth Medical Center and
Department of Medicine and Brain
  Research Institute
University of California Los Angeles
Los Angeles, California

Charles D. Ulrich II, M.D.
Center for Basic Research in Digestive
  Diseases
Mayo Clinic and Foundation
Rochester, Minnesota

Norman Weisbrodt, Ph.D.
Department of Physiology
University of Texas Medical School
Houston, Texas

Charles D. Wood, Ph.D.
Department of Pharmacology
Louisiana State University Medical School
Shreveport, Louisiana

TABLE OF CONTENTS

1 Methods for Assessing Gastric Secretion

Terez Shea-Donohue

"And if one considers . . . the adjacent viscera, like a lot of burning hearths around a great cauldron - . . . you may believe what an extraordinary alteration it is which occurs in the food taken into the stomach." Galen (second century A.D.)

HISTORICAL APPROACHES TO THE STUDY OF DIGESTION

THE ANCIENTS

Some of the first insights into gastric function were provided by Eraristratus, a member of the Greek Alexandrian school, in the third century B.C. His crude metabolic experiments attributing hunger to an empty stomach, however, were the result of a philosophical rather than scientific inquiry and must be interpreted as such. The ancients used the term "pneuma" or life force as a way of elevating man above the rest of the animal life. Air, taken in through the lungs, was refined in the heart becoming a vital spirit distributed to all parts of the body including the brain. In the brain, however, the pneuma was further purified into a psychic spirit for higher activities and distributed to the rest of the body by the nerves. In the second century A.D., Galen (131 - >210 A.D.), a Greek of the Alexandrian school who migrated to Rome and prospered under the patronage of Marcus Aurelius, expanded the idea of pneuma to include the alimentary tract as a source of life. Food was changed by the liver into blood imbued with the natural spirit. Galen believed that every organ was ideal for a particular bodily function. His treatise entitled "On the Natural Faculties"[1], contained a lively criticism of the principles of Eraristratus, and assigned four functions to the stomach, *facultas attratix, facultas retentrix, facultas alteratrix,* and *facultas expultrix*. These qualities were responsible for the "attraction" of food to the stomach where there was an interaction between two bodies, the stronger mastering the weaker. Galen claimed that Eraristratus was incorrect in his assumption that digestion was merely a mechanical process, rather, the mastery of the stomach over food produced an alteration which was aided by the addition of gastric juice, bile, pneuma and innate heat. Galen was also the first to consider abnormal function of the stomach. His writings include a reference to ulceration, the treatment of the day being coral powder (calcium carbonate). Heat, however, played the most important role in impaired function.

For the next several centuries, the widespread social instability was incompatible with scientific research. There were some 50 emperors in as many years post Galen. Mohammed came in 622 A.D., and by 722 A.D. the Moslems had conquered half of the known world. Arabic was the scientific language of the East while Latin and Greek were used in the West. Astrology exerted a tremendous influence on thought throughout the Middle Ages and was considered as

0-8493-8304-8/96/$0.00+$.50

1

much of a science as Medicine and Law. The beliefs of St. Augustine in the fifth century were typical of the Chistian world at this time in that all diseases were ascribed to the work of demons.

> "One of the first experiments that ought to be tried with this fluid . . . would be to make it dissolve meat in a vessel just as it dissolves it in the stomach. Actual digestion of aliments taking place under such abnormal conditions would be a most singular and interesting pheniomenon."
> R. A. F. Reaumur (1752)

THE SCHOLARS

Following the establishment of universities in the twelfth century, scientific research was concentrated in these centers of higher learning. The study of human anatomy relied on the work of Galen which had been translated and changed over the centuries. However, Galen had made his observations on animals, not humans, and the extrapolation of his observations to humans was not always accurate. Despite these handicaps, by the fourteenth century the general belief was that the stomach churned food and prepared it for passage into the lower abdominal by a process described as concoction. Dorland's Medical dictionary defines this as 1) a mixture of medicinal substances prepared by the aid of heat, 2) the digestive process. Heat was responsible for digestion but the source of the heat was not ingested food. The gastric juices were thought to come from the spleen.

With the fall of Constantinople in the mid-fifteenth century, there was a reemergence of original Latin and Greek texts with the flight of Eastern scholars to the West. There was also a renewed interest in Galen's work. Phillipus Aureolus Theophastus Bombast von Hehenheim (1493–1541), alias Paracelsus, was called the "Luther of Medicine" because of his disagreement with the Galenic tradition. An alchemist and a mystic, in the Christian sense, he is hailed as the first pharmacologist, introducing the elements of sulphur, mercury, and salt into pharmaceutical chemistry. In addition, he proposed that there were several varieties of foodstuffs which were handled in different ways during digestion. Despite this forward thinking, he did not forsake entirely the Galenic contribution of vital forces to the digestive process. Paracelsus put forth the principle of *Arachaeus,* a vital force in the stomach which separated useless from useful food. Failure of this process resulted in the accumulation of deleterious tartar which was the source of many illnesses. Cathartics were prescribed to purge this unwanted material.

The final break with the principles of Galen were attributed to Andreus Vesalius (1514–1564) who published his second edition of *Fabrica*[2] in 1555. His major contribution to research lies in his support of a novel approach to scientific inquiry. Essentially, observation was held above interpretation, ensuring the immortality of the results rather than the discussion section of published papers. The invention of movable type during the Rennaissance made a greater dissemination of scientific knowledge possible.

Further knowledge of gastric function awaited the arrival of chemistry. Jean Baptiste Van Helmont (1577–1644) a spiritualist and Paracelcian, studied philosophy, law, and medicine all before the age of 22. He introduced two new words into digestion, *blas* and *gas. Blas* was similar to the *Archaeus* of Paracelsus but *gas* is what we know as carbon dioxide. The term fermentation was used to describe digestion but the process was spiritual rather than physical. Food passed through a series of "digestions" using different ferments. Thus, the first digestion began in the stomach using the ferment of gastric juice which came from the spleen. The second digestion was in the duodenum using ferment in the bile brought from the liver. The sixth and last digestion used an innate ferment specific for each place, a process now called metabolism in its most basic form. It was Francois de la Boe, known as Franciscus Sylvius (1614–1672) who removed fermentation from the spiritual realm and placed it at the level of bench-top chemistry. The process no longer had a character of its own that was distinguishable from chemical events.

While Van Helmont introduced the concept of individual organs processing their own food, Santorio Santorio (1561–1636) applied this concept to the entire body. Best known for his study of insensible perspiration, he recognized the value of precision instruments and multiple measurements. He performed the simple experiment of weighing himself in a special chair before and after various activities. Insensible perspiration was used to explain differences in body weight that could not be accounted for by more visible bodily functions of eating, sweating, or defecation. Reports of his experiments published in *Ars de statica medicina*[3], however, were not made for the sake of science, but were a series of aphorisms to help men live by the rule.

During the seventeenth century, the iatrochemical and iatrophysical schools of thought espoused the idea that digestion was primarily a chemical or a mechanical event respectively. However, publication of the *Institutiones Medicae*[4] in 1708 by Herman Boerhave (1668–1738) consolidated the two views, declaring that solid food was brought into a state of solution assisted by mechanical titration. In this century there would be a number of important discoveries about digestion in the stomach. Rene de Reaumur (1683–1757), elected to the *Academie Francais* at the age of 25, made several important observations on the properties of gastric juice in birds. In an article entitled *"Sur la digestion des oiseaux"*[5], Reaumur recounts experiments using his pet kite, a type of buzzard that conveniently vomited all inedible food. The bird would be fed a sponge to which a string was attached. When it was brought up, Reaumur isolated the gastric juice and examined its properties. Unfortunately, the death of the pet during the course of his experiments forced Reaumur to consider less cooperative birds such as ducks and chickens. His contribution lies in the observation that the gastric juice was capable of digesting food outside the body, reducing the importance of pancreatic juice which was thought to be the source of digestion, aided by saliva and bile.

Lazaro Spallanzani (1729–1799) repeated the experiments of Reaumur using himself as a subject. In his work *Dissertazioni di fisica animale e vegetabile*[6], he eloquently described the need for observations in humans. He confirmed the observation of the solvent powers of gastric juice, but mistakenly concluded that the gastric juice was neutral. In 1777, Edward Stevens concluded that gastric juice contained an active component that was necessary for the assimilation of food.[7]

John Hunter published an article entitled *"On the Digestion of the Stomach After Death"*[8] in which he concluded that the gastric juice was acidic but only after death. Then, in 1803, John Young (1782–1804), published his thesis work on digestion entitled *"An Experimental Inquiry into the Principles of Nutrition and the Digestive Process."*[9] In it he states that:

> "We were first lead to suppose, the acid was only present when the viscus was in the morbid state; but experiments proved to us the contrary . . . being thus fully persuaded the acid, in the digested food of frogs, did not arise from a fermentation, but was to be referred to their gastric juice, we were lead by analogy to suppose, the acid of our own stomachs was to be attributed to the same origin."

At last, gastric digestion was no longer considered to be a process of heat, fermentation, or putrefaction. Unfortunately, Young concluded that the acid was phosphoric acid and we are left to wonder that if not for his untimely death in 1804, this gifted young scientist might have ultimately corrected his mistake.

The close relationship between chemistry and gastric physiology took a giant step in 1824 with the publication of *"On the nature of the acid and saline matters usually existing in the stomachs of animals"*,[10] by William Prout (1785–1850). He is credited with the identifying the free acid in gastric juice as hydrochloric acid. At the same time, William Beaumont (1785–1853), began his legendary studies of the stomach. On June 6, 1822, a fur trapper by the name of Alexis St. Martin was wounded accidently in the abdomen by a shot gun fired at close range. Beaumont was the military surgeon called to tend St. Martin who was not expected to survive his injury. Surprisingly, St. Martin recovered but was left with a 2.5 inch hole in his abdomen opening directly into the stomach. The repeated efforts of Beaumont over two years to close the wound were unsuccessful but gave Beaumont time to realize the potential for experimentation. During four extended periods of observation over the next ten years Beaumont was able to study the digestion of food over time, the effect of exercise, weather and emotion on the stomach, and to observe the effects of extracted gastric juice on various foods. His most important contributions include: an accurate and complete description of gastric juice; that hydrochloric acid was the important acid in the stomach along with another substance, later termed pepsin by Theodor Schwann (1810–1882) in 1855; that mucus and acid were secreted separately; and that there was a profound influence of mental disturbances on gastric secretion and digestion. He erroneously concluded that food was necessary for the secretion of acid, initiated by the mechanical action of food on the mucosa. His work was published in full in 1833.[11]

MODERN APPROACHES TO THE STUDY OF GASTRIC SECRETION

Despite the major interruption of non-military scientific research by the two major world wars of the twentieth century, work in the area of gastric secretion progressed exponentially. The gradual recognition that acid secretion was a complex interaction of neural, hormonal, and local factors fueled the development of techniques that preserved normal physiological conditions. On the other hand, attempts to answer the question regarding the mechanism of acid secretion required development of *in vitro* techniques. The first issue of Gastroenterology published in 1943 contained a symposium on the the mechanism of acid secretion with reviews by Davenport, Hollander, and Gray, three of the leading authorities in the field at the time.

IN VIVO TECHNIQUES

Ideally, an *in vivo* technique should provide an accurate estimation of acid secretion under conditions that closely mimic normal conditions. Gastric secretion is regulated by hormonal, neural and luminal factors all of which must be considered. The unknowing or uncontrolled elimination or modulation of one or more factors which control acid secretion can dramatically alter the results of a study.

Gastric Fistulas

In recognition of the importance of the studies of Beaumont, the cannulated gastric fistula was applied to the study of acid secretion in animals.[12] It remains a good alternative because of the minimal surgery required, the preservation of normal digestive function, and the ability to evaluate gastric secretion in conscious animals in a chronic preparation. It is useful for the collection of gastric juice in response to physiological or pharmacological stimuli. The cannula, however, suffers from some of the same problems as the aspiration method and does not permit the evaluation of acid response to solid material. The latter drawback likely contributed to Pavlov's design of the gastric pouch.

Gastric Pouches

One of the first physiological animal models to emerge as a novel scientific approach to the study of acid secretion were the gastric pouches, devised initially to collect pure gastric juice. A detailed explanation of the various pouch preparations, including surgical procedures, was published by Emas et al.[13] While the dog is the animal of choice, a brief discussion of the suitability of cats, rats and monkeys is also provided.

In 1878, Rudoplph Heidenhain (1834–1897) developed a denervated small pocket, surgically separated from the rest of the stomach which drained by a fistula to the outside. Although vagally denervated, this pouch retained some sympathetic innervation coursing with the splenic and other residual blood vessels (Figure 1A). Several modifications of Heidenhain's original method were introduced over the years. Briefly, the greater curvature is stretched with two non-crushing clamps delineating the pouch and a third hemostatic clamp across the vessels supplying the pouch area (Figure 1B). A lengthwise incision is made and the pouch sutured across the entire thickness. To limit constriction of the lumen, a transverse closure is recommended for the incision in the main stomach. Over the years, attempts were made to produce a completely denervated preparation, but success was elusive. Heidenhain first proposed that the composition of normal gastric parietal cells was constant,[14] a hypothesis which became incorporated into Pavlov's theory that the acid secretion had a constant normality. These concepts later formed the basis for modern theories on acid secretion.

The denervated pouch was refined by Ivan Petrovich Pavlov (1849–1936), who studied under Heidenhain and Ludwig. Pavlov found the crude preparation of Heidenhain unsuitable for studies applying his theory of "nervism" to the control of gastric secretion. Adhering to the

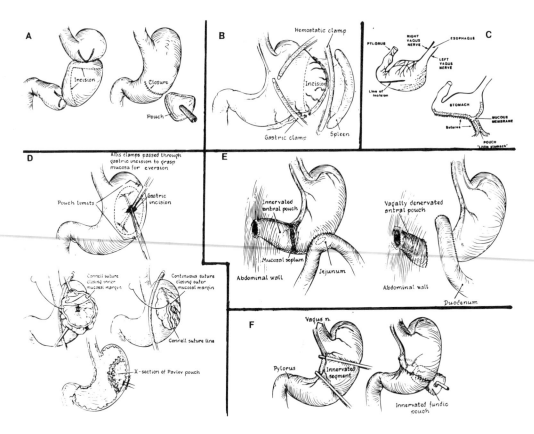

FIGURE 1 Pouch preparations and their modifications. A. Orginal Heidenhain pouch; B. Modification of the Heidenhain pouch; C. Original Pavlov pouch or "little stomach; D. Modification of the Pavlov pouch; E. Vagally innervated and denervated antral pouches; F. Vagally innervated funedic pouch. (A, B and D–F reprinted from Emas et al., *Handbook of Physiology,* Sect. 6, Vol. 2, Code, C., Chapter 42, 1967. With permission. C reprinted from Pare, W. Pavlov and his neurological investigations of the viscera, *Annals of the New York Academy of Science,* 597; 1990, 1–13.)

principles set forth by Claude Bernard on the importance of the internal milieu, Pavlov used his ambidexterity and extraordinary surgical skills to develop a chronic preparation, creating a miniature pouch attached to the main stomach that retained it's vascular and nerve supply (Figure 1C). Preservation of the vagal input requires careful placement of the incision. While Pavlov's incision was some 10 cm long, with improved anatomical information about vagal innervation, this was modified to a 3 cm cut along the anterior wall of the greater curvature.[15] Several clamps are inserted through the incision and circular section of mucosa is pulled through the opening (Figure 1D). The excised mucosa outlined by the clamps is sutured first along the inner edge and then the outer edge to form the inner and outer mucosal septa respectively. The pouch is accessed by placing a cannula in the dependent portion. Incomplete approximation of the inner mucosal septum is evidenced by the appearance of gastric contents in the cannula. In place of a cannula, direct access to the stomach can be achieved by creation of a cutaneous esophagostomy—a 5 cm midline incision in the cervical portion of the esophagus. Continuity of the esophagus is maintained so that there is little interference with normal oral feeding. This one step procedure is appropriate to use in aspiration or instillation of solutions. A two step procedure is recommended when the esophagostomy is also used for diversion of food during sham feeding.[16,17]

Pavlov was critical of acute experimentation and his pouch preparation enabled him to study gastric secretion chronically in healthy animals with normal function. The book, *The Work of the Digestive Glands*[12] published in 1902, was the product of nine years of research and earned him the Nobel prize in 1904. His contributions include: 1) the vagus is the secretory nerve of the gastric glands and 2) food in the stomach, but not in the intestine, stimulated acid secretion and the rate and quality of the secretion varied for different foods. In essence, he described the cephalic and gastric phases of acid secretion. In addition, in agreement with the theory that every organ is subject to opposing neural control, he proposed that the vagal stimulation resulted in both stimulatory and inhibitory effects. Pavlov's most important contribution, however, was the discovery of "psychic" secretion stimulated by "sham feeding" dogs with Pavlov pouches and esophagostomies. This validated the earlier observations of Beaumont on the effects of emotion of gastric function. It was shown that in dogs with salivary fistulas, the sight of food resulted in increased secretion of the glands, a reflex which could then be associated or paired with a neutal stimuli, such as a bell, to elicit a similar response. This revolutionary concept of a "conditioned reflex" so intrigued Pavlov that he subsequently focused his research on psychic reflexes leaving the digestive system to others.

Pavlov had already observed that acid secretion was scant in the denervated Heidenhain pouch. Acid secretion in response to insulin, 2-deoxyglucose or sham feeding, are all vagally mediated via induction of hypoglycemia which affects hypothalamic receptors. These tests are considered reliable indicators of the completeness of surgical vagal denervation. Surgical techniques continued to be refined in animals, especially in dogs, expanding the number of research models available to study acid secretion *in vivo*. The total gastric pouch was used to study the intestinal phase of acid secretion.[18] In this preparation, the esophagus is connected to the duodenum and the stomach drained through a cannula in the pylorus. Other pouch preparations include a pouch derived from the lesser curvature of the stomach[19] and the fundic pouch[20] both of which retain their vagal innervation but the surgical technique is difficult. In addition, there are the vagally innervated[21] and denervated[22] antral pouches (Figure 1E and F) and the innervated fundic pouch (Figure 1G).

These modifications of the Pavlov and Heidenhain pouches were used in the antrum to distinguish between neural and hormonal mechanisms of acid secretion. Such refinements contributed to the landmark work of Morton Grossman on the role of the long vago-vagal cholinergic and short parasympathetic reflexes in the control of acid secretion.[23] Combinations of antral and fundic pouches were also used in the same preparation. Instillation of a pH 7 solution into an antral pouch elicited an increase in gastric acid secretion in an adjacent denervated pouch of the fundus. If a pH 2 solution was introduced there was no increase in acid, indicating that contact of acid with the antral mucosa inhibits secretion of acid by the fundus. Distension of a denervated antral pouch elicited a secretory response in the proximal denervated fundic pouch, indicating that in the absence of neural connections, a hormonal substance was responsible. This was subsequently attributed to an inhibition of gastrin release from the antrum. To compare acid secretion simultaneously under denervated and innverated conditions in the same animal,[24] an innervated Amdrup pouch was used.[25] In this preparation, a pear shaped section taken from the anterior wall of the stomach with the base in the corporeal part of the lesser curvature, was combined with the denervated Heidenhain pouch, taken from the corporo-fundic portion of the stomach.

In 1967 when Emas et al.[13] published their work, they predicted a good survival of pouch preparations; after all, they had been sucessfully used for over half a century. Unfortunately, the need for good surgical skills, the sophistication of *in vitro* techniques, and the cost and difficulty of using large animals requiring chronic care has greatly reduced the popularity of pouch preparations. The total gastric pouch has endured because of its sucessful adaptation for use in small animals such as rats.[26]

Gastric Aspiration Techniques

By 1910, the accepted doctrine of "no acid, no ulcer" propelled clinical research towards elucidating the mechanism of acid secretion in an effort to improve medical therapy. Hypersecretion or hyperacidity was thought to be the common cause of ulcer. In the early part of the century, treatment was based on the "free acidity" that was measured after a test meal. A volume of solution (e.g. 50 mls) was injected into the stomach, left for a period of time (e.g. 15 min) and then withdrawn. The aspirates were then analyzed for H^+ and other ions. The equation "free acid" + "combined acid" = "total acid" was based on the theory that acid existed in a free form and in combination with proteins or other acid-binding substances. These fractions were thought to be distinguishable by the use of indicators. It is now known that indicators reflect only a change in pH rather than in a form of acid.

Methods introduced in the 1930's and 1940's to measure ion concentrations in gastric juice were improved over the years and many are now capable of microanalysis with computer storage of data. The concentration of H^+ in the clear supernatant of the gastric juice samples is determined *in vitro* by end point titration to pH 7.0 (physiochemical neutrality) or 7.4 (plasma pH) with a base such as NaOH or $NaHCO_3$. Acid concentration can also be assessed by determining the pH, a measure of H^+ activity, of the gastric juice. There are a number of conversion tables based on the concept that pH is the negative log of the H^+ concentration. Na^+ and K^+ concentrations are measured using a flame photometer and Cl^- concentration is determined by amperometric titration. Osmolality is measured by freezing point depression in an osmometer.

Simple Aspiration

Gastric aspiration was the first technique used in the clinical assessment of gastric acid secretion and remains the easiest and most universal method. Continuous aspiration of the gastric contents was performed first manually and then mechanically. In 1957, Hunt[27] modified the aspiration technique by using the indicator dye, phenol red, to determine acid secretion in response to serial test meals. Currently, the technique is performed using a double lumen nasaogastric tube placed fluoroscopically in the most dependent part of the stomach and connected to a suction pump (−5–10 mm Hg, −40 cm H_2O). If fluoroscopy is impossible or undesirable, the nasogastric tube can be inserted gently until a slight resistance is felt. Proper positioning of the tube can be verified by demonstrating that after injecting 20 ml of water into a previously emptied stomach, the total volume can be recovered.[28] This technique can be used to assess acid secretion either basally or in response to stimulation. Morton Grossman emphasized the importance of maximal secretory tests which first used histamine, then histalog and finally pentagastrin. The correct meaning of the the the term "maximal acid secretion" is the peak acid output (PAO) in response to the particular stimulant and not the highest rate possible by the parietal cells. PAO is thought to reflect the total parietal cell mass.

Measurement of acid secretion by gastric aspiration has several limitations. Dilution of the dye through endogenous secretion cannot be accounted for and may be a large source of error when used with meals or agents that enhance secretion. It does not correct for loss of gastric secretion through the pylorus which has been estimated to be as much as 50%.[29] In experimental animals, ligation of the pylorus has been used to circumvent the loss of fluid through the pylorus. The increase in secretion due to distension by the accumulated volume[30], however, must be considered. Continuous aspiration may further underestimate acid secretion as a result of back diffusion of hydrogen ions or neutralization of H^+ by alkaline secretions. Another complication is an increase in bile reflux from the duodenum due to the constant application of negative pressure, particularly when the aspiration is mechanical. This can be avoided, in part, by aspirating samples intermittently. Samples should be collected over 5 -or 10-minute intervals. Salivary contamination can be limited by the use of dental aids such as insertion and frequent changing of dental cotton, aspiration devices, and by delaying the start of the experiment for 30 to 60 minutes after the intubation procedure to allow salivary secretion to return to lower levels.

Measurement of HCO_3

The aspiration technique has been modified to measure HCO_3^- output.[31] Using the assumptions that the H^+ concentration of the parietal secretion is 160 mmol/l, that the osmolality of the parietal secretion is 1.06 times plasma osmolality, and that the osmolarity of the non-parietal component is identical to that of plasma, HCO_3^- can be calculated from the formula

$$HCO_3^- \text{ secretion} = V_{gj} \, 160 \, \triangle \text{ osmol} - K \triangle H / 320 - K$$

where V_{gj} is the volume of the gastric juice in liters, $\triangle$ osmol is the assumed osmolality of the gastric juice ($1.6 \times$ plasma osmol) less the measured osmolality of the gastric juice (mosmol/l), K is the assumed osmolality of the parietal component less the assumed osmolality of the non-parietal component, and $\triangle H$ is 160 mmol/l less the measured $\triangle H^+$ concentration of the gastric juice. Other techniques allow the determination of HCO_3^- in gastric juice collected from antral pouches[32] and fundic pouches after inhibition of acid secretion by vagotomy and antrectomy.[33] Histamine H_2 blockers have been used successfully to measure HCO_3^- in fundic pouches drained by fistulas (Figure 2) perfused with acidified saline (pH 6.0)[34] taking care to consider the possible inhibitory effects on alkalinization caused by the accumulation of CO_2 formed by the acid reaction with the secreted HCO_3. In closed pouches (Figure 2) HCO_3^- secretion can be determined using the Henderson-Hasslebach equation after measurement of intraluminal and CO_2 tension.[35] In this calculation, the pKa of CO_2 is assumed to be 6.09 and the solubility coefficient, 0.03. For the latter technique, it is also assumed that permeability to CO_2 is low so that the primary source of CO_2 is the reaction of H^+ and HCO_3^-.

Intragastric Titration

One of the most important physiological stimuli to the secretion of acid is food. Therefore, an alternate method of assessing gastric acid secretion, intragastric titration in vivo, was introduced in 1973 by Fordtran and Walsh[36] to measure acid secretion in response to a meal. The meal could be eaten normally or liquified and given intragastrically. The pH of the gastric juice is measured at 2–3 minute intervals and adjusted back to the pH of meal solution by the addition of a base.

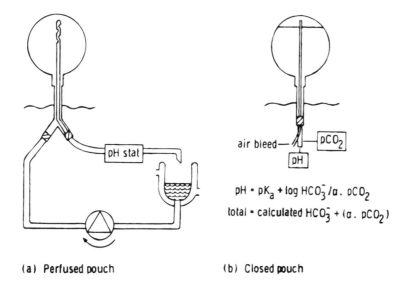

$$pH = pK_a + \log HCO_3^- / a \cdot pCO_2$$
$$total = calculated \; HCO_3^- + (a \cdot pCO_2)$$

(a) Perfused pouch   (b) Closed pouch

FIGURE 2 Methods used to determine alkaline secretion in the canine gastric pouch. (Reprinted from Garner and Hurst, *Basic Mechanisms of Gastrointestinal Mucosal Cell Injury and Cytoprotection,* Chapter 19, 1981. With permission.)

This technique does not permit the calculation of secretion of water or ions other than H^+. In addition, maintenance of the stomach at a constant pH, usually 5.5, removes the inhibitory feedback of acid entering the duodenum and produces elevated serum gastrin levels. A comparison of acid secretion in healthy subjects determined by gastric aspiration versus intragastric titration showed that gastric secretory rates were significantly higher when measured by the latter technique.[37] This was attributed to the gastric secretory response to even small amounts of fluid present during intragastric titration.

The Marker-Dilution Technique

In 1977, the ability to measure acid secretion *in vivo* was further improved with a novel adaptation of the marker-dilution technique by Dubois et al.[28] In recognition of the gastric and duodenal regulation of acid secretion, this technique addressed the physiological relationship between gastric emptying and secretion. Using the original contributions of Hildes and Dunlop[38] and George et al.,[39] this method is based on the principle that gastric volume reflects the processes of secretion and emptying and allows the simultaneous measurement of gastric volumes, ion and fluid secretion and emptying (Figure 3). This point is important as intragastric volume influences gastric acid secretion and intragastric H^+ concentration regulates, in part, gastric emptying. A sample of gastric juice is taken after mixing the gastric contents thoroughly for a 1-minute interval. The amount sampled is roughly proportional to the volume estimated during the 1-minute mixing period (approximately 2.5 ml sampled per 15 ml of gastric juice). During the next 1-minute interval, a volume of the test solution, twice that of the gastric sample, is instilled into the stomach and thoroughly mixed with the gastric contents and a second sample of gastric juice, equal in volume to the first, is taken (Figure 4). A test solution can be administered over a measured period of time and the gastric sampling repeated at 5, 10 and every 10 minutes thereafter until the end of the experiment. All solutions instilled into the stomach should be kept at 37° C since temperature affects gastric emptying (cold increases while heat decreases). Intragastric volumes of fluid (V_1, V_2 ...) and amounts of marker (phenol red or 99m-DTPA) are calculated using the marker dilution principle. Emptying rate (g) is determined for each

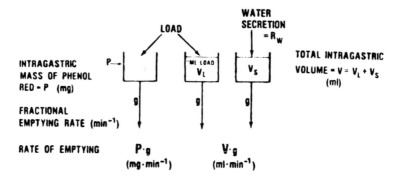

FIGURE 3 Principle of the marker dilution technique. The stomach contents may be divided into three compartments: (1) gastric marker; (2) gastric water volume injected with the load (V_L, "ml load"); and (3) gastric water volume secreted (V_S) by the stomach at a rate R_W (ml/min). (Reprinted from Dubois et al. *Am. J. Dig. Dis.,* 23, 993, 1981. With permission.)

10-minute interval (t) between two dilutions (**M** = concentration of marker), assuming that emptying is a first order (exponential) process during short intervals and using the equation:

$$g = -\log_e (M_2/M_1)/t$$

Net rate of fluid output (R_v) is determined for each 10-minute interval (t) between two dilutions assuming that it remains constant over the given interval and using the equation:

$$R_v = [V_2 - V_1 \cdot \exp (-g \cdot t)] \cdot g/[1 - \exp(-g \cdot t)]$$

The intragastric masses of H^+ (H_1, H_2, ...) are determined by multiplying the intragastric H^+ concentration by the corresponding intragastric volume. Net H^+ output is then calculated using the equation:

$$R_H = [H_2 - H_1 \cdot \exp (-g \cdot t)] \cdot g/[1 - \exp (-g \cdot t)]$$

Net gastric outputs of other ions (Na^+, K^+, or Cl^-) as well as the osmolality of the gastric

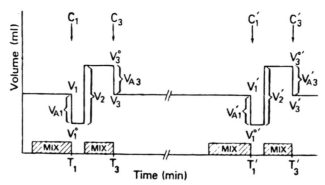

FIGURE 4 Schematic illustration of the marker dilution technique to simultaneously determine gastric secretion and emptying. (Reprinted from Dubois et al. *Am. J. Dig. Dis.,* 23, 993, 1981 with permission. V_1 is the volume in the stomach before the dilution procedure, C_1 is the concentration of the marker in the first aspirated sample of which the volume is V_{A1}, V_2 is the volume of the marker solution which is exactly twice that of V_{A1}, C_2 is the concentration of the marker in this solution, C_3 is the concentration of the marker in V_{A3} aspirated after mixing the V_2 thoroughly with the gastric contents.)

juice can also be measured using this formula, substituting the appropriate ion concentrations or osmolalities.

In contrast to earlier methods, this version corrected for any changes in the above parameters during the 1-minute mixing interval and allowed the measurement of acid secretion basally, as well as in response to stimulants or inhibitors. The accuracy of the model depends upon several assumptions: 1) the marker is neither absorbed nor secreted, the marker can be throughly mixed with the gastric contents during the 1-minute interval, 2) the marker leaves the stomach at a rate proportional to the intragastric concentration of the marker, 3) the gastric contents remain homogenous during the the interval between gastric samplings (5 or 10 min), 4) secretion and emptying remain constant during the time between samplings, and 5) there is no duodenogastric reflux. The first and second assumptions have been verified experimentally.[39,40,41] The third and fourth assumptions have not been validated, but intuitively, the calculation of gastric secretion and emptying independently over short intervals (5–10 minutes) should be superior to using a single estimation over a longer interval (30–60 minutes). The final assumption can be validated directly by determining the amount of intragastric bile or indirectly by measuring sodium concentration which should be stable over time, if attributable to only non-parietal secretion, and not bile salt contamination.

This model has been used extensively to evaluate gastric function in conscious subjects in response to physiological and pharmacological agents[42,43,44,45] as well as under conditions such as irradiation exposure[46] and stress.[47] In addition, the gastric response to a number of physiological liquid test meals can be determined along with the quantity of acid, osmoles, or calories delivered to the duodenum. The technique has been adapted for use in dogs, after surgical construction of an esophagostomy, and in guinea pigs with a gastric fistula.[48]

A major advantage of the marker-dilution technique is its ability to discern whether alterations in intragastric volume are due to changes in secretion or emptying. This is particularly useful in judging the effectiveness of potential antisecretory agents. For example, using gastric aspiration, it was concluded that the decrease in gastric volume following adminstration of a prostaglandin E_2 (PGE$_2$) analog was due to an inhibition of fluid secretion.[49] In contrast, the marker dilution technique revealed that fluid secretion was normal after the PGE$_2$ analog, and the loss of volume was via an increase in gastric emptying.[42] The antisecretory effect of PGF$_{2\alpha}$ analog was also demonstrated by this technique,[43] clarifying previous results using pylorus ligation indicating the lack of an effect of this prostaglandin on acid secretion.[50] Clinical abnormalities in gastric function can be similarly evaluated. Thus, patients with gastric retention and outlet obstruction have an elevated gastric fluid secretion in addition to delayed gastric emptying.[44] Zollinger Ellison syndrome, a disease characterized by gastric acid hypersecretion, was also associated with high intragastric volumes and gastric emptying rates.[28] An early disadvantage of the marker-dilution technique was the necessity for a computer capable of handling the complex program of iterative fitting. However, the program can now be performed by most IBM-compatible personal computers. The accuracy of the technique depends greatly upon the efficiency of the 1-minute mixing, which may be more difficult at larger volumes. Finally, the need to rapidly mix the gastric contents with the marker limits the model to the study of liquid meals.

The Double Marker Dilution Technique

The attempt to quantitate gastric function in response to a physiological meal led to the development of double-marker dilution techniques by Malegelada and others at the Mayo Clinic.[51] A sump tube is inserted in the the most dependent part of the stomach for the repeated sampling of gastric contents after the administration of a meal containing a nonabsorbable marker (^{14}CrPEG, 30 µCi, specific activity 0.5 µCi/mg). A triple-lumen tube is placed in the duodenum with a perfusion site proximally and an aspiration site with an air vent 20 cm distally

METHOD

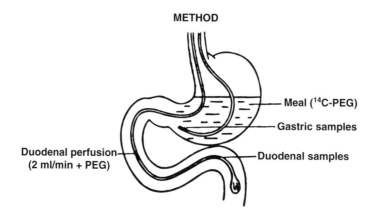

FIGURE 5 Gastric and duodenal tubes are located in their respective positions. Gastric marker is [^{14}C] polyethylene glycol ingested with the meal. The duodenal marker is polyethylene glycol constantly perfused into the duodenum. (Reprinted from Malagelada et al., *Gastroenterology,* 70, 203, 1976. With permission.)

(Figure 5). The duodenum is perfused at a constant rate (2 ml/min) with normal saline containing a second nonabsorbable marker (PEG 4000, 5g/l). Gastric emptying is quantitated by the rate of marker leaving the stomach and intragastric volume by dividing the amount of marker in the stomach (g ingested/g emptied) by its concentration (g/ml) at the time of the sample. The product of the intragastric volume and the concentration of H$^+$ calculated over each sampling interval gives the rate of acid secretion. The technique was modified for use in dogs, replacing the gastric tube with a cannula placed on the body of the stomach between the greater and lesser curvatures and a catheter placed in the lumen of the fundus (Figure 6).[52] Duodenal samples are taken 5 minutes after gastric samples to allow for the transit of the meal.

There are several fundamental assumptions which affect the accuracy of the technique: 1) the marker is uniformly distributed in the total volume within the stomach and duodenum, 2) measurements are based on a steady-state flow of fluid in the duodenum, and 3) the gastric meal marker is completely recovered from the duodenum. The first assumption may be valid with homogenous liquid meals, but homogenates or solids may elude quantification by the dilution technique due to separation of the marker into the bulk liquid phase. It has been argued that sampling of small suspended particles is proportional to the liquid phase and that larger particles contribute little to the overall gastric volume.[53] Differences in the meal consistency and content may also affect the accuracy of the second assumption and use of this model in the non-steady state has been addressed by Levitt and Bond.[54] Finally, the total recovery of the marker has not been achieved and there is a consistent underestimation of approximately 10%

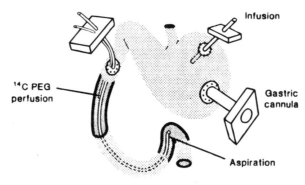

FIGURE 6 Diagrammatic representation of canine model, showing placement of acid infusion and aspiration devices. (Reprinted from Kholief et al., *Dig. Dis. Sci.,* 28, 633, 1983. With permission.)

in dogs[52] and 14% in humans.[51] Contrary to initial concerns, there appears to be little derangement of gastric emptying or secretion arising from placing a tube across the pylorus.[55]

At its best, this technique comes closest to a physiological evaluation of gastric acid secretion and emptying in response to a variety of meals (liquids, homogenates or solids). The many clinical and experimental studies performed have provided valuable insight on the subtleties of the interaction between the small bowel and the stomach, particularly on the intestinal phase of acid secretion which had been previously unappreciated. For example, differences in the magnitude and pattern of gastric, pancreatic and biliary responses to a meal given intragastrically as an homongenate, versus solid/liquid meals eaten conventionally, emphasized the importance of the route of ingestion.[53] One disadvantage of the double sampling method is its complexity. Errors can be compounded if there is incomplete mixing in any one of the compartments especially after meals containing solids. Despite these problems, the significance of the information obtained with this model has endured.

Other Techniques

Adaptations of early techniques were applied to study acid secretion in smaller animals, primarily rodents. In acute studies in animals, collection of the gastric juice after ligation of the pylorus prevents the exit of stomach contents into the duodenum. Indeed, pylorus ligation was developed as a model of hypersecretion in rats and is often referred to as the Shay preparation.[56] In anesthetized animals, the pylorus is ligated and the stomach flushed with saline by a catheter inserted orally. The animal is allowed to recover. In rats, gastric acid secretion is significantly elevated by 4 hours and is maximal by 7 hours at which time the animal is reanesthetized and the stomach removed and the gastric volume and acid concentration are determined. To eliminate distension by accumulated secretion, the stomach can be drained by a catheter placed in the ligated pylorus.[57] The model is also appropriate for mice.

A second technique for use in rodents was used by Garner and Flemstrom[35] for assessment of HCO_3 secretion but is equally appropriate for acid secretion (Figure 7). Briefly, in anesthetized animals, a catheter (see figure inset) is passed through the duodenum into the stomach and secured by placing a ligature around the pylorus. The catheter is pulled through the opening created in the abdominal wall. At the upper end of the stomach, a tube is placed down the esophagus into the cardiac regions and secured with a ligature around the neck region to prevent flow of saliva into the stomach. The experimental procedures involves filling the stomach with nondistending volumes of fluid followed by replacement with air.

The vivi-perfused stomach is another alternative to determine gastric secretion.[58,59] In this method, a conscious animal is used as a blood donor for an excised stomach from an anesthetized animal (Figure 8). This early preparation is handicapped tremendously by the need for large animals, the difficulty of the surgical preparation, and the possible complications arising from using a donor blood supply.

At the same time as the introduction of the dilution methods was the development of the single scan technique,[60] as a less laborious, more convenient, and non-invasive alternative to measure acid secretion. Earlier studies demonstrated that intravenously administered ^{99m}Tc (sodium pertechnetate) was cleared by the gastric mucosa in proportion to acid secretion. Technically there are many problems including the clearance of the ^{99m}Tc by non-parietal cells, the loss of ^{99m}Tc by gastric emptying, the need of a gamma camera, and the exposure of the patient to radioactive materials. Moreover, the clearance of the isotope after stimulation of acid secretion is likely related to changes in blood flow and may be accurate only under those conditions in which acid secretion is associated with an increase in mucosal blood flow. The method is best suited to measurement of peak acid output and may be convenient for the simple categorizing patients into hyper- or hyposecretors.

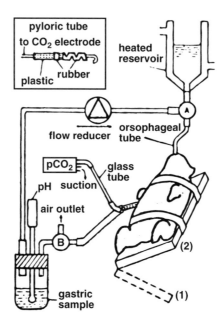

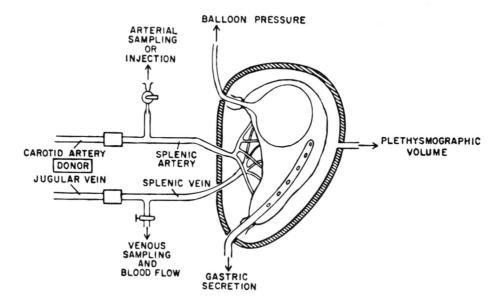

FIGURE 7 Diagram of apparatus used to collect gastric samples from guinea pig. Animal tilted 60 degrees between position 1 (filling stomach) and position 2 (emptying stomach); otherwise the animal is placed horizontally. Inset shows a diagram of pyloric outlet tube and position of cannula used to remove intragastric samples for measurements of P_{CO2} levels. (Reprinted from Garner and Flemstrom, *Am. J. Physiol.*, 234, E535, 1978. With permission.)

FIGURE 8 Viviperfused whole stomach preparation. (Reprinted from Emas et al., *Handbook of Physiology*, Sect. 6, Vol. 2, Code, C., Chapter 42, 1967. With permission.)

THE TRANSITION TO *IN VITRO* TECHNIQUES

The concept of pH and the ability to measure it emerged from the 1930's, opening up new lines of investigation centered around acid secretion as a movement of ions. In this manner, for some electrolytes the stomach was viewed as a large dialysis membrane separating the gastric lumen from the blood[61] (Figure 9). Gradually there was the realization that acid secretion was a matter of "ion accumulation," a term adopted from botanists studying potassium uptake by plants from the soil. Borrowing electrochemistry terms from Overton, Planck and Nernst, formulas for ion mobility and diffusion were introduced into the physiology of acid secretion. Interest in ions other than H^+ arose from the limited ability of the measurement of acid alone to serve as a discriminating diagnostic tool. At low secretory rates, the acidity of the gastric juice is low and the concentration of sodium is high. This proportion is inverted at high rates of secretion. The variability of the H^+ content of the gastric juice could not be accounted for by the Pavlov's original hypothesis that parietal cell secretion was constant.[62] If acid secretion was fixed then it must be modified once in the lumen either by dissipation or diffusion into the mucosa. Experiments were conducted to answer the questions on the cause of the variability of gastric juice composition, the decreased acid concentration in response to chemical irritants, the disappearance of acid intraluminal instillates, and the low acid secretion in gastric ulcer patients.

By the end of World War II, there were two major theories accounting for the changes in electrolyte composition of gastric secretion. The first was the "diffusion theory" of Torsten Teorell in which a primary parietal secretion was modified by the back diffusion of H^+ which was replaced by Na^+.[61,63,64] The driving force was the concentration gradient of each ion on either side of the mucosa. In addition, it was assumed that the diffusion took place in the form of the ion pairs NaCl and HCl in accordance with the Guggenheim approximation and Fick's law of molecular diffusion. It represented the last physiochemical solution to gastric secretion before the advent of membrane transport. The second was the "two component" theory of Hollander in which the final gastric juice was an admixture of a parietal and a non-parietal component.[65,66,67] The parietal component included H^+ and Cl^- and their outputs were increased by stimulation. The non-parietal component was composed of everything else and was secreted

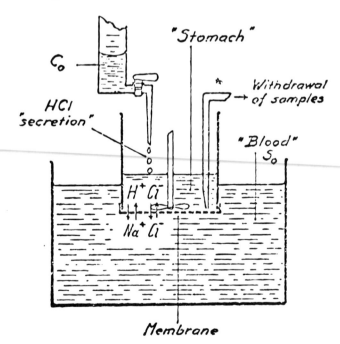

FIGURE 9 Principle of model demonstrating stomach interdiffusion. The stomach consists of a vessel separated from a large volume of NaCl solution by a dialysis membrane of a constant area. Acid secretion into the stomach can be imitated by allowing a HCl solution to flow in from a reservoir. The rate of "secretion" can be varied and the stomach can be emptied by suction. (Reprinted from Teorell, *Gastroenterology*, 9, 425–443, 1947. With permission.)

at a constant rate. The two theories were similar with respect to H^+ but differed in their consideration of Na^+. In both, H^+ was the primary secretion and had a constant concentration. However, stimulation of acid secretion under the back-diffusion hypothesis increased the volume of secretion and under the two component theory increased the HCl (with fluid) output. In addition, Na^+ enters the lumen passively down its concentration gradient in the diffusion model, while Na^+ enters as part of the bulk secretion in the two component model.

The back diffusion hypothesis was based primarily on data collected from instillation experiments in which solutions containing a known quantity of acid were placed in the stomach, left for a period of time, and then recovered. Similar experiments were conducted in animals using fundic or antral pouches or sheets of gastric muocsa in order to exclude salivary or bile contamination. For the most part, the acid concentration in the recovered juice was less, as predicted by back diffusion. Moreover, experimental results showing a parallel increase in acid with volume of secretion, the strong negative curvilinear correlation between H^+ and Na^+ and the increase in total Cl^- with increased acid, supported the hypothesis. Davenport's[68] proposal of a gastric mucosal barrier also confirmed Teorell's work. Gastric mucosal injury increased the normal amount of back diffusion by making the barrier leakier, accounting for the low acid, high sodium concentration in gastric ulcer disease. Conversely, conditions in which acid loss was negligible were presumed to reflect a state of balance between acid secretion and diffusion. In addition to some of the more obvious theoretical problems, there were two technical drawbacks: 1) the instillation procedure increased acid secretion via distension and 2) gastric emptying was assumed to be insignificant in the period between instillation and recovery of the acid solution.

The two component theory relied more on data collected by gastric aspiration. Theoretical relations between composition and volume were confirmed by experimental data showing that the negative relationship between H^+ and Na^+ was linear at all rates of secretion and by evaluating electrolyte secretion under steady state conditions. Improved methods to assess intragastric volume, such as those described in the previous section, indicated that instillation of fluid into the stomach increased volume and produced a net gain in Na^+, which was in excess of the loss of H^+. Rejection of the elegantly simple diffusion theory began with the application of Frederick Donnan's (1870–1956) theories on the distribution of ions across a membrane to the gastric acid secretion shifting H^+ movement away from the idea of "ion accumulation" to one of ion transport. Indeed, the secretion of hydrochloric acid was one of the first active transport processes identified and finally explained the ability of the stomach to accumulate such high concentrations of H^+. The demonstration that gastric epithelial cells secrete HCO_3^- provided the fundamental evidence that non-parietal secretion is the product of specific cells.

IN VITRO TECHNIQUES

Despite the significant advances made in the twentieth century in the measurement of gastric secretion *in vivo,* there was a gradual move away from studies in the whole animal. Experiments in intact tissue were unable to resolve the source of energy, the ionic mechanisms, or the electrical events involved in acid secretion. Isolated tissues had the advantage of minimizing or eliminating complicating factors such as neural control, diffusion barriers and variations in blood flow.

The entire excised mouse stomach (Figure 10) model was used by Davenport and Chavre[69] to assess acid secretion in response to a number of physiologic and pharamacologic agents. The stomach is removed, filled with phosphate buffered saline, ligated at each end, placed in a weighing bottle which is then set in a brass bomb. Neural and paracrine pathways remain intact. This method is deceptive in its simplicity since determination of acid secretion is made with attention to a set of exacting experimental conditions including regulation of temperature,

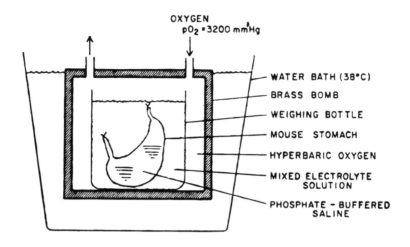

FIGURE 10 *In vitro* whole stomach preparation. (Reprinted from Emas et al., *Handbook of Physiology,* Sect. 6, Vol. 2, Code, C., Chapter 42, 1967. With permission.)

electrolyte balance, stomach distension, and pH of the solution applied to the stomach interior. An additional complication to this system is the need for hyperbaric oxygen at near toxic concentrations in order to penetrate the stomach muscle and oxygenate the interior mucosa. This preparation has been modified[70,71] so that catheters are inserted in each end of the stomach, the stomach washed with 15 ml of saline and then incubated in 20 ml of a buffered serosal solution gassed with 95% O_2/5% CO_2. The lumen is perfused at 1 ml/min with an unbuffered solution of similar composition to that bathing the serosa and gassed with 100% O_2. These changes solve the problem of maintaining a high O_2 supply to the mucosa. Using this technique one can measure the secretion of acid, various gastric hormones, during a basal state, in response to physiological and pharamacological agonists and antagonists or to electrical field stimulation. The result of constant perfusion with high O_2 is unknown. Furthermore, the secretory capacity of the *in vitro* stomach is generally less than in the *in vivo* stomach. This may be due to the interrupted blood supply.

Isolated Gastric Mucosa

The first experiments of the gastric mucosa *in vitro* were conducted by Delrue[72] in 1930. The mucosal is gently dissected from the serosa and muscle layer and mounted on a plastic chamber (Figure 11). In 1932 there was the recognition of a potential difference (PD) across the stomach,[73] with the lumen negative respective to the blood. Early studies in isolated gastric mucosa demonstrated a decrease in the PD upon the stimulation of acid secretion. It is now known that in the resting stomach the potential is between -60 and -80 mV and is due primarily to Cl^- secretion by both parietal and surface epithelial cells against its electrochemical gradient. During acid secretion, the PD falls to -30 or -40 mV with H^+ moving down its electrical gradient and promoting its transport against a large chemical gradient. The introduction of the dog flap preparation[74] in 1945 permitted the direct assessment of acid secretion, ion flux and PD (Figure 12). In this preparation, the blood supply from the donor animal is maintained and permits sampling for blood gases and nutrients. In 1950 Rehm[75] proposed a theory on the formation of HCl by the stomach based on the electrophysiologic properties across the stomach wall, setting the precedent for continued work on the active transport of H^+ and Cl^-.

The Ussing chamber further modified the flap preparation, adding the ability to access both serosal and mucosal sides of the stomach and improving short-circuit measurements.[76] Transmucosal or transmural electrical PD is measured by two matched calomel electrodes

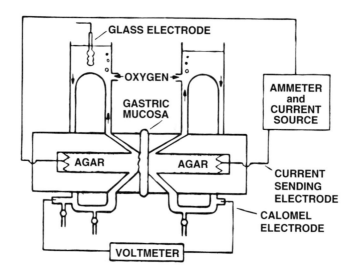

FIGURE 11 Apparatus for the study of gastric mucosal segment. Epithelial surface is on the left. Circulation is provided by oxygen gassing of the solutions. The glass electrode permits continuous measurement of pH. (Reprinted from Emas et al., *Handbook of Physiology,* Sect. 6, Vol. 2, Code, C., Chapter 42, 1967. With permission.)

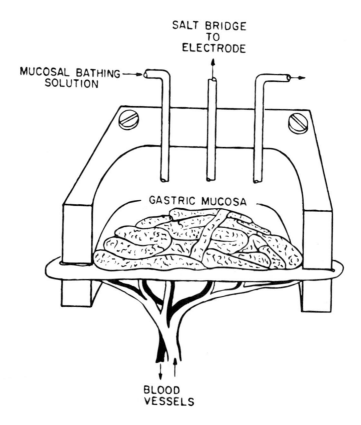

FIGURE 12 *In vivo* chambered stomach. Blood vessels are connected to the anesthetized animal. (Reprinted from Emas et al., *Handbook of Physiology,* Sect. 6, Vol. 2, Code, C., Chapter 42, 1967. With permission.)

connected to the mucosal and serosal sides by agar KCl bridges. Short circuit current (I_{sc}) is delivered to each side using Ag-AgCl electrodes in a tube of 3% agar in saturated KCl. The chambers are precalibrated with unbuffered Krebs in the absence of tissue and air flow adjusted to insure uniform and even gassing. In addition, instrument calibration for assymetrical voltage between electrodes (tip potential) and fluid resistance should be made. Difficulties at this point arise from air bubbles, breaks in the agar bridges, or bad electrodes. The chambers are then emptied completely by suction.

The tissue to be mounted is quickly dissected from the animal and placed in preoxygenated Krebs buffer containing glucose. Mucosa may be separated from the muscle layers for (transmucosal) or left intact (transmural). The ease of separation is largely dependent upon the size of the animal used. The tissue can be stretched out on a Sylgard® coated plate using several dissecting needles and subsequently "impaled" upon the chamber pins. Alternately, for smaller animals, the tissue is opened lengthwise a little at a time and carefully stretched over the chamber pins. The size of the exposed mucosal area is usually 1.8 cm^2 although smaller chambers are available. Tissue should be prepared quickly for mounting to reduce the chances of anoxia. Once in the chamber, the tissue is bathed with 5–10 mls salt solution by means of a gas lift and maintained at 37°C by a water jacket connected to a circulating pump. With the tissue voltage clamped at zero transmural PD, the resistance (ohm-cm^2) can be calculated by measuring the change in I_{sc} in response to a fixed voltage (e.g. 1 mV) and using Ohm's law to determine $R = 1 \text{ mV/change in } I_{sc}$. Healthy tissues with low resistances indicate a leaky epithelia due to poor preparation, anoxia, or incorrect mounting and should be replaced.

The nutrient (serosal) side contains a buffered solution while the secretory (luminal) side solution is unbuffered. The amount of 5 mM HCl or 10 mM NaOH added to the secretory side to maintain the pH at 7.4 can be used to calculate the amount of acid or base transported into the lumen. When measuring base secretion only, tissue should be incubated in the presence of an inhibitor of acid secretion. An early observation using this method was the 1:1 movement of H^+ into the mucosal solution accompanied by an OH^- into the serosal side.[77] In addition, at short circuit currents there was a flux of Cl^- towards the lumen and Na^+ towards the serosa which was taken to indicate an active transport of both of these ions.[78] While true for Na^+, patch clamp studies indicate that Cl^- transport into the lumen is not active. Initially used in amphibian gastric mucosa, the technique has been applied to the study of gastric acid secretion in mammals with variable degrees of success. This move to mammalian models may be reflected in the gradual change in the use of the term "oxyntic", describing amphibian cells which secrete acid and contain zymogen granules, to the more modern term "parietal" to describe mammalian cells which secrete acid only.

Ussing chambers are considered a somewhat outdated technique by many and are more often associated with studies in the intestine. It remains, however, a valuable and relatively simple way to assess gastric ion movement. Indeed, Ussing chambers have been used in medical student laboratories to illustrate the properties of epithelial transport[79] and have been modified to concurrently monitor smooth muscle function.[80] Potential limitations are the greater deterioration of mammalian tissue over time when compared to amphibian tissue. In addition, tissue is studied at or near maximal stretch, when in reality, transporting epithelia are rarely flat.

The development of microelectrodes sensitive to sodium, potassium, chloride, hydrogen and calcium, made possible measurement of the activities of individual ions within the intact mucosa. The permeability of the basal membrane to both K^+ and Cl^- and the scant paracellular movement of ions in the stomach were demonstrated using microelectrodes.[81] Surface cells are more readily accessible than the deeper parietal cells. Other technical difficulties include an interference from surface mucus which may obscure the underlying cells and the need to confirm recordings from parietel cells histologically using marker dyes. Microelectrodes have also been inserted in the wall of the fundus to ascertain intramural pH.[82] The relationship between intramural pH and intraluminal acid concentration,[82] and changes in intramural pH in response to mucosal ulceration,[83] or hemorrhagic shock[26] were defined with this technique.

In 1964, Davenport proposed, that under normal conditions the lining of the stomach acted as a barrier to the movement of H^+ and Na^+.[68] Exposure of the mucosa to the barrier breaker, eugenol, destroyed the integrity of this barrier allowing a leakage of H^+ back into the mucosa and a return flux of Na^+ into the juice. These fluxes were associated with a change in PD. The interpretation of these alterations in PD have evolved over the years. Exposure to damaging agents such as ethanol,[84] bile salts,[85] or aspirin[86] was consistently associated with a reduction in PD. This was found to be caused by an inhibition of active ion transport rather than of H^+ secretion and Na^+ absorption. Mucosal damage ensued as a result of an increase in permeability.[87] Conversely, an increase in PD indicated a protective effect on the mucosa. However, later studies found that decreases in PD associated with active acid secretion were not always associated with gastric damage. Moreover, protective agents such as PGE_2 analogs, reduced PD without altering mucosal permeability.[88] Thus, alterations in PD may be multifactoral and must be interpreted carefully.

Studies on isolated tissue must be credited with providing much of the early evidence of the effects of single stimulants. That histamine stimulation of acid secretion was mediated by an increase in cyclic AMP (cAMP) was shown first in the isolated frog gastric mucosa. However, the ability to study acid secretion in a more controlled system introduced a new set of problems in comparing results obtained *in vitro* and *in vivo*. Isolated stomachs of dogs, cats monkeys, and humans, secreted acid basally,[89] but, there were differences in the response to secretagogues. In dogs, histamine increased acid secretion *in vivo*,[90] but not *in vitro*.[91] In addition, ethanol decreased acid secretion *in vivo*,[68] increased it *in vitro*.[91] The applicability of *in vitro* observations to those *in vivo* was complicated further by species differences. H^+ output was increased in rabbits *in vitro*,[92] decreased in rats *in vivo*,[93] and unchanged in dog *in vivo*.[94] Moreover, the active transport of Na^+ from the serosa to the mucosa in isolated rabbit gastric mucosa was not observed in other species.[92] Addressing these discrepancies, Ekblad et al.,[95] studied the isolated piglet gastric mucosa, which appears to have similar electrical and secretory responses to mammals *in vivo*. Overall, studies in isolated mucosa are limited by the heterogenity of the cell population which limits identification of a single response with a specific cell.

Isolated Gastric Glands and Parietal Cells

The knowledge that acid secretion *in vivo* was under the influence of endocrine, neural, and paracrine pathways, and that these routes were interdependent, led to the development of techniques to evaluate the effects of a single stimulant. The cellular physiology of acid was elucidated using three major preparations, isolated fundic glands, isolated parietal cells and isolated vesicles from parietal cells. Glands represent a more "intact" system as gland preparations retain intercellular connections, cell appearance, gap junctions and polarity. In addition, the fewer isolation steps in preparing glands increases the viability of the resulting cells. Finally, isolated glands provide a greater concentration of parietal cells per volume than intact tissue. However, as with isolated mucosa, the major drawback to gland preparations is the heterogeneity of the cell population limiting its use to parietal cell functions which are easily distinguished from other cells.

A comprehensive critique of the major methods used to disperse isolated fundic glands and mucosal cells was made by Soll and Berglindh.[96] Although specifically addressed in this review, the ease with which the mucosa can be separated from the underlying muscle varies among species. It is accomplished with relatively few problems in dogs. In rabbits and pigs, however, the animal is anesthetized, the abdomen opened, the aorta cannulated and ice cold phosphate buffered saline injected under pressure. This step greatly facilitates the subsequent scraping of the gastric mucosa after the stomach is removed and opened. Other equally important factors to consider are the age of the animal, the concentration and type of digestive enzymes used in the dispersion, the use of calcium chelators, and the length of incubation. The effectiveness of the initial digestion should be assessed before the addition of mechanical steps to improve digestion. The heavier gastric glands can be separated from other elements by centrifugation. Further separation of glands into individual cells can be accomplished by velocity or density. Velocity exploits the larger cell size of the parietal cell using unit sedimentation velocity, elutriation or the less satisfactory method of repeated centrifugation. The resulting enriched fraction of parietal cells (50–90%) must then be separated from the persistent remaining glands. Density techniques use a variety of media whose osmolality and effects on cell function must be weighed individually. Identification of all cell types present in the preparation is of paramount importance and efforts to enrich the yield of parietal cells from subpopulations of cells are worthwhile.

Studies using isolated gastric glands and parietal cell provided the first evidence of the mechanisms controlling acid secretion at the level of the parietal cell.[97] Most isolated gland and cell preparations responded well to histamine and acetylcholine. However, in order to observe a response to gastrin in rabbits, glands require treatment with a phosphodiesterase inhibitor such as isobutylmethylxanthine to inhibit the breakdown of cAMP, or a sulfhydryl reducing agent such as dithiothreitol, to increase the sensitivity of the parietal cell to histamine.[98] Acetylcholine is a weak stimulant in rabbits but is the most potent of the three stimuli in dogs.

Acid secretion cannot be measured directly in isolated glands since the generation of H^+ produces an equivalent production of base. Changes in oxygen consumption, morphology, aminopyrine uptake and glucose oxidation are taken as evidence of acid secretion. Indeed, at one time oxygen consumption was the best indicator of the activity of the hydrogen ion pump. Using the knowledge that weak bases accumulate in compartments with a low pH, the acid secretion in gastric glands can be assessed indirectly. The cellular uptake of the base reflects the amount of acid sequestered intracellularly and is taken as a index of acid secretion. The pK_a of each weak base must be considered with regard to the expected pH gradient as the entry of base is limited to compartments in which the pH is lower than the pK_a of the base. For this reason, bases with a high pK_a should be used when the acidity is low. The ideal base should also be lipid soluble in its unprotonated form, but once in the acid compartment, the protonated form should be lipid-impermeable so it will remain there. Finally, the intracellular dye should bind with intracellular components so that its efflux is slow. With a pK_a of 5, ^{14}C-aminopyrine satisfies most of the above criteria and has been used extensively to quantitate acid secretion, particularly after stimulation. Acridine orange[99] and 9-aminoacridine[100] have also been used to measure the acid secretion based on their color change when sequestered. In addition, these bases have been used with Nomarski optics or fluorescent microscopy to visualize the morphological transformation of parietal cells during stimulation. Berglindh et al.[101] and Malinkowski et al.[102] used isolated glands permeabilized by electric shock or digitoxin exposure and then treated with oligomycin to inhibit oxidative phosphorylation. Under these conditions, they showed that aminopyrine uptake (H^+ secretion) was dependent upon the addition of ATP. It should be noted that there may be an uneven uptake of indicator dyes especially in a heterogenous cell population. In addition, the distribution of the dye within the cell is unknown and thus, pH values represent an average of all intracellular compartments. Finally, indicator dyes give a reasonable estimate of H^+ uptake for a short period but cannot be used to assess H^+ uptake continuously.

The use of isolated glands and tissue was crucial in elucidating the mechanism of action of the three major stimulants of acid secretion: histamine, acetylcholine, and gastrin. Sir Henry Dale discovered histamine, but in 1920, Popilelski showed its involvement in parietal cell acid secretion. Kamorov[103] later separated the actions of gastrin from histamine, leading to the early theory that histamine was the final common mediator for acid secretion.[104] The other two major secretoagogues, gastrin and acetylcholine, were thought to increase acid secretion by releasing histamine. There were problems, however, in assigning histamine as an obligatory intermediate. Both pentagastrin and acetylcholine were more potent stimulants of acid secretion per mole in a variety of species.[88,105] Moreover, atropine blocked the secretory response to pentagastrin, 2-deoxyglucose, which acts via vagal stimulation, and to food, but not to histamine.[106] Finally, gastrin and acetylcholine increased histamine release in rabbits, but there was no evidence that the amount of histamine was altered during acid secretion in humans. In addition to species differences, the evidence was inconclusive regarding the source of histamine in individual species. Thus, the most important source of histamine appears to be mast cells in dogs and humans, but enterochromaffin-like cells (ECL) in rats and rabbits.

For a brief time, gastrin emerged as the frontrunner for the primary stimulant of acid secretion.[107] However, the discovery that analogs of 4-methylhistamine antagonized gastric histamine receptors[108] led to the development of H_2 receptor antagonists. These H_2 antagonists blocked acid secretion in response to all physiological stimuli[106] providing strong support for the histamine theory. Finally, the independent action of gastrin, histamine and acetylcholine were demonstrated in studies in dispersed parietal cells.[109] Soll et al. published numerous results demonstrating the site and specificity of histamine, gastrin and acetylcholine receptors on the parietal cell. The three receptors all activate acid secretion, but via different intracellular messengers. In this multiple response system, histamine is proposed to act as a potentiator of acetylcholine and gastrin rather than as a final common mediator.[96] The interdependence and potentiation among the three secretagogues occurs beyond binding at the receptor.

There are several disadvantages in studying isolated cells in culture. The first is the question of the influence of *in vitro* conditions on cell function and the application of data from a single cell to *in vivo* observations. In addition, species differences have been observed, particularly between data obtained in rabbits and dogs. Finally, preparations of pure parietal cells were rarely possible and it is important to characterize other cells in the preparation. For example, mucus secreting cells could be stained by periodic acid Schiff reagent. At no time were the limitations of these studies more evident than with the publication of the study in rats by Mezey and Palkovits[110] in 1992 based on molecular biology techniques. *In situ* hybridization histochemistry was used to visualize cells making protein for the receptors for the three major secretagogues. Suprisingly, they found no receptors in the epithelial cell layer which contained the gastric glands, but receptors were located on immunocytes contained in the lamina propria. Previous results showing receptors on the parietal cells were derived largely from pharmacological studies showing receptor agonist binding and competitive inhibition by specific antagonists. Mezey and Palkovits concluded that contamination of the isolated cell preparations with other cells, including immunocytes, may have accounted for the secretory response to histamine and acetylcholine, rather than a direct effect on the parietal cell itself as presumed. These results have neither been confirmed nor denied, and their clinical implications have not been fully addressed. However, application of molecular biology to the study of acid secretion continues. Ideally, data obtained from isolated cells should be interpreted carefully and verified when possible using other preparations.

Isolated Gastric Vesicles

Isolated vesicles have been used primarily to study the enzyme reactions and transport properties of the parietal cell. Arguably, the most important finding to emerge from this technique was the isolation of the enzyme, H^+/K^+ ATPase, on the apical membrane of parietal cells. The clinical importance of this discovery was realized with the development of the substituted benzimidazoles, such as omeprazole, which inhibit this enzyme,[111] the final step in acid secretion. Unlike Na^+/K^+ ATPase, this enzyme is insensitive to oubain and is confined to the secretory portion of the gastric mucosa. It is specifically on the tubovesicle in the resting cell and in the secretory canaliculi in the secreting cell. Based on initial data in frog mucosa, it was thought to be electrogenic,[112] but subsequent studies in mammalian vesicles discarded this idea in favor of an electroneutal exchange.

Vesicles may be prepared by dissecting the fundus away from the antrum and cardiac regions. The fundus is then flooded with 3 M NaCl to produce an exfoliation of most surface epithelial cells which are then removed by wiping the mucosa.[113] The remaining mucosa is scraped and suspended in cold 0.25 M sucrose, and 20 mM tris-HCl buffer (pH 7.4). The tissue is homogenized briefly and centrifuged for 30 minutes at 20,000 g. The resultant pellet is washed once and the entire supernatant centrifuged for 60 minutes at 78,000 g. The crude microsomal pellet is then fractionated by ficoll-sucrose density gradient density centrifugation. This produces several classes of membranes which may vary in their content of enzyme.

Vesicles prepared from isolated parietal cell membranes are oriented inside-out so that the outer surface of the vesicle reflects the cell interior. The basic principle behind vesicular H^+ transport is that in the absence of ATP, vesicles have a low permeability to either K^+ or Cl^- and a small but measurable H^+ conductance. In the presence of ATP and K^+ inside the vesicle, H^+ moves into the interior of the vesicle in exchange for the K^+, leaving hydroxyl ion on the outside. Acid transport into the gastric vesicles was first demonstrated by Lee et al.[114] showing that, in the presence of ATP, the suspending medium was alkalinized. The process was reversed when the vesicles were disrupted by the addition of detergents. Lyophilization of the vesicles or addition of a K^+ ionophore also reverses the H^+ gradient.

Vesicles (0.25−0.3 mg/ml) are normally incubated for 2 hours at room temperature or for longer periods at 4°C in 150 mM KCl, 2 mM $MgCl_2$ and kept on ice until used, ideally within 3 hours.[115] Subsequent dilution of the vesicle preparation in osmotic media such as 386 mM mannitol or isotonic sucrose enhances the KCl gradient by reducing the intravesicular space and elevating the K^+ concentration which can be used in exchange for H^+. Rehydration of the intravesicular space is dependent upon the permeability of the vesicle membrane to the solute used to create the osmotic gradient. Equilibration in KCl or K_2SO_4 for long periods (24–72 hrs) at 4°C to maintain function yields a greater intravesicular K^+. Uptake of H^+ in response to ATP is dependent upon both the concentration of KCl and the duration of the preincubation.[116] There is a progressive loss in the osmotic sensitivity of H^+ transport with longer periods of incubation with KCl.

The dependency of acid secretion of extracellular K^+ was demonstrated early on in isolated gastric mucosa[117] and later confirmed in gastric glands.[118] The mechanism, however, which operated to increase parietal cell permeability to K^+ in vivo remained one of the unsolved mysteries of vesicle research. Significant uptake of H^+ into the resting vesicle could only be demonstrated if the vesicle interior was preloaded with K^+ by long term incubation with KCl. In addition, a slow uptake was possible in the presence of a K^+ channel ionophore. Studies by Wolosin and Forte[119], however, showed that differences in H^+/K^+ activity result from isolation of vesicles from parietal cells in the basal versus the stimulated state. In the resting state, vesicles have a low interior K^+ content and the membrane permeability to K^+ is low. There is however, a small basal Mg^{2+} ATPase activity and a slight increase in H^+ movement in the presence of K^+. Luminal K^+ (lumen = vesicle interior) is needed for H^+ transport because H^+/K^+ is stimulated by luminal K^+ which is then used in exchange for H^+ in the parietal cell (cell interior = vesicle medium). Addition of valinomycin, a K^+ ionophore, or of nigericin (at certain concentrations) or gramicidin, neutral H^+/K^+ exchange carriers, stimulates H^+ entry by increasing the entry of K^+ into the vesicle.[120] The gradient is then reversed by nigericin (or gramicidin).

In stimulated vesicles, incubation with KCl or addition of valinomycin is not needed for ATP-induced H^+ transport. Once the HCl gradient is formed, addition of ionophores such as nigericin (Figure 19, both tracings) reverse the gradient. In addition, the protonophore, tetrachlorosalicylanide (TCS) allows the back leak of HCl and is often used in combination with valinomycin, the K^+ ionophore to dissipate the gradient. Vesicles taken from stimulated mucosa have an increased enzyme activity and a high K^+ and Cl^- permeability suggesting that

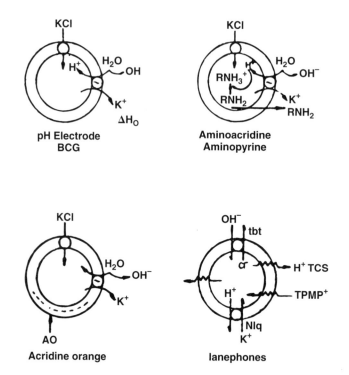

FIGURE 13 Models illustrating the mechanism of the different probes used to monitor pH changes and the different ionophores used to modify the signals. BCG, bromocresol green; R, NH_2, 9 aminopyrine or aminoacridine; tbt, tributyltin, an anion (OH^-/Cl^-) exchange ionophore; TCS, tetrachlorsalicylanilide. (Reprinted from Rabon et al., *Proc. Symp. Gastric Ion Transport,* 1977, 409. With permission.)

there is a K^+ entry pathway in stimulated cells that is absent in the basal state. The increased enzyme activity and intravesicular K^+ is associated with an altered membrane conductance to K^+ and Cl^- and a decreased resistance facilitated, in part, by the enlarged apical surface area which occurs following stimulation of acid secretion. Recent evidence from patch clamp studies indicates that receptor-mediated activation of the second messenger cAMP (via histamine) or Ca^{2+} (via gastrin or acetylcholine) increases K^+ conductance via two distinct K^+ channels in the basolateral membrane.[121]

Several techniques have been employed to study ion transport in membrane vesicles, the most popular being pH electrodes (electrometric) and pH sensitive dyes (spectrophotometric). It should be noted, however, that many of these dyes have an inhibitory effect on ATPase activity. Probes can be used to detect either changes in the pH of the medium (external) or in the vesicle space (internal). Electrodes and the pH indicator dye, bromocresol green, can be used to measure changes in external pH which are usually very slight. The suspending medium is traditionally maintained at 6.1, a point at which the acid generated during the hydrolysis of the ATP in the medium is less than that accumulated intravesicularly. Alkalinization as a result of H^+ transport is verified by the addition of small amounts of HCl to the medium. Electrodes have a slow response and are unable to measure the actual pH gradient formed and, therefore, they should be selected for the lowest electrical noise and the fastest response. Monitoring of external pH is helpful when the kinetics of the response are rapid.

Internal pH can be measured using several probes: 1) fluorescent, spectrophometric, or radioactive detection of weak bases which accumulate in the vesicular space such as 9-aminoacridine and unlabelled or labelled (^{14}C) aminopyrine; 2) pH indicator dyes such as malachite green; 3) negative (oxonol dyes) and positively charged probes (carbocyanine dyes); and 4) dyes that bind to the membrane as a function of changes in pH (acridine orange). Generally, the movement of each of these internal probes from the external medium to the vesicle interior is monitored by a change in absorbance or fluorescence using a scanning spectrophotometer or fluorimeter. In the case of labelled bases, suspensions of the vesicles are placed on filter paper, washed and counted. Weak bases are trapped inside the intravesicular space as a consequence of the low pH. Measurement is made of the color change or fluoresecent quenching upon conversion of the unprotonated to the protonated form. The electroneutrality of the H^+/K^+ exchange was elucidated using lipid permeable ions to assess possible changes in potential in response to stimulation by ATP. These probes are usually given in the presence of ionophores to establish gradients which allow accumulation of the probe. Thus, in the presence of valinomycin to create a K^+ gradient (high K^+ inside), the anionic oxonol dyes such as 8-anilino-napthalenesulfonate (ANS) or SCN-undergo a change in absorbance in response to ATP giving evidence of a positive internal potential. Alternately, in the presence of ATP to generate a H^+ gradient (high H^+ inside), cationic carbocyanines such as diethyoxocarbocyanine or di-S-C_3-5 undergo no change in optical signal indicating the absence of an interior negative potential contributing to H^+ movement during acid secretion. Addition of the protonophore TCS induces a back leak of the H^+ leaving the cation dyes trapped on the interior of the vesicle which then induces an alteration in fluorescence showing an internal negative potential. The mechanism of the various internal and external probes used to analyse changes in pH in the vesicles is illustrated in Figure 13.[122]

Vesicle preparations have provided valuable insight into the mechanism of H^+ secretion, particularly the kinetics of the H^+/K^+ ATPase and the entry of KCl. The recognition of a change in the vesicular membrane during the stimulated state eliminated much of controversy over variability in results. It must be remembered, however, that acid secretion *in vivo* is a mutifactoral system and acid concentration in vesicles does not reach the physiological maximum. In addition, the differences between responses in vesicles versus those obtained in more intact preparations (glands) would indicate that vesicles are an important, but not complete, model of acid secretion, lacking perhaps such factors as carbonic anhydrase.

MECHANISMS OF GASTRIC ACID SECRETION

EARLY THEORIES OF ACID SECRETION

No discussion of acid secretion would be complete without addressing the various models proposed for acid secretion over the years. Indeed, modifications of previous mechanisms were often a direct result of new techniques. Most of the early models were derived from *in vivo* studies which could only imagine events at the cellular level. *In vitro* techniques are justly credited with our current understanding of the mechanism of acid secretion.

The Precursor Theory

Although it was known since Prout that the stomach acid was HCl, the source was unclear. An early theory of acid secretion involved a hydrolyzable precursor which was converted to acid in the lumen. From histological studies, gastric acid was proposed to come from cells in the fundus called acidophiles because of their ability to take up acidic dyes like eosin. The location of acid to these cells was somewhat accidental and was later attributed to the large number of mitochondria rather than to acid secretion. Using isolated glands, Bradford and Davies[123] subsequently confirmed that the primary secretion of the parietal cell was acid thereby eliminating the precursor theory.

The Redox Reaction

Data obtained from the *in vivo* methods that predominated in the early part of the twentieth century were consistent with H[+] secretion as a redox reaction based on the separation of protons and electrons.[124] *In vitro* methods demonstrating the oxygen-dependence of acid secretion[125] supported an electrogenic redox model.

The Carbonic Anhydrase Theory

The next advance came with Davenport's demonstration of carbonic anhydrase in the gastric mucosa. He proposed that the parietal cell reaction was a chloride shift similar to that observed in erythrocytes, but in reverse. This explanation of acid secretion used a known simple passive transport system; however, the mechanism by which H[+] exited the cell was unknown. In 1946, Davenport retracted his theory in the famous obituary entitled *In memorium: the carbonic anhydrase theory of gastric secretion.*[126] Although this model could not explain energy-dependence of generating a large H[+] gradient, basic concepts such as the "alkaline tide" have endured.[127]

The Two Component Theory

The mechanism of HCl secretion associated with the "two component" theory introduced by Hollander in the 1940's involved two chemical reactions occuring in the wall of the intracellular cannaliculi.[128] In this model there was a permeability to water, H[+], and Cl[-] on the apical side of the cell and to water and alkaline buffers on the basolateral side. The reactions at the wall of the intracellular cannaliculus were:

$$NaCl + H_2O = HCl + NaOH$$

$$NaOH + NaH_2PO_4 = H_2O + Na_2HPO_4$$

Based on data obtained from *in vitro* studies addressing the electrophysiological properties of the gastric mucosa,[75] Hollander proposed that electrical energy generated by the membrane regulated acid secretion and that the source of the H[+] was a biochemical action.

MODERN THEORIES OF ACID SECRETION

The movement of H[+] into the lumen occurs in the face of a tremendous concentration gradient. Cl[-] also moves against a gradient, albeit much smaller. In the 1960's, the uphill transport of these two ions into the lumen were viewed as two separate active processes. This view was later modified to include a symport for the apical exit of K[+] with Cl[-] as well as a separate channel for Cl[-].[129]

Application of electrophysiology techniques to the study of acid secretion in gastric glands demonstrated that both active and passive transport processes are involved in acid secretion. It was not until the mid–1980's that the mechanism of activation of H[+]/K[+], of K[+] entry into the lumen and of Cl[-] permeability were unraveled. Measurements of enzyme activity and pH sensitive dyes have contributed to the current model of acid secretion in which the basolateral membrane contains an energy dependent Na[+]/K[+] pump and a passive Na[+]/H[+] and Cl[-]/OH[-] exchangers. On the apical side there is an active H[+]/K[+] pump which is somehow linked to increased KCl permeability.[130] Bethanechol, which increases intracellular Ca[2+], and cAMP stimulate acid secretion inducing morphological changes in the parietal secretion primarily translocation of the tubulovesicles to the apical surface. Coincidently, these agents also activate two distinct inward rectifying basolateral K[+] channels, which facilitate K movement out of the cell.[121] Activation of these channels was depressed by omeprazole, but the effect appeared to be indirect. In addition, it is possible that the hyperpolarization resulting from the loss of K^+ may also promote Cl^- exit at the apical membrane. It is likely that the 1990's will provide the steps linking receptor mediated stimulation of parietal cell with the ultrastructural and biochemical changes leading to acid secretion.

THE FUTURE

As with many other areas, studies of gastric secretion will likely take advantage of computer technology and molecular biology. Computer modelling of metabolic systems requires certain assumptions about the dynamics of the system and as long as the assumptions are correct, the model is accurate. Licko and Ekblad[131] conceived of a single-state nonlinear mathematical model of acid secretion based both on experimental and simulated data. Their model is based on a two step hypothesis of acid secretion in which the generation and secretion of HCl are distinct sequential processes separated by an acid storage pool. At this point, acceptance of the model requires a similar view. An "elemental" model accounts for the observation that brief exposure to a high concentration of a stimulant elicits a prolonged maximal rate of acid secretion when compared to a similar exposure to a low concentration of the same stimulus. From this they conclude that acid secretion is a saturable process limited by the amount of stored acid available for release rather than to the concentration of the stimulus. The "augmented" model includes subsystems to account for the time delay following stimulation and the mechanism of action of the stimulant. If the mathematical models are defensible by empirical data, computer modelling offers a new and exciting tool for the study of acid secretion.

The exponential growth in the application of molecular biology techiques has already impacted the study of gastric acid secretion. During the last 25 years, the development of nucleic acid sequencing methods, restriction enzymes, and plasmids has resulted in an elucidation of the factors involved in the gene regulation of gastrointestinal peptides particularly of the gastrin/cholecytokinin, glucagon/secretin, and pancreatic polypeptide/neuropeptide Y/peptide YY families of hormones. For an individual peptide or hormone, isolation and characterization of the mRNA, construction of the corresponding cDNA and screening of the cDNA library, amplification of the cDNA using polymerase chain reaction, and isolation of the cloned genes illustrate just a few of the methods of this complex process.[132] Hopefully, the understanding of the gene expression of gut peptides will bring greater insight into their function.

SUMMARY AND CONCLUSIONS

Most of our knowledge of digestion, specifically of acid secretion, was gained in the twentieth century. Table 1 summarizes commonly used techniques. Data obtained from pouch preparations fostered an appreciation of the complexity of acid secretion. Comparison of acid secretory responses in the denervated Heidenhain pouch with those of the innervated Pavlov pouch, or in modifications of these pouches, allowed for the discrimination between the neural and humoral components of acid secretion. Clinical assessment of gastric acid secretion was propelled by the close association of acidity and ulceration. The use of a tube to collect gastric juice was the basis for subsequent gastric aspiration techniques. Continuous or intermittent aspiration was first modified by Hunt to include an indicator dye to measure gastric acid in response to a series of test meals. The method of intragastric titration was developed to expand the repertoire of stimulants to include solids. The desire to improve accuracy of the measurements led to the technique of Dubois et al.,[28] which allowed the simultaneous measurement of acid

TABLE 1
Methods for Assessing Gastric Acid Secretion

Technique	Advantages	Disadvantages	Comments
In vivo			
Gastric fistula	Simple surgery, conscious animals, chronic preparation, normal gastric function retained	Error due to loss of acid by gastric emptying or dilution by secreted fluid, liquid meals only	Can be adapted for small animals
Gastric pouches	Various modifications allow separation of neural and hormonal factors, conscious animals, chronic preparation	Need large animals, requires advanced surgical skills	Can be adapted for sham feeding experiments in dogs by constructing esophagostomies
Continuous aspiration	Simple to perform, no surgical intervention, conscious subjects	Nasogastric intubation eliminates use in many species, eliminates normal feedback from duodenum, reflux may result from continuous suction, liquid meals only	Can be adapted to other species by constructing fistulas or esophagostomies
Intragastric titration	No surgical intervention, conscious subjects, liquid and solid meals.	Artificial maintenance of intragastric pH to fixed value interferes with normal feedback mechanisms, error due to loss of acid by gastric emptying or dilution by secreted fluid	
Dye dilution technique	Corrects for loss of acid by gastric emptying or dilution by secreted fluid, normal gastric function retained	Nasogastric intubation eliminates use in many species, requires specific computer program, liquid meals only, acute studies	Can be used to determine secretion of other components of gastric juice (e.g. Na^+, K^+, Cl^-, mucus)
Double marker technique	Normal gastric function retained, allows study of intestinal regulation,	Nasogastric intubation eliminates use in many species, requires specific computer program, requires technical expertise, acute studies	
Shay preparation (pylorus ligation)	Easy to perform, eliminates loss of acid through pylorus, used in small animals	Increase in gastric volume alters secretion, eliminates normal feedback from duodenum, inappropriate for large animals, acute preparation	Often used in combination with other methods
Chambered stomach	Allows measurement of ion flux, potential difference, blood supply intact, access to secretory surface	Need large animals, requires surgical skills, acute preparation	

TABLE 1
(*continued*)

Technique	Advantages	Disadvantages	Comments
In vitro			
Excised stomach	Easy to perform, need small animals, appropriate to measure acid in response to hormones, nerve stimulation and exogenous agents, intact mucosa, eliminates complications of variations in blood flow	Requires constant perfusion of stomach, maximum acid secretion less than *in vivo,* blood supply interrupted	
Ussing chamber	Allows measurement of ion transport, potential difference, short circuit currents, tissue resistance, access to nutrient and secretory surfaces, intact mucosa	Blood supply interrupted, mucosa is stretched,	Attachment of strain gauge allows simultaneous measurement of muscle function
Microelectrodes	Measure activities of individual within intact mucosa, intramural pH, access to surface cells,	Interference by mucus	
Isolated glands	Retain cell polarity and cell to cell connections	Heterogenous cell population, acid secretion measured indirectly	
Isolated parietal cell	Measure response specific to parietal cell	Acid secretion measured indirectly, loss of cell polarity and cell to cell connections, contamination by other cells	Immunohistochemical study questions location of receptors of major stimulants of acid secretion
Isolated vesicles	Measure enzyme activity and ion transport, resting and stimulated states	Acid secretion measured indirectly, predicted accumulation of H^+ less than *in vivo*	

and fluid secretion as well as gastric emptying. Each refinement in the aspiration technique was made in consideration of the numerous physiological controls of gastric secretion, culminating in the double-marker dilution method of Malagelada et al.[51] Performance of the more novel aspiration techniques was marred by the increasing amount of time and computer expertise needed to collect and analyze the results. Unfortunately, the ability to perform these techniques was at times confined to the centers at which they were developed. This has been remedied with the tremendous advancements in computer technology allowing most of these programs to be run on a personal computer.

The inability of *in vivo* techniques to discern the source of energy, the ionic mechanisms, or the electrical events involved in acid secretion led to the development of methods using isolated tissues. These methods had the advantage of minimizing or eliminating complicating factors such as neural control, diffusion barriers and variations in blood flow. The isolated dog flap preparation was one of the first methods to examine such parameters as potential difference and ion flux. Isolated tissue in a Ussing chamber enabled accurate measurements of short circuit current, illustrating the 1:1 movement of H^+ into the mucosal solution accompanied by OH^- into the serosal side. Isolated mucosa was also important in elucidating the response to single stimulants, particularly histamine. However, the heterogeneity of the cell population, compounded by problems with species differences, limited the use isolated mucosa in its ability to identify a single response with a specific cell type.

The cellular physiology of acid secretion was investigated using isolated gastric glands, parietal cells, and vesicles. Glands are the most 'intact' of these three preparations, retaining their intercellular connections, cell appearance, gap junctions and polarity but also contain a heterogenous cell population. Isolated cells acid secretion cannot be measured directly in isolated cells and glands. Instead, sequestration of weak bases, like aminopyrine, reflect the amount of acid sequestered intracellularly and are used as a index of acid secretion. These preparations were invaluble in elucidating the mechanism of action of the three major stimulants of acid secretion *in vivo,* histamine, gastrin, and acetylcholine. Studies in isolated parietal cells revealed the presence of three distinct receptors and demonstrated an interdependence and potentiation among the three secretagogues. These classic observations have been questioned, however, by recent immunohistochemical studies which failed to visualize any receptors on the parietal cell.

Membrane vesicle preparations were used to isolate the H^+/K^+ ATPase, which fuels the apical H^+/K^+ exchanger, the final step in acid secretion. Assessment of acid secretion is indirect requiring the use of probes which monitor changes in pH or ion potential. Although the K^+ dependency of acid secretion was well documented, vesicles showed that stimulated parietal cells undergo an increase in enzyme activity accompanied by an alteration in K^+ conductance. Patch clamp studies suggest that basolateral K^+ channels are activated in response to cAMP and Ca^{2+}, important second messengers of receptor-mediated acid secretion.

It is certain that future studies will take advantage of two major weapons: the power of the computer modelling and the burgeoning arsenal of molecular biology techniques. Mathematical modelling of acid secretion has been attempted and research into the gene regulation of several of the major families of hormones is progressing rapidly. There is certainly room to improve current methods or develop new techniques to study gastric acid secretion. The complex control of acid secretion insures the continuance of *in vivo* approaches. However, *in vitro* techniques will invariably provide more detailed information regarding the workings of the parietal cell, with molecular biology in a supportive role. If this seems like an endorsement for using a combination of both *in vivo* and *in vitro* techniques; it is.

REFERENCES

1. **Galen,** *On the Natural Faculties,* English translation Brock, A. J., Harvard University Press, Cambridge, 1963.
2. **Vesalius, A.,** *Fabrica,* 1555.
3. **Santorio, S.,** *Ars de statica medicina,* Translation by Quincy, J., William Newton, London, 1712.
4. **Boerhave, H.,** *Institutiones Medicae,* 1708.
5. **Reaumur, R.,** *Sur la digestion des oiseaux,* Mem. Acad. Roy. Sci., Paris, 1752.
6. **Spallanzani, L,** *Dissertations Relative to the Natural History of Animals and Vegetables,* translated from the Italian of the Abbe Spallanzani, J. Murray, London, 1784.
7. From an English translation of a thesis by Edward Stevens contained in Spallanzani, *Dissertations Relative to the Natural History of Animals and Vegetables,* London, J. Murray, 1784.

8. **Hunter, J.,** *On the Digestion of the Stomach After Death,* Philosophical Transactions, 1772.

9. **Young, J.,** *An Experimental Inquiry into the Principles of Nutrition, and the Digestive Process,* Eaken & Mecum, Philadelphia, 1803.

10. **Prout, W.,** *On the Nature of the Acid and Saline Matters Usually Existing in the Stomachs of Animals,* Phil. Trans., 114, 45, 1824.

11. **Beaumont, W.,** *Experiments and Observations on the Gastric Juice and the Physiology of Digestion,* Plattsburgh, N. Y., F. G. Allen, 1833.

12. **Pavlov, I. P.,** *The Work of the Digestive Glands,* Thompson, W. H., Translator, London, Charles Griffin and Co., 1902.

13. **Emas, S., Swan, K. G., and Jacobson, E. D.,** Methods of studying gastric secretion, in *Handbook of Physiology. Section 6: Alimentary Canal, Volume II,* Code, C. F., Ed., American Physiological Society, Washington, D. C., 1967, chapter 42.

14. **Heidenhain, R.,** *Uber die Absonderung der Fundusdrusen des Magens,* Pflugers Arch. Ges. Physiol., 19, 148–166, 1879.

15. **Thomas, J. E.,** A simplified procedure for preparing an improved Pavlov pouch, *Proc. Soc. Exptl. Biol. Med.,* 50, 58, 1942.

16. **Komorov, S. A. and Marks, I. N.,** Esophagostomy in the dog allowing natural feeding, *Proc. Soc. Exptl. Biol. Med.,* 97, 574, 1958.

17. **Olbe, L.,** Esophageal cannula fog, a simple mode of preparation for sham feeding experiments, *Gastroenterlogy,* 37, 460, 1959.

18. **Lim, R. K., Ivy, A. C., and McCarthy, J. E.,** Contributions to the physiology of gastric secretion, *Quart. J. Exptl. Physiol.,* 15, 13, 1925.

19. **Armour, J.,** A lesser curvature gastroplasty, *Can. Med. Assoc. J.,* 23, 756, 1930.

20. **Perry, J. F., Salmon, P., Griffin, W. O., Root, H. D., and Wangensteen, O. H.,** A simple technique for preparing vagally innervated gastric pouches in dogs, *Surgery,* 45, 937, 1959.

21. **Uvnas, B., Andersson, S., Elwin, C. E., and Malm, A.,** The influence of exclusion of the antrum-duodenum passage or the HCl secretion in Pavlov pouch, *Gastroenterology,* 30, 790, 1956.

22. **Grossman, M. I., Robertson, C. R., and Ivy, A. C.,** Proof of a hormonal mechanism for gastric secretion—The humoral transmission of the distension stimulus, *Am. J. Physiol.,* 152, 1, 1948.

23. **Grossman, M. I.,** Secretion of acid and pepsin in response to distension of vagally innervated fundic gland area in dogs, *Gastroenterology,* 42, 718–721, 1962.

24. **Guldvog, I.,** Vagally innervated and denervated gastric pouch in one and the same dog—a new model, *Scand. J. Gastroenterol.,* 15, 921, 1980.

25. **Goldvog, I. and Gedde-Dahl, D.,** Comparison of physiological and pharmacological stimulation of acid secretion in vagally innervated and denervated gastric pouches in the same dog, *Scand. J. Gastroenterol.,* 15, 929, 1970.

26. **Kivilaakso, E.,** High plasma HCO_3^- protects gastric mucosa against acute ulceration in the rat, *Gastroenterology,* 81, 921, 1981.

27. **Hunt, J. N. and MacDonald, I.,** The relation between the volume of a test meal and the gastric secretory response, *J. Physiol.,* 117, 289, 1952.

28. **Dubois, A., Van Eerdewegh, P., and Gardner, J. D.,** Gastric emptying and secretion in Zollinger-Ellison Syndrome, *J. Clin. Invest.,* 59, 255, 1977.

29. **Johansson, C.,** Studies of gastrointestinal interactions, *Scand. J. Gastroenterol.,* 9 (suppl 28), 1, 1974.

30. **Brodie, D. A.,** The mechanism of gastric hyperacidity produced by pyloric ligation in the rat, *Am. J. Dig. Dis.,* 11, 231, 1966.

31. **Feldman, M.,** Gastric H^+ and HCO_3 secretion in response to sham feeding in humans, *Am. J. Physiol.,* 248, G188, 1985.

32. **Grossman, M. I.,** The secretion of the pyloric glands of the dog, *Proc. Int. Congr. Physiol. Sci. 21st,* Buenos Aires, 1959, 226.

33. **Hollander, F.,** The two-component mucus barrier, *Arch. Int. Med.,* 94, 107, 1954.

34. **Garner, A. and Hurst, B. C.,** Gastric bicarbonate secretion and mucosal cell loss in the dog, in *Basic Mechanisms of Gastrointestinal Mucosal Cell Injury and Cytoprotection,* Harmon, J. F., Ed., Williams and Wilkins, Baltimore, MD, 1981, chapter 19.

35. **Garner, A. and Flemstrom, G.,** Gastric HCO_3^- secretion in the guinea pig, *Am. J. Physiol.,* 234, E535, 1978.

36. **Fordtran, J. S. and Walsh, J. S.,** Gastric acid secretion rate and buffer content of the stomach after eating. Results in normal subject and in patients with duodenal ulcer, *J. Clin. Invest.,* 52, 645, 1973.

37. **Feldman, M.,** Comparison of acid secretion rates measured by gastric aspiration and by *in vivo* intragastric titration in healthy human subjects, *Gastroenterology,* 76, 954, 1979.

38. **Hildes, J. A. and Dunlop, D. L.,** A method for estimating the rates of gastric secretion and emptying, *Can. J. Med. Sci.,* 29, 83, 1951.

39. **George, J. D.,** New clinical method for measuring the rate of gastric emptying: the double sample test meal, *Gut,* 9, 237, 1968.

40. **Hunt, J. N.,** Gastric emptying and secretion in man, *Physiol. Rev.,* 39, 491, 1959.

41. **Hunt, J. N.,** A modification of the method of George for the study of gastric emptying, *Gut,* 15, 812–813, 1974.

42. **Nompleggi, D., Myers, L., Castell, D. O., and Dubois, A,** Effect of a prostaglandin E_2 analog on gastric emptying and secretion in rhesus monkeys, *J. Pharmacol. Exp. Ther.,* 212, 491, 1980.

43. **Shea-Donohue, T., Nompleggi, D., Meyers, L., and Dubois, A.,** Effect of a prostaglandin $F_{2\alpha}$ analog on gastric emptying and secretion in rhesus monkeys, *J. Pharmacol. Exp. Ther.,* 219, 287, 1981.

44. **Dubois, A., Price, S. F., and Castell, D. O.,** Gastric retention in peptic ulcer disease. A reappraisal, *Am. J. Dig. Dis.,* 23, 993, 1978.

45. **Dubois, A., Gross, H. A., Ebert, M. H., and Castell, D. O.,** Altered gastric emptying and secretion in primary anorexia nervosa, *Gastroenterology,* 77, 319–323, 1979.

46. **Danquechin-Dorval, E., Mueller, G. P., Eng, R. R., Durakovic, A., Conklin, J. J., and Dubois, A.,** Effect of ionizing radiation on gastric secretion and gastric motility in monkeys, *Gastroenterology,* 89, 374, 1985.

47. **Dubois, A. and Natelson, B. H.,** Habituation of gastric function suppression in monkeys after repeated free-operant avoidance sessions, *Physiological Psychology,* 6, 524, 1978.

48. **Weichbrod, R. H., Harmon, J. W., Batzri, S., Cisar, C. F., and Dubois, A.,** A chronic *in vivo* model for the measurement of gastric function in the awake guinea pig, *Lab Animal Sci.,* 35, 550A, 1985.

49. **Nylander, B. and Andersson, S.,** Gastric secretory inhibition by three methyl analogs of prostaglandin E_2 administered intragastrically to man, *Scan. J. Gastroenterol.* 9, 751–758, 1974.

50. **Robert, A., Nezamis, J., Lancaster, C., and Hanchar, A. J.,** Cytoprotection by prostaglandins in rats. Prevention of gastric necrosis produced by alcohol, HCl, NaOH, hypertonic NaCl, and thermal injury, *Gastroenterology,* 77, 433–443, 1979.

51. **Malagelada, J. -R., Longstreth, G. F., Summerskill, W. H. J., and Go, V. L. W.,** Measurement of gastric function during digestion of ordinary solid meals in man, *Gastroenterology,* 70, 203, 1976.

52. **Kholief, H., Larach, J., Thomforde, G. M., Dozois, R. R., and Malagelada, J. -R.,** A canine model for the study of gastric secretion and emptying after a meal, *Dig. Dis. Sci.,* 28, 633, 1983.

53. **Malagelada, J. -R., Go, V. L. W., and Summerskill, W. H. J.,** Different gastric, pancreatic, and biliary responses to solid-liquid or homogenized meals, *Am. J. Dig. Dis.,* 24, 101–110, 1979.

54. **Levitt, M. D. and Bond, J.,** Use of the constant perfusion technique in the non-steady state, *Gastroenterology,* 73, 1450–1453, 1977.

55. **Longstreth, G. F., Malagelada, J. -R., and Go, V. L. W.,** The gastric response to a transpyloric duodenal tube, *Gut,* 16, 777–780, 1975.

56. **Shay, H., Sun, D. C. H., and Gruenstein, M.,** A quantitative method for measuring spontaneous gastric secretion in the rat, *Gastroenterology,* 26, 906, 1954.

57. **Donald, D. E. and Code, C. F.,** A study of gastric secretion in fasting rats, *Gastroenterology,* 20, 298, 1952.

58. **Lim, R. K. S., Necheles, H., and Ni, T. G.,** The vasomotor reactions of the vivi-perfused stomach, *Chinese J. Physiol.,* 1, 381, 1927.

59. **Ni, T. G. and Lim, R. K. S.,** The gas and sugar metabolism of the vivi-perfused stomach, *Chinese J. Physiol.,* 2, 45, 1928.

60. **Taylor, T. V., Holt, S., McLoughlin, G. P., and Heading, R. C.,** A single scan technique for estimating acid output, *Gastroenterology,* 77, 1241–1244, 1979.

61. **Teorell, T.,** Electrolyte diffusion in relation to the acidity regulation of the gastric juice, *Gastroenterology,* 9, 425–443, 1947.

62. **Pavlov, I. P.,** *The Work of the Digestive Glands* Edition 2, Lippincourt, Philadelphia, 1910.

63. **Teorell, T.,** On the primary acidity of the gastric juice. *J. Physiol.,* London, 97, 308–315, 1940.

64. **Teorell, T.,** On the permeability of the stomach for acids and some other substances, *J. Gen. Physiol.,* 23, 263–274, 1939.

65. **Hollander, F.,** The composition of pure gastric juice, *Am. J. Dig. Dis.,* 1, 319–329, 1934.

66. **Hollander, F.,** Factors which reduce gastric acidity, *Am. J. Dig. Dis.,* 5, 364–372, 1938.

67. **Hollander, F.,** Gastric secretion of electrolytes, *Fed. Proc. Am. Soc. Exp. Biol.,* 11, 706–714, 1952.

68. **Davenport, H. W.,** Gastric mucosal injury by fatty and acetyl-salicyclic acids, *Gastroenterology,* 46, 245–253, 1964.

69. **Davenport, H. W. and Chavre, V. J.,** Conditions affecting acid secretion by mouse stomachs *in vitro, Gastroenterology,* 15, 467, 1950.

70. **Bunce, K. T. and Parsons, M. E.,** A quantitative study of metiamide, a histamine H_2-antagonist, on the isolated whole rat stomach, *J. Physiol.,* London, 258, 453, 1976.

71. **Shubert, M. L., Hightower, J., Coy, D. H., and Maklouf G. M.,** Regulation of acid secretion by bombesin/GRP neurons of the gastric fundus, *Am. J. Physiol.,* 260, G156, 1991.

72. **Delrue, G.,** Etude de secretion acide de l'estomac, *Arch. Int. Physiol.,* 33, 196–216, 1930.

73. **Durbin, R. P.,** Electrical potential difference of the gastric mucosa, In: *Handbook of Physiology. Section 6: The Gastrointestinal System, Volume 2,* Code, C.F., Ed., American Physiological Society, Bethesda, MD, 1967, chapter 49.

74. **Rehm, W. S.,** The effect of electric current on gastric secretion and potential, *Am. J. Physiol.,* 144, 115–125, 1945.

75. **Rehm, W. S.,** A theory on the formation of HCl by the stomach, *Gastroenterology,* 14, 401–417, 1950.

76. **Ussing, H. H. and Zerahn, K.,** Active transport of sodium as the source of electrical current in the short circuit isolated frog skin, *Acta Physiol. Scand.,* 23, 110, 1951.

77. **Rehm, W. S.,** Ion permeability and electrical resistance of the frog's gastric mucosa, *Fed. Proc.,* 26, 1303–1313, 1967.

78. **Hogben, C. A. M.,** Active transport of chloride by isolated frog gastric epithelium; origin of the gastric mucosal potential, *Am. J. Physiol.,* 180, 641–649, 1955.

79. **Hegel, U., Fromm, M., Kruesel, K. M., and Wiederholt, M.,** Bovine and porcine large intestine as model epithelia in a student lab course, *Adv. Physiol. Education,* 10, S10, 1993.

80. **Li, Y. F., Weisbrodt, N. W., Harari, Y., and Moody, F.,** Use of a modified Ussing chamber to monitor intestinal epithelial and smooth muscle function, *Am. J. Physiol.,* 261, G166, 1991.

81. **Spenney, J. G., Saccomani, G., Spitzer, H. L. and Sachs, G.,** Composition of gastric cell membranes and polypeptide fractionation using ionic and non-ionic conductance pathways, *Arch. Biochem. Biophys.,* 161, 456, 1974.

82. **Kivilaakso, E., Fromm, D., and Silen, W.,** Effect of the acid secretory state on intramural pH of the rabbit gastric mucosa, *Gastroenterology,* 75, 641, 1978.

83. **Kivilaasko, E., Fromm, D., and Silen, W.,** Relationship between ulceration and intramural pH of gastric mucosa during haemorrhagic shock, *Surgery,* 84, 70, 1978.

84. **Shanbour, L. L., Miller, J., and Chowdhury, T. K.,** Effects of alcohol on active transport in the rat stomach, *Am. J. Physiol.,* 226, 397–400, 1974.

85. **Kuo, Y. J., and Shanbour, L. L.,** Inhibition of ion transport by bile salts in canine gastric mucosa. *Am. J. Physiol.,* 231, 1433–1437, 1976.

86. **Kuo, Y. J., and Shanbour, L. L.,** Mechanism of action of aspirin on canine gastric mucosa, *Am. J. Physiol.,* 230, 762–767, 1976.

87. **Davenport, H. W.,** Ethanol damage to canine oxyntic glandular mucosa, *Proc. Soc. Exp. Biol. Med.,* 126, 657, 1967.

88. **Tepperman, B. L., Tepperman, F. S., Fang, W. F., and Jacobson, E. D.,** Effects of 16, 16-dimethyl prostaglandin E_2 on ion transport by isolated rabbit gastric mucosa and rat intestinal epithelial cells, *Can. J. Physiol. Pharmacol.,* 56, 834–839, 1978.

89. **Kitahara, S., Fox, H. R., and Hogben, C. A. M.,** Acid secretion, Na^+ and the origin of the potential difference across isolated mammalian stomachs, *Am. J. Dig. Dis.,* 14, 221, 1969.

90. **Hanson, M. E., Grossman, M. I., and Ivey, A. C.,** Doses of histamine producing minimal and maximal secretory responses in dog and man, *Am. J. Physiol.,* 153, 242, 1948.

91. **Kuo, Y. J., Shanbour, L. L., and Sernka, T. J.,** Effect of ethanol on permeability and ion transport in the isolated dog stomach, *Dig. Dis.,* 19, 818, 1974.

92. **Fromm, D., Schwartz, J. H., and Quijano, R.,** Transport of H^+ and other electrolytes across isolated gastric mucosa of the rabbit, *Am. J. Physiol.,* 228, 166, 1975.

93. **Taft, R. C. and Sessions, J. T.,** Inhibition of gastric acid secretion by dibutryl cyclic adenosine-3′,5′-monophosphate, *Clin. Res.,* 20, 43.

94. **Mao, C. C., Shanbour, L. L., Hodgins, D. S., and Jacobsen, E. D.,** Adenosine-3′,5′-monophosphate (cyclic AMP) and secretion in the canine stomach, *Gastroenterology,* 63, 427, 1972.

95. **Ekblad, E. B. M., Machen, T. E., Licko, V., and Rutten, M. J.,** Histamine, cyclic AMP and the secretory response of the piglet gastric mucosa, in *Proc. Symp. Gastric Ion Transport, Uppsala 1977,* Obrink, K. J. and Flemstrom, G., Eds., Almqvist & Wiksell International, Stockholm, 1977, 69.

96. **Soll, A. H. and Berglindh, T.,** Physiology of isolated gastric glands and parietal cell: receptors and effectors regulating function, in *Physiology of the Gastrointestinal Tract, Second Edition,* Johnson, L. R., Ed., Raven Press, New York, 1987, 883.

97. **Berglindh, T., Helander, H. F., and Obrink, K. J.,** Effects of secretagogues on oxygen consumption, aminopyrine accumulation and morphology in isolated gastric glands, *Acta Physiologica, Scand.,* 87, 21A–22A, 1976.

98. **Chew, C. S. and Hersey, S. J.,** Gastrin stimulation of isolated gastric glands, *Am. J. Physiol.,* 242, G504–G512, 1982.

99. **Berglindh, T. and Hansen, D.,** Characterization of isolated gastric glands from the dog, *Fed. Proc.,* 43, 996, 1984.

100. **Rottenberg, H. and Lee, C. P.,** Energy dependent hydrogen ion accumulation in submitochondrial particles, *Biochemistry,* 14, 2675–2680, 1975.

101. **Berglindh, T., Dibona, D. R. Pace, C. S., and Sachs, G.** ATP dependence of H^+ secretion. *J. Cell Biol.,* 85, 392–401, 1980.

102. **Malinkowska, D. H., Koelz, H. R., Hersey, S. J. and Sachs, G.,** Properties of the gastric proton pump in unstimulated permeable gastric glands, *Proc. Nat. Acad. Sci. USA,* 78, 5908, 1981.

103. **Komorov, S. A.,** Gastrin, *Proc. Soc. Exp. Biol. Med.,* 38, 514, 1938.

104. **McIntosh, J. G.,** Histamine as a normal stimulant of gastric secretion, *Q. J. Exp. Physiol.,* 28, 87, 1938.

105. **Kasebekar, D. K., Rehm, W. S. and Sachs, G.,** Eds., Marcel Dekker, New York, 1976, 212.

106. **Grossman, M. I. and Konturek, S. J.,** Inhibition of acid secretion in dog by metiamide, a histamine antagonist acting on H_2 receptors, *Gastroenterology,* 66, 517, 1974.

107. **Johnson, L. R.,** Control of gastric acid secretion. No room for histamine, *Gastroenterology,* 61, 105, 1971.

108. **Black, J. W, Duncan, W. A. M, Durant, C. J., Ganellin, C. R., and Parsons, E. M.,** Definition and antagonism of histamine H_2 receptors, *Nature* (London), 232, 385, 1972.

109. **Soll, A. H.,** The actions of secretagogues on oxygen uptake by isolated mammalian parietal cells, *J. Clin. Invest.,* 61, 370–380, 1978.

110. **Mezey, E. and Palkovits, P.,** Localization of targets for anti-ulcer drugs in cells of the immune system, *Science,* 258, 1662–1665, 4 December 1992.

111. **Fellenium, E., Berglindh, T., Sachs, G., Olbe, L., Elander, E., Sjostrand, S., and Wallmark, B.,** Substituted benzimidazoles inhibit gastric acid secretion by blocking (H^+/K^+) ATPase, *Nature,* 290, 159, 1981.

112. **Rehm, W. S.,** in *Metabolic Transport,* Hokin, L. E., Ed., Academic Press, New York, 1972, 197.

113. **Saccomani, G., Chang, H. H., Mihas, A. A., Crago, S., and Sachs, G.,** An acid transporting enzyme in human gastric mucosa. *J. Clin. Invest.,* 64, 627, 1979.

114. **Lee, J., Simpson, G., and Scholes, P.,** An ATPase from the dog gastric mucosa: changes of outer pH in suspensions of membrane vesicles accompanying ATP hydrolysis, *Biochim. Biophys. Acta,* 60, 825, 1974.

115. **Rabon, E., Chang, H., and Sach, G.,** Quantitation of hydrogen ion and potential gradients in gastric membrane vesicles, *Am. Chem. Soc.,* 17, 3345, 1978.

116. **Michelangeli, F. and Proverbio, F.,** *Acta Physiol. Scand. Special Suppl.,* 1978

117. **Rehm, W. S., Sanders, S. S., Rutledge, J. R., Davies, T. L., Kurfees, J. F., Keesee, D. C., and Bajandas, F. J.,** Effect of removing external K^+ on frog's staomach in Cl^--free solution, *Am. J. Physiol.,* 210, 689, 1966.

118. **Koelz, H. R., Sachs, G., and Berglindh, T.,** Cation effects on acid secretion in rabbit gastric glands, *Am. J. Physiol.,* 241, G431, 1981.

119. **Wolosin, J. M. and Forte, J. G.,** Changes in the membrane environment of the $(K^+ + H^+)$-ATPase following stimulation of the gastric oxyntic cell, *J. Biol. Chem.,* 256, 3149, 1981.

120. **Sachs, G., Kaunitz, J., Mendlein, J., and Wallmark, B.,** Biochemistry of gastric acid secretion: H^+-K^+-ATPase, in *Handbook of Physiology Section 6: The Gastrointestinal System,* Scultz, S. G., Forte, J. G., and Rauner, B. B., American Physiological Society, Bethesda, MD, 1989, chapter 12.

121. **Mieno, H. and Kajiyama, G.,** Electrical characteristics of inward-rectifying K^+ channels in isolated bullfrog oxyntic cells, *Am. J. Physiol.,* 24, G206, 1991.

122. **Rabon, E., Chang, H. H., Saccomani, G., and Sachs, G.,** Transport parameters of gastric vesicles, in *Proc. Symp. Gastric Ion Transport.* Obrink, K. J. and Flemstrom, G., Eds., Almquist & Wiksell International, Stockholm, Sweden, 1977, 409.

123. **Bradford, N. M. and Davies, R. E.,** The site of hydrochloric acid production in the stomach as determined by indicators, *Biochem. J.,,* 46, 414, 1950.

124. **Davenport, H. W.,** Metabolic aspects of gastric acid secretion, in *Metabolic Aspects of Transport Across Cell Membranes,* Murphy, Q. R., Ed., University of Wisconsin Press, Madison, 1957, 295.

125. **Davies, R. E.,** Hydrochloric acid production by isolated gastric mucosa, *Biochem. J.,* 42, 609, 1948.

126. **Davenport, H. W.,** In memorium: the carbonic anhydrase theory of gastric acid secretion, *Gastroenterology,* 7, 374, 1946.

127. **Davenport, H. W.,** *Physiology of the Digestive Tract,* Ed. 2, Year Book, Chicago, 1966.

128. **Hollander, F.,** The chemistry and mechanics of hydrochloric acid formation in the stomach. *Gastroenterology* 1:401, 1943.

129. **Sachs, G.,** The gastric proton pump: The H^+-K^+-ATPase, in *Physiology of the Gastrointestinal Tract,* Johnson, L. R., Ed., Raven Press, New York, 1987, chapter 28.

130. **Forte, J. G. and Soll, A.,** Cell biology of hydrochloric acid secretion, in *Handbook of Physiology Section 6: Alimentary Canal, Volume II,* Code, C. F., Ed., American Physiological Society, Washington, D. C., 1967, chapter 11.

131. **Licko, V. and Ekblad, E. B. M.,** Dynamics of a metabolic system: what single-action agents reveal about acid secretion, *Am. J. Physiol.,* 262, G581, 1992.

132. **Haun, R. S., Minth, C. D., Andrews, P. C., and Dixon, J. E.,** Molecular biology of gut peptides, in *Handbook of Physiology, Section 6: Alimentary Canal, Volume II,* Code, C. F., Ed., American Physiological Society, Washington, D. C., 1967, chapter 1.

133. **Sachs, G.,** The gastric proton pump: The H^+-K^+-ATPase, in *Physiology of the Gastrointestinal Tract,* Johnson, L. R., Ed., Raven Press, New York, 1981, chapter 28.

2 Brain Control of Gastric Acid Secretion: Experimental Methods of Approach

Vicente Martínez and Yvette Taché

INTRODUCTION

Central modulation of gastric acid secretion has been recognized since the early 1800s when the French physiologist, Pierre Jean Georges Cabanis,[1] made the pre-scientific observation that emotion modified gastrointestinal function. Later, in 1833 the army surgeon William Beaumont[2] brought the first objective evidence that emotional states could influence gastric acid secretion in his fistulous subject, Alexis Martin. Approximately 100 years later, Pavlov's pioneer experimental work provided the first experimental demonstration that the central nervous system (CNS) alters gastric acid secretion. He established that the anticipation of eating, as well as visual and gustative stimuli increase gastric acid secretion through vagal dependent pathways in dogs.[3] These findings established the existence of the cephalic or "psychic" phase of gastric secretion as the vagally mediated acid response to the sight and smell of food. Thereafter, electrical stimulation or lesions of brain nuclei pointed out possible areas in the hypothalamus, limbic system, and medulla which would influence gastric acid secretion (review in[4,5]).

During the 1970s, many of the peptides originally detected in the gut were also discovered to be present in the CNS[6] where they exert a potent regulatory action on the autonomic nervous system.[7] Taken together these findings suggested that brain peptides could be involved in the extrinsic modulation of gut function.[8,9] Convergent evidence, which accumulated over the past 15 years, clearly established that the central vagal and sympathetic regulation of gastric acid secretion involved brain peptides.[10–17] This was demonstrated by delivering into the cerebrospinal fluid (CSF) or brain nuclei neuropeptides and related stable analogs as well as antagonists.

This chapter will focus on methodological approaches which are suitable to investigate the role of the CNS in the control of gastric acid secretion. It will describe the animal models and techniques available to localize active structures and transmitters in the CNS which regulate gastric secretion.

ANIMAL MODELS

Although the initial demonstration of a role of the CNS in the control of gastric acid secretion came from experiments performed in the dog,[3] this species has subsequently been selected mostly to study peripheral mechanisms regulating gastric secretion.[18] During the last decade, advance knowledge obtained on the brain circuitries and transmitters modulating gastric acid secretion and the peripheral mechanisms conveying the information from the brain to the stomach resulted from investigations performed in the rat.[19]

The advantage of this experimental model to explore the CNS control of gastric acid secretion is several fold: 1) unlike the dog or cat, the rat is readily available and cost-effectively housed under standard laboratory conditions; 2) the laboratory rat breeding techniques insure constant genetic conditions among animals; 3) most importantly, there is an extensive knowledge of rat brain anatomy and reliable coordinates are available to allow reproducible access to discrete brain nuclei[20,21] while this is a major impediment in the dog; 4) rats are sturdy enough to tolerate multiple surgeries and chronic cannulation with a resistance to infection which is well superior to other species such as guinea pigs or hamsters; and 5) findings on the effects of CSF injection of peptides on gastric secretion obtained in the rat[5,19,22] have been confirmed also in the cat[23–25] and the dog[26–29] attesting to the relevance of this rodent model to study the brain regulation of gastric acid secretion.

Therefore, this review will be focused mainly on techniques and data reported in the rat.

MEASUREMENT OF GASTRIC ACID SECRETION

Changes in gastric secretion induced by manipulations of the CNS can be easily monitored by determining the variations in acid secretion by the parietal cells of the fundic (oxyntic) mucosa of the rat stomach. Secretion collected from the gastric lumen by different techniques allow monitoring of the following parameters: 1) volume of secretion; 2) pH; 3) concentration of acid expressed in mmol/l and measured by titration of a known volume of sample juice with a base (commonly 0.01 N NaOH) until a set pH (commonly 7.0 or 5.5); and 4) the acid output, expressed in μmoles of acid per unit of time, and calculated by multiplying the acid concentration by the volume of secretion collected over a set period of time. When gastric secretion is collected by flushing or perfusing the stomach over time, acid output is directly calculated by titration of the perfusate.

Several techniques permit rapid and sensitive monitoring of acid secretory response in both conscious or anesthetized rats.

CONSCIOUS MODELS

CHRONIC GASTRIC FISTULA

Preparation

This technique developed early on in the dog[18] proved to be suitable when applied to rats as described in details by several groups.[30–32] Rats are anesthetized (pentobarbital or methohexital, 50 mg/kg, ip), the stomach is exteriorized through a median celiotomy and an incision is made into the non glandular portion. A stainless steel cannula of the type developed in Pavlov's laboratory and adapted to rats is most commonly used.[32] The cannula is inserted into the gastric corpus and tied in place with a purse-string suture. The distal end of the cannula is brought out through a left paramedian incision in the skin.

Collection and Assessment of Acid Secretion

In the interval after surgery, animals should be conditioned to the experimental procedure for collection of secretion performed under light restraint in Bollman cages.[33] This is achieved by placing the rat in Bollman cages for a few hours every day for at least 7 days before gastric secretory studies are begun. Basal gastric acid secretion is sensitive to ambient temperature[34,35] and presents circadian rhythmicity[36]. Therefore, when working with conscious animals, the experiments should always be done under controlled conditions of ambient temperature and at similar time of the day. In addition, hydratation of animals needs to be maintained by intravenous infusion of saline (1.5–2.5 ml/h) particularly during experiments that last over 2 hours or that involve stimulated acid secretion.

Two techniques are available in chronic gastric fistulae rats maintained in Bollman cages to monitor gastric acid secretion. After rinsing the stomach until clear with warm saline through the open fistula and a 30–45 minute period of stabilization has passed, gastric secretions are collected either by gravity drainage or perfusion.

By gravity drainage a polyethylene tube is usually placed into the stomach through the cannula to aid the continuous free drainage of secretion. This procedure is the only one that allows monitoring changes in volume of gastric juice secreted (1.5–2.5 ml/h under basal conditions).[31,37] However, because the volume of secretion over a short period of time (2–5 min) is small, it is not a method of choice to measure acid secretion at short time intervals. Values of acid output (8–10 μmol/10 min) obtained by free drainage are lower than when the stomach is perfused.[31,38]

Perfusion of the gastric lumen through a double lumen catheter positioned through the cannula can be achieved equally by two techniques: the flush technique which consists of flushing through the double lumen catheter 2–5 ml of warm saline (pH 7.0) followed by a bolus of 5 ml of air, at regular intervals of time (every 5–10 min or more)[31,39] (Figure 1); or continuous perfusion of the gastric lumen with warm saline using a peristaltic pump (flow rate 1–2.5 ml/min). The acid output is measured in the perfusate at set intervals[31] (Figure 2). Automatic titration in a reservoir can also be achieved with constant recording every 2 minutes.[40] Variations of NaOH concentration for titration of the perfusate can also increase the sensitivity of the titration.[31] This latter method has the advantage to better characterize the time of onset and duration of action of CNS-induced gastric changes since constant recording every 1–2 minutes can be achieved. Irrespective of the technique of perfusion, the values of acid output reached

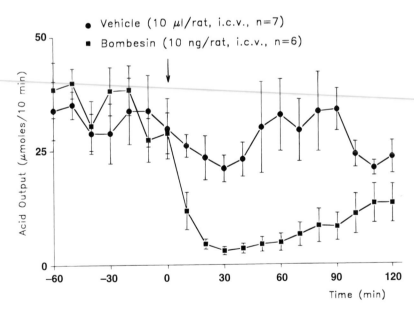

FIGURE 1   Inhibition of basal gastric acid secretion by icv injection of bombesin in conscious rats with chronic icv cannula and gastric fistula. Acid secretion was measured every 10 min by titration of the perfusate obtained by the flushing technique (5 ml saline + 5 ml air).

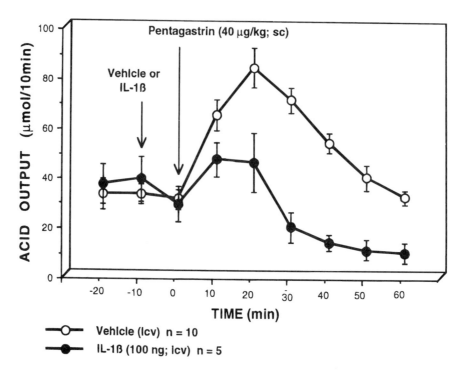

FIGURE 2 Inhibition of pentagastrin-stimulated gastric acid secretion by interleukin-1β (IL-1β) injected icv in conscious rats with chronic icv cannula and gastric fistula. Acid secretion was measured on fractions collected by constant perfusion of the stomach with saline (1 ml/min). (Reproduced from Saperas, E. and Taché, Y., *Life Sci.,* 52, 788, 1993. With permission.)[41]

20–30 μmol/10 min (Figures 1 and 2) and are higher than those collected by spontaneous dripping.[31,39,41] It has been related to a better recovery and not to mechanical stimulation of the gastric mucosa by the perfusion.[31]

Although basal acid secretion is generally steady over several hours within the same animal, variability is observed from one animal to the other[31,39] and each animal should serve as its own control. The acid secretion during the interdigestive phase observed in rats, unlike in dogs or humans,[18] reflects tonic vagal input.[42]

Advantages and Disadvantages

The advantages of this chronic conscious model are several fold. In reference to all parameters, it most closely mimics the physiological conditions related to the control of gastric secretion by avoiding interference from acute surgery and deep anesthesia on gastric function and central action of drugs. The chronic preparation can last for several weeks and animals can be subjected to (within a 3–4 day rest period) different experiments. Each animal can serve as its own control, reducing the variability of data and the number of animals. However, since gastric acid secretion is increased with the weight of the animals when experiments on the same animal are performed over months, acid output may be better expressed by unit body weight (100 g), particularly when the weight of the animal before surgery is below 200 g.[43] Since fasted rats equipped with chronic gastric fistulae secrete acid for several hours under basal conditions,[31,38,39,41] studies on the centrally mediated inhibition of acid secretion can be performed without the need to stimulate secretion (Figure 1). Centrally acting inhibitors of acid secretion can however be assessed under stimulated conditions (Figure 2). Gastric acid secretion might be increased by peripheral administration of pentagastrin (Figure 2), histamine, carbachol, intragastric perfusion of meal (usually 8% peptone meal), gastric distention or by increasing gastric vagal outflow[30,31,37,38,41,44,45] (Table 1). The acid response to intragastric peptone administration in rats has been recently characterized by Lloyd et al.[46] The methodology must take into account that 10% of the titratable gastric acid response is not due to acid secretion but most likely related to intragastric digestion of peptone.[46]

One consideration of which the researcher must be aware is that in the chronic fistula rat, neither the cardia nor the pylorus are ligated and juice may be lost by drainage into the duodenum. However, the leakage of gastric secretion through the pylorus under basal conditions has been estimated to be only 7% by the phenol red method.[31] However, the possible increase of the loss of secretion when gastric emptying is stimulated concurrently with that of acid secretion by central injection of neurotransmitters such as thyrotropin-releasing hormone (TRH)[47] has not been assessed under these conditions. Contamination of gastric juice by saliva has also been reported to occur mainly when rats leaked themselves.[30] However, rats in Bollman cages sleep most of the time under basal conditions.[30] Since several centrally acting peptides increase grooming behavior,[48] the contamination by saliva of gastric secretion can be a potential factor of which the researcher must be aware. Reflux of duodenal contents in the stomach occurs in only 4% of the cases without causing consistent changes in acid content.[30,31]

CNS Assessment

In chronic conscious preparations, the CNS modulatory actions of treatments are usually assessed in rats that have, in addition to the chronic gastric fistula, intracerebroventricular (icv) cannulae. For instance, bombesin and interleukin-1β-inhibits basal and stimulated acid secretion in rats with chronic icv cannula and gastric fistula (Figures 1 and 2).[37,39,41] This model is also suitable for chronic implantation of cannulae into specific brain nuclei or into the cisterna magna.

TABLE 1
Methods Used to Stimulate Gastric Acid Secretion in Rats to Study Central action of Substances on Gastric Secretion

Animal models	References
CONSCIOUS	
Chronic gastric fistula	
Pentagastrin (16 μg/kg, iv; 40 μg/kg, sc)	39, 41
2-Deoxy-D-glucose (75 mg/kg, sc)	37
Meal (ig 8% peptone)	135
Pylorus Ligation	
TRH (1 μg, ic) or RX 77368 (30 ng, ic)	61, 85
2-Deoxy-D-glucose (3 mg, ic)	85
Histamine (32 mg/kg, sc)	85
ANESTHETIZED (Urethane)	
Electrical vagal stimulation	78
TRH (0.1–1 μg, ic) or RX 77368 (0.01–0.1 μg, ic)	61, 126
Baclofen (4 mg/kg, sc; 6 mg/kg/h, iv)	126, 133
Histamine (10 mg/kg, iv)	62, 136
Pentagastrin (250 μg/kg, sc; 10–16 μg/kg/h, iv)	62, 117, 129, 137
Meal (ig 8% peptone)	46

iv, intravenous; sc, subcutaneous; ig, intragastric; ic, intracisternal; TRH, Thyrotropin-releasing hormone.

PYLORIC LIGATION

Preparation

The preparation of pylorus-ligated rats or "Shay rats" has been described earlier in details by Shay et al.[43] Under a short anesthesia (diethyl ether, halothane or Brevital), a small middle incision extending from the xiphoid is performed. The duodenum is identified and the junction between the pylorus and duodenum is picked up and ligated. Special care must be taken not to occlude or damage major blood vessels and to have a consistent procedure to tighten the pyloric junction.[49] The incision is closed by suture. Animals regain the righting reflex within 5–15 minutes.

Measurement of Acid

After a set experimental period (2–4 h), conscious rats are euthanized, esophagus and duodenum are clipped and gastric secretion collected by opening the stomach. After centrifugation, volume, pH and concentration of acid in the supernatant can be easily measured. When pellet in secretion is over 0.3 ml, secretion should be disregarded due to contamination with food or feces.[43]

In 2–4 hours pylorus ligated rats, the acid secretion is stimulated compared with the basal rate in gastric fistula rats.[49] The acid response is not due to the release of gastrin but to vago-vagal dependent cholinergic stimulation brought on by the ligature placed around the pylorus.[40,49–51] Further evidence of a vagal mediation was shown by the fact that endogenous medullary TRH, which plays a major stimulatory role in the vagal regulation of gastric function[15,47] contributes to the acid response to pylorus ligation.[52]

Advantages and Disadvantages

The advantages of this preparation are several fold. Animals can be prepared quickly under short anesthesia that allows the investigator to perform simultaneous acute intracisternal (ic) injection and pylorus ligation. Experiments can begin immediately after pyloric ligation under awake conditions and simultaneous information on changes in volume, pH, acid concentration and output can be obtained (Figure 3). Because of the high basal rate of secretion, which is however submaximal, both the inhibitory and stimulatory action of centrally acting substances on both the volume of secretion and acidity can be demonstrated under these conditions (Figure 3). For instance, using this method of collection, we were able to show that corticotropin-releasing factor (CRF), microinjected into various hypothalamic sites, increases the volume of secretion while inhibiting the concentration of acid and that the increase in volume reflects a stimulation of bicarbonate secretion.[53,54] Likewise, as shown in Figure 3, peripheral prostaglandin E_2 (PGE_2) increases the volume of secretion while acidity is decreased and ic bombesin inhibits both parameters. In addition, during the last decade, reproducible information on the central action of peptides influencing acid secretion has been obtained in 2-hour conscious pylorus-ligated rats with a pattern of response which is similar to that observed in chronic gastric fistula.[5,19,41,55]

The obvious disadvantage is that this procedure does not allow repeated collections on the same animal. Rats cannot serve as their own control and the influence of treatment needs to be assessed by comparison with a control group. The anesthesia, even of short duration, and surgery exert an inhibitory effect on acid secretion particularly during the 60 minutes after pylorus ligation.[56,57] Care should be taken to control these parameters. In addition, although the experimental collection period of gastric secretion can last for several hours, times over 3 hours are not suitable because of pronounced gastric distention due to the accumulation of secretion over time, the occurrence of mucosal lesions and the lack of further accumulation of gastric

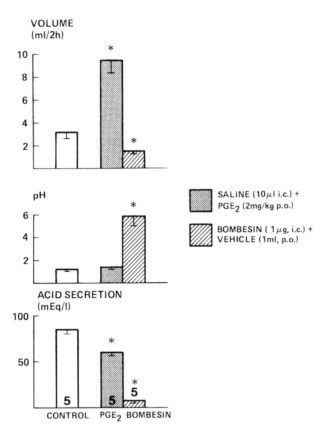

FIGURE 3   Effect of orally administered prostaglandin E_2 (PGE_2) and icv injected bombesin on gastric acid secretion (pH, volume, concentration of acid) in conscious 2 h pylorus-ligated rats. (Adapted from Taché, Y., *Peptides,* 6, Suppl. 3, 69, 1985.)[129]

juice.[43,51] The distension of the gastric wall and the diffusion of acid into the mucosa after 2–3 hours appear to stimulate "efferent function" of capsaicin sensitive fibers.[58] This induces the release of calcitonin gene-related peptide (CGRP) contained in sensory afferent nerves which inhibits acid secretion.[16,59]

CNS Assessment

The 2-hour pylorus-ligated rat preparation represents a standard technique to study the inhibitory and stimulatory influence of ic injection of peptides and peripheral mechanisms involved in the control of gastric secretion in conscious rats.[5,19] In particular, the demonstration that ic injection of bombesin, β-endorphin, CGRP, CRF and interleukin-1β inhibit[8,60–62] and that TRH and somatostatin[9,63] stimulate gastric acid secretion was initially observed in conscious 2-hour pylorus-ligated rats. However, other acute CNS methods of approach (lateral ventricle or specific brain nuclei) that required surgery and longer anesthesia compared with ic injection are not suitable in conjunction with monitoring acid secretion in pylorus-ligated rats. Brain surgery, indeed, acts as a stressful stimuli that potently inhibits acid secretion, through the central release of CRF.[57] Chronically implanted cannula into the lateral brain ventricle or specific brain sites have been used in conscious 2-hour pylorus-ligated rats to establish the hypothalamic sites of the inhibitory action of bombesin, CRF, CGRP, calcitonin and interleukin-1β (Figure 4).[13,53,64,65]

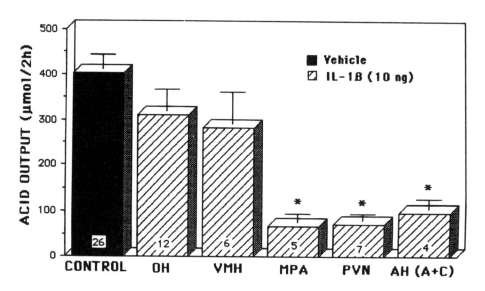

FIGURE 4 Inhibition of gastric acid secretion by intrahypothalamic microinjection of interleukin-1β (IL-1β) in conscious 2h pylorus-ligated rats with unilateral chronic cannula in the ventromedial hypothalamus (VMH), medial preoptic area (MPA), paraventricular nucleus of the hypothalamus (PVN), anterior hypothalamus (AH) and other nonresponsive hypothalamic sites (OH). (Reproduced from Saperas, E., et al., *Am. J. Physiol.,* 263, G414, 1992. With permission.)[64]

ANESTHETIZED MODELS

Preparation

Changes in gastric acid secretion in anesthetized animals are evaluated through intragastric cannulae acutely implanted. In this model, the whole stomach is transformed in a pouch-like preparation by ligating the pylorus and the esophagus (at the cervical level). Then, a double lumen cannula is placed into the gastric corpus through a small incision in the nonglandular portion of the stomach. Gastric juice can be collected by the flushing technique (2 boli of 5 ml of warm saline, pH 7.0, and 5 ml bolus of air at regular intervals of time) (Figure 5) or by continuous perfusion of the gastric lumen with a peristaltic pump which allows the monitoring of acid secretion every 2 minutes.[40] (Figure 6).

Measurement of Secretion

By these techniques only pH and acid output per time interval can be measured. Although, different anesthetics (diethyl ether, mebumal, chloral hydrate, pentobarbital, α-chloralose, urethane) are available, all markedly depress both basal and stimulated acid secretion.[31,66–68] For instance, urethane-anesthetized rats show a very low basal acid secretion (1–5 μmoles of acid/10 min) (Figures 5 and 6).[31,39,67] The low secretion of acid results from the increase in the synthesis and release of antral somatostatin induced by urethane.[67]

Advantages and Disadvantages

This model has the advantage of being very sensitive to vagal input. When the gastric vagal activity is increased (i.e. by TRH injected into the dorsal vagal complex or the cisterna magna, (Figures 5 and 6) acid secretion is potently stimulated by 300–500% over basal values and the modulatory action of other transmitters can be easily noticed[15,47] (Figure 5). In addition, the anesthetized rat preparation allows for the performance of acute brain surgery, particularly to

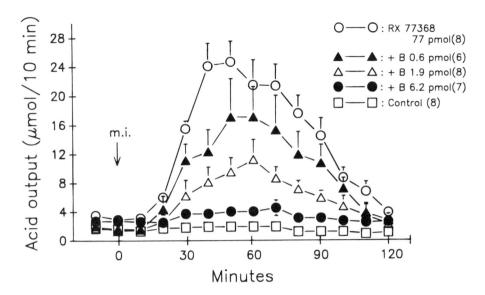

FIGURE 5   Inhibition of TRH analog, RX 77368, into the dorsal vagal complex-induced stimulation of gastric acid secretion by bombesin (B) microinjected (m.i.) simultaneously in urethane-anesthetized rats with acute gastric fistula. (Reproduced from Ishikawa, T. and Taché, Y., *Regul. Pept.,* 24, 187, 1989. With permission.)[106]

investigate the role of medullary nuclei involved in the vagal regulation of gastric function. This is because the dorsal vagal complex is not amendable to chronic cannulation.[15,19,47] Lastly, basal secretion is stable and kinetic studies over several hours can be easily performed on the same animal allowing the investigator to define the onset and duration of the response of centrally acting test substances[40] (Figure 5).

However, this model is not suitable to assess somatostatin-dependent gastric mechanisms involved in the inhibitory effect of substances injected centrally since the basal somatostatin release and synthesis are nearly maximally stimulated.[39,67] In addition, the central inhibitory

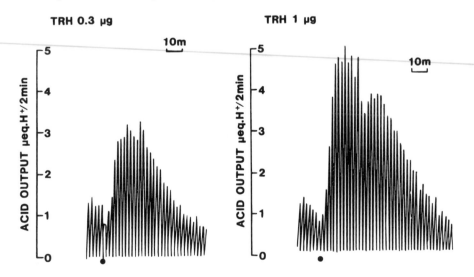

FIGURE 6   Stimulation of gastric acid secretion by intracisternal injection of TRH (black dot) on gastric acid secretion in urethane-anesthetized rats with constant perfusion and 2 min titration of the perfusate. (Reproduced from Taché, Y., et al., *Regul. Pept.,* 13, 21, 1985. With permission.)

influence on gastric acid secretion needs to be assessed under stimulated conditions due to the low basal rate of secretion. Stimulants of gastric acid secretion in urethane-anesthetized rats are listed in Table 1. One other limitation is the influence of anesthetics on the CNS which may modify the central action of compounds under study.

CNS Assessment

The urethane-anesthetized rats acutely implanted with gastric cannulae proved to be useful to study the CNS modulatory actions of peptides on gastric function by performing acute injection into the CSF or specific brain nuclei with a glass micropipette. The medullary sites of action of TRH, bombesin and CGRP have been established using this technique[19,22,47] (Figures 5 and 6).

VAGAL STIMULATION OF GASTRIC FUNCTION

Vagal efferent and afferent pathways mediate most of the central mechanisms involved in the control of gastric function. Gastric vagal afferent fibers terminating in the nucleus tractus solitarius arise primarily from cell bodies located in the nodose ganglion.[69,70] Gastric vagal efferent pathways originate mainly (90–95%) in the dorsal motor nucleus.[71,72] This organization supposes that most of the vagal control of gastric function is mediated by vago-vagal reflexes.[73,74] Simultaneously, the nucleus tractus solitarius and the dorsal motor nucleus receive numerous projections from other areas of the brain, mainly from the hypothalamus, central amygdala and raphe nuclei. This suggests that inputs from these areas can also modulate gastric function.[5] Vagally-stimulated acid secretion is a suitable model to study central and peripheral mechanisms involved in acid regulation.[75]

The acid response to vagal stimulation has been largely studied in urethane-anesthetized rats (Figure 5).[15,47] Several techniques are reliable to induce vagally mediated acid secretion.

ELECTRICAL FACTORS

The right cervical vagal nerve is usually exposed since it has been shown that to be slightly, but consistently, more efficient than the left cervical vagus in producing acid secretion in rats.[76] The distal cut end is fixed to a silver electrode.[76,77] Monitoring of acid secretion after cervical vagal stimulation at various frequencies indicates that small C-fibers are involved in mediating the response.[76,77] In consequence, optimal electrical parameters to induce sustained increase of gastric acid secretion in urethane- or thiopental-anesthetized rats are a stimulation of low frequencies (1–4 Hz pulses) generally of 0.1–1 msec duration with an intensity of 0.5–1 mA.[76–78]

The latency of the acid response under optimum conditions is about 2.5 minutes[76] and can produce an acid secretory response of comparable magnitude to that induced by gastrin or histamine.[76]

The disadvantage of this technique is its lack of selectivity; both efferent and afferent fibers (by antidromic response) are stimulated in the same proportion.[79] In addition, this method requires a surgical approach and an anesthetized preparation. Electrical vagal stimulation with both vagi cut has been used to demonstrate the nonvagal dependent inhibition of stimulated acid secretion induced by bombesin injected icv.[78]

CHEMICAL FACTORS

Hypoglycemic Substances

Hypoglycemia induced by insulin or analogs of glucose that cannot be metabolized, such as 2-deoxy-D-glucose, has long been recognized to induce vagal-dependent acid secretion in several species and in humans.[4] In rats, evidence that suggests that low blood glucose levels are detected in the hypothalamus leading to increase gastric vagal outflow and therefore gastric secretion are: a) microinjection of 2-deoxy-D-glucose in the lateral hypothalamus (but not elsewhere) stimulates gastric acid secretion; b) insulin-induced acid secretion is abolished by local anesthesia in the lateral hypothalamus.[80,81] The advantage of this procedure is that the central vagal stimulation of acid secretion can be achieved by peripheral injection (usually intravenous bolus injection).[55] It has also served as a test to verify the completeness of the vagotomy.[4,82] However, there is a delay of about 30–60 minutes in the onset of the acid response.[83] More importantly the degree of hypoglycemia at which vagal gastric secretory response occurs is not normally observed in animals, even when fasted, and there is a simultaneous activation of the sympathetic nervous system.[84] Stimulation of gastric acid secretion by 2-deoxy-D-glucose was shown to be inhibited by icv injection of gastrin releasing peptide (GRP) in pylorus ligated or chronic gastric fistula rats.[37,85]

Central TRH

In 1980, ic injection of TRH was reported to be a potent vagal stimulant of acid secretion in conscious pylorus-ligated rats.[9] Since then, TRH or its analog, RX 77368, as well as other analogs injected into the CSF or microinjected into medullary nuclei have been well established to be reliable stimulants of gastric acid secretion.[15,47,86] The onset of the response occurred within 4 minutes with a peak response at 10–30 minutes depending upon the experimental conditions of injection (Figures 5 and 6). The magnitude of the acid response is dose related and can reach the maximal acid response observed after histamine or pentagastrin.[47] The advantages of this method are several fold. It is highly reproducible in different experimental conditions of collection of gastric secretion (conscious pylorus-ligated or anesthetized rats with acute gastric fistula).[47] It is well characterized with respect to the central and peripheral mechanisms of action. In particular, TRH exerts a direct excitatory action on the dorsal motor nucleus neurons increasing vagal efferent activity to the stomach.[15,86] Moreover, convergent evidence indicates that endogenous medullary TRH plays a physiologically stimulatory role in the regulation of gastric function.[15,47,86,87] However, unlike 2-deoxy-D-glucose, it is not active upon peripheral administration and requires direct application into the CSF or the dorsal motor nucleus of the vagus.[47]

Gamma-Aminobutyric Acid (GABA) Mimetics

Goto et al. provided the first evidence in 1983 that the GABA mimetic, β-(p-chlorophenyl)-gamma-aminobutyric acid (PCP-GABA; Baclofen) given subcutaneously is a powerful stimulant of gastric acid secretion through central vagal dependent pathways in rats.[88–90] Under these conditions, acid secretion occurred within 10 minutes with a plateau response at 40 minutes which is long lasting and associated with enhanced vagal efferent activity.[89,90] The advantage of this procedure is that the GABA mimetic, baclofen can be injected either peripherally (subcutaneously or intravenously) (Figure 7) or centrally (ic or icv). However, the central and peripheral mechanisms of action have not yet been well characterized.[88–90] Moreover, the secretory response is sensitive to body temperature as it occurs only at 30°C and is abolished at 36–38°C in rats.[91]

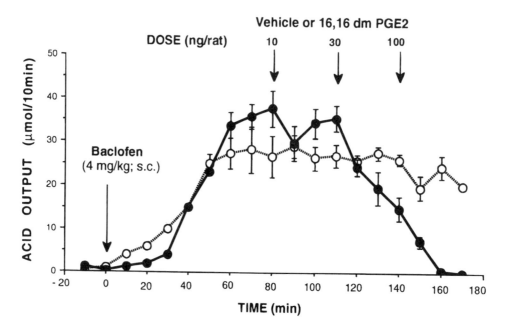

FIGURE 7 Stimulation of gastric acid secretion by subcutaneous injection of the GABA mimetic, baclofen, and reversal by intracisternal injection of stable PGE$_2$ analog, 16, 16 dimethyl PGE$_2$ (16, 16 dm PGE$_2$), in urethane-anesthetized rats with acute gastric fistula. (Reproduced from Saperas, et al., *Eur. J. Pharmacol.*, 209, 1, 1991. With permission.)[133]

CNS REGULATION OF GASTRIC SECRETION: METHODS OF APPROACH

Peripheral routes of administration have often been used to assess the effects of drugs on the CNS. However, many substances either do not or only weakly circumvent the blood-brain barrier. In addition, central and peripheral actions can be difficult to dissociate after peripheral administration.[92] Several techniques are available to assess the role of the CNS in the regulation of gastric function.[5] One approach that has gained recognition compared with electrical lesioning or stimulation of specific areas performed in earlier studies[4] is the delivery of transmitters or analogs into the CSF or specific brain areas. The techniques more commonly used to assess the role of the CNS on the control of gastric acid secretion in rats are summarized in Table 2.

Injection into the CSF

The delivery of drugs into the CSF allows testing their potential influence in the central control of gastric acid secretion in rats. Different sites of injection have been described depending upon the CNS areas to be explored. CSF injection sites (as far as ease of access in the rat) are the lateral brain ventricle (icv) and cisterna magna (ic) (Figure 8). However, injection into the third and fourth ventricles can also be performed (Figure 8) as well as the subarachnoidal space of the spinal cord (intrathecal).

SITES OF INJECTION

Intracerebroventricular Injection

Lateral ventricle injection allows substances to penetrate the brain from its inner surface. The guide and injection cannulae for icv cannulation are commercially available and, also,

TABLE 2
Experimental Techniques Used to Assess the CNS Regulation of Gastric Acid Secretion in Rats

Treatment	CNS Area	References
CSF-SPINAL INJECTIONS		
ICV (10 μl)	Ventricles + subarachnoid space	37,39,41,96,131
IC (10 μl)	Brain stem + upper cervical level	40,57,61,95,117
3RD or 4TH V (3 μl)	Ventricular system	96
Intrathecal (5–17 μl)	Spinal cord	97,108
BRAIN PARENCHYMA MICROINJECTION		
Hypothalamic nuclei (50–100 nl)	PVN, LH, VMH	53,54,64,65,110
Medullary nuclei (1–50 nl)	DVC, RP, NA, RO	86,87,106–108
Pontine nuclei (50–100 nl)	LC/SC	137
ELECTRICAL STIMULATION, LESION		
Hypothalamic nuclei		4,5,96,116
Coronal transection		96
Spinal cord transection		97,117,127

CSF: ceresbrospinal fluid; ICV: intracerebroventricular; IC: intracisternal; PVN: paraventricular nucleus of the hypothalamus; LH: lateral hypothalamus; VMH: ventromedial hypothalamus; DVC: dorsal vagal complex; RP: raphe pallidus; NA: nucleus ambiguus; RO: raphe obscurus; LC/SC: locus coeruleus/subcoeruleus.

many techniques for the preparation of inexpensive chronic cannulae have been described.[93,94] Rats are anesthetized and the head place in a stereotaxic instrument. The skull is cleaned and stainless steel mounting screws are placed (avoiding to penetration into the brain) in the four corners surrounding the Bregma (intersection of the coronal and sagittal skull sutures). Guide cannulae (22 gauge) are implanted using tridimensional coordinates from one of the brain atlases available. One of the most commonly referenced is that by Paxinos and Watson[21] in which coordinates are (mm from bregma): antero-posterior: −0.8; lateral ± 1.5; and dorsoventral: −3.5. The reference point for depth in most of the atlas readings is from the brain surface; one millimeter should be added when skull thickness is taken for reference. After localizing the cannula position the skull is drilled and the dura slit with a needle, then the cannula is inserted till the appropriate depth. The cannula is anchored with acrylic dental cement to the skull surface

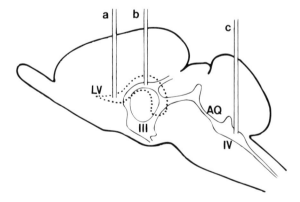

FIGURE 8 Schematic representation of the brain ventricular system showing the relative localization of lateral (i.c.v.) (a), third (b) and fourth (c) ventricles cannulae for injection. LV, lateral brain ventricle; III, third ventricle; IV, fourth ventricle; AQ, aqueduct.

and the mounting screws and plugged by stainless steel wire stylet. Skin closure is made with simple interrupted sutures bringing the skin tight against the cement cap. Experiments can be performed a few days after surgery. Animals with chronic icv cannulae can be injected repetitively for several weeks with a period of 3–4 days between consecutive injections depending upon the clearance of the substance. This model in combination with chronic gastric fistulae is suitable to study the influence of central inhibitors of acid secretion as shown for bombesin, GRP or interleukin-1β.[37,39,41] In this case, brain surgery is usually performed 2 days prior to the implantation of the gastric cannula.

Injections are performed with a stainless steel injection cannula (28 gauge) inserted into the guide cannula and attached to a polyethylene tubing (usually PE-50). In rats, the volume commonly injected is 10 µl, using a Hamilton syringe. Injection cannulae protrude 1 mm from the guide cannulae and this assures that the injected volume is effectively delivered into the CSF and does not remain in the lumen of the guide cannulae. The volume injected should be slowly delivered over 30–60 second periods and the injection cannula should be positioned for one extra minute to avoid any reflux of the CSF.

Intracisternal Injection

The injection into the cisterna magna is commonly performed acutely in anesthetized animals (either under short anesthesia with ether or halothane or in urethane-anesthetized animals). The head is fixed in a stereotaxic device and the neck flexed to expose the occipital region. The needle of a Hamilton syringe is inserted directly through the skin till the occipital membrane which is punctured and the injection performed. The withdrawal of CSF into the syringe indicates the accuracy of the injection site. Injection volume is usually 5–10 µl.

Intracisternal injection can be also performed in conscious animals chronically implanted into the cisterna magna with a cannulae, which consists of a polyethylene catheter (PE-10, ≈2 cm length) fitted into a PE-50 catheter (≈3 cm length). To perform the implantation of the cannula rats are anesthetized and the occipital membrane is exposed and sliced. Approximately 1–2 mm of the PE-10 catheter is inserted into the cisterna magna and stuck to the surface of the occipital membrane and the adjacent muscles. Muscles and skin are sutured surrounding the free portion of the cannula. The correct position of the cannula can be determined by the reflux of CSF; to avoid the continuous leakage of CSF, the cannula must be capped. These cannulae have a dead space of about 4 µl, therefore the injection of drugs should be made in a volume not higher than 5 µl, followed by another injection of 5 µl of sterile saline or artificial CSF to wash the cannula (final volume injected = 10 µl). Cannulation of the cisterna magna for acute injection can also be performed for experiments in which repeated injection will be performed.[95]

Injection into the Third and Fourth Ventricles

Cannulae are chronically implanted into the third or fourth ventricle with similar procedures to those described for the icv chronic cannulae (Figure 8). Acute injection, under short anesthesia, into the fourth ventricle of bombesin followed by pyloric ligation in rats results in inhibition of gastric acid secretion.[96]

Intrathecal Injection

Intrathecal injection are performed in urethane-anesthetized or conscious rats to assess the role of the spinal cord in the control of gastric secretion.[97] A polyethylene catheter (PE-10) is introduced into the subarachnoid space through a transverse incision in the atlanto-occipital membrane. The length of the catheter within the spinal cord varies with the spinal levels at which the injection is directed. When the length of the catheter is approximately 6 cm (7 µl dead space), its tip rests at vertebral levels T9–T10.[97] Similar chronic intrathecal preparations were originally reported to study analgesic properties of opiates.[98] Other techniques have been described that reduce the intrathecal length of the catheter by indirect insertion into the rachis lumbar segment.[99] The advantage in this method is that in chronic experiments, spinal compression occurs over a shorter length and less rats show signs of motor impairments.[99] Volumes injected intrathecally oscillate between 5 and 17 μl.[98]

CNS SITES OF ACTION

Validation of CSF Injection Sites

At the end of experiments, after the euthanasia of the animals, the CSF injection sites should be validated by determining the correct location of the cannulae. The injection of dye through the cannulae under the same conditions as for the substances tested allows the direct macroscopic visualization of the effectiveness of injection. The presence of dye staining the wall of the brain ventricles, the upper cervical cord (after ic injection) or the spinal cord at the level where the catheter was located (after intrathecal injection) indicate the correctness of the cannula location. In conscious animals, behavioral changes after the injection of peptides[48] (variations in the exploratory behavior in free moving animals and changes in grooming activity) can be an additional parameter to indicate that a drug has been effectively delivered in the CNS. However, the specific site of injection must be checked at the end of the experiments.

Central vs Peripheral Action: Leakage from the CSF into the Periphery

A drug injected into a lateral ventricle may act anywhere in the brain ventricular system (Figure 8) and in the subarachnoid space as well,[93] and the areas reached by the drug will depend upon the volume injected. In the rat, a drug injected icv in a 10 μl volume reaches the third ventricle without detectable changes on icv pressure. When drugs are delivered into the third ventricle a direct action on the caudate nuclei, septum, amygdala and hippocampus can be excluded; similarly, when drugs are injected into the fourth ventricle an action on thalamic and hypothalamic nuclei and on the periaqueductal gray matter can also be excluded.[93] Drugs injected ic do not enter the cerebral ventricles at all, and their action will be mainly on the outer surface of the brain, brain stem and upper cervical cord.[93]

To differentiate between the forebrain and hindbrain sites of action, there is a technique consisting of interrupting the communication between the ventricles.[96] Silicone grease or cold cream is injected through chronically or acutely implanted cannulae into the fourth ventricle. This technique can be used acutely in both awake and anesthetized rats.[96] For example, aqueductal plug, interrupting the communication between the third and fourth ventricles has been used to establish that the lateral and fourth brain ventricle injection of bombesin-induced inhibition of gastric acid secretion relates respectively to forebrain and hindbrain sites of action.[96] This procedure can only be performed acutely since the increase in intracranial pressure resulting from the interrupted CSF flux limits the applicability to chronic experiments.

Since drugs delivered into the CSF could diffuse rapidly, by a non-carrier mechanism, into the peripheral circulation,[92,100–104] further support for a central site of drug action is provided by: 1) the demonstration of higher potency following injection into the CSF compared with intravenous infusion—usually at 1/10th ratio for CSF vs iv infusion strongly supports a CNS action; 2) establishment of selective responsive nuclei by microinjection into the brain parenchyma; 3) maintenance of the biological action after CSF injection in the presence of circulating antibodies that will neutralize any active material leaking from the CSF into the general circulation. These three postulates have been fulfilled for several peptides, such as bombesin, CRF,

CGRP and interleukin-1β, that influence gastric acid secretion upon injection into both the CSF or the general circulation, insuring a centrally mediated action and not leakage into the periphery.[12,13,16,60,105]

MICROINJECTION INTO BRAIN NUCLEI

Microinjection techniques consist to deliver transmitters into the vicinity of a small population of neurons or specifically into brain nuclei well characterized morphologically. They allow for the establishment of the specific brain nuclei responsive to the transmitter shown to have an effect upon CSF injection. The choice of brain nuclei to be investigated may be determined based on the presence of receptors and nerve terminals for the transmitters under study, connection of the brain nuclei with autonomic centers and relative potency upon icv vs ic injections with or without acqueductal plug (Table 2).

Microinjection techniques are applicable to perform studies in both conscious animals with chronic cannulae or acute preparation in anesthetized animals.

METHODS OF MICROINJECTIONS

Chronic Preparation

Stainless-steel guide cannulae (26 gauge) with internal cannulae for injection (33 gauge) are commonly used in awake animals. The technique of implantation is the same as that described for the chronic icv cannulae. The coordinates of implantation will depend upon the brain nuclei to be explored, and they can be easily obtained from a stereotaxic atlas.[20,21] The cannula should be located in the near vicinity of the nuclei to be studied, to avoid any damage to its structure. For example, when studying the hypothalamic sites of action of interleukin-1β inhibiting acid secretion, chronic cannulae for microinjection were located 1 mm above the hypothalamic nuclei.[64]

Commonly, chronic cannulae are implanted unilaterally in either the right or the left nuclei since in most cases unilateral injection is enough to reproduce responses.[64,65] However, in blockade experiments to assess the role of endogenous transmitters in specific brain nuclei, the administration of the antagonist is performed bilaterally. Double cannula systems for bilateral chronic cannulation are commercially available, and methods to produce bilateral cannulae have been described by some authors.[94]

The microinjection is achieved with injectors connected to a polyethylene catheter and a 1 μl Hamilton syringe, using the technique of pressure ejection. Injections should be done in a 30–60 second period, and the injectors should be kept in the cannula for 2 more minutes.

Acute Microinjection

Acute microinjection in anesthetized models is suitable to assess the role of medullary nuclei (dorsal motor nucleus, nucleus of the solitary tract, raphe obscurus and raphe pallidus) which cannot be easily chronically cannulated.[106–108] Glass micropipettes with small tips are acutely inserted into the parenchyma according to the stereotaxic coordinates of the nuclei to be studied in rats that are acutely implanted with a gastric fistula. Glass micropipettes are connected to a polyethylene catheter filled with water or oil and the injection is commonly done by pressure ejection using a 1 μl Hamilton syringe. Microinjections are performed over 30–60 second period, and the micropipette should be left in place for 2 minutes before being withdrawn. Acute microinjection can be also done using barreled glass micropipettes by the technique of iontophoretic delivery. This procedure requires the application of continuous electrical currents to induce the release of electrically active substances contained in the micropipette. Iontophoretic injection is not efficient in cases where compounds are poorly soluble in water or not electrically charged. An extensive review on methodological aspects of pressure ejection and iontophoresis can be found in Stone.[109]

Volumes for Intraparenchymal Microinjection

The area of tissue in which a microinjected substance can diffuse depends upon the concentration and the volume injected. Small volumes should be microinjected in attempt to confine the drug to the targeted nucleus. In conscious animals, it has been shown that the volume of microinjection into structures of a diameter of 1 mm or less should not exceed 50 nl.[110] Larger volumes (200–500 nl) spread more diffusely into distant anatomical regions, thus potentially leading to a widespread rather than localized neuronal response.[110] In particular, the injection of excitatory substances that can produce neuronal damage should be reduced as much as possible to avoid the diffusion. For example, the activation of neuronal cell bodies with low doses of the neurotoxic agent, kainic acid, should be performed with volumes not larger than 30 nl to avoid the spread and the damage of the tissue.[87] Pressure ejection system have been developed that reached an accuracy in the picoliter and nanoliter range.[111–113] However in blockade and immunoneutralizing experiments, it is necessary to perform bilateral microinjection and the volumes injected are usually larger. This is related to the low potency of antagonists available (CRF antagonist, α-helical CRF$_{9-41}$) that required high concentrations of substances not easily soluble in a small volume.[87,114]

Validation of the Injection Sites and Specificity

After the experiments, the microinjection must be validated by the anatomical localization of the injection site. Commonly, brains are removed after the euthanasia and fixed in formalin and a cryoprotective solution. Cryostat sections (30–40 µm thickness) are obtained and stained with toluidine blue following an histological standard staining procedure. The sections are examined microscopically and the microinjection sites localized by the visualization of the point of fermination of the cannula or micropipette track. The precise injection sites are usually reproduced on plates obtained from one of rat stereotaxic atlases. In chronic preparations it is possible to mark the position of the tip of the injection cannula by the microinjection of a dye before removing the cannula. Dyes (alcian blue, pontamine sky blue) produce permanent extracellular spots in the site of injection, that can be easily localized during the microscopic examination of the sections. The rate of success for exact localization depends upon the nuclei under study. For instance the rate of success in the locus coeruleus (40%) is lower than in the paraventricular nucleus of the hypothalamus (60–70%) or lateral hypothalamus.[114,115]

The response observed after the microinjection of a drug can be due either to the non-specific stimulation of the area (for example by osmotic or pH changes) or to the spread of the drug into surrounding areas. The specificity of action has to be further assessed by the microinjection of the vehicle or other inactive analogs in the same area and by performing the microinjection into brain parenchyma surrounding but outside of the nucleus under study. The action can be considered drug-specific when it is not reproduced by the vehicle or other drugs injected in the same area; and site-specific when a lack of response is observed after the microinjection nearby but outside the nuclei studied.

ELECTRICAL STIMULATION AND LESION OF BRAIN NUCLEI

In earlier studies in rats, cats, dogs, and monkeys electrical stimulation or electrolytic lesions of specific brain nuclei was the main method of approach to study the influence of the CNS on gastric secretion (Table 2).[4] Results obtained brought considerable evidence to support the importance of the CNS regulation, but show a high disparity probably due to species-specific differences, animal preparations, stimulation parameters and lesion sizes.[4,96,116] The effectiveness of the lesions or electrical stimuli should be verified by histological examination of the brains at the end of the experiments, stating the location and extent of the lesions and the position of the electrodes.[96,116] The location of the CNS nuclei involved in the control of gastric function has also been assessed by brain and spinal cord transection at different levels. For example, the acute complete supracollicular transection or cervical cord transection have been used to establish that bombesin acts both in forebrain and hindbrain and spinal cord to inhibit acid secretion in rats.[96,117]

However, these experimental methods of approach have the disadvantage to lack specificity and to be cumbersome to perform compared with the chemical stimulation or blockade experiments.[5]

PERIPHERAL MECHANISMS MEDIATING CNS ACTIONS

Peripheral mechanisms underlying the central action of drugs affecting gastric acid secretion can be assessed by pharmacological, surgical, electrophysiological and endocrinological methods of approach. Neural pathways are commonly investigated by surgical deafferentation of the vagus, coeliac and mesenteric ganglia and adrenalectomy. Vagotomy can be performed either at subdiaphragmatic or cervical levels.[60,117,118] Since vagotomy delays gastric emptying of solids, experiments are mainly done acutely in anesthetized rats using a subdiaphragmatic vagotomy.[60,117] In chronic experiments, subdiaphragmatic vagotomy needs to be done in conjunction with pyloroplasty or animals need to be fed a liquid diet.[119] Also since there are adaptive changes in the vagus a few weeks after vagotomy,[120] experiments should be performed within one to two weeks following surgery. In addition to the surgical approach, a technique for recording efferent or afferent activity in the gastric branch of the vagus has recently been developed.[73] Changes in the gastric efferent activity are monitored in response to the ic injection of peptides influencing gastric acid secretion.[95,121] During the last few years, chemical deafferentation with capsaicin, selectively destroying type C sensory pathways, by local (perivagally or on the mesenteric and/or superior ganglia) or systemic treatment, has become a specific strategy to assess the role of sensory afferent fibers in the central control of gastric function.[122,123] Pharmacological blockade of neural action with selective receptor antagonists acting peripherally are additional tools to investigate neural mechanisms.[117,118,124]

The methodological approach to probe the involvement of the endocrine system involve measuring the serum or plasma levels of hormones, such as gastrin or somatostatin, by RIA techniques[40,125] and immunoneutralization of circulating and tissular peptides by the intravenous administration of specific antibodies.[39,126,127] The role of pituitary hormones can be assessed in hypophysectomized rats;[128] in general, the involvement of endocrine factors released peripherally can be investigated in cross-circulating experiments.[117] The peripheral release of prostaglandins is routinely evaluated as a mechanism mediating central inhibitory actions. The role of prostaglandins has been commonly assessed by pretreatment with indomethacin to inhibit prostaglandin generation.[61,129,130] In addition, gastric prostaglandin output can be measured in the interstitial space of the gastric mucosa using dialyses fibers implanted into the gastric wall.[130]

CNS REGULATION OF GASTRIC ACID SECRETION

The brain contains a large number of highly specific binding sites for many biochemical transmitters (both neuropeptides and classic neurotransmitters). Several of these substances have been found to influence gastric acid secretion when injected centrally.[5,17,22,86] The biological activity of many of these compounds has been also assessed by the injection of specific antagonists and antibodies and changes in gene expression in response to brain stimuli associated with the vagally mediated increase in gastric acid secretion.[15,57,131,132]

During the last few years central prostaglandins, mainly PGE_2 which inhibits acid[133] (Figure 7), have become important in mediating the potent inhibition of gastric acid secretion induced by interleukin-1 action in the hypothalamus.[105] Since the first reports that bombesin, TRH, β-endorphin, and somatostatin act in the brain to influence acid secretion,[8,9,63] the central action of over 40 peptides have been investigated.[5,22,134] Among these peptides, there are two for which convergent evidence indicates a physiological role in the central regulation of gastric acid secretion: TRH and CRF. Medullary TRH seems to play a physiological stimulatory role in the regulation of gastric vagal outflow, while central CRF mediates the inhibition of acid secretion in response to stress exposure. The establishment of the physiological relevance of the central action of many peptides, such as bombesin, calcitonin or CGRP is still to be investigated with the new development of specific antagonists.[5,17,22,86]

SUMMARY AND CONCLUSIONS

Although early on, several animals including dogs, monkeys, cats were experimental models of choice to study the CNS control of gastric acid secretion, the rat proved to be a relevant experimental model to enhance knowledge on the brain circuitry and underlying biochemical substrata regulating gastric acid secretion. Chronic gastric and intracerebral cannulae (either into the ventricular system or specific brain nuclei) allow rats to be studied under conscious conditions with respect of central and peripheral mechanisms involved in the regulation of basal and stimulated gastric acid secretion. More information has been gained by studying the CNS control of gastric function in 2h pylorus ligated rats. Acute preparations in anesthetized animals, usually with urethane, show a very low basal secretion and required stimulation by vagal or peripherally acting secretagogues to enhance acid secretion, so centrally acting inhibitors can be investigated. In this case the role of the CNS is commonly assessed by either microinjection of drugs into specific brain nuclei, or into the CSF. Validation of the injection sites, and the specificity of the responses obtained can be assessed by injecting other drugs, discarding peripheral actions due to leakage into the general circulation and microinjecting the drugs in the vicinity of the responsive nuclei. Peripheral neural pathways involved in the CNS control are dissected by surgical or chemical deafferentation and by specific pharmacological blockade, while the role of the endocrine system can be evaluated by RIA measurement of changes in serum levels of hormones and immunoneutralization of tissular and circulating hormones.

Using these techniques several peptides and classic transmitters have been established as acting in the brain to influence gastric acid secretion. Peptides appear to be important brain regulators of acid secretion and useful tools to unravel the pathways mediating brain-gut interactions.

ACKNOWLEDGMENTS

The authors's work was supported by the National Institute of Mental Health, grant MH-00663 and the National Institute of Arthritis Metabolism and Digestive Disease: grant DK-30110, DK-33061, and DK-41301 (Antibody and Animal Cores). Dr. Martínez is in receipt of a fellowship from the Ramón Areces Foundation (Madrid, Spain). Mr. P. Kirshbaum is acknowledged for helping in the preparation of the manuscript.

REFERENCES

1. **Cabanis, P. J. G.,** *On the Relations Between the Physical and Moral Aspects of Man,* Mora, G., Ed. Johns Hopkins University Press, Baltimore, 1981, 650.
2. **Beaumont, W.,** *Experiments and Observations on the Gastric Juice and the Physiology of Digestion,* Osler, W., Ed. Dover Publications Inc., New York, 1959.
3. **Pavlov, I.,** *The Work of The Digestive Glands. (English Translation by W. H. Thompson),* C. Criffin & Co, London, 1910.
4. **Brooks, F. P.,** Central neural control of acid secretion, in *Handbook of Physiology. Section 6: The Alimentary Canal,* Code, C. F., Ed. American Physiological Society, Washington, D. C., 1967, 805.
5. **Taché, Y.,** Central regulation of gastric acid secretion, in *Physiology of the Gastrointestinal Tract,* Johnson, L. R., Christensen, J., Jackson, M., Jacobson, E. D. and Walsh, J. H., Eds. Raven Press, New York, 1987, 911.
6. **Krieger, D. T.,** Brain peptides: what, where and why? *Science,* 222, 975, 1983.
7. **Brown, M., Taché, Y. and Fisher, D.,** Central nervous system action of bombesin: mechanism to induce hyperglycemia, *Endocrinology,* 105, 660, 1979.
8. **Taché, Y., Vale, W., Rivier, J. and Brown, M.,** Brain regulation of gastric secretion: influence of neuropeptides, *Proc. Natl. Acad. Sci.,* U. S. A., 77, 5515, 1980.
9. **Taché, Y., Vale, W. and Brown, M.,** Thyrotropin-releasing hormone-CNS action to stimulate gastric acid secretion, *Nature,* 287, 149, 1980.
10. **Taché, Y. and Wingate, D.,** *Brain-Gut Interactions,* CRC Press, Boca Raton, 1991.
11. **Taché, Y., Garrick, T. and Raybould, H.,** Central nervous system action of peptides to influence gastrointestinal motor function, *Gastroenterology,* 98, 517, 1990.
12. **Taché, Y., Ishikawa, T., Gunion, M. and Raybould, H.,** Central nervous system action of bombesin to influence gastric secretion and ulceration, *Ann. N. Y. Acad. Sci.,* 547, 183, 1988.
13. **Taché, Y. and Saperas, E.,** Potent inhibition of gastric acid secretion and ulcer formation by centrally and peripherally administered interleukin-1, *Ann. N. Y. Acad. Sci.,* 659, 353, 1992.
14. **Taché, Y., Mönnikes, H., Bonaz, B. and Rivier, J.,** Role of CRF in stress-related alterations of gastric and colonic motor function, *Ann. N. Y. Acad. Sci.,* 697, 233, 1993.
15. **Taché, Y., Yang, H. and Yoneda, M.,** Vagal regulation of gastric function involves thyrotropin-releasing hormone in the medullary raphe nuclei and dorsal vagal complex, *Digestion,* 54, 65, 1993.
16. **Taché, Y.,** Inhibition of gastric acid secretion and ulcers by calcitonin gene-related peptide, *Ann. N. Y. Acad. Sci.,* 657, 240, 1992.
17. **Taché, Y.,** Central mechanisms in control of acid secretion, *Curr. Opinion Gastro.,* 7, 842, 1992.
18. **Grossman, M. I.,** Neural and hormonal stimulation of gastric secretion of acid, in *Handbook of Physiology. Section 6: Alimentary Canal,* Code, C. F., Ed. American Physiological Society, Washington, D. C., 1967, 835.
19. **Taché, Y., Yang, H. and Yanagisawa, K.,** Brain regulation of gastric acid secretion by neuropeptides, in *Brain-Gut Interactions,* Taché, Y. and Wingate, D., Eds. CRC Press, Boca Raton, 1991, 169.
20. **Swanson, L. W.,** *Brain Maps: Structure of the Rat Brain,* Elsevier Sciences, Amsterdam, 1992,
21. **Paxinos, G. and Watson, C.,** *The Rat Brain in Stereotaxic Coordinates,* 2nd Ed., Academic Press, Orlando, 1986.
22. **Taché, Y. and Yang, H.,** Brain regulation of gastric acid secretion by peptides: sites and mechanisms of action, *Ann. N. Y. Acad. Sci.,* 597, 128, 1990.
23. **Feng, H. S., Lynn, R. B., Han, J. and Brooks, F. P.,** Gastric effects of TRH analogue and bicuculline injected into dorsal motor vagal nucleus in cats, *Am. J. Physiol.,* 259, G3210, 1990.
24. **Lynn, R. B., Feng, H.- S., Han, J. and Brooks, F. P.,** Gastric effects of thyrotropin-releasing hormone microinjected into the dorsal motor vagal nucleus in cats, *Life Sci.,* 48, 1247, 1991.
25. **White, R. L. Jr., Rossiter, C. D., Hornby, P. J., Harmon, J. W., Kasbekar, D. K. and Gillis, R. A.,** Excitation of neurons in the medullary raphe increases gastric acid and pepsin production in cats, *Am. J. Physiol.,* 260, G91, 1991.

26. **Pappas, T., Taché, Y. and Debas, H.,** Cerebro-ventricular somatostatin stimulates gastric acid secretion in the dog, in *Regulatory Peptides in Digestive, Nervous and Endocrine Systems. INSERM Symposium No. 25,* Lewin, M. J. M. and Bonfils, S., Eds. Elsevier Science Publishers BV, Amsterdam, 1985, 323.

27. **Lenz, H. J., Klapdor, R., Hester, S. E., Webb, V. J., Galyean, R. F., Rivier, J. E. and Brown, M. R.,** Inhibition of gastric acid secretion by brain peptides in the dog. Role of the autonomic nervous system and gastrin, *Gastroenterology,* 91, 905, 1986.

28. **Pappas, T., Hamel, D., Debas, H., Walsh, J. H. and Taché, Y.,** Cerebroventricular bombesin inhibits gastric acid secretion in dogs, *Gastroenterology,* 89, 43, 1985.

29. **Lenz, H. J.,** CNS regulation of gastric and autonomic functions in dogs by gastrin-releasing peptide, *Am. J. Physiol.,* 18, G298, 1988.

30. **Lane, A., Ivy, A. C. and Ivy, E. K.,** Response of chronic gastric fistula rat to histamine, *Am. J. Physiol.,* 192, 221, 1957.

31. **Borella, L. E. and Herr, F.,** A new method for measuring gastric acid secretion in unanesthetized rats, *Gastroenterology,* 61, 345, 1971.

32. **Komarov, S. A., Bralow, S. P. and Boyd, E.,** A permanent rat gastric fistula, *Proc. Soc. Exp. Biol. Med.,* 112, 451, 1963.

33. **Bollman, J. L.,** A cage which limits the activity of rats, *J. Lab. Clin. Med.,* 33, 1348, 1948.

34. **Witty, R. T. and Long, J. F.,** Effect of ambient temperature on gastric secretion and food intake in the rat, *Am. J. Physiol.,* 219, 1359, 1970.

35. **Arai, I., Muramatsu, M. and Aihara, H.,** Body temperature dependency of gastric regional blood flow, acid secretion and ulcer formation in restraint and water-immersion stressed rats, *Jpn. J. Pharmacol.,* 40, 501, 1986.

36. **Larsen, K. R., Moore, J. G. and Dayton, M. T.,** Circadian rhythms of acid and bicarbonate efflux in fasting rat stomach, *Am. J. Physiol.,* 260, G610, 1991.

37. **Dubrasquet, M., Roze, C., Ling, N. and Florencio, H.,** Inhibition of gastric and pancreatic secretions by cerebroventricular injections of gastrin-releasing peptide and bombesin in rats, *Regul. Pept.,* 3, 105, 1982.

38. **Mulvihill, S. J., Pappas, T. N. and Debas, H. T.,** Characterization of in vivo acid secretory responses of rabbit with comparison to dog and rat, *Dig. Dis. Sci.,* 34, 895, 1989.

39. **Martínez, V., Yang, H., Wong, H. C., Walsh, J. H. and Taché, Y.,** Somatostatin antibody does not influence bombesin-induced inhibition of gastric acid secretion in rats, *Peptides,* 16, 1, 1995.

40. **Taché, Y., Goto, Y., Hamel, D., Pekary, A. and Novin, D.,** Mechanisms underlying intracisternal TRH-induced stimulation of gastric acid secretion in rats, *Regul. Pept.,* 13, 21, 1985.

41. **Saperas, E. and Taché, Y.,** Central interleukin-1β-induced inhibition of acid secretion in rats: specificity of action, *Life Sci.,* 52, 785, 1993.

42. **Alphin, R. S. and Lin, T. M.,** Preparation of chronic denervated gastric pouches in the rat, *Am. J. Physiol.,* 197, 257, 1959.

43. **Shay, H., Sun, D. C. H. and Gruenstein, M.,** A quantitative method for measuring spontaneous gastric secretion in the rat, *Gastroenterology,* 26, 906, 1954.

44. **Emas, S., Nylander, G. and Wallin, B.,** Comparison of the dose-response curves for acid output to pentagastrin determined by two techniques in chronic gastric fistula rats, *Digestion,* 22, 94, 1981.

45. **Lloyd, K. C. K., Holzer, H. H., Zittell, T. T. and Raybould, H. E.,** Duodenal lipid inhibits gastric acid secretion by vagal, capsaicin-sensitive afferent pathways in rats, *Am. J. Physiol.,* 264, G659, 1993.

46. **Lloyd, K. C. K., Raybould, H. E., Taché, Y. and Walsh, J. H.,** Role of gastrin, histamine, and acetylcholine in the gastric phase of acid secretion in anesthetized rats, *Am. J. Physiol.,* 262, G747, 1992.

47. **Taché, Y., Stephens, R. L. and Ishikawa, T.,** Central nervous system action of TRH to influence gastrointestinal function and ulceration, *Ann. N. Y. Acad. Sci.,* 553, 269, 1989.

48. **Cowan, A., Khunawat, P., ZuZhu, X. and Gmerek, D. E.,** Effects of bombesin on behavior, *Life Sci.,* 37, 135, 1985.

49. **Brodie D. A.,** The mechanism of gastric hyperacidity produced by pylorus ligation in the rat, *Am. J. Dig. Dis.,* 11, 231, 1966.

50. **Vallgren, S., El Munshid, H. A., Hedenbro, J., Rehfeld, J. F. and Hakanson, R.,** Mechanism of gastric acid response to pylorus ligation: effect of nephrectomy, *Scand. J. Gastroenterol.,* 18, 491, 1983.

51. **Hakanson, R., Hedenbro, J., Liedberg, G., Sundler, F. and Vallgren, S.,** Mechanisms of gastric acid secretion after pylorus and oesophagus ligation in the rat, *J. Physiol.,* 305, 139, 1980.

52. **Hernandez, D. E., Jennes, L. and Emerick, S. G.,** Inhibition of gastric acid secretion by immunoneutralization of endogenous brain thyrotropin-releasing hormone, *Brain Res.,* 401, 381, 1987.

53. **Gunion, M. W. and Taché, Y.,** Intrahypothalamic microinfusion of corticotropin-releasing factor inhibits gastric acid secretion but increases secretion volume in rats, *Brain Res.,* 411, 156, 1987.

54. **Gunion, M. W., Kauffman, G. L. and Taché, Y.,** Intrahypothalamic microinfusion of corticotropin-releasing factor elevates gastric bicarbonate secretion and protects against cold-stress ulceration in rats, *Am. J. Physiol.,* 258, G152, 1990.

55. **Taché, Y. and Gunion, M.,** Central nervous system action of bombesin to inhibit gastric acid secretion, *Life Sci.,* 37, 115, 1985.

56. **Paré, W., Vincent, G. P. and Isom, K. E.,** Comparison of pyloric ligation and pyloric cuff techniques for collecting gastric secretion in the rat, *Lab. Anim. Sci.,* 29, 218, 1979.

57. **Stephens, R. L., Yang, H., Rivier, J. and Taché, Y.,** Intracisternal injection of CRF antagonist blocks surgical stress-induced inhibition of gastric secretion in the rat, *Peptides,* 9, 1067, 1988.

58. **Holzer, P.,** Local effector functions of capsaicin-sensitive sensory nerve endings: involvement of tachykinins, calcitonin gene-related peptide and other neurotransmitters, *Neuroscience,* 24, 739, 1988.

59. **Kato, K., Yang, H., Wong, H. C. and Taché, Y.,** Role of calcitonin gene-related peptide (CGRP) in the regulation of gastric acid secretion and mucosal integrity in the rat, *Gastroenterology,* 104, A114, 1993.

60. **Taché, Y., Goto, Y., Gunion, M. W., Vale, W., Rivier, J. and Brown, M.,** Inhibition of gastric acid secretion in rats by intracerebral injection of corticotropin-releasing factor, *Science,* 222, 935, 1983.

61. **Saperas, E., Yang, H., Rivier, C. and Taché, Y.,** Central action of recombinant interleukin-1 to inhibit acid secretion in rats, *Gastroenterology,* 99, 1599, 1990.

62. **Taché, Y., Gunion, M., Lauffenberger, M. and Goto, Y.,** Inhibition of gastric acid secretion by intracerebral injection of calcitonin gene related peptide in rats, *Life Sci.,* 35, 871, 1984.

63. **Taché, Y., Rivier, J., Vale, W. and Brown, M.,** Is somatostatin or a somatostatin-like peptide involved in central nervous system control of gastric secretion? *Regul. Pept.,* 1, 307, 1981.

64. **Saperas, E., Yang, H. and Taché, Y.,** Interleukin-1β acts at hypothalamic sites to inhibit gastric acid secretion in rats, *Am. J. Physiol.,* 263, G414, 1992.

65. **Gunion, M. W. and Taché, Y.,** Bombesin microinfusion into the paraventricular nucleus suppresses gastric acid secretion in the rat, *Brain Res.,* 411, 156, 1987.

66. **Graffner, H., Ekelund, M. and Hakanson, R.,** Anesthetic agents suppress basal and stimulated gastric acid secretion, *Scand. J. Gastroenterol.,* 26, 1200, 1991.

67. **Yang, H., Wong, H., Wu, V., Walsh, J. H. and Taché, Y.,** Somatostatin monoclonal antibody immunoneutralization increases gastrin and gastric acid secretion in urethane-anesthetized rats, *Gastroenterology,* 99, 659, 1990.

68. **Hwei, Y. and Thompson, J. H.,** Effect of anesthetic agents on maximal histamine-induced gastric secretion in Shay rats, *Am. J. Physiol.,* 213, 1331, 1967.

69. **Rinaman, L., Card, J. P., Schwaber, J. S. and Miselis, R. R.,** Ultrastructural demonstration of a gastric monosynaptic vagal circuit in the nucleus of the solitary tract in rat, *J. Neurosci.,* 9, 1985, 1989.

70. **Berthoud, H. R., Jedrzejewska, A. and Powley, T. L.,** Simultaneous labeling of vagal innervation of the gut and afferent projections from the visceral forebrain with DiI injected into the dorsal vagal complex in the rat, *J. Comp. Neurol.,* 301, 65, 1990.

71. **Berthoud, H. R., Fox, E. A. and Powley, T. L.,** Abdominal pathways and central origin of rat vagal fibers that stimulate gastric acid, *Gastroenterology,* 100, 627, 1991.

72. **Berthoud, H. R., Carlson, N. R. and Powley, T. L.,** Topography of efferent vagal innervation of the rat gastrointestinal tract, *Am. J. Physiol.,* 260, R200, 1991.

73. **Wei, J. Y., Taché, Y. and Kruger, L.,** Sources of anterior gastric vagal efferent discharge in rats: an electrophysiological study, *J. Aut. Nerv. Syst.,* 37, 29, 1992.

74. **Davison, J. S. and Grundy, D.,** Modulation of single vagal efferent fibre discharge by gastrointestinal afferents in the rat, *J. Physiol.,* 284, 69, 1978.

75. **Taché, Y.,** Vagal regulation of gastric secretion, in *Control of Acid Secretion,* Mignon, M. and Galmiche, J. -P., Eds. John Libbey Eurotext, Paris, 1988, 13.

76. **Berthoud, H. R., Laughton, W. B. and Powley, T. L.,** Vagal stimulation-induced gastric acid secretion in the anesthetized rat, *J. Auton. Nerv. Syst.,* 16, 193, 1986.

77. **Berthoud, H. R. and Powley, T. L.,** Characteristics of gastric and pancreatic responses to vagal stimulation with varied frequencies: evidence for different fiber calibers? *J. Auton. Nerv. Syst.,* 19, 77, 1987.

78. **Okuma, Y., Yokotani, K. and Osumi, Y.,** Sympatho-adrenomedullary system mediation of the bombesin-induced central inhibition of gastric acid secretion, *Eur. J. Pharmacol.,* 139, 73, 1987.

79. **Thiefin, G., Raybould, H. E., Leung, F. W., Taché, Y. and Guth, P. H.,** Capsaicin-sensitive afferent fibers contribute to gastric mucosal blood flow response to electrical vagal stimulation, *Am. J. Physiol.,* 259, G1037, 1990.

80. **Kadekaro, M., Timo-Iaria, C. and Valle, L. E. R.,** Neural systems responsible for the gastric secretion provoked by 2-deoxy-D-glucose cytoglucopoenia, *J. Physiol. (Lond.),* 252, 565, 1975.

81. **Collin-Jones, D. G. and Himsworth, R. L.,** The location of the chemoreceptor controlling gastric acid secretion during hypoglycaemia, *J. Physiol. (Lond.),* 206, 397, 1970.

82. **Sylvestre, J. L.,** Validation tests of completeness of vagotomy in rats, *J. Auton. Nerv. Syst.,* 9, 301, 1983.

83. **Webber, D. E. and Morrissey, S. M.,** Separate hypoglycaemic thresholds for gastric acid and pepsin secretion following insulin or posterior hypothalamic stimulation, *Can. J. Physiol. Pharmacol.,* 57, 1283, 1979.

84. **Scheurink, S. and Ritter, S.,** Sympathoadrenal responses to glucoprivation and lipoprivation in rats, *Physiol. Behav.,* 53, 995, 1993.

85. **Taché, Y., Marki, W., Rivier, J., Vale, W. and Brown, M.,** Central nervous system inhibition of gastric secretion in the rat by gastrin-releasing peptide, a mammalian bombesin, *Gastroenterology,* 81, 298, 1981.

86. **Taché, Y. and Yang, H.,** Role of medullary TRH in the vagal regulation of gastric function, in *Innervation of the Gut: Pathophysiological Implications,* Taché, Y., Wingate, D. L. and Burks, T. F., Eds. CRC Press, Boca Raton, 1993, 67.

87. **Yang, H., Ohning, G. and Taché, Y.,** TRH in dorsal vagal complex mediates acid response to excitation of raphe pallidus neurons in rats, *Am. J. Physiol.,* 265, G880, 1993.

88. **Goto, Y. and Debas, H. T.,** GABA-mimetic effect on gastric acid secretion. Possible significance in central mechanisms, *Dig. Dis. Sci.,* 28, 56, 1983.

89. **Goto, Y., Taché, Y., Debas, H. and Novin, D.,** Gastric and vagus nerve response to GABA agonist baclofen, *Life Sci.,* 36, 2471, 1985.

90. **Hara, N., Hara, Y., Natsume, Y. and Goto, Y.,** Direct evidence indicating that a GABA-mimetic stimulates acid secretion through central mechanisms, *Jpn. J. Pharmacol.,* 53, 271, 1990.

91. **Takeuchi, K., Nishiwaki, H., Niida, H. and Okabe, S.,** Body temperature-dependent action of baclofen in rat stomach, *Dig. Dis. Sci.,* 35, 458, 1990.

92. **Banks, W. A. and Kastin, A. J.,** Peptide transport systems for opiates across the blood-brain barrier, *Am. J. Physiol.,* 259, E1, 1990.

93. **Feldberg, W. S.,** *Fifty Years on: Looking Back on Some Developments in Neurohumoral Physiology,* Liverpool Univeristy Press, Liverpool, 1982, 31.

94. **Elliott, P. J.,** A reliable, rapid and inexpensive method for producing and implanting chronic cannulae into brains of small animals, *Pharmacol. Biochem. Behav.,* 24, 1809, 1986.

95. **Yoshida-Yoneda, E., Wei, J. Y. and Taché, Y.,** Bombesin acts in the brain to decrease gastric vagal efferent discharge in rats, *Peptides,* 14, 339, 1993.

96. **Gunion, M. W. and Taché, Y.,** Fore- and hindbrain mediation of gastric hypoacidity after intracerebral bombesin, *Am. J. Physiol.,* 15, G675, 1987.

97. **Yang, H., Cuttitta, F., Raybould, H. and Taché, Y.,** Intrathecal injection of bombesin inhibits gastric acid secretion in the rat, *Gastroenterology,* 96, 1403, 1989.

98. **Yaksh, T. L. and Rudy, T. A.,** Analgesia mediated by a direct spinal action of narcotics, *Science,* 192, 1357, 1976.

99. **Martin, H., Kocher, L. and Chery-Croze, S.,** Chronic lumbar intrathecal catheterization in the rat with reduced-length spinal compression, *Physiol. Behav.,* 33, 159, 1984.

100. **Passaro, E. Jr., Debas, H., Oldendorf, W. and Yamada, T.,** Rapid appearance of intraventricularly administered neuropeptides in the peripheral circulation, *Brain Res.,* 241, 335, 1982.

101. **Pekary, A., Stephens, R., Simard, M., Pang, X. -P., Smith, V., Distephano, J. J., III and Hershman, J. M.,** Release of thyrotropin and prolactin by a thyrotropin-releasing hormone (TRH) precursor, TRH-Gly: conversion to TRH is sufficient for in vivo effects, *Neuroendocrinology,* 52, 618, 1990.

102. **Tannenbaum, G. S. and Patel, Y. C.,** On the fate of centrally administered somatostatin in the rat: massive hypersomatostatinemia resulting from leakage into the peripheral circulation has effects on growth hormone secretion and glucoregulation, *Endocrinology,* 118, 2137, 1986.

103. **Clark, R. G., Jones, P. M. and Robinson, I. C. A. F.,** Clearance of vasopressin from cerebrospinal fluid to blood in chronically cannulated Brattleboro rats, *Neuroendocrinology,* 37, 242, 1983.

104. **Morimito, T., Okamoto, M., Nakamuta, H., Stahl, G. L. and Orlowski, R. C.,** Intracerebroventricular injection of 125I-salmon calcitonin in rats: fate, anorexia and hypocalcemia, *Jpn. J. Pharmacol.,* 37, 21, 1985.

105. **Taché, Y. and Saperas, E.,** Central actions of interleukin 1 on gastrointestinal function, in *Neurobiology of Cytokines Part B,* De Souza, E. B., Ed. Academic Press Inc., San Diego, 1993, 169.

106. **Ishikawa, T. and Taché, Y.,** Bombesin microinjected into the dorsal vagal complex inhibits vagally stimulated gastric acid secretion in the rat, *Regul. Pept.,* 24, 187, 1989.

107. **Yang, H., Stephens, R. L. and Taché, Y.,** TRH analogue microinjected into specific medullary nuclei stimulates gastric serotonin secretion in rats, *Am. J. Physiol.,* 262, G216, 1992.

108. **Ishikawa, T., Yang, H. and Taché, Y.,** Medullary sites of action of the TRH analogue, RX 77368, to stimulate gastric acid secretion in the rat, *Gastroenterology,* 95, 1470, 1988.

109. **Stone, T. W.,** *Microiontophoresis and Pessure Ejection,* Wiley and Sons, New York, 1985.

110. **Vanhof, S., Siren, A. L. and Feuerstein, G. Z.,** Volume-dependent spatial distribution of microinjected thyrotropin-releasing hormone (TRH) into the medial preoptic nucleus of the rat: an autoradiographic study, *Neurosci. Lett.,* 113, 187, 1990.

111. **Shipley, M. T.,** A simple, low cost hydraulic pressure device for making microinjections in the brain, *Brain Res. Bull.,* 8, 237, 1982.

112. **Rogers, R. C.,** An inexpensive picoliter-volume pressure ejection system, *Brain Res. Bull.,* 15, 669, 1985.

113. **Rogers, R. C. and Hermann, G. E.,** Dorsal medullary oxytocin, vasopressin, oxytocin antagonist, and TRH effects on gastric acid secretion and heart rate, *Peptides,* 6, 1143, 1985.

114. **Mönnikes, H., Schmidt, B. G. and Taché, Y.,** Psychological stress-induced accelerated colonic transit in rats involves hypothalamic corticotropin-releasing factor, *Gastroenterology,* 104, 716, 1993.

115. **Mönnikes, H., Schmidt, B. G., Tebbe, J., Bauer, C. and Taché, Y.,** Microinfusion of corticotropin releasing factor into the locus coeruleus/subcoeruleus stimulates colonic motor function in rats, *Brain Res.,* 644, 101, 1994.

116. **Gunion, M. W., Taché, Y., Walsh, J. H. and Novin, D.,** Suppression of gastric acid secretion by intracisternal bombesin does not require the ventromedial hypothalamus, *Life Sci.,* 35, 1769, 1984.

117. **Taché, Y., Lesiege, D. and Goto, Y.,** Neural pathways involved in intracisternal bombesin-induced inhibition of gastric secretion in rats, *Dig. Dis. Sci.,* 31, 412, 1986.

118. **Taché, Y., Lesiege, D., Vale, W. and Collu, R.,** Gastric hypersecretion by intracisternal TRH: dissociation from hypophysiotropic activity and role of central catecholamine, *Eur. J. Pharmacol.,* 107, 149, 1985.

119. **Mönnikes, H., Schmidt, B. G., Raybould, H. E. and Taché, Y.,** CRF in the paraventricular nucleus mediates gastric and colonic motor response to restraint stress, *Am. J. Physiol.,* 262, G137, 1992.

120. **Powley, T. L., Prechtl, J. C., Fox, E. A. and Berthoud, HR,** Anatomical considerations for surgery of the rat abdominal vagus: distribution, paraganglia and regeneration, *J. Auton. Nerv. Syst.,* 9, 79, 1983.

121. **Wei, J. Y. and Taché, Y.,** Alterations of efferent discharges of the gastric branch of the vagus nerve by intracisternal injection of peptides influencing gastric function in rats, *Gastroenterology,* 98, A531, 1990. (Abstract)

122. **Raybould, H. E., Holzer, P., Reddy, N. S., Yang, H. and Taché, Y.,** Capsaicin-sensitive vagal afferents contribute to gastric acid and vascular responses to intracisternal TRH analog, *Peptides,* 11, 789, 1990.

123. **Plourde, V., Wong, H. C., Walsh, J. H., Raybould, H. E. and Taché, Y.,** CGRP antagonists and capsaicin on celiac ganglia partly prevent postoperative gastric ileus, *Peptides,* 14, 1225, 1993.

124. **Druge, G., Raedler, A., Heiner, G. and Lenz, J.,** Pathways mediating CRF-induced inhibition of gastric acid secretion in rats, *Am. J. Physiol.,* 256, G214, 1989.

125. **Wong, H. C., Walsh, J. H., Yang, H., Taché, Y. and Buchan, A. M.,** A monoclonal antibody to somatostatin with potent in vivo immunoneutralizing activity, *Peptides,* 11, 707, 1990.

126. **Yang, H., Wong, H. C., Walsh, J. H. and Taché, Y.,** Effect of gastrin monoclonal antibody 28.2 on acid response to chemical vagal stimulation in rats, *Life Sci.,* 45, 2413, 1989.

127. **Kato, K., Yang, H. and Taché, Y.,** Role of peripheral capsaicin-sensitive neurons and CGRP in central vagally mediated gastroprotective effect of TRH, *Am. J. Physiol.,* 266, R1610, 1994.

128. **Taché, Y. and Collu, R.,** CNS mediated inhibition of gastric secretion by bombesin: independence from interaction with brain catecholaminergic, and serotoninergic pathways and pituitary hormones, *Regul. Pept.,* 3, 51, 1982.

129. **Taché, Y.,** Intracisternal bombesin induced inhibition of gastric secretion is not mediated through prostaglandin or opioid pathways, *Peptides,* 6, Suppl. 3, 69, 1985.

130. **Yoneda, M. and Taché, Y.,** Vagal regulation of gastric prostaglandin E2 release by central TRH in rats, *Am. J. Physiol.,* 264, G231, 1993.

131. **Lenz, H. J., Raedler, A., Greten, H., Vale, W. W. and Rivier, J. E.,** Stress-induced gastrointestinal secretory and motor responses in rats are mediated by endogenous corticotropin-releasing factor, *Gastroenterology,* 95, 1510, 1988.

132. **Yang, H., Wu, S. V., Ishikawa, T. and Taché, Y.,** Cold exposure elevates thyrotropin-releasing hormone gene expression in medullary raphe nuclei: relationship with vagally mediated gastric erosions, *Neuroscience,* in press, 1994.

133. **Saperas, E., Kauffman, G. and Taché, Y.,** Role of central prostaglandin E_2 in the regulation of gastric acid secretion in the rat, *Eur. J. Pharmacol.,* 209, 1, 1991.

134. **Licinio, J., Wong, M. -L. and Gold, P. W.,** Localization of interleukin-1 receptor antagonist mRNA in rat brain, *Endocrinology,* 129, 562, 1991.

135. **Lloyd, K. C. K.; Holzer, H. H., Zittel, T. T. and Raybould, H. E.,** Duodenal lipid inhibits gastric acid secretion by vagal, capsaicin-sensitive afferent pathways in rats, *Am. J. Physiol.,* 264, G659, 1993.

136. **Yanagisawa, K., Yang, H., Walsh, J. H. and Taché, Y.,** Role of acetylcholine, histamine and gastrin in the acid response to intracisternal injection of TRH analog, RX 77368, in the rat, *Regul. Pept.,* 27, 161, 1990.

137. **Mönnikes, H., Eichhorn, A., Bauer, A., Tebbe, J. and Taché, Y.,** CRF microinfused into the locus coeruleus complex (LCC) inhibits gastric acid secretion in rats, *Gastroenterology,* 104, A840, 1993.

3 Gastroduodenal Mucosal Protection Studies

Gregory S. Smith, Jose C. Barreto, and Thomas A. Miller

INTRODUCTION

A variety of models are available to the investigator who wishes to determine whether a given experimental insult causes damage to the gastroduodenal mucosa, and, correspondingly, whether a putative protective substance or change in experimental protocol can prevent such injury. It must be emphasized at the outset that no one model is superior to all others in studying mucosal protection. Some models are best utilized for acute studies whereas others are more suitable when chronic considerations are being addressed. Further, many models are best suited to study gastric injury and protection, while others can be adapted to study these parameters in both the stomach and duodenum. *In vivo* models are generally more physiologic than those performed under *in vitro* conditions. However, the *in vivo* model usually gives an "overall picture" of the specific consideration being studied, whereas an *in vitro* model is much more mechanistic. Of equal note, some models are more readily undertaken in a particular species and less adaptable to others. Finally, all models assessing mucosal protection have certain inherent advantages and disadvantages. For all of these reasons, considerable confusion may be encountered in selecting a particular model to study a particular component or consideration referable to mucosal protection.

It is the aim of this chapter to highlight for the reader the most popular models currently in use for assessing mucosal injury and protection involving the stomach and duodenum, to point out the obvious advantages as well as obvious and sometimes not so obvious disadvantages associated with a specific experimental approach, and to familiarize the reader with the precise experimental techniques required to effectively carry out meaningful studies with these models. While various classification systems can be employed to accomplish this discussion, the present chapter will consider experimental approaches carried out under *in vivo* circumstances and compare those with other models that are performed under *in vitro* conditions. At the very least, *in vivo* means that the blood supply has been maintained. For *in vitro* experiments, all connections of the tissue have been severed with the host animal so that circulatory, humoral, and neural inputs are no longer operational.

IN VIVO MODELS

While various animal species have been employed to study mucosal protection under *in vivo* conditions, rats have been a particularly attractive animal model as evidenced by the fact that this animal is chosen for experimental use 14 times more often than all other laboratory animals combined.[1] The popularity of this animal for gastroduodenal research continues to the present and exists for several reasons. First, rats are relatively inexpensive and easy to house

0-8493-8304-8/96/$0.00+$.50
© 1996 by CRC Press, Inc.

compared to larger vertebrates. This economic benefit directly allows preliminary pilot experiments to be carried out at a very modest cost. Secondly, the small size of rats and their relative ease in handling allows for large groups to be studied in a single experimental setting so that multiple components of a more complex physiologic process can be examined simultaneously, if so desired. Thirdly, findings in the rat are generally extrapolatible physiologically to what exists in the human stomach. Finally, since rats are normally not considered the ideal human pet, their use in gastrointestinal research does not engender the same emotional response by animal activists that other species, such as the dog and cat, can invoke. For these reasons, more attention will be given to rats as experimental models than other animal species.

MODELS IN WHICH THE STOMACH AND DUODENUM
HAVE NOT BEEN PHYSIOLOGICALLY DISTURBED

A large body of experimental data has been obtained in gastroduodenal protection studies using intact animals in which the stomach or duodenum has not been physiologically disturbed. The rat has been particularly popular for this type of study, although larger animals have at times been utilized. In studies assessing the damaging effect of a particular substance on the gastric epithelium and its prevention or attenuation by a putative protective agent, the intact animal model has proved especially popular. For studies of this nature, unanesthetized, but fasted (usually 18–24 hour fast) rats are lightly restrained by placing the investigator's hand around the back of the animal so that the index and middle fingers of his hand pass around the neck and thereby lightly restrict movement of the clavicles from the front. The animal is then lifted from the place it is standing and is rotated so that its body is at a 90° angle with the floor. A metal or hard plastic orogastric or oroesophageal tube attached to a syringe containing the putative damaging agent is then inserted into the rear of the oropharynx which initiates a swallowing response in the animal. This tube is advanced carefully into the esophagus and then down into the stomach of the rat. The test solution is then easily administered directly to the surface of the gastric mucosa under slight pressure. At varying periods after the administration of the test solution (ranging from 5 minutes to 1–3 hours), animals are sacrificed at which time the stomach can be removed, and various morphologic and biochemical parameters measured. Just prior to sacrifice, the animal is anesthetized using a rapidly acting substance, such as ether or the inhalation anesthetic, methoxyflurane. Upon anesthetization, the abdomen is opened through a vertical incision following which clamps are placed on the distal esophagus and proximal duodenum at the level of the pyloric sphincter. The stomach is then rapidly separated from its vascular, neural, and fascial attachments with scissors dissection. The animal is subsequently killed via anesthetic overdose or cervical dislocation.

Depending upon the goals of the study undertaken, the removed stomach can be opened and examined for the presence or absence of macroscopic injury, usually depicted by the presence of linear hemorrhagic lesions or petechiae. Such lesions can be quantitated by measuring their length and width or determining the percentage surface area of the gastric mucosa involved using digitized planimetry. If only the incidence of lesions is of interest, the number of lesions formed is simply counted. When microscopic evaluation of injury is to be determined, the stomach is usually filled with a fixative, such as Karnovsky's solution,[2] prior to opening it. This preparation for histologic analysis can be done before the stomach is actually removed from the animal, but after clamping it at the esophageal and pyloric regions, or can be done upon its immediate removal. In either case, a small needle (usually 27 gauge) attached to a syringe filled with fixative is injected into the forestomach (Figure 1) of the rat so that even distribution of the fixative occurs throughout the stomach. After applying such a fixative, the stomach is immersed in a solution of similar fixative for an additional 24–48 hours following its removal. Specimens of stomach can then be taken after such fixation and prepared for

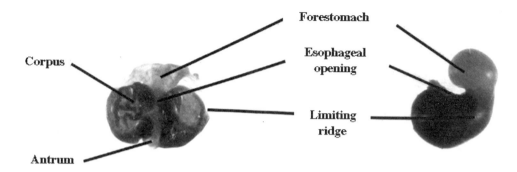

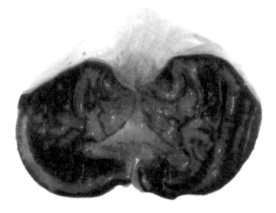

FIGURE 1   Comparative view of a normal intact rat stomach (right) and a similar stomach which has been opened along the greater curvature to expose its mucosal surface (left). Note the anatomical landmarks.

histologic assessment using routine techniques.[3-4] The magnitude of histologic injury can then be determined using previously published scoring techniques.[3-6]

The aforementioned experimental approach has been utilized extensively to characterize the damaging effects of various topically applied damaging agents to the gastric epithelium.[3-8] Among damaging agents evaluated in this fashion have been various concentrations of ethanol, bile salts, aspirin, other nonsteroidal anti-inflammatory compounds, as well as strong acids and alkali. The injury produced by these xenobiotic substances consists of hemorrhagic band-like lesions (Figure 2) usually confined to the glandular (acid-secreting portion and antrum—Figure 1) stomach if the damaging substance is ethanol or strong acid or base, or more petechiae-like lesions if the damaging agent is a bile salt, aspirin, or other nonsteroidal anti-inflammatory compound.

In addition to determining morphologic correlates of gastric injury, specimens of gastric mucosa can also be conveniently sampled for measurement of various biochemical parameters. Examples of such parameters would be tissue levels of prostaglandins, leukotrienes, DNA or RNA, and various energy substrate metabolic compounds, such as ATP, AMP, glucose, pyruvate, and lactate. Measurement of such biochemical substances has been commonly carried out with this model in an attempt to link the magnitude of gastric injury with a perturbation in a particular biochemical substance of interest.

In addition to using this model to study the dynamics of gastric injury following the oral administration of a damaging agent, it has also been adapted to evaluate the potential protective

FIGURE 2   Photograph of an injured rodent stomach which has been opened along the greater curvature. This particular stomach was exposed to a combination of 150 mM HCl and 50% ethanol. Note the numerous hemorrhagic streaks which run parallel to the long axis of the stomach.

capability of a putative protective agent. When performing protection studies, the approach to inducing damage is identical, but prior to administering the damaging substance, the protective agent being evaluated is given. It may be administered orally, like the damaging agent, using the same orogastric tube, or given parenterally. If the latter approach is used, the protective agent is usually given subcutaneously or intraperitoneally, or less often intravenously. If a protective agent is given, it is usually administered 15–30 minutes prior to the damaging substance. Protection studies using this model have formed the basis of much of the prostaglandin cytoprotection research that has been carried out over the past 15 years. The reader interested in this type of research should consult references 3 through 10 for more details.

The obvious advantage of this intact rat stomach model in studying mucosal protection relates to the fact that the physiology of the stomach has remained unperturbed and the animal is conscious during the administration of the damaging agent or following its administration after pretreatment with a putative protective agent, such as prostaglandin. This model closely resembles the human condition in the sense that injury and its prevention or alleviation occur under conditions when humoral and neural influences are left intact as well as the stomach's vascular supply. Secondly, animals employed in such studies are exposed to a minimum of stress so that the investigator can be reasonably assured that the observed experimental results are due directly to the effect of the test agent in question and not in response to some extraneous surgical, physical, or other chemical manipulation. Thirdly, this type of experimental approach creates mucosal injury which is rapid, easy to induce, consistent and reproducible, and associated with virtually no mortality. The lesions formed under these experimental conditions can usually be quantified macroscopically and further evaluated microscopically with relative ease.

From a procedural standpoint, a minor disadvantage of this model stems from problems associated with the physical intubation of the animal to insure that the damaging agent reaches the stomach. Occasionally, the orogastric tube can be misdirected into the trachea whereupon the damaging agent is infused incorrectly into the respiratory tract. On even rarer occasions, the orogastric tube can be inserted into the throat of the animal with such force that it either perforates the esophagus or the wall of the proximal stomach. These minor disadvantages are greatly attenuated with experience and practice. The major disadvantage of this model is the problem with all *in vivo* models, namely, that the precise events that give rise to injury and/or are responsible for protection against such injury at the cellular level cannot be defined and will usually require some type of *in vitro* preparation.

In addition to the model just described, the intact, conscious rat has also been commonly used experimentally to induce stress-related gastric and duodenal ulcers and to evaluate possible protective agents against such ulcer formation. Several means have been used by investigators to induce stress. These have included injections of high concentrations of agents such as corticosteroids and reserpine that commonly induce gastric injury[11–12] and the sulfhydryl containing compound, cysteamine, which commonly induces duodenal injury.[13] Other approaches have involved the placement of rats in plexiglass or stainless steel restraint cages which severely limit their free bodily movements[14–16] (Figure 3). This restraint has been carried out at both room temperature as well as under cold conditions, such as 4°C, for varying periods of time. Usually the animal has to be restrained for at least 3–4 hours before any visible lesion formation can be demonstrated upon inspection of the stomach or duodenum. An alternative approach to inducing stress ulcer formation has involved the placement of animals in specially designed cages so that they are actually positioned in an upright posture. Animals are then immersed in cold water to the level of the ziphoid process which is held constant at 20–23°C for varying periods of time ranging from as short as one hour to as long as 24 hours.[17–18] Usually, the longer the immersion period, the more likely that visual lesion formation will supervene. The cold water immersion stress model has been used to produce both gastric and duodenal lesions in rats,[17] and gastric lesions in guinea pigs.[18] When such models have been employed, it has generally been recommended that a rectal thermometer be used to measure core body temperature

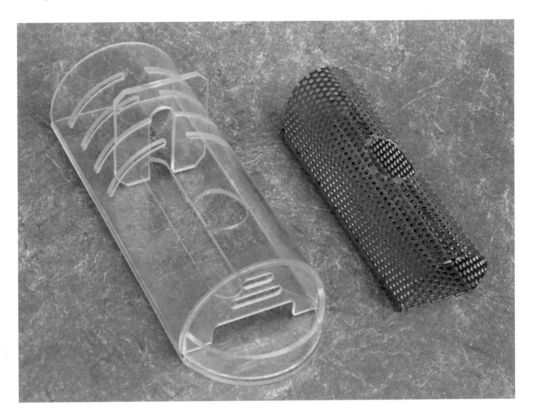

FIGURE 3 A comparative view of the modern plexiglass rodent restraint cage (left) and its older stainless steel prototype (right).

in these animals to insure maintenance of the desired target temperature. With all of these models, the animals are anesthetized at the completion of stress at which time their stomachs are removed and visible lesions quantified. Similar to studies with xenobiotic agents, specimens can also be obtained at the time of sacrifice for microscopic evaluation of injury or biochemical analysis of some mucosal substance.

Any of the stress models just mentioned are relatively easy to perform with virtually no mortality. The major disadvantage is that the gastroduodenal injury produced is much more subtle than that encountered with chemical damaging agents, and the majority of injury is manifest as discrete punctate lesions rather than clear cut hemorrhagic streaks. Consequently, it is often more difficult to quantitate this type of damage without additional histologic assessment. Further, in contrast to chemically induced injury which is limited to the stomach and involves its glandular portion, stress injury may involve the stomach or duodenum or both, and when involving the stomach may include the nonglandular forestomach or glandular stomach alone or both in combination. Another relative disadvantage is that the protocols are much more time consuming than with chemically induced injury, requiring on average at least 4 hours of stress and not infrequently longer periods. Protocols of 24 hours duration are not uncommon with these types of stress models. Finally, the level of pain that animals may experience during these protocols is uncertain, and many animal care committees are less likely to approve these protocols than those using more rapid-acting chemically induced models of injury.

PYLORUS LIGATION MODEL OF GASTRIC INJURY

One of the oldest models to induce acute gastric injury is the pylorus ligation model first described by Shay and colleagues in the 1940s.[19] Accordingly, this model is commonly referred to as the "Shay ulcer model". For this experimental preparation, fasted rats are anesthetized with an appropriate anesthetic and the abdomen is then opened via a midline incision. After removing the surrounding connective tissue components with blunt dissection, the pylorus of the stomach is visualized. Subsequent mobilization of the pylorus is then carried out and a 4-0 silk ligature is passed around the pylorus and gently ligated in place, taking care not to damage accompanying blood vessels or to place excess traction on the stomach. With the animal still anesthetized, an orogastric tube is then inserted into the oropharynx and is advanced through the esophagus into the proximal stomach. Up to 4 ml of prewarmed saline is then injected through this tube into the lumen of the stomach to serve as a rinse and then the entire volume is recovered by gentle aspiration through this same tube. After removal of the tube, the muscle and skin of the abdominal wall are closed and the animal is allowed to recover from anesthesia. Animals are then placed in cages with wide mesh bottoms to prevent coprophagia. The continual secretion of acid by the rat stomach over the ensuing hours results in a reproducible model of gastric injury, involving primarily the glandular epithelium.[19–20] Usually, a minimum of 4 hours is necessary after pylorus ligation to insure consistent, reproducible injury. At sacrifice, the stomach is removed, opened along the greater curvature and examined for the presence or absence of macroscopic injury. Using some type of scoring technique, examples of which have been previously described, the number of macroscopic lesions is then quantified. In addition to this gross determination of injury, the stomach may be fixed at the time of sacrifice and examined for the presence or absence of histologic injury. Further, samples of mucosa can be taken at sacrifice for analysis of mucosal biochemical substances, if so desired.

The Shay ulcer model has been very popular over the years for investigators studying various aspects of gastric pathophysiology. An attractive feature of this preparation is the relative ease with which it can be carried out. The entire preparation, for example, can be performed in 5–10 minutes with minimum stress to the animals involved. Thus, unwanted long term effects of general anesthesia are avoided with this model. Additionally, there is no damage to either the gastric blood or nerve supply with this preparation so that these components of normal gastric function remain undisturbed. Another advantage of the pylorus ligation model is that it allows the investigator the opportunity to collect residual stomach contents at the termination of the experiment. Since this model of gastric damage is dependent on acid secretion under *in vivo* conditions, sampling of the residual volume and its subsequent titration to neutrality allows the investigator the opportunity to actually calculate acid secretion and to correlate the extent of acid concentration with the extent of injury that is produced under these conditions. Another feature to which this model lends itself is that a putative protective agent can be given at the time of pylorus ligation, either by infusing it directly into the stomach or administering it through a parenteral means and thereby determining at the time of animal sacrifice whether the agent elicited its protective effect by inhibition of acid production or by some independent action. Some investigators have even used this preparation to determine the potential synergistic effects of both acid and a gastric irritant in inducing injury. For this type of study, a known amount of a potential gastric ulcerogen, such as alcohol, is infused into the stomach after pylorus ligation, and the effect of this ulcerogen in combination with acid production on gastric injury assessed at the time of sacrifice. A putative protective agent may also be given with this type of ulcer preparation when the pylorus is ligated and its ability to prevent injury assessed at the time of animal sacrifice.

Many investigators have chosen to use the pylorus ligation model not as a means of inducing injury, but rather to assess the antisecretory property of a particular agent. Since acid is continually secreted by rats, the secreted acid that collects after pylorus ligation can be evaluated both with and without a putative antisecretory agent. By using different doses of the suspected antisecretory substance(s), usually administered parenterally, a dose response analysis can be carried out. For these types of studies, the animals are usually sacrificed 2–3 hours after pylorus ligation before the accumulated acid has an opportunity to directly damage the gastric epithelium.

The only major disadvantage of the pylorus ligation model is the longer time frame (at least 4 hours) required to induce gastric injury, if this is the reason the model is being employed. Further, since this preparation does involve some degree of surgical skill, a small mortality may be associated with it due to anesthetic overdose or less commonly poor surgical technique.

CHAMBERED STOMACH MODELS

Another model to induce acute gastric injury is the chambered stomach preparation. This model was originally described in dogs by Rehm,[21] but more recently has been adapted by Morris and colleagues,[6,22] for use in the rat. With the increasing cost of using dogs for laboratory research and the strong emotions engendered by animal activists when employing such an animal experimentally, more and more research in recent years has utilized the rat for chambered stomach work. Regardless of whether rats, dogs, or other species are employed, the basic experimental preparation is the same. Thus, after an overnight fast and insuring an adequate level of anesthesia, a midline laparotomy is performed and the stomach exposed. When dogs are used, a segment of the gastric corpus with its vasculature intact is mounted between the rings of a lucite chamber in such a fashion that the mucosa is exposed and can be examined throughout experiments (Figure 4). With such a large animal, as much as 36 cm^2 of exteriorized surface can be exposed. This large surface area can be studied as a whole or, if desired, divided into roughly two equal sections with a lucite bar that is part of the chamber apparatus (Figure 5). The advantage of the latter feature, first developed by Moody and Durbin,[23] is that one half of the stomach can serve as control and the other half as the experimental test side. With smaller animals, such as the rat, most of the stomach is mounted in the chamber apparatus after freeing it from its surrounding connective tissue. It too, however, retains its vascular attachment to the host animal. The overall surface area of the exposed stomach when using a rat, however, is considerably less and averages approximately 1.5 cm^2. While a lucite bridge can also be placed

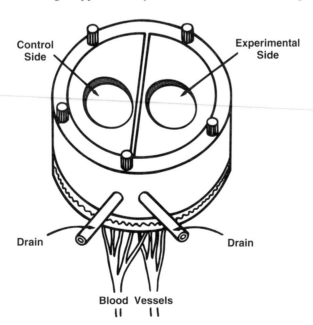

FIGURE 4 Schematic diagram of a canine gastric chamber preparation which allows an exteriorized segment of stomach to be viewed constantly throughout the duration of the experimental period without compromising its blood supply.

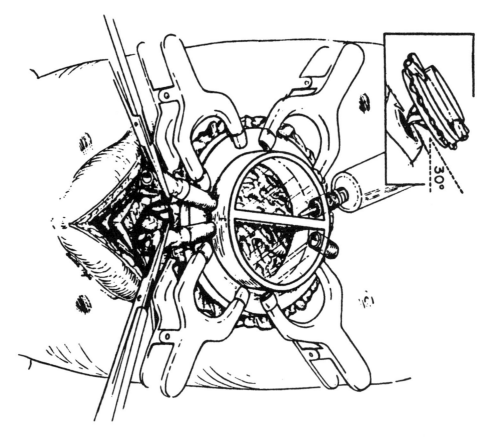

FIGURE 5   Schematic diagram of an exteriorized canine stomach preparation. The plexiglass crossbar in this preparation divides the gastric mucosa into two equal halves, commonly called a "Moody Chambered Stomach". Thus, one side of this gastric chambered preparation serves as its own control. Note that this preparation also allows the exteriorized stomach to be tilted, allowing for easy gravity drainage of the reservoir contents. (Reprinted with permission from Moody and Durbin, *Am. J. Physiol.* 209(1):122–126, 1965.)

across this exposed surface so that it likewise can be divided into two halves, this is more difficult than with the dog and has not found much favor with most investigators.

After securing the mounted stomach in the lucite chamber, the exposed mucosal surface is initially bathed with some type of buffered solution to keep it moist and to prevent it from drying. This volume is usually fixed and can be replaced with fresh solution at varying time periods throughout the experiment. If a dog stomach is chambered, as much as 20 ml of a solution can be placed on the mucosal surface. With rat stomachs, however, this amount usually does not exceed 2–3 ml. After allowing the preparation to stabilize following mounting, various damaging substances can be added directly into the bathing solution and their injurious effects examined over time. Depending on the goals of the experiment, the length of study may vary from 30 minutes up to 2–3 hours.

The notable advantage of this experimental model is that the exposed gastric epithelium can be visually inspected throughout the study and effects of various perturbations on lesion formation directly assessed at the same time that blood flow to the stomach is maintained. Less certain is the intactness of the nerve supply to this preparation. Because a wedge of stomach is separated from the rest of this organ and mounted, almost certainly many vagal nerve fibers are severed upon such mounting. In fact, many investigators believe that this preparation is a totally vagally denervated model. Sympathetic neural components, however, are felt to remain undisturbed.

Despite this potential drawback, the chambered stomach preparation does allow the investigator to study temporal events relevant to the pathogenesis of gastric injury. This is possible because the investigator can actually see what is occurring in "real time" to the mounted gastric epithelium. Further, this approach standardizes experiments since the surface area of the gastric mucosa as well as the volumes of test solutions which are employed in these studies are held constant for all animals used. Since the investigator has access to the luminal contents in this preparation, aliquots may be conveniently removed for subsequent biochemical analysis of an interesting parameter and can easily be replaced as required throughout the experimental time course. Additionally, with minor modifications made to the chamber, electrodes can be placed directly on the mucosal surface so that potential difference measurements can be carried out in "real time" while the stomach is exposed to various combinations of gastroprotective or damaging compounds. Since measurement of potential difference has been shown to correlate with the integrity of the gastric mucosa (see Discussion under Ussing chamber), acquisition of this additional electrophysiologic information allows another means of assessing injury to the surface epithelium with this preparation.

Another interesting advantage of the chambered stomach is that it allows the investigator exclusive control over how much of the surface area of the mounted stomach is to be exposed to the luminal bathing solution. Thus, as pointed out previously, particularly with respect to the dog, one side of the chamber can serve as control and the other side as test. Because this is less easily accomplished in the rat, than the dog, various modifications have been employed to enable a portion of the exteriorized mucosa to serve as a control. One interesting approach has been used by Morris and associates.[24] These investigators, after mounting the rat stomach in the lucite chamber, have rotated the animal's torso and thereby tilted the chambered portion of the stomach so that one portion of the exposed epithelium is more readily in contact with the luminal bathing solution than the other portion. This has enabled a damaging agent to be in contact with one part of the stomach but not another so that appropriate comparisons can be made. Further, in assessing the phenomenon of adaptive cytoprotection,[25-26] a mild irritant, (a low dose of a damaging substance that is not damaging by itself but becomes damaging when administered in a higher concentration), can then be applied to the surface of the gastric mucosa that is rotated so that it covers only one half of the chambered epithelium. After the desired pretreatment period is completed, the mild irritant is removed, and the chambered stomach is rotated back to its normal horizontal position. A damaging agent is then applied to the gastric mucosa which is now fully exposed to the entire surface. In carrying out experiments in this fashion, the portion of the stomach pretreated with the mild irritant, and subsequently exposed to a damaging substance, can be compared with the portion that was not exposed to this substance. Thereby, assessments can be made with respect to the efficacy of the mild irritant as a protective agent.

Other features that make the chambered stomach an attractive experimental preparation are that sampling of the mucosa either throughout the experiment, or more commonly at the end of experiment, can be taken for histologic analysis or determination of some biochemical substance that may have been perturbed by the injurious process. Further, catheters have been placed in branches of the splenic artery that directly perfuse the chambered stomach so that administration of various drugs can be directly administered to the mounted stomach to alter blood flow, inhibit acid production, prevent injury from a particular damaging agent, or any combination of these effects[27-28] (Figure 6).

Notwithstanding these considerations, there are certain disadvantages which accompany this type of protocol. First, since this is an invasive surgical preparation, particular care must be taken in the selection of the anesthetic. Compounds such as pentobarbital which have profound effects on splanchnic blood flow should probably be avoided altogether, in favor of others such

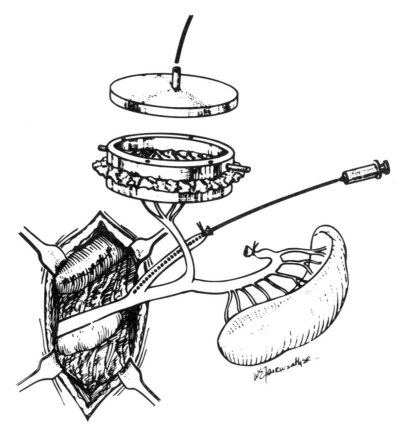

FIGURE 6   Schematic diagram of a modified *ex vivo* canine stomach preparation which allows for the simultaneous intra-arterial infusion of various test solutions. (Reprinted with permission from Ritchie, W. P., *Gastroenterology* 68:699, 1975.)

as methoxyflurane or chloralose-urethane which do not exhibit these effects. Secondly, some mortality can be expected with this type of model due to poor surgical technique or anesthetic overdose. These problems, however, greatly decrease as experience with this technique is gained.

PERFUSED STOMACH PREPARATION

For this model, fasted animals are anesthetized following which they are subjected to laparotomy. After exposing the stomach, a catheter is placed in the proximal portion through the animal's mouth which is then secured by a ligature around the distal esophagus. Care is taken in placing this catheter so as not to injure blood vessels or the vagus nerve. A second catheter is placed via the duodenum into the distal stomach and secured by a ligature in that location. By connecting these two catheters to an infusion pump, a damaging agent can be continuously perfused through the stomach for whatever time period is desired.[29] In addition to this feature, the perfused stomach model enables various physiologic studies to be performed, such as the flux of a marker across the mucosa as an index of gastric damage. A common marker used to assess damage is chromium radiolabelled EDTA as described by Kvietys and associates.[30] Another feature of this model is that if substances need to be chronically infused intravenously to assess their ability to prevent injury, or the impact of various neural components (e.g. vagotomy) are being evaluated in terms of altering gastric defense, this model is quite adaptable to those capabilities. The major disadvantage of this preparation is that anesthesia needs to be given to carry out the experiments, which may alter gastric function to some degree so that findings are not entirely comparable to what would be obtained in the intact, nonanesthetized circumstance. Further, some degree of surgical skill is required to construct this model for experimental use.

ISCHEMIA/REPERFUSION MODELS OF GASTRIC INJURY

The recent interest in oxygen-derived free radical induced injury to the gastrointestinal tract secondary to ischemia/reperfusion has led to the development of a number of closely related models of acute gastric injury in the rat. All of these models share a basic design in that each of them contains components of ischemia and reperfusion. It is the interaction of these components that is believed to induce the injury noted in these models.

One of the most convenient models of studying ischemia/reperfusion injury to the stomach is to subject a rat to a period of severe hypovolemic shock followed by reperfusion of shed blood for varying periods of time. For these studies, fasted rats are anesthetized and either a femoral artery or carotid artery is cannulated with a polyethylene cannula (PE-50 to PE-90). This cannula is then attached to a physiologic transducer to enable monitoring of the animal's blood pressure. One such model initially described by Itoh and Guth[31] has been used by a number of investigators to study ischemia/reperfusion injury in the stomach. With their model, the rat is subjected to a midline laparotomy and the pylorus is visualized and then ligated with a 4-0 silk suture. A catheter is then placed through a puncture wound in the distal esophagus and secured in place with another ligature. Prewarmed normal saline is then introduced into the gastric lumen to rinse it free of any contents. After evacuating the lumen through this catheter, hydrochloric acid (0.1 N HCl/100 gm body weight) is then introduced into the lumen at a volume of 1 ml. An alternative approach is to pass an oroesophageal tube into the stomach and secure it in place with a ligature at the gastroesophageal junction. The pylorus is then cannulated with another catheter (PE-280) to serve as a collecting conduit. A circuit is then established and maintained, such that 0.1 N HCl at a rate of 1 ml/min is introduced through the oroesophageal tube and then collected via the pyloric cannula. Regardless of the particular model chosen for study, each animal should be injected with heparin at a dose of 100 units/ 100 g body weight to prevent the clotting of blood in the cannulas or the transducers. After insuring that the blood pressure has stabilized and represents true baseline values, the animal is bled through the previously placed carotid or femoral arterial catheter to induce shock to the level of the target value desired. For most of these studies, the target value is a mean arterial blood pressure between 25 and 30 mm Hg. The blood pressure is then maintained at this level to insure ischemia for varying time periods by removing or reinfusing shed blood as required. The experiment may be terminated at any time to evaluate effects of ischemia alone on gastric mucosal integrity, or following complete or incomplete reinfusion of shed blood to assess effects of ischemia and reperfusion in combination. At the time of animal sacrifice, the stomach can be evaluated for gross lesion formation and samples obtained for further analysis microscopically.

These models can also be adapted to assess the protective capabilities of putative gastroprotective agents. The agent can be introduced directly into the stomach along with the acid solution at the commencement of study or administered separately through a parenteral route. Further, a noxious substance such as bile or ethanol can also be introduced into the stomach at the time acid is originally placed to see what effect the acid/damaging agent combination has on inducing injury to the stomach in the context of shock and reperfusion.

Although the aforementioned studies can be employed in a large animal such as the dog, the cost of such a study is usually prohibitive. For that reason, most investigators have used these models in small animals like the rat.

CHRONIC MUCOSAL INJURY MODELS

The models previously described all involve experimental approaches to inducing injury over fairly short time periods, i.e. minutes to hours. Although human gastric injury can express itself in a similar time frame with damaging agents such as ethanol and aspirin, the gastric damage produced in true gastric ulceration requires a much longer time period to express itself. At least two different models have been developed to evaluate a more chronic form of gastric and/or duodenal injury, thereby simulating more closely the human form of chronic acid peptic disease. Both models have utilized rats to conduct these experiments.

The first model involves the application of acetic acid to the serosal side of either the stomach or the duodenum.[32] For these studies, fasted rats are anesthetized and undergo a midline laparotomy. The serosal surface of the desired organ is then isolated and a round metal mold of a fixed size is placed tightly against the gastric wall of the lesser curvature or along the greater curvature below the limiting ridge of the stomach. Conversely, the mold may be directly applied to the serosal surface of the duodenum with even more ease. Seventy μl of 100% acetic acid are then placed into the mold and is allowed to remain in contact with the serosa for approximately 60 seconds to induce the production of gastric damage. Duodenal injury is induced by a 30-second application of the same acid solution to the duodenal serosa. After these brief exposures, the fluid is removed and the tissue is lightly wiped with absorbent paper. The abdomen is then closed and the animal returned to its cage. Animals subjected to these procedures are then allowed food and water ad libitum and are sacrificed at varying time periods thereafter to follow the development of ulcer formation.

Within 30 minutes after removal of acetic acid from the serosa, necrosis can be demonstrated within the gastric mucosa. Twenty-four hours after removal of the acetic acid solution, discrete mucosal ulcerations are apparent with this preparation. The damage produced by this model increases with time and by three days after acetic acid removal, it is not uncommon to observe transmural perforations through the gastric wall. These same results can be expected with the application of acetic acid to the duodenum, with the notable exception that duodenal ulcers produced with this model tend to be histologically deeper than gastric fundic or antral ulcers produced under similar damaging conditions.

A second model of chronic gastric injury involves physically wounding the gastric mucosa as described by Wong and Loewenthal.[33] Fasted rats are again anesthetized and undergo a midline laparotomy. The stomach is mobilized from its surrounding connective tissue by blunt dissection and an incision is made in the nonsecreting forestomach. The gastric contents are generally aspirated and then a glandular portion of the gastric mucosa is everted through the incision in the forestomach. A chalazian clamp is applied to the mucosal surface and the area enclosed by the rings of the clamp and the rough edges are electrocoagulated. The clamp is removed from the damaged portion of the stomach and the everted mucosa is returned to its original orientation. The incision in the forestomach is closed with absorbable suture following which the muscle and skin layers of the abdominal wall are closed. Animals are then returned to their cages and allowed to consume both water and food as they desire. As with the other model, animals are sacrificed at varying time periods and the gastric mucosa examined for the presence or absence of injury.

Both approaches just described utilize physical "molds" so that the injury which is produced under these conditions (average size 7 mm) is reproducible and little interexperimental variation occurs. Thus, this consistent injury is ideal for following healing processes *in vivo*. Compounds which are thought to help speed the healing of deep ulcers can be easily administered to these animals by various means and their effects on lesion size can be directly determined. Since most of the gastric wall components are involved in the damaging process with these models, this type of injury closely parallels that encountered in true gastric ulceration in humans. Thus, damage to the submucosal compartment, muscularis externa, and the muscularis mucosa which is commonly seen in gastric ulcers can be mimicked with these techniques. The same can be said with the duodenal ulcer model outlined above.

There are distinct disadvantages with these preparations as well. First, since they involve invasive surgical techniques, a certain degree of mortality can be expected which is influenced by the surgical skills of the investigator. In addition, with the acetic acid model, damage is more pronounced in the first few days following its induction than occurs later so that studies aimed at examining initial healing processes must be timed appropriately. A further criticism that can be directed at both of these methods is that physical trauma is used to inflict damage to gastroduodenal tissues raising the question of whether these preparations are truly suitable for studies investigating the physiologic basis for gastroduodenal injury.

MISCELLANEOUS *IN VIVO* PREPARATIONS

Left Gastric Artery Infusion Model

The purpose of this preparation is to provide a means of directly infusing substances into the stomach wall itself and in so doing alter a particular physiologic process that under normal conditions would be necessary to maintain gastric mucosal integrity. The best arterial bed to accomplish this goal is that supplied by the left gastric artery. For this preparation, animals are first anesthetized and then through a midline laparotomy incision, the left gastric artery is carefully exposed from its connective tissue sheath which runs just posterior to the caudal esophagus at the gastroesophageal junction. Particular care must be taken not to damage either the left gastric vein or the vagus nerve fibers which traverse this junction along with this artery. Once exposed, the artery is ligated where it arises from the celiac axis and is then cannulated distal to the ligature with a 23 gauge teflon cannula which is secured in place with a second ligature. The cannula is then attached to a silicon connector and an infusion cannula which is either attached to a syringe through which the given test agent can be manually infused or to an actual infusion pump (see Figure 7). A flashback of blood into the cannula after its insertion is an appropriate indication of patent cannulation.

Although manual infusion of drugs into the left gastric arterial circulation can be readily accomplished with this preparation it is generally easier to directly attach the cannula to a calibrated infusion pump whereby drugs are infused at constant rates so that an even volume of infusion can be achieved. At the conclusion of these experiments, the animals are sacrificed and stomachs removed and examined for the presence or absence of macroscopic injury, microscopic injury when appropriate, or the retrieval of mucosal samples that can subsequently be prepared for the measurement of any number of relevant biochemical parameters.

The major advantage of this technique is the ability to directly infuse substances into the gastric wall and determine effects on gastric pathophysiology. Several investigators have used this approach to evaluate the roles of various substances in promoting gastric injury. An example would be the work of Esplugues and Whittle[34] in which platelet activating factor (PAF) was studied in a dose response fashion to determine its role in inducing gastric injury. Stein and colleagues[35] have also adapted this preparation to infuse the oxygen derived free radical generating system xanthine/xanthine oxidase in an effort to determine what role oxygen radicals might play in producing experimental gastric lesions.

Disadvantages of this preparation include the need to have animals fully anesthetized throughout experiments. Thus, it remains desirable to select an anesthetic which has minimal effects on systemic arterial blood pressure which in and of itself could make the gastric mucosa more susceptible to injury than would occur otherwise. Procedurally, the left gastric artery cannulation is difficult to carry out and the use of a stereo microscope is mandatory in order to minimize technical problems associated with this cannulation. Investigators who are facile at surgical techniques can employ this preparation without undue difficulty. Others, however,

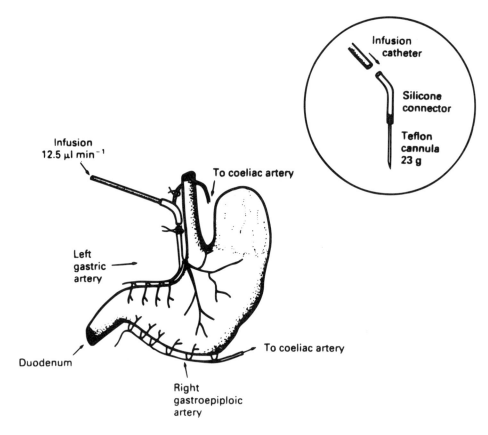

FIGURE 7 Schematic diagram of the technique required for the local intra-arterial infusion of test solutions directly into the rat gastric vasculature through the left gastric artery. (Reprinted with permission from Esplugues et al., *B. J. Pharm.* 93:222–218, 1993.)

would probably find the surgical skill necessary to prepare this model sufficiently cumbersome that the practicality of using it is prohibitive.

Vascular Ligation Models

It is well established that an adequate blood supply to the stomach is mandatory if the gastric mucosa is to remain healthy and intact. Taking advantage of this observation, a number of models have been utilized over the years to induce gastric injury by ligating various vascular beds that supply the stomach. The damage resulting from the vascularly compromised area has then been compared with normal epithelium in terms of metabolism, cellular turnover, and ability to withstand an injurious insult such as that induced by a topical damaging agent like alcohol or aspirin. For these types of studies, fasted rats have routinely been used and subjected to midline laparotomy after being adequately anesthetized. To induce vascular compromise to a given portion of the stomach, the blood vessels of interest supplying that region are identified and ligated after which the abdominal wall is closed. Animals are then allowed to recover from surgery for periods up to 24 hours. Depending upon the vascular bed ligated, severe damage can result to the region of the stomach deriving its blood supply from that bed. Such damage is usually evident within 24 hours and not infrequently leads to gastric perforation.

While this technique to induce gastric injury has been around for decades, its popularity has weaned over the years. One reason for the decline in interest is that it makes intuitive sense that if one compromises the blood supply to any organ, a deleterious effect on normal homeostasis and integrity will result. Thus, it is not surprising that ligating vessels in the rat stomach leads to mucosal injury. Further, questions can be raised regarding extrapolation of information found in these models to the human situation. In contrast to the rat stomach, compromise of blood flow to a single vascular bed in the human stomach does not always lead to reproducible injury. This relates to the pronounced collateralization of blood flow in the human stomach that is not as well developed in the rat. Of equal note, when ligating a given vascular bed in the rat stomach, the resultant damage is quite unpredictable. This damage may range from simple hyperemia to fulminating and penetrating ulcers in animals within the same experimental group. Thus, it is not always easy to predict the extent of injury produced by this model, even when experimental conditions are standardized. This intra-experimental variation is probably reason enough to rule out this model for routine studies involving gastric injury and repair.

IN VITRO MODELS

While a large body of important information has been generated regarding the pathogenesis of gastroduodenal injury and its prevention or attenuation by various protective agents using the *in vivo* models reviewed thus far in this chapter, it must be noted that *in vitro* models have also contributed greatly to our understanding of damage and protection. The immediate disadvantage of using an *in vitro* model, however, is the fact that the cells of the tissue being studied are unavoidably perturbed once removed from their environment, and may in fact be in an altered physiologic state relative to their *in vivo* existence. Accordingly, *in vitro* models should be used cautiously and primarily to answer a specific question that cannot be adequately addressed under *in vivo* conditions. Once that decision is made, the great advantage of *in vitro* preparations is gained, namely their simplicity. Furthermore, in contrast to *in vivo* models, a very focused hypothesis can be tested with great precision when studied *in vitro*.

CELL CULTURE TECHNIQUES

Conceptually, but not necessarily technically and procedurally, the "simplest" *in vitro* model is cell culture. This experimental approach involves the isolation of pure cells from gastric or duodenal epithelium, allowing them to grow, and then perturbing their environment with various experimental manipulations to study both physiologic and pathophysiologic responses to a given perturbation. While a number of investigators have used this technique to unravel important information relative to the pathogenesis of gastroduodenal injury and the means by which protective agents prevent such injury, culturing cells has generally proven to be a difficult exercise because of the thick adherent mucus that covers the luminal surface of the gastroduodenal epithelium resulting in masses of cells sticking together in a manner that makes separation of a pure cell type quite problematical. Also, no immortal cell lines are available for gastric or duodenal cells so that all the work has to be done with primary cultures. Nonetheless, primary cultures of cells have been used to develop a confluent monolayer of acid resistant cells and to answer key questions concerning the role that a particular chemical substance might play in gastric or duodenal defense. To overcome some of the difficulties encountered with cell culture techniques, other investigators have studied functional "clumps" of cells such as isolated gastric glands. Even this technique has proved cumbersome and has only been used with success by a small number of investigators. Because the procedures employed to prepare functional clumps of cells or isolate pure cells from gastric or duodenal tissue for cell culture are sufficiently complex and sophisticated so as to require elaborate description and detail, further discussion will not be undertaken. The reader who wishes to learn more about these techniques should consult references 36 to 41.

Sheets of Cells

Compared to cell culture techniques, sheets of cells have been commonly used by investigators to study various components of gastroduodenal injury and protection. For such experiments, the Ussing chamber preparation has dominated the field. This method is of such importance in studying gastroduodenal physiology and pathophysiology that a comprehensive discussion of its use in mucosal defense research is in order.

The "Ussing chamber",[42,43] already discussed in Chapter 1, will be discussed in some added detail here. Perhaps the most useful attribute of the Ussing chamber is that it makes possible the measurement of potential difference (PD) across the tissue being studied,[44] a parameter which has been related to tissue viability.[45] Since measurement of this electrical parameter is so important in Ussing chamber work, a brief introduction to the genesis of the PD in tissue follows.

The simplest method for generating a PD across two compartments is with the type of battery known as the concentration cell. To understand this arrangement, one needs to imagine two compartments in which unequal NaCl concentrations are separated by a membrane which is somewhat permeable to chloride, but impermeable to sodium. Chloride, being more diffusible than sodium, will initially diffuse down its concentration gradient. Charge separation is therefore created across the membrane, a condition exactly analogous to the charging of a capacitor. The amount of charge separation and the time of charge-up is dependent on the capacitance of the membrane, the permeability of the ion, and the magnitude of the gradient. As the potential difference across the compartment builds up, chloride entry slows, because the increasing charge separation retards chloride movement. At some point, the gradient driven rate of chloride entry into one compartment is opposed by the electrically driven rate of chloride exit from the other compartment and net chloride flux ceases. When this circumstance occurs, equilibrium has been established across the membrane and a peak voltage is reached which now remains constant. The voltage equilibrium is given by the Nernst equation[44-45] and is solely dependent on the ratio of chloride in the two compartments. It is important to stress that the amount of charge separation across the membrane is trivial with respect to the total ions in solution in an Ussing chamber. In fact, this situation is true for biological systems in general. Therefore, bulk solution electrode neutrality is always maintained in both compartments.

The origin of PD in gut mucosa is infinitely more complex than this simple example outlined above, because many ions of varying permeabilities traverse a multi-component barrier by taking a multitude of paths. Compounding the problem of interpreting PD in gut mucosa is the fact that some ions are being actively transported, a crucial difference from the example above, which deals only with passive diffusion. Nevertheless, if treated as a "black box", a net one way flux of charge across gut mucosa (which can be the sum of many ion movements or controlled by one ion) yields a PD which can be measured with an amplifier and a voltmeter just as easily as in the simplest concentration cell; therein lies the real power of the Ussing methodology in assessing tissue injury and protection. All cells maintain ion asymmetries with respect to their external environment; indeed, the ability to utilize energy to maintain an internal milieu is the hallmark of life itself. In many of the studies reviewed in this chapter, the underlying premise is that dead, dying, or injured tissue will not be able to perform its normal function with respect to maintaining ion asymmetry, and reductions in PD will occur. Accordingly, therefore, PD is a functional index of tissue viability. In support of this premise, the PD of dead tissue is zero, both in theory and in practice.

It is possible to measure both the voltage and current when performing an Ussing chamber experiment. Since voltage (V) is the multiple of current (I) and resistance (R), it is possible to compute the resistance in the circuit as well. Resistance values in tissue imply an impediment to the flow of ions and in gastric mucosa, particularly, it is considered that resistance measurements yield valuable information with regard to the breakdown of the gastric mucosal barrier.

Unfortunately, investigators have reported decreases in resistance during injury, immediately followed by recovery to control values followed by further decreases. Such results do not inspire confidence with regard to predicting injury by measuring total tissue resistance and are usually supplemented by morphologic assessments of injury. In an Ussing chamber, it is also possible to clamp the PD to zero, by imposing a voltage of opposite polarity, to measure the short circuit current, a parameter that has also been used as an index of tissue viability.

One important study by Svanes and colleagues[46] used frog gastric mucosa as the experimental tissue in an Ussing chamber model. This study was the first to characterize mucosal repair. Briefly, frog gastric mucosa was damaged by adding hypertonic sodium to the luminal compartment and electrophysiologic parameters were used to follow the extent and time course of the damage. Subsequently, the tissue was allowed to recover in the chamber and at the time of completion of study, tissues were removed for morphologic assessment of damage. This study illustrates several important uses to be derived from Ussing chamber work. Electrophysiologic (i.e. functional) assessment of damage and recovery were determined with a damaging agent in the luminal compartment. This work was possible because tissue polarity (lumen to serosa) was maintained and control tissues were not damaged by residing in the chamber. This functional assessment of damage and recovery could then be correlated with its morphologic counterparts after removing the tissue upon completion of study and examining it histologically.

The versatility of this preparation can be further highlighted by several other examples. Thus, the investigator's ability to manipulate the composition of the two compartments was utilized in a study which demonstrated that serosal bicarbonate was required to ameliorate acid damage in chambered sheets of cells of rat esophagus.[47] In another study, chambers were used to investigate contact angle measurements as an index of aspirin damage in dog gastric mucosa.[48] The time course and extent of aspirin damage were determined in the chamber by following PD and resistance changes. Upon completion, the tissue was removed and prepared for contact angle analysis and correlations were made between chamber parameter indices of damage and the contact angle of the tissue.

A further example of the adaptability of the Ussing chamber preparation followed the work of Folkman and associates[49] who reported that basic fibroblast growth factor (b-FGF) enhanced healing in a duodenal model of injury. Angiogenesis was invoked as the key event in the healing that was stimulated by the presence of b-FGF. Subsequently, it was shown that b-FGF enhanced restitution of frog gastric mucosa in an Ussing chamber model.[50] Since this latter experiment was performed *in vitro,* and on a short time scale, angiogenesis and wound contraction could be ruled out as factors enhancing restitution, a powerful demonstration of the simplifying power of this *in vitro* preparation.

In recent years, the Ussing chamber technique has been adapted so that cell micropuncture experiments can also be performed.[51] For these studies, the gastric mucosa of the necturus was used. This amphibian stomach has giant cells which enables an operator using a microscope and micromanipulator to impale surface cells of necturus antrum with a pH and/or PD sensitive electrode. The applicability of the technique is limited by the fact that some technical skill is required along with expensive and sophisticated equipment. Nonetheless, the experiments which can be performed are extremely powerful and events can be observed which affect luminal or basolateral membrane resistance and PD. Similar to Ussing chamber experiments in which sheets of cells are mounted, damaging agents can be added to the luminal aspect of the tissue, but unlike these other experiments, the effect of damage can be observed upon an individual cell. The effect of luminal acid on the acidification of a luminal surface cell has also been studied in an experiment which directly tested the presence of a gastric mucosal barrier at the surface of the gastric lumen.[51] In other microelectrode work using necturus cells, nutrient bicarbonate was noted to attenuate changes in cell membrane potentials caused by luminal exposure of the cell to aspirin.[52] Finally, Li and associates[53] have developed an *in vitro* model using the Ussing chamber in which the intestinal mucosa and muscularis can be studied functionally as a unit. This technique can easily be adapted to study gastric mucosa and muscle in the same fashion.

The foregoing discussion highlights the tremendous adaptability of the Ussing chamber preparation to study mechanisms of mucosal defense. The number of different mucosae that can be mounted in this preparation is almost limitless. Thus, rat, dog, rabbit, cat, guinea pig, and amphibian gastric and duodenal mucosae have all been studied with this technique. Usually the muscular component of the gastric or duodenal wall is separated from the mucosa prior to its mounting, but in mucosae in which the gastric wall is relatively thin, such as the rat, this separation may prove difficult; in this case, the entire thickness of the gastric wall is commonly mounted. Further, tissue viability can usually be maintained for several hours when mounted in Ussing chambers so that it is not unusual to conduct experiments that are 2 to 4 hours in duration.

WHOLE STOMACH PREPARATION

The last *in vitro* preparation to be considered in ascending order of physiologic complexity is the whole organ bath preparation. For this experimental method, the stomach is removed intact after ligating the blood vessels that supply it and transecting the distal esophagus and proximal duodenum. The remaining remnant of esophagus in continuity with the stomach is ligated and a stoppered plastic cannula is passed through the pyloric sphincter via the small remnant of duodenum attached to the stomach. The stomach prepared in this fashion is then placed in a buffered (i.e. Krebs) nutrient solution maintained at 37°C and vigorously bubbled with oxygen. This procedure makes the luminal contents accessible for sampling since aliquots of the intraluminal contents can be readily withdrawn through a syringe that is connected to the stoppered cannula (see Figure 10, Chapter 1). With this preparation, experiments can generally be conducted for several hours.

A typical example of the type of studies that can be carried out with this preparation is described by Whittle and Steel[54] who used this experimental approach to measure the release of various tissue enzymes during ethanol damage. This *in vitro* model was especially suited for this type of study as it enabled repetitive sampling of intragastric contents for enzyme analysis after ethanol challenge. With an intact stomach under *in vivo* conditions, this type of information could not have been readily obtained since orally administered ethanol could not have been withdrawn from the stomach and any enzymes released during damage would most likely have been denatured by the previously administered ethanol. It should be emphasized that concomitant placement of a cannula through the esophageal remnant and into the forestomach, in addition to that already placed through the pyloric sphincter, provides a means of continually perfusing the luminal surface of the stomach with this preparation, even though this approach was unnecessary for the study just described.

ACKNOWLEDGMENT

This work was supported by Research Grant DK 25838 awarded to Dr. Miller from the National Institutes of Health.

REFERENCES

1. **Shively, M. J.,** Biology of laboratory animals, in *Veterinary Anatomy: Basic, Comparative, and Clinical,* Texas A&M University Press, College Station, Texas, 1984, 507.

2. **Karnovsky, M. J.,** A formaldehyde-glutaraldehyde fixative of high osmolality for use in electron microscopy, *J. Cell Biol.,* 27, 137A, 1965.

3. **Schmidt, K. L., Henagan, J. M., Smith, G. S., Hilburn, P. J., and Miller, T. A.,** Prostaglandin cytoprotection against ethanol-induced gastric injury in the rat, *Gastroenterology,* 88, 649, 1985.

4. **Lacy, E. T. and Ito, S.,** Microscopic analysis of ethanol damage to rat gastric mucosa after treatment with a prostaglandin. *Gastroenterology,* 83, 619, 1982.

5. **Guth, P. H., Paulsen, G., and Nagata, H.,** Histologic and microcirculatory changes in alcohol-induced gastric lesions in the rat: Effect of prostaglandin cytoprotection, *Gastroenterology,* 87, 1083, 1984.

6. **Wallace, J. L., Morris, G. P., Krausse, E. J., and Greaves, S. E.,** Reduction by cytoprotective agents of ethanol-induced damage to the rat gastric mucosa: A correlated morphologic and physiologic study, *Can. J. Physiol. Pharmacol.,* 60, 1686, 1982.

7. **Robert, A.,** Cytoprotection by prostaglandins, *Gastroenterology,* 77, 761, 1979.

8. **Robert, A., Nezamis, J. E., Lancaster, C., and Hanchar, A. J.,** Cytoprotection by prostaglandins in rats: Prevention of gastric necrosis produced by alcohol, HCl, NaOH, hypertonic NaCl and thermal injury, *Gastroenterology,* 77, 433, 1979.

9. **Szabo, S., Trier, J. S., and Frankel, P. W.,** Sulfhydryl compounds may mediate gastric cytoprotection, *Science,* 214, 200, 1981.

10. **Konturek, S. J., Radecki, T., Brozozowski, T., Piastucki, I., Dembinska-Kiec, A., and Zmuda, A.,** Gastric cytoprotection by prostaglandins, ranitidine, and probanthine in rats: Role of endogenous prostaglandins, *Scand. J. Gastroenterol.,* 16, 7, 1981.

11. **Robert, A., Nezamis, J. E., and Phillips, J. P.,** Effect of prostaglandin E_1 on gastric secretion and ulcer formation in the rat, *Gastroenterology,* 55, 481, 1968.

12. **Lee, Y. H., Cheng, W. D., Bianchi, R. G., Mollison, K., and Hansen, J.,** Effects of oral administration of PGE_2 on gastric secretion and experimental peptic ulcerations, *Prostaglandins,* 3, 29, 1973.

13. **Robert, A.,** The inhibitory effects of prostaglandins on gastric secretion: Their possible role in the treatment of gastric hypersecretion and peptic ulcer, in *Progress in Gastroenterology,* Vol III, Glass, G. B. J., ed., Grune & Stratton, New York, 1977, 777.

14. **Hanson, H. M. and Brodie, D. A.,** Use of restrained rat technique for study of the antiulcer effect of drugs, *J. Appl. Physiol.,* 15, 291, 1960.

15. **Boyd, S. C., Caul, W. F., and Bowen, B. K.,** Use of cold-restraint to examine psychological factors in gastric ulceration, *Physiology & Behavior,* 18, 865, 1977.

16. **Basso, N., Materia, A., Forlini, A., and Jaffe, B. J.,** Prostaglandin generation in the gastric mucosa of rats with stress ulcer, *Surgery,* 94, 104, 1982.

17. **Itoh, M., Yokoyama, Y., Miyamato, T., Imai, S., Joh, T., Matsusako, K., Iwai, A., and Takeuchi, T.,** Gastric mucosal injury by water-immersion restraint stress in the rat: Role of active oxygen species, in *Free Radicals in Digestive Diseases,* M. Tsuchiya et al., eds., Elsevier Press, New York, 1988, 99.

18. **Shibuya, D., Ohara, T., Eda, K., Sasaki, R., Asaki, S., and Goto, Y.,** Role of free radicals in experimental gastric ulcers in guinea pigs, in *Free Radicals in Digestive Diseases,* M. Tsuchiya et al., eds., Elsevier Press, New York, 1988, 81.

19. **Shay, H., Komarov, S. A., Fels, S. S., Meranze, D., Gruenstein, M., and Siplet, H.,** A simple method for the uniform production of gastric ulceration in the rat, *Gastroenterology,* 5, 43, 1945.

20. **Shay, H., Sun, D. C. H., and Gruenstein, M.,** A quantitative method for measuring spontaneous gastric secretion in the rat, *Gastroenterology,* 26, 906, 1954.

21. **Rehm, W. S.,** The effect of histamine and HCl on gastric secretion and potential, *Am. J. Physiol.,* 141, 537, 1944.

22. **Morris, G. P. and Wallace, J. L.,** The roles of ethanol and acid in the production of gastric mucosal lesions in rats, *Virchows Arch.,* 38, 23, 1981.

23. **Moody, F. G., and Durbin, R. P.,** Effects of glycine and other instillates on concentration of gastric acid, *Am. J. Physiol.,* 209, 122, 1965.

24. **Morris, G. P., Donaldson, C. L., Holitzner, C. A., Tufts, K. H., and Williamson, T. E.,** Local and referred protection in the gastric mucosa: Prostaglandin-independent and prostaglandin-dependent mechanisms, in *Mechanisms of Injury, Protection, and Repair of the Upper Gastrointestinal Tract,* Garner, A. and O'Brien, P. E., eds., John Wiley and Sons, New York, 1991, 371.

25. **Chaudhury, T. K. and Robert, A.,** Prevention by mild irritants of gastric necrosis produced in rats by sodium taurocholate, *Dig. Dis. Sci.,* 25, 830, 1980.

26. **Robert, A., Nezamis, J. E., Lancaster, C., Davis, J. P., Field, S. O., and Hanchar, A. J.,** Mild irritants prevent gastric necrosis through "adaptive cytoprotection" mediated by prostaglandins, *Am. J. Physiol.,* 245, G113, 1983.

27. **Ritchie, W. P. Jr.,** Acute gastric mucosal damage induced by bile salts, acid, and ischemia, *Gastroenterology,* 68, 699, 1975.

28. **Cheung, L. Y. and Newton, W. T.,** Cyclic guanosine monophosphate response to acetylcholine stimulation of gastric alkaline secretion, *Surgery,* 86, 156, 1979.

29. **Smith, S. M., Grisham, M. B., Manci, E. A., Granger, D. N., and Kvietys, P. R.,** Gastric mucosal injury in the rat: Role of iron and xanthine oxidase, *Gastroenterology,* 92, 950, 1987.

30. **Kvietys, P. R., Twohig, B., Danzell, J., and Specian, R. D.,** Ethanol-induced injury to the rat gastric mucosa: Role of neutrophils and xanthine oxidase-derived radicals, *Gastroenterology,* 98, 909, 1990.

31. **Itoh, M. and Guth, P. H.,** Role of oxygen-derived free radicals in hemorrhagic shock-induced gastric lesions in the rat, *Gastroenterology,* 88, 1162, 1985.

32. **Okabe, S., Roth, J. L. A., and Pfeiffer, C. J.,** A method for experimental, penetrating gastric and duodenal ulcers in rats: Observations on normal healing, *Digestive Diseases,* 16, 277, 1971.

33. **Wong, J. and Loewenthal, J.,** Chronic gastric ulcer in the rat produced by wounding at the fundo-antral junction, *Gastroenterology,* 71, 416, 1976.

34. **Esplugues, J. V. and Whittle, B. J. R.,** Gastric mucosal damage induced by local intra-arterial administration of Paf in the rat, *Br. J. Pharm.,* 93, 222, 1988.

35. **Stein, H. J., Esplugues, J., Whittle, B. J. R., Bauerfeind, P., Hinder, R. A., and Blum, A. L.,** Direct cytotoxic effects of oxygen radicals on the gastric mucosa, *Surgery,* 106, 171, 1989.

36. **Soll, A. H.,** Specific inhibition by prostaglandins E_2 and I_2 of histamine stimulated (^{14}C)-aminopyrine accumulation and cyclic adenosine monophosphate generation by isolated canine parietal cells, *J. Clin. Invest.,* 65, 1222, 1980.

37. **Terano, A., Ota, S., Mach, T., Hirashi, H., Stachura, J., and Ivey, K. L.,** Prostaglandin protects against taurocholate-induced damage to rat gastric mucosal cell culture, *Gastroenterology,* 92, 669, 1987.

38. **Terano, A., Mach, T., Stachura, J., Tarnawski, A., and Ivey, K. H.,** Effect of 16,16 dimethyl PGE^2 on aspirin-induced damage to rat gastric epithelial cells in tissue culture, *Gut,* 25, 19, 1984.

39. **Tarnawski, A., Brozozowski, T., Sarfeh, I. J., et al.,** Prostaglandin protection of human isolated gastric glands against indomethacin and ethanol injury: Evidence for direct cellular action of prostaglandin, *J. Clin. Invest.,* 81, 1989, 1988.

40. **Hiraishi, J., Terano, A., Ota, S. I., Ivey, K. J., and Sugimoto, T.,** Oxygen metabolite-induced cytotoxicity to cultured rat gastric mucosal cells, *Am. J. Physiol.,* 253, G40, 1987.

41. **Olson, C. E.,** Glutathione modulates toxic oxygen metabolite injury of canine chief cell monolayers in primary culture, *Am. J. Physiol.,* 254, G49, 1988.

42. **Ussing, H. H. and Zerahn, K.,** Active transport of sodium as the source of electric current in the short-circuited isolated frog skin, *Acta Physiol. Scand.,* 23, 110, 1951.

43. **Schultz, S. G. and Zalusky, R.,** Ion transport in isolated rabbit ileum. I. Short circuit current and Na refluxes, *J. Gen. Physiol.,* 47, 567, 1964.

44. **Schultz, S. G.,** Electrical potential differences and electromotive forces in epithelial tissues, *J. Gen. Physiol.,* 59, 794, 1972.

45. **Kitahara, S., Fox, K. R., and Hogben, C. A.,** Acid secretion, Na^+ absorption, and the origin of the potential difference across isolated mammalian stomachs, *Dig. Dis. Sci.,* 14(4), 221, 1969.

46. **Svanes, K., Itoh, S., Takeuchi, K., Silen, W.,** Restitution of the surface epithelium of the *in vitro* frog gastric mucosa after damage with hyperosmolar sodium chloride, *Gastroenterology,* 82, 1409, 1982.

47. **Tobey, N. A., Powell, D. W., Schreiner, V. J., and Orlando, R. C.,** Serosal bicarbonate protects against acid injury to rabbit esophagus. *Gastroenterology,* 96(6), 1466, 1989.

48. **Goddard, P. J., Hills, B. A., and Lichtenberger, L. M.,** Does aspirin damage canine gastric mucosa by reducing surface hydrophobicity? *Amer. J. Physiol.,* 252, 6421, 1987.

49. **Folkman, J., Szabo, S., Stovroff, M., McNeil, P., Li, W., and Shing, Y.,** Duodenal ulcer: Discovery of a new mechanism and development of angiogenic therapy which accelerates healing, *Ann. Surg.,* 214, 414, 1991.

50. **Paimela, H., Goddard, P. J., Carter, K., Khabee, R., McNeil, P. L., Ito, S., and Silen, W.,** Restitution of frog gastric mucosa in vitro: Effect of basic fibroblast growth factor, *Gastroenterology,* 104, 1337, 1993.

51. **Kiviluoto, T., Paimela, H., Mustonen, H., and Kivilaakso, E.,** Intracellular pH in isolated necturus antral mucosa exposed to luminal acid, *Gastroenterology,* 98, 901, 1990.

52. **Soybel, D. I., Davis, M. B., and West, A. B.,** Effects of aspirin on pathways of ion permeation in Necturus antrum: Role of nutrient HCO_3-. *Gastroenterology,* 103(5), 1475, 1992.

53. **Li, Y. F., Weisbrodt, Harari, Y., and Moody, F. G.,** Use of a modified Ussing chamber to monitor intestinal epithelial and smooth muscle functions. *Am. J. Physiol.,* 261, G166, 1991.

54. **Whittle, B. J. R. and Steel, G.,** Evaluation of the protection of rat gastric mucosa by a prostaglandin analogue using cellular enzyme marker and histologic techniques, *Gastroenterology,* 88, 315, 1985.

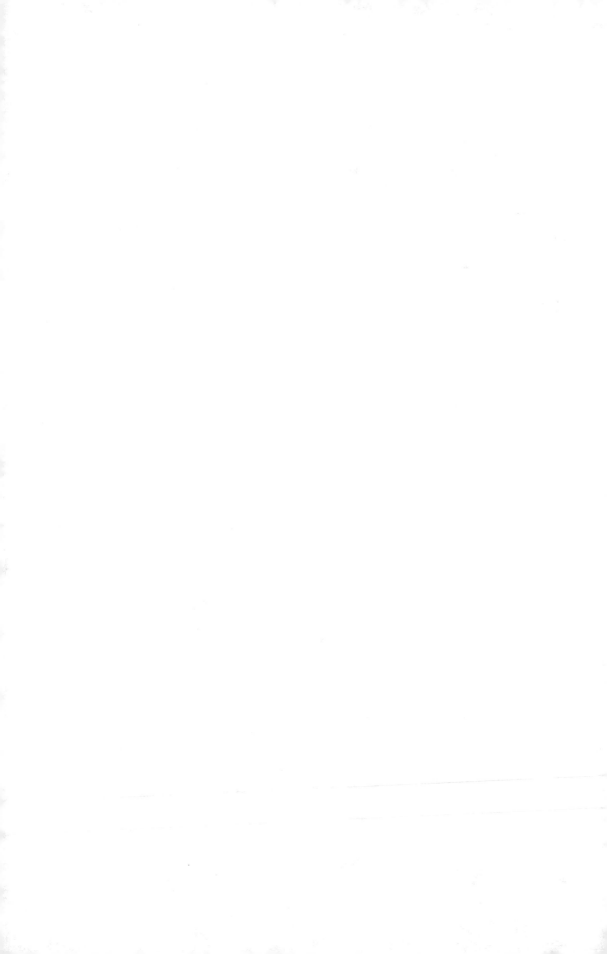

4 Intestinal Absorption and Secretion: *In Vivo* Studies

Philip L. Smith

INTRODUCTION

The gastrointestinal tract from the stomach to the anus contains the same basic structure. On the luminal surface there is a single layer of columnar epithelial cells with specialized cells (e.g. goblet cells, endocrine cells, M cells) as appropriate for its function of digesting and absorbing nutrients, water and electrolytes. In different regions of the gastrointestinal tract, structural features (e.g. gastric glands, villi, microvilli and crypts) together with unique cell types provide for optimal coordination of digestive and absorptive processes. Directly beneath the epithelial cell layer is the *lamina propria,* a region of loose connective tissue which contains blood and lymph vessels as well as a variety of cell types (e.g. lymphocytes and eosinophils). Propulsion of material along the length of the gastrointestinal tract and mixing of contents within segments of the intestine is accomplished through the concerted efforts of the muscularis mucosa, circular and longitudinal muscles. Neuronal control of digestion and absorption is exerted by both intrinsic (submucosal or Meissner's plexus, myenteric or Auerbach's plexus, Henle's plexus) and extrinsic (sympathetic and parasympathetic) elements. Neurotransmitters which exert regulatory control of gastrointestinal functions in addition to acetylcholine and norepinephrine include a number of biogenic amines and peptides (e.g. vasoactive intestinal peptide, dynorphin, calcitonin gene related peptide, substance P, cholecystokinin, somatostatin, 5-hydroxytryptamine, enkephalin and neuropeptide Y). In this chapter, focus will be on models for studying gastrointestinal absorption and secretion including some models which have been developed to mimic pathophysiological conditions. Methods for assessing gastric acid secretion, neurohumoral regulation or motility will not be discussed since these are the subject of other chapters in this volume.

For the ensuing discussions, it is helpful to provide a common description of the processes involved in absorption and secretion. The absorptive process in this chapter will refer to the transfer of molecules from the lumen of the gastrointestinal tract to the mesenteric circulation. Systemic availability will refer to the absorption of a molecule from the lumen to the systemic circulation. Therefore, for a molecule to be absorbed and become systemically available, there are a number of physical and biological barriers which it must overcome. The physical factors include solubility and chemical stability while the biological factors include permeability, liver extraction and metabolic stability. The secretory process describes the case in which the luminal volume of all or some segment of the gastrointestinal tract is increased through movement of fluid and electrolytes from the blood.

The literature is replete with descriptions of models for studying gastrointestinal functions. These include ingenious use of circumstances such as the pioneering work of William Beaumont who in the 1820s took advantage of the gun shot wound gastric fistula formed in a patient,

0-8493-8304-8/96/$0.00+$.50
© 1996 by CRC Press, Inc.

Alexis St. Martin, to study the composition and functions of gastric juice, gastric motility and neuronal control of gastric function[1] to the isolated loop methods for determining intestinal absorption established by Thiry[2] and subsequently modified by Vella[3] in the middle to late 1800s.

ANIMAL MODELS FOR STUDYING ABSORPTION

THIRY-VELLA LOOP MODEL

In its most basic approach, absorption has been studied by determining the amount of a molecule appearing in the feces following oral administration. More elaborate methods have also been established to determine regional differences in the absorption of a molecule from the intestine or stomach. In the Thiry-Vella loop model,[2,3] a segment of intestine with its blood and lymph supply intact was exteriorized while the remainder of the intestine was anastomosed. A solution of the substrate to be studied was then introduced into the exteriorized loop and at subsequent time intervals the loop was emptied and the amount of substrate remaining in the solution determined. Infusion of solutions through the loop has also been employed to study the transport of calcium and fluid in the intestine or effects of secretagogues.[4-6]

For this and a number of experimental techniques employed, absorption is evaluated by the principal of mass balance. Accordingly, the molecule of interest is introduced into the gastrointestinal tract either by mouth or by a port system and at some time later, the amount not absorbed is recovered and determined. Determination of the amount recovered is often difficult due to an inability to sample from the gastrointestinal tract or due to our lack of understanding of the processes responsible for disappearance of material from the gastrointestinal lumen (e.g. metabolism within the lumen, adherence to the gut wall) or appearance in the gastrointestinal lumen (e.g. secretion in the bile). To aid in the determination of the amount of a molecule remaining in the intestinal lumen, marker molecules have been employed. These markers are in fact measuring the intestinal volume and providing a measure of net intestinal fluid absorption or secretion occurring during the time period of the study. By comparing the concentration of the marker molecule and the test molecule at the beginning and end of the study, the absorption of the test molecule can be calculated. Obviously, for this method to be successful, the marker molecule must not be absorbed, metabolized or otherwise lost in the lumen of the intestine and it must also be accurately measured preferably by a simple analytical technique. Additionally, the marker molecule should have characteristics similar to those of the test molecule to avoid problems which could be associated with differences in partitioning in aqueous and lipid environments of the intestinal lumen. From the ensuing discussion, it will be seen that this approach has been refined but is still the basis for a number of animal models in use today. Animal models have been employed for studying gastrointestinal physiology and pathophysiology, determining the sites of absorption of molecules within the gastrointestinal tract, determining the bioavailability of molecules and aiding in the design and selection of dosage forms for molecules. However, it should be kept in mind that there are a number of differences in the anatomy and physiology of different animal models and that results from these studies are not always predictive of the fate in man. A comparison of the anatomy and physiology of different animal models will not be considered here but the interested reader is referred to the review of Dressman and Yamada.[7]

GASTRIC POUCH

For the majority of molecules, the stomach is not a major site of absorption. However, there are a number of molecules which have been reported to be absorbed across the gastric mucosa[8-11] and techniques for studying gastric absorption have been developed. The contribution of gastric absorption to the total systemic availability of a molecule will be dependent on a number of factors including gastric residence time which varies in the fed and fasted states and physicochemical properties of the molecule including dissolution rate, ionization constant and lipophilicity. In 1983, Worland and coworkers[8] described a method for isolating the stomach to evaluate gastric absorption. In this model, a cannula was placed in the left gastric vein to collect blood samples for determination of gastric absorption. However, since relatively few molecules are absorbed to a significant extent from the stomach and with the development of scintigraphic techniques (see below) to evaluate gastric residence time and the potential for gastric absorption, these *in situ* techniques are not commonly employed.

ISOLATED LOOPS

The Thiry-Vella loop method[2,3] has undergone many modifications over the years. In a simplified approach employing anesthetized animals, the abdomen is opened and a loop of the intestine is ligated. The intestine is then filled with a volume of solution containing the substrate of interest and at the appropriate time the intestinal segment is drained and the concentration of substrate determined[9,12–15] Absorption in this model can be expressed in terms of intestinal length or tissue weight. Subsequently, this absorption model was refined to include proximal and distal cannula for perfusing and collecting effluent from the intestinal segment.[16–25]

Although these methods have been extensively employed to provide information regarding intestinal permeability of molecules and differences in their regional absorption, the major limitation of this model is that disappearance is assumed to equate to systemic absorption. However, since a number of factors can complicate interpretation of results from these studies including binding and metabolism within the gut wall and/or hepatic first pass extraction or metabolism, modification of this technique to provide for systemic blood sampling and sampling from the portal vein can provide a more accurate evaluation of the rate and extent of absorption and systemic availability. In addition, these animal models involve the use of anesthetics which may alter intestinal absorption.[25,26]

Systemic blood sampling can be accomplished via repeated venous puncture or through chronic catheterization of a vein such as the jugular or femoral. For jugular catheterization in rats, an indwelling catheter is inserted through an incision in the neck exposing the jugular vein and the catheter is then exposed at the nape of the neck and plugged with a stainless steel pin. To maintain patency, the catheter can be filled with a 50% dextrose solution containing heparin (200 units/ml). With this technique, appearance of molecules in the blood can be determined and the relative systemic availability of different molecules or the effects of formulation approaches on the systemic availability of molecules compared in the same animal. By comparing the plasma levels of a molecule following intestinal administration with the plasma levels following intravenous administration, bioavailability can be determined.[27] Calculation of the bioavailability of a molecule, does not allow a determination of the relative contributions of absorption in the intestine and clearance/extraction by the liver. To determine the relative contributions of these two processes, determination of hepatic clearance/extraction or intestinal absorption *per se* is required. One technique for determining the contribution of hepatic clearance/extraction to the systemic availability of a molecule is to directly administer the molecule to the portal vein and subsequently determine the appearance of the molecule in the systemic circulation. Comparison of the systemic availability of a molecule following intraportal administration *vs* intraintestinal administration allows calculation of the relative contributions of intestinal absorption and hepatic clearance/extraction. Administration of molecules to the hepatic vein of animals can be accomplished through direct injection in smaller animals or through the use of indwelling portal catheters in larger animals.[28,29] Indwelling catheters in animals can also be employed for sampling the portal blood to determine absorption.[30]

For studying the absorption of lipids, methods have been developed for cannulation and collection of lymph.[31–33] These techniques have been applied to a variety of studies of intestinal absorption including effects of bile, fatty acids and pH on retinol absorption,[34] absorption of salicylates[35] and the effect of age on the absorption of vitamin E.[36]

CHRONIC MODELS

RAT MODEL

For chronic absorption studies in rodents, Fejes-Toth and coworkers[37] have described a catheterization procedure via the ventral and/or lateral tail vein which allows blood sampling or administration of molecules in conscious, unrestrained animals. In addition, a modification of the Thiry-Vella loop model has been described in which an intestinal segment of a rat with the blood supply and innervation intact is isolated.[38] The connection of the remaining length of intestine is restored through anastomosis. The isolated intestinal segment is then connected to a pair of teflon cannulas which are attached to the abdominal wall and are accessible for administration or collection of solutions through silicon perfusion tubes. Although a permanent silicone catheter inserted into the inferior vena cava via the femoral vein was employed for blood sampling, a combination of the modified Thiry-Vella loop model with the chronic catheterization described by Fejes-Toth et al.[37] may provide an advantage by reducing stress to the animals. The modified Thiry-Vella loop technique has the advantages of providing a conscious animal model in which the segment of intestine to be examined can be selected (e.g. regioselective absorption) and cross-over studies can be conducted. In this model, systemic availability data is derived from appearance in the systemic circulation and is done in conscious animals. Thus, issues associated with anesthesia are avoided. However, this model does not provide for sampling from the portal vein and thus does not allow a separation of the absorption of a molecule and the contribution of first pass liver effects.

CANINE MODEL

Chronic models for intestinal absorption/systemic availability have developed over the past two decades through the use of plastic materials such as teflon and silastic. These materials are flexible and generally inert as well as being rugged. Rubinstein and coworkers[39] have reported on a method for implantation of cannulae in the duodenum and/or ileum of the dog which allows for perfusion of an intestinal segment and collection of the perfusate or for the administration of dosage forms either solid or liquid thereby bypassing the stomach and the influence of gastric retention/emptying and gastric pH on absorption (a comparison of systemic availability following oral administration and intraduodenal administration would provide information regarding the potential for stomach absorption/degradation). This model has been employed in several studies designed to investigate the influence of gastrointestinal motility on solid dosage form transit through the intestine.[40] The major advantages of this model include the ability to perform experiments in conscious animals and the ability to maintain and use these animals for extended periods of time (> 1.5 years) thereby minimizing the number of animals employed.

A variation on this model has been recently developed in which the intestinal cannula is a vascular access port with the dome of the port implanted under the upper flank of the animal and the distal end of the catheter placed into the intestinal segment of interest.[41–43] Animals with intestinal ports have been employed to investigate regional differences in absorption thereby providing information not only on the effects of gastric emptying and gastric pH but also on the feasibility of developing modified release formulations or of increasing the efficiency of absorption through colonic delivery. This model like the model of Rubenstein and coworkers[39] has the advantage of being a chronic model which can be studied without anesthesia. However, this model does not allow evaluation of solid dosage forms or removal of perfusion solutions.

ANIMAL MODELS FOR STUDYING SECRETION

THIRY-VELLA LOOP MODEL

In addition to its use as a model for studying intestinal absorption, the Thiry-Vella loop model has been employed to investigate the mechanisms involved in secretory diarrhea. Carpenter and coworkers[4] employed the Thiry-Vella loop model to study the effect of *Vibrio cholerae* enterotoxin in the absence or presence of glucose on fluid and electrolyte transport by both jejunal and ileal loops prepared in the same animals. Studies designed to determine the effects of prostaglandins and theophylline as well as cholera enterotoxin were conducted with the Thiry-Vella loop model.[44] In these studies, the investigators employed a superior mesenteric artery catheter to infuse prostaglandins or theophylline in an attempt to mimic administration at the physiologic site of production or action of these agents.[44] Comparison of results obtained following intrajejunal or superior mesenteric artery administration of prostaglandin E_1 demonstrated that at constant infusion rates, changes in jejunal fluid transport were always greater following superior mesenteric artery infusion.[44] The mesenteric artery catheter was passed to a self-sealing steel and Dacron valve which was accessible through an incision in the skin.[44] However, as noted by the authors, insertion of the superior mesenteric artery catheter resulted in an increased mortality in the animals.[44] The Thiry-Vella loop model has also been employed to demonstrate the antidiarrheal effect of drugs (e.g. chlorpromazine, lidamidine) in animals challenged with dexoycholate to induce secretion.[45] Together, these studies elegantly illustrate the utility of the Thiry-Vella loop model for studying intestinal secretion. Although the model is reproducible and can provide information regarding the potential antisecretory effect of molecules, the resources required for maintenance of this model have provided the impetus for investigators to develop alternate small animal models.

ISOLATED LOOPS/ENTEROPOOLING

Models employing anesthetized animals in which the abdomen is opened via a midline incision and a segment of intestine is either cannulated for evaluating fluid secretion by perfusion with a volume marker or by tying off a loop of intestine which has been filled with an appropriate amount of solution and the volume of solution evaluated subsequently have been described for hamsters, rabbits, rats, gerbils, guinea pigs, chinchilla, cats, mice, dogs and also miniature pigs.[46-52] In all these models, care is taken not to compromise the intestinal blood supply. Administration of intestinal secretagogues has been accomplished through perfusion/administration in the intestinal loop or through intra-arterial infusion. In rats, the method for intra-arterial infusion involves feeding a catheter through the left common carotid artery into the aorta.[53] In rabbits, intra-arterial infusion is accomplished via an arterial catheter inserted into the femoral artery to a position above the level of the mesenteric artery.[54-56] Direct intra-arterial infusion provides a method for administering agents which are normally produced and released in the blood or subepithelial tissues. Thus, these molecules will have access to their physiological receptors as opposed to intra-intestinal administration where access to the relevant site(s) for receptor interaction may be limited. This technique has been employed to investigate the effects of α-2 adrenergic inhibition of intestinal secretion elicited by prostaglandin E_1 or vasoactive intestinal peptide in the rat[53] and the effects of prostaglandins and leukotrienes on intestinal motility in the rabbit.[54–56]

The intestinal loop model provides a rapid method for assessing intestinal secretion and together with direct intra-arterial administration of agents, it can be employed to evaluate the effects of putative mediators of intestinal secretion on changes in fluid movement in the intestine and intestinal motility. However, this is an acute model in which the animal is anesthetized and this model does not easily allow antisecretory agents to be evaluated following the initiation and attainment of a steady-state rate of secretion.

Another rapid method for evaluating intestinal secretagogues *in vivo* was reported in 1976.[57] In this model, prostaglandins were administered either orally or subcutaneously to rats and at various times (up to five hours) following dosing, the small intestine was removed from the animals and the fluid accumulated in the small intestine was drained and quantitated. In developing this model, a number of variables were evaluated in addition to the optimal time post dosing in an attempt to increase the sensitivity of the "enteropooling" assay. These included the effects of fluid loading, fasting and anticholinergic agents. From these studies, it was demonstrated that prostaglandins (as well as carbachol, magnesium sulphate, phenolphthalein, castor oil and sodium taurocholate or sodium taurochenodeoxycholate) reproducibly stimulate fluid secretion into the lumen of the small intestine (but not the cecum or colon). This fluid accumulation is dose related, maximal at 30 minutes and not altered by prior fluid loading. Although this model allows evaluation of the secretory potential of putative intestinal secretagogues, it is an acute model in which a single animal is required for each data point and the effects of antidiarrheal agents must be evaluated from pretreatment of animals which is not the normal treatment regimen.

CECECTOMIZED RAT

In 1990, Fondacaro and coworkers[58] adapted the cecectomized rat model for use in studying intestinal secretion and the effects of potential antidiarrheal drugs. This model, originally reported by Ambuhl et al.[59] to study the role of the cecum in protein digestion involves surgical resection of the cecum of the rat thereby avoiding the variability in diarrheal output observed in the normal rat. In their studies, Fondacaro and coworkers[58] demonstrated that fluid accumulated in the small intestine and cecum following oral administration of cholera toxin but no fluid accumulation was observed in the colon. Thus, these studies suggest that the cecum acts to ameliorate diarrhea of small intestinal origin. Cecectomy did not produce any changes in body weight gain, serum sodium concentration or hematocrit over a 30-day period following surgery.[58] In addition, food intake, stool consistency and output and activity were all reported to be normal.[58] In cecectomized but not sham operated animals, oral administration of 16,16-dimethyl prostaglandin E_2, carbachol or cholera toxin resulted in a reproducible increase in fecal output.[58] The increased fecal output associated with oral administration of 16,16-dimethyl prostaglandin E_2 was reversed by oral administration of three antidiarrheal agents, chlorpromazine, clonidine and morphine.[58] This model was subsequently employed to evaluate the antidiarrheal effects of α-2 adrenoceptor agonists and correlated with results from *in vitro* studies and enteropooling assays.[60]

Advantages of the cecectomized rat model for studying diarrhea and the development of antidiarrheal agents include the smaller size of the animal and thus compound requirements and the ability to conduct experiments chronically without anesthesia, restraint or associated cannula. Additionally, the reproducibility of the response allows evaluation of potential antisecretory agents during a diarrheal episode rather than prior to induction of intestinal secretion.

STUDIES IN MAN

LUMINAL PERFUSION

Mass balance experiments for determining intestinal absorption have been conducted in man employing a variety of techniques including double or triple lumen intubation tubes. The technique employs balloons for occluding an intestinal segment and the test solution is introduced and sampled from the intestinal segment with separate tubes.[61] Concern over the possibility that the balloons could alter intestinal absorptive and secretory processes resulted in the development of a technique in which an intubation tube was swallowed and as the tube moved along the gastrointestinal tract, samples of intestinal fluid could be taken via aspiration.[62,63] With this method, the site of absorption was estimated from the length of tube intubated. A modification of this luminal perfusion technique was reported by Borgstrom and coworkers in 1957,[64] in which the perfusion tube was designed with openings at a specificied distance for aspiration of luminal contents and also the marker, polyethylene glycol was employed. Continuous sampling of the infused solution has been accomplished by siphoning or suction.[65] Using this technique, absorption of substrates (e.g. D-xylose[65]) can be assessed. In 1966, Cooper and coworkers[66] reported on a triple lumen intubation tube for evaluating intestinal absorption or secretion. With this technique, test solutions are introduced through the most proximal intubation tube and sampled at both the middle and most distal intubation tubes. The major advantage of this additional tube is that it allows for correction of fluids secreted into the intestinal segment being studied. Using this technique, mechanisms involved in the absorption and secretion of salts (e.g. sodium, bicarbonate and chloride) and the permeability characteristics of the human small intestine have been determined.[67–70] In the mechanistic studies of Fordtran and coworkers,[69] these investigators also employed a system for measuring the electrical potential difference between the intestinal lumen (using an interenteric electrode attached to the intubation tube) with reference to a skin electrode. Both the chemical and electrical driving forces for movement of salts across the gastrointestinal mucosa could be determined. Effects of intestinal secretagouges such as vasoactive intestinal polypeptide and secretin on the active and passive transport of electrolytes have been investigated with these techniques.[71–73] In a variation on these techniques, the mechanisms of antidiarrheal action of loperamide have been investigated by introducing a single lumen tube into the stomach for administration of solutions and a rectal tube for colletion of fluid.[74] These studies have in general supported the conclusions from animal studies or have provided a basis for selecting appropriate animal models to be used in assessing gastrointestinal absorption and secretion.

SCINTIGRAPHIC METHODS

The major criticism of any experimental method which is designed to describe gastrointestinal absorption or secretion is the degree to which it deviates from the normal physiological condition. The most physiologic technique would therefore not involve invasive procedures or anesthesia and would allow the subject to conduct routine activities to avoid psychological factors. No technique can meet all of these criteria but the introduction of scintigraphic methods has provided a procedure whereby the normal physiologic condition can be closely mimicked. Gamma scintigraphy has advantages over the use of X-ray methods[75,76] in that patients are not exposed to such high radiation doses and that quantitative monitoring can be done continuously.

Gamma scintigraphy has been applied to a variety of measurements of esophageal and gastrointestinal transit of pharmaceutical dosage forms.[77-89] Simultaneous monitoring of plasma and/or urine drug concentrations with quantification of a drug in different regions of the gastrointestinal tract can provide information regarding sites and extent of absorption and any changes in these parameters which may occur as a result of altering the dosage form. These studies have also evaluated the effect of physiological factors on gastrointestinal transit of dosage forms[78,79,90-93] and changes in gastrointestinal transit occurring as a result of pathophysiological conditions such as inflammatory bowel disease, constipation and diarrhea.[94-97] Kaufmann and coworkers[93] employed scintigraphic techniques to demonstrate that opiates decrease colonic transit in the proximal colon and that these effects are reversed by the opiate receptor antagonist, naloxone. In recent studies of Barrow and coworkers, scintigraphic techniques were employed together with an experimental model of diarrhea to assess the antidiarrheal effects of codeine in man.[98,99] From their studies, it was demonstrated that codeine delays the mouth to cecum transit in general and produces an additional delay in the transit through the ascending colon.[98] The conclusions of the studies by Barrow and coworkers[98] are in agreement with those of Schiller and colleagues[74] who investigated the antidiarrheal effects of loperamide by monitoring polyethylene glycol concentrations in the intestinal effluent following rapid intragastric infusion of an electrolyte solution. The antidiarrheal effect of loperamide was shown to result from a change in the motor function of the intestine thereby delaying the intestinal transit time without any effect on the rate of absorption by intestinal cells.[74]

A limited number of radionuclides possess the appropriate characteristics for scintigraphic studies. Limitations in the use of radionuclides are related to the energy range (50–400 keV) which is optimum for imaging by gamma cameras. Radionuclides with higher-energy gamma emissions are not appropriate due to degraded images and the presence of alpha or beta emissions which expose patients to unacceptable doses of radiation. Radionuclides commonly employed for gamma scintigraphic studies include indium[113m] and technetium[99m] which have half-lifes of 1.7 and 6 hours, respectively and gamma emissions of 393 and 140 keV, respectively. For studies requiring longer periods of imaging (e.g. colonic transit times, modified release dosage forms, absorption in the colon), indium[111] can be employed (half-life of 67 hours and gamma emissions of 173 and 247 keV). Erbium[171] (half-life of 7.5 hours and gamma emissions of 112, 296 and 308 keV) and samarium[153] (half-life of 47 hours and a gamma emission of 103 keV) also have appropriate characteristics for scintigraphic studies. For gastrointestinal transit studies, the radionuclides are incorporated into a nonabsorbable marker. This has been accomplished by chelation with ethylenediaminetetraacetic acid (EDTA) or diethylenetriaminepentaacetic acid (DTPA) or by adsorption to a cation exchange resin such as Amberlite. Alternatively, a nonradioactive marker (e.g. samarium oxide enriched with samarium[152] isotope) can be incorporated into a dosage form and subsequently exposed to neutron bombardment in a nuclear reactor to produce the gamma emitting radionuclide. A drawback to this latter procedure is that neutron activation may produce damaging effects on the dosage form being evaluated or that other radionuclides may be produced by the activation process.

PERMEABILITY STUDIES

Permeability of the gastrointestinal tract refers to the presence of pores which allow compounds to traverse the epithelial layer thereby gaining access to the vasculature. A major route for many small water soluble molecules to gain access to the vasculature across the intestinal epithelium is the paracellular pathway via the "tight junctional" complexes or zonula occludens. These junctional complexes are a dynamic system which are regulated to open and close thereby providing a permeability for a variety of nutrients, small molecules and fluid.[100-103] Furthermore, studies have demonstrated that the linear density of tight junctions varies in different locations of the intestine. Marcial and coworkers[104] have reported that the linear density of the tight junctions in the crypt region of the small intestine is 77 m/cm^2 compared to a much smaller linear density in the villus region of only 22 m/cm^2. In addition, the number of strands in the tight junctional complex which has been reported to correlate with the conductance of the junctional complex has been shown to be greater in the villus region of the small intestine than in the crypt region (6 vs 4.4).[104] Determination of intestinal permeability of molecules and changes in intestinal permeability under a variety of physiological and pathophysiological conditions have been studied in man and animals using both radiolabelled and non-radiolabelled probes. However, caution in interpretation of these results is required since a variety of factors such as the nutritional state of the subject (e.g. fed *vs* fasted), the size and shape of the permeability probe employed and the integrity of the gastrointestinal tract (e.g. in patients with celiac sprue in which the villus epithelium is absent thereby allowing direct access to the crypt region) will directly affect permeability measurements.

Non-radiolabelled markers

The characteristics of molecules which make them appropriate as non-radiolabelled markers for clinical studies to assess intestinal permeability include: 1) having the ability to be administered orally; 2) being both inactive and nonreactive; 3) having a low molecular weight; 4) being water soluble and having limited absorption; 5) being rapidly cleared by the kidneys and excreted into the urine in an amount which is directly proportional to the amount transported across the intestinal epithelium. Permeability markers which have been extensively employed include the sugar alcohol, mannitol and the mono- and disaccharides, rhamnose, lactulose and cellobiose with cross-sectional diameters of 6.7, 8.3, 9.5 and 10.5 angstroms and the polymer, polyethylene glycol 400 which has a cross-sectional area of 5.3 angstroms. As reported by Laker and coworkers[105] and further evaluated by Blomquist and coworkers,[106] mannitol permeability values when assessed by urinary excretion may be influenced by the presence of this compound in normal urine. Thus, the variability observed in studies conducted with non-radiolabelled mannitol may be a reflection of these 'extra' sources of mannitol. Furthermore, markers like lactulose may undergo degradation by colonic bacteria which can influence permeability assessment of the colon. Despite these potential problems, these probes have been employed alone or in combination (e.g. lactulose/mannitol) to demonstrate that intestinal permeability is increased in a variety of pathophysiologic conditions including cystic fibrosis,[107] acute gastroenteritis,[108] celiac disease[109–111] and Crohn's disease.[109, 112–114] Although these studies are helpful in monitoring intestinal permeability and identifying changes which occur in pathophysiological conditions, the major drawback of these methods is that the sites and mechanisms of altered permeability cannot be determined without the use of invasive procedures such as intestinal infusion.[112]

Radiolabelled markers

Chromium^{51}-EDTA and technetium^{99m}-DPTA have been been extensively investigated as probes for gastrointestinal permeability.[115–127] These molecules are non-metabolized and have cross-sectional diameters of approximately 11 angstroms which is similar to the non-radiolabelled marker cellobiose. In addition to these radiolabelled probes, other molecules such as mannitol and polyethylene glycol can be radiolabelled with ^{14}C or ^{3}H and have been used either alone or in combination with other probes to assess gastrointestinal permeability.[128] As with non-radiolabelled markers, these probes can be administered to patients orally and monitored in the urine to assess intestinal permeability and changes in intestinal permeability resulting from pathophysiological or chemical effects.

SUMMARY AND CONCLUSIONS

From these discussions, it is obvious that there are a myriad of techniques described for assessing oral absorption and secretion. Selection of the most suitable method is dependent on the questions which are being addressed. However, it is also apparent that animal models cannot address more basic questions regarding the mechanisms involved in transepithelial transport. For these issues, application of *in vitro* techniques together with molecular biological approaches are required. The advancement of gamma scintigraphic techniques has dramatically increased our understanding of gastrointestinal transit and absorption in human subjects. Despite this increase in human investigation, there will continue to be a great demand for reliable methods for determining gastrointestinal absorption and systemic availability in the development of new therapeutics and in providing models for assessing changes associated with gastrointestinal diseases.

REFERENCES

1. **Beaumont, W.,** *Experiments and observations on the gastric juice and the physiology of digestion,* Dover Publishers, Inc., New York, 1955.
2. **Thiry, L.,** Uber eine neue methode den dunndarm zu isolieren, *Sitzungsber Akad Wiss Wien Kl. I,* 50, 77, 1864.
3. **Vella, L.,** Nuovo methodo per avere il succo enterico puro e stabilirne le proprieta fisiologiche, *Mem. Acad. Sci. Inst. Bologna. Ser.,* 42, 515, 1880.
4. **Carpenter, C. C. J., Sack, R. B., Feeley, J. C., and Steenberg, R. W.,** Site and characteristics of electrolyte loss and effect of intraluminal glucose in experimental canine cholera, *J. Clin. Invest.,* 47, 1210, 1968.
5. **Cramer, C. F.,** *In vivo* intestinal transport of calcium and water from solutions recycled through healed gut loops in dogs, *J. Nutrit.,* 84, 118, 1964.
6. **Cramer, C. F. and Dueck, J.,** *In vivo* transport of calcium from healed Thiry-Vella fistulas in dogs, *Am. J. Physiol.,* 202, 161, 1962.
7. **Dressman, J. B., and Yamada, K.,** Animal models for oral drug absorption, *Pharmaceutical Bioequivalence,* Dighe, S. V., Welling, P. G., and Tse, F. L. S., Eds., Marcel Dekker, 1990, 235.
8. **Worland, P. J., Drummer, O. H., and Jarrott, B.,** An *in situ* gastric pouch technique for direct measurement of the gastric absorption of drugs in the rat, *J. Pharmacol. Methods,* 10, 215, 1983.
9. **Doluisio, J. T., Billups, N. F., Dittert, L. W., Sugita, E. T., and Swintosky, J. V.,** Drug absorption I: An *in situ* rat gut technique yielding realistic absorption rates, *J. Pharm. Sci.,* 58, 1196, 1969.
10. **Welling, P. G.,** Influence of food and diet on gastrointestinal drug absorption: A review, *J. Pharmacokinet. Biopharm.,* 5, 291, 1977.
11. **Crouthamel, W. G., Tan, G. H., Dittert, L. W., and Doluisio, J. T.,** Drug absorption IV: Influence of pH on absorption kinetics of weakly acidic drugs, *J. Pharm. Sci.,* 60, 1160, 1971.
12. **Hober, R., and Hober, J.,** Experiments on the absorption of organic solutes in the small intestine of rats, *J. Cell Physiol.,* 10, 401, 1937.
13. **Doluisio, J. T., Tan, G. H., Billups, N. F., and Diamond, L.,** Drug absorption II: Effect of fasting on intestinal drug absorption, *J. Pharm. Sci.,* 58, 1200, 1969b.
14. **Hisaka, A., Kasamatsu, S., Takenaga, N., and Ohtawa, M.,** Absorption of a novel prodrug of L-DOPA, L-3-(3-hydroxy-4-pivaloyloxyphenyl)alanine (NB-355): *In vitro* and *in situ* studies, *Drug Metab. Disp.,* 18, 621, 1990.
15. **Park, J. Y., Ho, N. F. H., and Morozowich, W.,** Physical model approach to gastrointestinal absorption of prostaglandins II: *In situ* rat intestinal absorption of dinoprost, *J. Pharm. Sci.,* 73, 1588, 1984.
16. **Taylor, D. C., Pownall, R., and Burke, W.,** The absorption of β-adrenoceptor antagonists in rat *in-situ* small intestine; the effect of lipophilicity, *J. Pharm. Pharmacol.,* 37, 280, 1985.
17. **Horvath, I., and Wix, G.,** Hormaonal influences on glucose resorption from the intestine, *Acta Physiol. Acad. Sci. Hung.,* 2, 435, 1951.

18. **Higaki, K., Takechi, N., Kato, M., Hashida, M., and Sezaki, H.,** Effect of medium-chain glycerides on the intestinal absorption of phenol red: Studies on mechanisms of the promoting effect, *J. Pharm. Sci.,* 79, 334, 1990.

19. **Fullerton, P. M., and Parsons, D. S.,** Absorption of sugars and water from the rat intestine *in vivo, Q. J. Exp. Physiol.,* 41, 387, 1956.

20. **Csaky, T. Z., and Ho, P. M.,** Intestinal transprot of D-xylose, *Proc. Soc. Exp. Biol. Med.,* 120, 403, 1965.

21. **Friedman, D. I., and Amidon, G. L.,** Intestinal absorption mechanism of dipeptide angiotensin converting enzyme inhibitors of the lysyl-proline type: Lisinopril and SQ 29,852, *J. Pharm. Sci.,* 78, 995, 1989.

22. **Johnson, D. A., and Amidon, G. L.,** Determination of intrinsic membrane transport parameters from perfused intestine experiments: A boundary layer approach to estimating the aqueous and unbiased membrane permeabilities, *J. Theor. Biol.,* 131, 93, 1988.

23. **Hu, M., Sinko, P. J., DeMeere, A. L. J., Johnson, D. A., and Amidon, G. L.,** Membrane permeability parameters for some amino acids and β-lactam antibiotics: Application of the boundary layer approach, *J. Theor. Biol.,* 131, 107, 1988.

24. **Komiya, I., Park, J. Y., Kamani, A., Ho, N. F. H., and Higuchi, W. I.,** Quantitative mechanistic studies in simultaneous fluid flow and intestinal absorption using steroids as model solutes, *Int. J. Pharm.,* 4, 249, 1980.

25. **Coupar, I. M.,** Choice of anesthetic for intestinal absorption and secretion experiments using rats, *J. Pharmacol. Meth.,* 13, 331, 1985.

26. **Yuasa, H., Matisuda, K., and Watanabe, J.,** Influence of anesthetic regimens on intestinal absorption in rats, *Pharm. Res.,* 10, 884, 1993.

27. **Rowland, M., and Tozer, T. N.,** *Clinical Pharmacokinetics,* 2nd ed,, Lea & Febiger, Philadelphia, 1989.

28. **Shoemaker, W. C., Walker, W. F., Van Itallie, T. B., and Moore, F. D.,** A method for simultaneous catheterization of major hepatic vessels in a chronic canine preparation, *Am. J. Physiol.,* 196, 311, 1959.

29. **Shoemaker, W. C.,** Measurement of hepatic blood flow in the unanesthetized dog by a modified bromosulphalein method, *J. Appl. Physiol.,* 15, 473, 1960.

30. **Rosenberg, S. H., Spina, K. P., Woods, K. W., Polakowski, J., Martin, D. L. Yao, Z., Stein, H. H., Cohen, J., Barlow, J. L., Egan, D. A., Tricarico, K. A., Baker, W. R. and Kleinert, H. D.,** Studies directed toward the design of orally active renin inhibitors 1. Some factors influencing the absorption of small peptides, *J. Med. Chem.* 36, 449, 1993.

31. **Warshaw, A. L.,** A simplified method of cannulating the intestinal lymphatic of the rat, *Gut,* 13, 66, 1972.

32. **Bollman, J. L., Cain, J. C., and Grindlay, J. H.,** Techniques for the collection of lymph from the liver, small intestine, or thoracic duct of the rat, *J. Lab. Clin. Med.,* 33, 1349, 1948.

33. **Bollman, J. L., Flock, E. V., Cain, J. C., and Grindlay, J. H.,** Lipids of lymph following feeding of rat: experimental study, *Am. J. Physiol.,* 163, 41, 1950.

34. **Hollander, D.,** Retinol lymphatic and portal transport: influence of pH, bile, and fatty acids, *Am. J. Physiol.,* 239, G210, 1980.

35. **Sudo, L. S.,** Lymphatic transport of salicylates in dogs, *Gen. Pharmac.,* 20, 779, 1989.

36. **Hollander, D., and Dadufalza, V.,** Lymphatic and portal absorption of vitamin E in aging rats, *Dig. Dis. Sci.,* 34, 768, 1989.

37. **Fejes-Toth, G., Naray-Fejes-Toth, A., Ratge, D., and Frolich, J. C.,** Chronic arterial and venous catheterization of conscious, unrestrained rats, *Hypertension,* 6, 926, 1984.

38. **Polema, F. G. J., and Tukker, J. J.,** Evaluation of a chronically isolated internal loop in the rat for the study of drug absorption kinetics, *J. Pharm. Sci.,* 76, 433, 1987.

39. **Rubinstein, A., Li, V. H. K., Gruber, P., Bass, P., and Robinson, J. R.,** Improved intestinal cannula for drug delivery studies in the dog, *J. Pharmacol. Meth.,* 19, 213, 1988.

40. **Gruber, P., Rubinstein, A., Li, V. H. K., Bass, P., and Robinson, J. R.,** Gastric emptying of nondigestible solids in the fasted dog, *J. Pharm. Sci.,* 76, 117, 1987.

41. **Marcello, J., Gosnell, J., Orner, D., Meunier, L. D., Nichols, A., Vasko, J., Barone, F., Perri, J., and Smith, P. L.,** Peptide absorption from small and large intestine determined in conscious dogs employing a chronic intestinal access port model, *Pharm. Res.,* 9, S-179, 1992.

42. **Meunier, L. D., Kissinger, J. T., Jenkins, E. L., Cobb, R. L., Billetta, T. K., Barone, F. C., and Smith, P. L.,** A chronic intestinal access port model in conscious dogs, *Am. Assoc. Lab. Anim. Sci. Bull.,* 30, 26, 1991.

43. **Smith, P. L., Yeulet, S. E., Citerone, D. R., Drake, F., Cook, M., Wall, D. A., and Marcello, J.,** SK&F 110679: Comparison of absorption following oral or respiratory administration, *J. Cont. Rel.,* 28, 67, 1994.

44. **Pierce, N. F., Carpenter, C. C. J. Jr., Elliott, H. L., and Greenough, W. B. III,** Effects of prostaglandins, theophylline, and cholera exotoxin upon transmucosal water and electrolyte movement in the canine jejunum, *Gastroenterology,* 60, 22, 1971.

45. **Gullikson, G. W., Dajani, E. Z., and Bianchi, R. G.,** Inhibition of intestinal secretion in the dog: A new approach for the management of diarrheal states, *J. Pharmacol. Exp. Ther.,* 219, 591, 1981.

46. **Hecklye R. J., Wolochow, H., and Christiansen, C.,** *Vibrio cholerae* enterotoxin in miniature pigs, *J. Bacteriol.,* 100, 1140, 1969.

47. **Basu, S., and Pickett, M. J.,** Reaction of *Vibrio cholera* and choleragenic toxin in ileal loop of laboratory animals, *J. Bacteriol.,* 100, 1142, 1969.

48. **Taub, M., Bonorris, G., Chung, A., Coyne, M. J., and Schoenfield, L. J.,** Effect of propranolol on bile acid- and cholera enterotoxin-stimulated cAMP and secretion in rabbit intestine, *Gastroenterology,* 72, 101, 1977.

49. **Burrows, W., and Musteikis, G. M.,** Cholera infection and toxin in the rabbit ileal loop, *J. Infec. Dis.,* 116, 183, 1966.

50. **Leitch, G. J., Iwert, M. E. and Burrows, W.,** Experimental cholera in the rabbit ligated ileal loop: Toxin-induced water and ion movement, *J. Infect. Dis.,* 116, 303, 1966.

51. **Cline, W. S., Lorenzsonn, V., Benz, L., Bass, P., and Olsen, W. A.,** The effects of sodium ricinoleate on small intestinal function and structure, *J. Clin. Invest.,* 58, 380, 1976.

52. **Guerrant, R. L., Chen, L. C., and Sharp, G. W. G.,** Intestinal adenylcyclase activity in canine cholera: Correlation with fluid accumulation, *J. Infect. Dis.,* 125, 377, 1972.

53. **Nakaki, T., Nakadate, T., Yamamoto, S., and Kato, R.,** *Alpha-*2 adrenergic inhibition of intestinal secretion induced by prostaglandin E_1, vasoactive intestinal peptide and dibutyryl cyclic AMP in rat jejunum, *J. Pharmacol. Exp. Ther.,* 220, 637, 1982.

54. **Burakoff, R., and Percy, W. H.,** Studies *in vivo* and *in vitro* on effects of PGE_2 on colonic motility in rabbits, *Am. J. Physiol.,* 262, G23, 1992.

55. **Burakoff, R., Nastos, E., Won, S., and Percy, W. H.,** Comparison of the effects of leukotrienes B_4 and D_4 on distal colonic motility in the rabbit *in vivo, Am. J. Physiol.,* 257, G860, 1989.

56. **Burakoff, R., Nastos, E., and Won, S.,** Effects of $PGF_{2\alpha}$ and of indomethacin on rabbit small and large intestinal motility *in vivo, Am. J. Physiol.,* 258, G231, 1990.

57. **Robert, A., Nezamis, J. E., Lancaster, C., Hanchar, A. J., and Klepper, M. S.,** Enteropooling assay: A test for diarrhea produced by prostaglandins, *Prostaglandins,* 11, 809, 1976.

58. **Fondacaro, J. D., Kolpak, D. C., Burnham, D. B., and McCafferty, G. P.,** Cecectomized rat: A model of experimental secretory diarrhea in conscious animals, *J. Pharmacol. Methods,* 24, 59, 1990.

59. **Ambuhl, S., Williams, V. J., and Senior, W.,** Effects of caecectomy in young adult female rat on digestibility of food offered *ad libitum* and in restricted amounts, *Aust. J. Biol. Sci.,* 32, 205, 1979.

60. **Fondacaro, J. D., McCafferty, G. P., Kolpak, D. C., and Smith, P. L.,** Antidiarrheal activity of *alpha-*2 adrenoceptor agonist SK&F 35886, *J. Pharmacol. Exp. Ther.,* 249, 221, 1989.

61. **Miller, T. G.,** Intubation studies of the human small intestine. XXVI. A review of a ten-year experience, *Gastroenterology,* 3, 141, 1944.

62. **Nicholson, J. T. L., and Chornock, F. W.,** Intubation studies of the human small intestine. XXII. An improved technic for the study of absorption; its application to ascorbic acid, *J. Clin. Invest.,* 21, 505, 1942.

63. **Blankenhorn, D. H., Hirsch, J., and Ahrens, E. H.,** Transintestinal intubation: Technic for measurement of gut length and physiologic sampling at known loci, *Proc. Soc. Exper. Biol. Med.,* 88, 356, 1955.

64. **Borgstrom, B., Dahlquist, A., Lundh, G., and Sjovall, J.,** Studies of intestinal digestion and absorption in the human, *J. Clin. Invest.,* 36, 1521, 1957.

65. **Fordtran, J. S., Soergel, K. H., and Ingelfinger, J.,** Intestinal absorption of D-xylose in man, *New Eng. J. Med.,* 267, 274, 1962.
66. **Cooper, H., Levitan, R., Fordtran, J. S., and Ingelfinger, F. J.,** A method for studying absorption of water and solute from the human small intestine, *Gastroenterology,* 50, 1, 1966.
67. **Davis, G. R., Santa Ana, C. A., Morawski, S., and Fordtran, J. S.,** Active chloride secretion in the normal human jejunum, *J. Clin. Invest.,* 66, 1326, 1980.
68. **Fordtran, J. S., Rector, F. C. Jr., Ewton, M. F., Soter, N., and Kinney, J.,** Permeability characteristics of the human small intestine, *J. Clin. Invest.,* 44, 1935, 1965.
69. **Fordtran, J. S., Rector, F. C. Jr., and Carter, N. W.,** The mechanisms of sodium absorption in the human small intestine, *J. Clin. Invest.,* 47, 884, 1968.
70. **Turnberg, L. A., Fordtran, J. S., Carter, N. W., and Rector, F. C. Jr.,** Mechanism of bicarbonate absorption and its relationship to sodium transport in the human jejunum, *J. Clin. Invest.,* 49, 548, 1970.
71. **Davis, G. R., Santa Ana, C. A., Morawski, S. G., and Fordtran, J. S.,** Effect of vasoactive intestinal polypeptide on active and passive transport in the human jejunum, *J. Clin. Invest.,* 1687, 1981.
72. **Hicks, T., and Turnberg, L. A.,** The influence of secretin on ion transport in the human jejunum, *Gut,* 14, 485, 1973.
73. **Krejs, G. J., Fordtran, J. S., Bloom, S. R., Fahrenkrug, J., De Muckadell, O. B. S., Fisher, J. E., Humphrey, C. S., O'Dorisio, T. M., Said, S. I., Walsh, J. J., and Shulkes, A. A.,** Effect of VIP infusion on water and ion transport in the human jejunum, *Gastroenterology,* 78, 722, 1980.
74. **Schiller, L. R., Santa Ana, C. A., Morawski, S. G., and Fordtran, J. S.,** Mechanism of the antidiarrheal effect of loperamide, *Gastroenterology,* 86, 1475, 1984.
75. **Steinberg, W. H., Frey, G. H., Masci, J. N., and Hutchins, H. H.,** Methods for determining *in vivo* tablet disintegration, *J. Pharm. Sci.,* 54, 747, 1965.
76. **Evans, K. T., and Roberts, G. M.,** The ability of patients to swallow capsules, *J. Clin. Hosp. Pharm.,* 6, 207, 1981.
77. **Robertson, C. S., and Hardy, J. G.,** Oesophageal transit of small tablets, *J. Pharm. Pharmacol.,* 40, 595, 1988.
78. **Coupe, A. J., Davis, S. S., Evans, D. F., and Wilding, I. R.,** Correlation of the gastric emptying of non-disintegrating tablets with gastrointestinal motility, *Pharm. Res.,* 8, 1281, 1991.
79. **Coupe, A. J., Davis, S. S., and Wilding, I. R.,** Variation in gastrointestinal transit of pharmaceutical dosage forms in healthy subjects, *Pharm. Res.,* 8, 360, 1991.
80. **Davis, S. S., Hardy, J. G., Taylor, M. J., Stockwell, A., Whalley, D. R., and Wilson, C. G.,** The *in-vivo* evaluation of an osmotic device (Osmet) using gamma scintigraphy, *J. Pharm. Pharmacol.,* 36, 740, 1984.
81. **Davis, S. S., Khosia, R., Wilson, C. G., and Washington, N.,** The gastrointestinal transit of a controlled release pellet formulation of tiaprofenic acid, *Int. J. Pharm.,* 35, 253, 1987.
82. **Davis, S. S., Christensen, F. N., Khosia, R., and Feely, L. C.,** Gastric emptying of large single unit dosage forms, *J. Pharm. Pharmacol.,* 40, 205, 1988.
83. **Davis, S. S., Hardy, J. G., and Fara, J.,** The intestinal transit of pharmaceutical dosage forms, *Gut,* 27, 886, 1986a
84. **O'Reilly, S., Wilson, C. G., and Hardy, J. G.,** The influence of food on multiparticulate dosage forms, *Int. J. Pharm.,* 34, 213, 1987.
85. **Khosla, R. C., and Davis, S. S.,** The effect of tablet size on the gastric emptying of nondisintegrating tablets, *Int. J. Pharm.,* 62, R9, 1990.
86. **Hardy, J. G., Wilson, C. G., and Wood, E.,** Drug delivery to the proximal colon, *J. Pharm. Pharmacol.,* 37, 874, 1985.
87. **Parker, G., Wilson, C. G., and Hardy, J. G.,** The effect of capsule density on transit through the proximal colon, *J. Pharm. Pharmacol.,* 40, 376, 1988.
88. **Price, J. M. C., Davis, S. S., and Wilding, I. R.,** The effect of fibre on gastrointestinal transit times in vegetarians and omnivores, *Int. J. Pharm.,* 76, 123, 1991.
89. **Bechgaard, H., Christensen, F. N., Davis, S. S., Hardy, J. G., Taylor, M. J., Whalley, D. R., and Wilson, C. G.,** Gastrointestinal transit of pellet systems in ileostomy subjects and the effect of density, *J. Pharm. Pharmacol.,* 37, 718, 1985.
90. **Ollerenshaw, K. J., Norman S., Wilson, C. G. and Hardy, J. G.,** Exercise and small intestinal transit, *Nucl. Med. Commun.,* 8, 105, 1987.

91. **Mundy, M. J., Wilson, C. G., and Hardy, J. G.,** The effect of eating on transit through the small intestine, *Nucl. Med. Commun.,* 10, 45, 1989.

92. **Price, J. M. C., Davis, S. S., and Wilding, I. R.,** Characterization of colonic transit of nondisintegrating tablets in healthy subjects, *Dig. Dis. Sci.,* 38, 1015, 1993.

93. **Kaufman, P. N., Krevsky, B., Malmud, L. S., Maurer, A. H., Somers, M. B., Siegel, J. A., and Fisher, R. S.,** Role of opiate receptors in the regulation of colonic transit, *Gastroenterology,* 94, 1351, 1988.

94. **McLean, R. G., Smart, R. C., Gaston-Parry, D., Barbagallo, S., Baker, J., Lyons, N. R., Bruck, C. E., King, D. W., Lubowski, D. Z., and Talley, N. A.,** Colon transit scintigraphy in health and constipation using oral iodine-131-cellulose, *J. Nuc. Med.,* 31, 985, 1990.

95. **Hardy, J. G., Davis, S. S., Khosla, R., and Robertson, C. S.,** Gastrointestinal transit of small tablets in patients with ulcerative colitis, *Int. J. Pharm.,* 48, 79, 1988.

96. **Davis, S. S., Robertson, C., and Wilding, I. R.,** Gastrointestinal transit of a multiparticulate tablet formulation in patients with active ulcerative colitis, *Int. J. Pharm.,* 68, 199, 1991.

97. **Roberts, J. P., Newell, M. S., Deeks, J. J., Waldron, D. W., Garvie, N. W., and Williams, N. S.,** Oral [^{111}In]DTPA scintigraphic assessment of colonic transit in constipated subjects, *Dig. Dis. Sci.,* 38, 1032, 1993.

98. **Barrow, L., Steed, K. P., Spiller, R. C., Maskell, N. A., Brown, J. K., Watts, P. J., Melia, C. D., Davies, M. C., and Wilson, C. G.,** Quantitative, noninvasive assessment of antidiarrheal actions of codeine using an experimental model of diarrhea in man, *Dig. Dis. Sci.,* 38, 996, 1993.

99. **Barrow, L., Steed, K. P., Spiller, R. C., Watts, P. J., Melia, C. D., Davies, M. C., and Wilson, C. G.,** Scintigraphic demonstration of accelerated proximal colonic transit by lactulose and its modification by gelling agents, *Gastroenterology,* 103, 1167, 1992.

100. **Madara, J. L.,** Tight junction dynamics: is paracellular transport regulated?, *Cell,* 53, 497, 1988.

101. **Madara, J. L.,** Loosening tight junctions—lessons from the intestine, *J. Clin. Invest.,* 83, 1089, 1989.

102. **Madara, J. L., and Pappenheimer, J. R.,** Structural basis for physiological regulation of paracellular pathways in intestinal epithelia, *J. Membr. Biol.,* 100, 149, 1987.

103. **Pappenheimer, J. R., and Reiss, K. Z.,** Contribution of solvent drag through intercellular junctions to absorption of nutrients by the small intestine of the rat, *J. Membr. Biol.,* 100, 123, 1987.

104. **Marcial, M. A., Carlson, S. L., and Madara, J. L.,** Partitioning of paracellular conductance along the ileal and crypt-villus axis: a hypothesis based on structural analysis with detailed consideration of tight junction structure-function relationships, *J. Membr. Biol.,* 80, 59, 1984.

105. **Laker, M. F., Bull, H. J., and Menzies, I. S.,** Evaluation of mannitol as a probe marker of gastrointestinal permeability in man, *Eur. J. Clin. Invest.,* 12, 485, 1982.

106. **Blomquist, L., Bark, T., Hedenborg, G., Svenberg, T., and Norman, A.,** Comparison between the lactulose/mannitol and ^{51}Cr-ethylenediaminetetraacetic acid/^{14}C-mannitol methods for intestinal permeability: Frequency distribution pattern and variability of markers and marker ratios in healthy subjects, *Scand. J. Gastroenterol.,* 28, 274, 1993.

107. **Leclercq-Foucart, J., Forget, P. P., and Vancustem, J.,** Lactulose/rhamnose intestinal permeability in children with cystic fibrosis, *J. Pediatr. Gastroenterol. Nutr.,* 6, 66, 1987.

108. **Isolauri, E., Juntunen, M., Wiren, S., Vuorinen, P., and Koivula, T.,** Intestinal permeability changes in acute gastroenteritis: effects of clinical factors and nutritional management, *J. Pediatr. Gastroenterol. Nutr.,* 8, 466, 1989.

109. **Pearson, A. D. J., Eastham, E. J., Laker, M. F., Craft, A. W., and Nelson, R.,** Intestinal permeability in children with Crohn's disease and coeliac disease, *Br. Med. J.,* 285, 20, 1982.

110. **Hamilton, I., Cobden, I., Rothwell, J., and Axon, A. T. R.,** Intestinal permeability in coeliac disease: the response to gluten withdrawal and single dose gluten challenge, *Gut,* 23, 240, 1982.

111. **Juby, L. D., Rothwell, J., and Axon, A. T. R.,** Lactulose/mannitol test: An ideal screen for celiac disease, *Gastroenterology,* 96, 79, 1989.

112. **Chadwick, V. S., Phillips, S. F., and Hoffman, A. F.,** Measurement of intestinal permeability using low molecular weight polyethylene glycols (PEG 400). II. Application to normal and abnormal permeability states in man and animals, *Gastroenterology,* 73, 247, 1977.

113. **Magnusson, K.-E., Sundqvist, T., Sjoedahl, R., and Tagesson, C.,** Altered intestinal permeability to low molecular weight polyethylene glycols (PEG 400) in patients with Crohn's disease, *Acta Chir. Scand.,* 149, 323, 1983.

114. **Jenkins, R. T., Goodacre, R. L., Rooney, P. J., Bienenstock, J., Sivakumarin, T., and Walker, W. H. C.,** Studies of intestinal permeability in inflammatory diseases using polyethylene glycol 400, *Clin. Biochem.,* 19, 298, 1986.

115. **Bjarnason, I. C., Levi, A. J., and Peters, T. J.,** Absorption of 51-chromium-labelled ethylenediaminetetraacetate in inflammatory bowel disease, *Gastroenterology,* 85, 318, 1983.

116. **Ainsworth, M., Eriksen, J., Rasmussen, J. W., Schaffalitzky, D. E., and Muckadell, O. B.,** Intestinal permeability of ^{51}Cr-labelled ethylenediaminetetraacetic acid in patients with Crohn's disease and their healthy relatives, *Scand. J. Gastroenterol.,* 24, 993, 1989.

117. **Teahon, K., Smethurst, P., Pearson, M., Levi, J. A., and Bjarnason, I.,** The effect of elemental diet on intestinal permeability and inflammation in Crohn's disease, *Gastroenterology,* 101, 84, 1991.

118. **Issenman, R. M., Jenkins, R. T., and Radoja, C.,** Intestinal permeability compared in pediatric and adult patients with inflammatory bowel disease, *Clin. Invest. Med.,* 16, 187, 1993.

119. **O'Morain, C., Abelow, A. C., Chervu, L. R., Fleischner, G. M., and Das, K. M.,** Chromium^{51} ethylenediaminetetraacetate test: a useful test in the assessment of inflammatory bowel disease, *J. Lab. Clin. Med.,* 108, 430, 1986.

120. **Jenkins, R. T., Jones, D. B., Goodacre, R. L., Collins, S. M., Hunt, R. H., and Bienenstock, J.,** The reversibility of increased intestinal permeability ot ^{51}Cr-EDTA in patients with inflammatory gastrointestinal diseases, *Am. J. Gastroenterol.,* 82, 1159, 1987.

121. **Jenkins, R. T., Ramage, J. K., Joones, D. B., Goodacre, R. L., Collins, S. M., and Hunt, R. H.,** Small bowel and colonic permeability to ^{51}Cr-EDTA in patients with inflammatory bowel disease, *Clin. Invest. Med.,* 11, 151, 1988.

122. **Jenkins, R. T., Rooney, P. J., Jones, D. B., Bienenstock, J. and Goodacre, R. L.,** Increased intestinal permeability in patients with rheumatoid arthritis: a side-effect of oral nonsteroidal anti-inflammatory drug therapy?, *Br. J. Rheumatol.,* 26, 103, 1987.

123. **Van Der Meer, S. B., Forget, P. P., and Heidendal. G. A. K.,** Small bowel permeability to ^{51}Cr-EDTA in children with recurrent abdominal pain, *Acta Pediatr. Scand.,* 79, 422, 1990.

124. **Forgot, P., Sodoyes-Goffaux, F., and Zappitelli, A.,** Permeability of the small intestine to [^{51}Cr] EDTA in children with acute gastroenteritis or eczema, *J. Pediatr. Gastroenterol. Nutr.,* 4, 393, 1985.

125. **Casellas, F., Aguade, S., Soriano, B., Accarino, A., Molero, J., and Guarner, L.,** Intestinal permeability to ^{99}m-Tc-diethylenetriaminopentaacetic acid in inflammatory bowel disease, *Am. J. Gastroenterol.,* 81, 767, 1986.

126. **Peled, Y., Watz, C., and Gilat, T.,** Measurement of intestinal permeability using ^{51}Cr-EDTA, *Am. J. Gastroenterol.,* 80, 770, 1985.

127. **Resnick, R. H., Royal, H., Marshall, W., Barron, R., and Werth, T.,** Intestinal permeability in gastrointestinal disorders. Use of oral [^{99m}Tc] DTPA, *Dig. Dis. Sci.,* 35, 205, 1990.

128. **Behrens, R. H., Szaz, K. F., Northrop, C., Elia, M., and Neale, G.,** Radionucleide tests for the assessment of intestinal permeability, *Eur. J. Clin. Invest.,* 17, 100, 1987.

5 Assessment of Intestinal Electrolyte Transport *In Vitro*

Scott M. O'Grady

INTRODUCTION

A variety of *in vitro* techniques have been used to investigate the mechanisms, regulation and pharmacology of electrolyte transport across intestinal epithelia. These techniques have provided a greater understanding of the cellular mechanisms which underlie fluid transport and regulation of luminal fluid ionic composition within the gastrointestinal tract. In most cases, the success of these techniques is directly linked to the degree to which driving forces for ion movements across individual membranes and the intact epithelium can be controlled. In this chapter, some of the commonly used techniques for measuring electrolyte transport across epithelial tissues will be addressed with specific reference to studies conducted with native intestinal epithelia. The use of isolated crypts for study of ion transport is also discussed. The goal of this review is to provide background about the types of experiments that can be performed with these techniques and to give some examples of how the results of such experiments have contributed to our understanding of electrolyte transport in intestinal epithelia. The focus will be on transepithelial electrical measurements and flux studies that can be used to investigate the properties of intact intestinal epithelia. It should be pointed out that detailed reviews on electrophysiological techniques (e.g. intracellular microelectrode techniques[1,2] and patch clamp recording[3,4]) have been recently published and will not be discussed in this review.

TRANSEPITHELIAL ELECTRICAL MEASUREMENTS

This section describes procedures for tissue preparation and measurement of electrical properties of intact epithelia mounted in Ussing chambers. The voltage clamp technique originally developed by Hans Ussing for the study of Na absorption across frog skin has been extensively used to investigate mechanisms and regulation of ion transport across intestinal epithelia from a variety of species.[5-8] The technique is versatile and provides information about net ion movements across the tissue. It has also been used in combination with blocker compounds for identification and localization of specific transport pathways in both apical and basolateral membranes.

TISSUE PREPARATION

Preparation of Tissues for Ussing Chamber Experiments

Studies using native intestinal epithelia have shown that removal of the submucosal muscle layers prior to mounting tissues in Ussing chambers improves the viability and accessibility of

0-8493-8304-8/96/$0.00+$.50
© 1996 by CRC Press, Inc.

the basolateral membrane to various drugs, hormones and neurotransmitters.[9–13] It also eliminates sporadic muscle contractions that alter the electrical properties of the epithelium. Removal of submucosal muscle can be accomplished by blunt dissection using either a dissecting microscope or magnifying glass. Alternatively, the mucosa can be stripped away from most of the lamina propria using the edge of a glass microscope slide.[9,10,13] The glass slide stripping procedure eliminates the Isc response to neuronal depolarization indicating that submucosal nerves have been removed from the epithelium.[10] In addition, the response time of the tissue to secretagogues added to the serosal solution is reduced compared with tissues prepared by blunt dissection (Figure 1). Following the removal of submucosal muscle, the epithelium and remaining lamina propria can be mounted in commercially available Lucite® chambers and connected to a reservoir system for circulation of Ringer solution on both mucosal and serosal sides of the epithelium. In some cases, Sylgard® rings have been used to reduce edge damage to the epithelium. It may also be useful to support the tissue with a nylon mesh screen if hydrostatic pressure differences between mucosal and serosal solutions produce significant damage to the epithelium.[14] For most studies, a temperature controlled gas lift recirculating reservoir system provides an efficient means for oxygenating the tissue and mixing solution contents with the epithelial surface. For mammalian tissues, a mixture of 95% O_2/5% CO_2 gas is used in combination with bicarbonate buffering (25 mM HCO_3) to provide adequate oxygenation and control of solution pH. It is also possible to set up a flow-through perfusion system to provide a continuous supply of fresh Ringer solution to the tissue. For tissues where Na-dependent glucose carriers are present in the apical membrane, it is important to substitute mannitol for glucose in the mucosal solution to avoid activation of this transport pathway. It is worth noting that the current response of the tissue following addition of glucose (1–5 mM) to the mucosal solution can provide a useful means of assessing tissue viability.

Epithelial monolayers in culture have also been used in Ussing chambers to study transepithelial electrolyte transport.[15–18] Perhaps the most extensively used intestinal cells for these experiments has been the T_{84} human colonic carcinoma cell line. In general, cells are seeded on

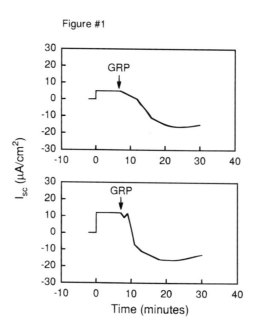

FIGURE 1   Comparison of the time course effects of gastrin releasing peptide (GRP) on porcine distal colon Isc. Tissues were prepared by either blunt dissection (top tracing) or by the glass slide stripping procedure (bottom tracing).

specially designed culture dish inserts that possess a permeable nucleopore membrane as the supporting surface for the cells. The membrane can be coated with collagen or other matrix material to improve cell attachment. Cells are allowed to grow to confluency and to develop a transepithelial resistance that will allow for reliable measurements of potential difference (PD) and short circuit current (Isc). The design of the insert allows culture media to access both apical and basolateral surfaces of the epithelium as the cells grow. Usually 4–6 days are required to achieve a tissue resistance useful for ion transport studies (about $1000 \ \Omega \ cm^{-2}$). The nucleopore membrane has a conductance of approximately $100 \ \Omega \ cm^{-2}$ and therefore is not a significant barrier to electrolyte movement relative to the epithelium.[19]

Potential Difference, Resistance and Short-Circuit
Current Measurements

To eliminate chemical driving forces for the movement of ions across the epithelium, identical Ringer solutions are used on both the mucosal and serosal sides of the tissue. To control the electrical driving force, current is passed across the epithelium to nullify the spontaneous transepithelial potential.[5,11] Commercially available Ussing chambers are fitted with ports for voltage sensing and current passing agar bridges. Agar bridges can be constructed using polyethylene tubing containing agar (4% solution) dissolved in Ringer solution. The voltage sensing bridges are placed in close proximity to the epithelium and connected to either calomel electrodes or $Ag/AgCl_3$ pellets immersed in 3M KCl solution. The current passing bridges are fitted at the opposite ends of the chamber and connected to either $Ag/AgCl_3$ pellets or chloride coated silver wire electrodes immersed in saturated KCl solution. It is important to note that over time, the agar becomes permeated with KCl solution so periodic replacement of the agar bridges may be required to reduce contamination of chamber solutions with KCl.

Epithelial voltage clamps can be constructed by the investigator or obtained from commercial suppliers for measuring transepithelial potential difference and for passing current. Tissue conductance is then calculated using Ohm's law. The fluid resistance compensation circuitry of the voltage clamp serves to subtract out fluid resistance so that the current applied across the epithelium is sufficient to nullify the spontaneous transepithelial PD. This current is referred to as the short circuit current (Isc) and is equal to the sum of the net ion movements that occur across the tissue. For most experiments, it is convenient to automate the acquisition of Isc and PD data by linking the current and voltage recording outputs of the voltage clamp to a microcomputer. If tissues are to be continuously short circuited, an analog output signal from the computer can be used to briefly pass a current pulse so that periodic PD measurements and conductance calculations can be made. The digitized data can then be exported to a variety of graphics software packages to produce hardcopy records of the data. Alternatively, the voltage clamp outputs can be connected to a chart recorder for continuous recording of Isc or PD. In this case manual switching of the clamp from short to open circuit settings is required to obtain PD and conductance data.

The problem of achieving complete short-circuiting of intestinal and colonic epithelia is complicated by the presence of an uncompensated series resistance associated with the crypt lumen. From impedance analysis of rabbit descending colon, the crypt lumen resistance was estimated to be $17 \pm 0.7 \ \Omega \ cm^2$.[20] Hence, if the Isc is equal to $-50 \ \mu A$, the lack of compensation for crypt resistance would result in a transepithelial potential of -0.85 mV ($V_T = R_c$ Isc). It is important to note that this potential difference will be localized to the crypt epithelium, not the surface cells. In rabbit colon it was estimated that the existence of this potential would result in a net K flux equal to $0.09 \ \mu Eq/cm^2$ hr ($2.5 \ \mu A$). Net K secretion across the epithelium was 4 times greater ($0.39 \ \mu Eq/cm^2$ hr) indicating that active K secretion is present in descending colon.[21] Thus, the presence of an uncompensated series resistance will limit the accuracy of transepithelial flux measurements. However, the relative effects of secretagogues and transport inhibitors should not be significantly affected.

MEASUREMENTS OF MEMBRANE Na PERMEABILITY AND PUMP CURRENT

Apical Membrane Na Permeability

To measure Na permeability of the apical membrane, current-voltage relationships can be determined using K-depolarized tissues mounted in Ussing chambers.[22–24] To produce depolarization of the basolateral membrane, the serosal solution is replaced with a high K Ringer solution. The mucosal solution is essentially identical to normal Ringer solution except that K salts are replaced with Na salts when different luminal Na concentrations are required. Near instantaneous current-voltage curves can be recorded as previously described.[22–24] The "shunt" I-V curves are obtained following replacement of all mucosal Na with K and waiting for decay of the resulting outward current transient. Alternatively, amiloride or benzamil can be used to dissect the transcellular Na current from paracellular and diuretic-insensitive components of the total I_{Na}. The I_{Na}-V curve will be obtained from subtraction of the shunt current at a given voltage from those obtained in the presence of normal $[Na]_o$ in the luminal solution. P_{Na} and $[Na]_i$ can then be calculated by fitting the I_{Na}-V curve with the constant field equation[22]:

$$I_{Na} = P_{Na}(F^2 V/RT/1 - \exp(-FV/RT)) [[Na]_o - ([Na]_i \exp(-FV/RT))] \qquad (1)$$

where P_{Na} = apical membrane Na permeability
   $[Na]_o$ and $[Na]_i$ = extracellular and intracellular Na concentrations
   F = Faraday's constant
   V = transmembrane voltage (presumably equal to the transepithelial voltage)
   R = gas constant
   T = absolute temperature

Experiments with toad urinary bladder[25,26] and rabbit descending colon[20,27,28] have shown that the I-V relation is well described by the constant field equation. A non-linear least squares fit of the experimental data using equation #1 will yield an estimate of P_{Na} and $[Na]_i$. An increase in P_{Na} produced by hormonal stimulation for example, is reflected as an increase in slope of the I_{Na}-V plot. Any change in $[Na]_i$ is reflected as a shift in the reversal potential. In previous experiments where this approach was used to study the effects of antidiuretic hormone (ADH) on toad urinary bladder epithelium, a 2 fold increase in P_{Na} was reported.[25] Similar experiments with aldosterone (ALD) treated bladders produced a four fold increase in P_{Na}.[26] This technique has also been applied to studies of Na permeability in rabbit distal colon.[27] In this study I_{Na}-V relationships from basolateral membrane depolarized tissues were compared with I_{Na}-V relationships obtained from experiments where Na current across the apical membrane was plotted as a function of apical membrane voltage (Ψ_a) as determined using conventional microelectrodes (Figure 2). The I_{Na}-V relationships using these two techniques were nearly identical and supports the previously reported observation that the basolateral membrane is primarily K selective[20,21,28] and that high serosal [K] reduces the basolateral membrane voltage to near zero. Under these conditions, the implicit assumption that Ψ_a is equal to the transepithelial PD is reasonable and thus provides direct support for the use of this technique for studies of Na transport across the apical membrane.[22] However, estimates of P_{Na} with K-depolarized tissues were found to be 40% lower than obtained from experiments where microelectrodes were used to directly measure Ψ_a. A possible explanation for this effect is that removal of Na from the

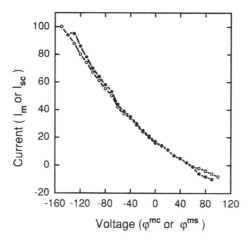

FIGURE 2 Comparison of the I-V relations of the amiloride-sensitive pathway in rabbit descending colon plotted as either the change in Isc as a function of φ^{ms} (transepithelial potential) O, or as I_{Na} vs. φ^{mc} (apical membrane potential) ●. (Reproduced from Thompson et al., *J. Memb. Biol.,* 66, 41, 1982. With permission.)

serosal solution inhibits the activity of Na-Ca exchangers that are known to exist in the basolateral membrane.[29] The consequence is an increase in intracellular calcium that inhibits Na entry across the apical membrane. Thus, it is important to note that K depolarization of the basolateral membrane may produce secondary effects that may affect the accuracy of P_{Na} determinations using this technique.

Errors Associated With K-Depolarized Epithelia

K-depolarized epithelial preparations studied to date maintain active Na transport. This conclusion is inferred from the effects of amiloride, ouabain and metabolic inhibitors on Isc and by the effects of hormones such as ADH and aldosterone to produce stimulation of transcellular Na transport. However, there are some important sources of error that must be considered when using this approach.[30] First of all, incomplete depolarization of the basolateral membrane potential will produce errors in the estimates of apical membrane conductance as well as intracellular Na activity. The actual apical membrane Na conductance ($^{a}g_{Na}$) is related to the measured conductance ($^{m}g_{Na}$) by:

$$(^{a}g_{Na})/(^{m}g_{Na}) = 1 + (R_{bl}/R_{a}) \tag{2}$$

Where: (R_{bl}/R_{a}) = the ratio of basolateral to apical resistance. From previous impedance analysis studies[31,32], (R_{bl}/R_{a}) is at most 1:4 and probably less than 1:10 for tight or moderately tight epithelia. For many experiments this degree of error is acceptable. In contrast, measurement of intracellular Na concentration is more susceptible to error. The existence of a series potential difference (V_{S}) will produce a shift in the measured I-V curve along the voltage axis so that an error in the estimate of reversal potential will occur. The relationship between the actual cell Na concentration ($[^{a}Na_{i}]$) and the measured Na concentration ($[^{m}Na_{i}]$) is:

$$([^{a}Na_{i}])/([^{m}Na_{i}]) = \exp(FV_{s}/RT) \tag{3}$$

Where: R,T and F have their usual meanings. Thus, if $V_{S} = 10$ mV (cell negative with respect to the serosal solution), then $[^{a}Na_{i}]$ will be underestimated by 33%. However, relative changes in $[^{m}Na_{i}]$ will still be qualitatively correct.

In addition to the errors mentioned above, it has been shown in toad bladder epithelia that K depolarization eliminates at least one mechanism for regulation of Na absorption. In this tissue it was observed that in the presence of normal NaCl Ringer solution on the serosal side, a −10 mV voltage step produced a transient Isc overshoot that rapidly decayed to a steady-state level within 10–15 seconds.[33] This overshoot and subsequent decay in Isc was not observed when the serosal solution was replaced with high KCl-sucrose solution. This result implied that Na entry down-regulates the Na permeability of the apical membrane and that this effect is not seen following K-depolarization. The precise nature of this regulatory mechanism is not completely understood. It may involve increases in Ca^{2+} uptake across the basolateral membrane that could reduce apical Na permeability as suggested in the previous section.

Measurement of Pump Current

Pump current can be measured using intact epithelial tissues when the apical membrane resistance to Na and K ions is eliminated with pore-forming antibiotics such as nystatin or amphotericin B.[27,34–36] To perform these experiments, the apical and basolateral surface of the epithelium is bathed with K-methanesulfonic acid Ringer solution, and either amphotericin (10 μM) or nystatin (30 μg/ml) are added to the mucosal solution. This procedure causes the transepithelial PD to depolarize to approximately zero mV. Equal aliquots of NaCl solution are then added to both sides of the tissue to produce a [Na] vs PD concentration-response relationship. From the total epithelial resistance (determined by passing a periodic current pulse of known magnitude across the epithelium and measuring the change in PD) and the transepithelial PD values, the Isc can be calculated from Ohm's law. This protocol can then be repeated in the presence of ouabain (100 μM) using the same tissue so that the ouabain-dependent changes in current can be calculated. A similar series of experiments can be conducted with Na-benzenesulfonate Ringer as the initial solution on both sides of the epithelium.[35] In this case K-methanesulfonate Ringer solution is added back to the tissue to produce a [K] vs PD concentration-response relationship before and after addition of ouabain. From these relationships it is possible to gain information about the Na and K affinities of the ouabain-sensitive current and to demonstrate the dependency of this current on the presence of both ions.[36] Information about the Na:K stoichiometry of the pump can also be obtained with amphotericin permeabilized tissues. In studies with the turtle colon, transepithelial Na and K fluxes were determined along with Isc. The change in net Na flux relative to the change in Isc was then compared to the change in net K flux relative to Isc; the ratio for Na:K was 3.01 to 2.21.[35] This result confirmed the ionic basis for ouabain-dependent current changes produced by amphotericin. The observation that the [Na] vs PD plot shows a sigmoid relationship for both rabbit colon and urinary bladder[28,34] also suggests multiple binding sites for Na and that some cooperativity between binding sites exists.

TRANSMURAL ELECTRICAL STIMULATION OF SUBMUCOSAL NERVES

Stimulation of Submucosal Nerves

Electric transmural stimulation (ETS) of submucosal nerves is most effectively performed on tissues where the muscle layers have been removed by blunt dissection so that a significant portion of submucosa remains associated with the epithelium. Glass slide stripping generally produces a preparation that is poorly responsive to ETS.[10] Tissues are mounted in Ussing chambers as previously described. Rectangular, bipolar pulses of electric current are passed across the epithelium through aluminum foil electrodes that are positioned diagonally on opposite sides of the tissue.[37–39] A stimulator such as the Grass model S-88 connected in series with a stimulus isolation unit (model SIU 5B, Grass Instruments, Quincy, MA) to reduce stimulus artifacts serves well for activating submucosal nerves (300 pulses from 0.5–10 Hz, 5 msec pulse duration). By varying frequency, it is possible to release different types of neurotransmitters.[40] Low frequency stimulation (0.5 Hz) presumably releases non-peptide neurotransmitters, whereas high frequency (10 Hz) stimulation releases peptide and certain classical neurotransmitters.[40] ETS generally produces rapid changes in Isc that quickly return to basal levels.[37–39,41,42] It is important to note that the metabolic activity of submucosal nerves is generally high, so it is important that an adequate supply of glucose (5–10 mM) is provided in the serosal solution for these experiments. For most studies, peak changes in current are recorded and compared to various treatment conditions. However, if detectable changes in duration of the Isc response is observed, it is possible to quantitate the effect by integrating the change in Isc from the beginning of the response to complete recovery so that total charge transfer for that time interval is recorded. In all cases it is important to determine whether tachyphylaxis to successive ETS occurs. If so, it is important that appropriate time control experiments are performed using paired tissues (paired on the basis of conductance and basal Isc within 10–15%) to correct for the decrease in responsiveness of the epithelium (Figure 3).

Identification of Neurotransmitters Released
Following Nerve Stimulation

To verify that the evoked Isc response of the epithelium is due to neurotransmitter release and not to some direct effect of electric stimulation on the epithelium, tissues can be pretreated with tetrodotoxin (TTX, 100 nM) to block neuronal Na channels.[37–42] This serves to inhibit conduction of nerve fiber depolarization to the terminals and attenuates the release of neurotransmitters. The net result is to inhibit the increase in Isc and thus verify that functional nerves within the preparation are required to observe an effect of ETS. Another toxin that is useful for blocking neurotransmitter release from nerve terminals is ω conotoxin (CgTX, 100nM).[43–45] This toxin is known to block N and L class voltage gated calcium channels that appear to be involved in calcium influx and neurotransmitter release at the nerve terminal.[43,44] The effects of these toxins on ETS evoked increases in Isc in porcine distal colon is shown in Figure 4. To prove that TTX or CgTX are not toxic to the epithelium, the effects of glucose or a known secretagogue can be tested to verify that the epithelium is still viable and responsive to nutrient and hormonal stimulation.

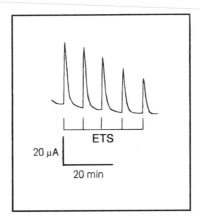

FIGURE 3   Effects of repetitive electric transmural stimulation (ETS) of submucosal nerves in the porcine distal colon epithelium. Note the decrease in Isc amplitude at each point of stimulation. This result indicates tachyphylaxis to repeated exposure of neurotransmitters released by electrical stimulation.

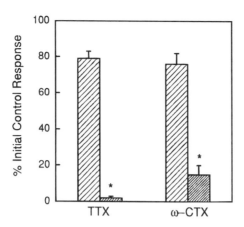

FIGURE 4   Effects of TTX and omega conotoxin on EFS evoked increases in Isc in the porcine distal colon epithelium.

To functionally identify specific neurotransmitters that are released following ETS, two approaches have been used. The first and most commonly used approach is to test various antagonists to specific neurotransmitter receptors that may exist on the epithelium or on neurons that directly innervate epithelial cells. There are several studies that have shown that a significant fraction of the ETS evoked increase in Isc is blocked by atropine and other cholinergic antagonists.[41,42,46] These results imply that acetylcholine is released following ETS and that muscarinic receptors appear to mediate its effects on Isc.[47] Recently, nicotinic receptors presumably located on neuronal cell bodies were also found to play some role in mediating cholinergic responses of the porcine distal jejunum since hexamethonium was shown to produce significant inhibition (about 80%) of the ETS evoked Isc response.[39] The second approach used to identify neurotransmitters following ETS is to pretreat the tissue with the neurotransmitter of interest to induce tachyphylaxis. The tissue is then subjected to a second dose of the transmitter substance to ensure that tachyphylaxis has occurred prior to ETS. Such experiments have been performed using substance P (SP) in porcine intestine. Although tachyphylaxis to SP was achieved, no significant effect on the ETS evoked Isc was observed.[39]

In many species the increase in Isc produced by ETS is presumably due to stimulation of Cl secretion. This conclusion is based on the effects of Cl substitution and on the effects of inhibitors such as furosemide or bumetanide. The simplest interpretation of the results from these studies is that replacement of Cl or treatment with loop diuretic compounds produces inhibition of Cl secretion without altering the response of submucosal nerves to ETS. However it is possible that Cl replacement or the presence of loop diuretics changes the responsiveness of submucosal nerves to electrical stimulation. Thus the decrease in the Isc response may not result from direct inhibition of Cl secretion. The most reliable method for determining the ionic basis of the Isc change is to perform flux measurements. For example, in porcine jejunum it was observed that ETS stimulated net Cl secretion in some tissues while in others there was an increase in Cl absorption with a substantial increase in the residual flux.[39] This observation suggested that the effects of ETS on ion transport may be different depending upon the basal state of the tissue and on the condition of the nerve plexuses that remain associated with the epithelium.

FLUCTUATION ANALYSIS

Properties of the Amiloride Sensitive Na Channel

Previous studies with frog skin,[48–51] toad and rabbit urinary bladder,[14,20] hen coprodeum[52] and turtle colon[53,54] have shown that statistical analysis of the fluctuations in Isc produced by interaction of the diuretic drug amiloride (or related compounds) with Na channels can be used to determine the single channel current (i) and the number (N) of functional channels present in the apical membrane of these tissues. The method assumes a population of channels each behaving independently of the others and existing in only two states: open (p = open probability) or closed (q = 1 − p, denoting the probability of being closed). The total macroscopic current is:

$$I = ipN \tag{4}$$

To induce measurable fluctuations between open and closed states of the channel, an analog of amiloride (CDPC, available from Aldrich Chemical Co.) can be used that allows for measurement of microscopic rate constants with less variability than those previously reported with amiloride.[51,53] This is because CDPC is a relatively weak blocker of Na channels so that it induces clearly identifiable Lorentzian spectra with little inhibition of transepithelial Na transport. In addition CDPC is electroneutral over a wide range of pH, which reduces the effect of membrane potential on the rate coefficients for the blocking reaction.[53] It is assumed that the interaction between CDPC and the Na channel (C_{Na}) follows the model for open channel block represented below:

$$[CDPC] + C_{Na} \overset{k_1}{\underset{k_2}{\rightleftarrows}} [CDPC]\, C_{Na} \tag{5}$$

where k_1 and k_2 are the association and dissociation rate constants respectively and C_{Na} represents the unblocked open channels. If the CDPC concentration greatly exceeds the number of channels $N = (C_{Na} + CDPC\, C_{Na})$, the chemical reaction rate (τ) will be equal to the sum of the association and dissociation rate constants such that:

$$\tau = (k_1\, [CDPC] + k_2)^{-1} \tag{6}$$

At equilibrium, $k_1\, [CDPC]\, [C_{Na}] = k_2\, [CDPC\, C_{Na}]$ so that the probabilities p or q that the channel is open or blocked are respectively:

$$p = [C_{Na}]/N = k_2/(k_1\, [CDPC] + k_2) \tag{7}$$

$$q = [CDPC\, C_{Na}]/N = k_1\, [CDPC]/(k_1\, [CDPC] + k_2) \tag{8}$$

The macroscopic current can now be written as:

$$I = ipN = iNk_2/(k_1\, [CDPC] + k_2) \tag{9}$$

Since the variance (σI^2) in current for a single channel is proportional to the product of p and q, the variance of the fluctuations in macroscopic current for all N channels will be:

$$(\sigma I^2) = Ni^2p - Ni^2p^2 = Ni^2p(1-p) = i^2pq = Iqi = Iik_1[CDPC]/(k_1\, [CDPC] + k_2) \tag{10}$$

Thus the variance of the macroscopic current can be related to the association and dissociation rate constants for CDPC block of the channel. It is possible to determine the chemical reaction rate (τ) by calculating the single sided power density spectrum S(f) of the current fluctuations:

$$S(f) = S_o/[1 + (f/f_c)^2] \tag{11}$$

where f = frequency, S_o = the plateau value of S(f) at low frequencies and f_c = corner frequency which is equivalent to τ but expressed as an angular frequency:

$$f_c = 1/2\pi\tau = 1/2\pi \ (k_1 \ [CDPC] + k_2) \tag{12}$$

The plateau value is proportional to the variance of the current fluctuations (σI^2):

$$S_o = 4iAIk_1[CDPC]/(k_1 \ [CDPC] + k_2)^2 \tag{13}$$

where A = membrane area. Of the three unknowns to be determined, i and N are assumed to be independent of the CDPC concentration while p varies with concentration according to Eq #7. To determine these unknowns the power density spectrum is measured at different CDPC concentrations and S(f) fit to extract the corner frequency and plateau values. This procedure, in effect, gives the rate τ and the variance of the fluctuations (σI^2) at each concentration. Linear regression of $2\pi f_c$ as a function of [CDPC] gives the rate constants k_1 and k_2 as the slope and intercept respectively. Values for i at a given blocker concentration (i_{NaB}) can be calculated using the equation below:

$$i_{NaB} = S_o(2\pi f_c)^2/4Ik_1 \ [CDPC] \tag{14}$$

To obtain i_{Na} and N values in the absence of block, i_{NaB} is plotted as a function of [CDPC] and extrapolated to zero blocker concentration. N is then determined from equation 15:

$$N = I_{Na}/i_{Na} \tag{15}$$

The major advantage of fluctuation analysis is that it provides a non-invasive approach for investigating the properties of ion channels in an intact epithelial preparation. In intestinal epithelia, it has been used to study Na channels in rabbit descending colon,[20] hen coprodeum[52] and cholinergic regulation of Na channels in the turtle colon.[53] In rabbit colon, amiloride decreases Isc with half maximal inhibition at 0.2 μM. Examination of amiloride induced fluctuations in Isc revealed a single time-constant relaxation noise in the power density spectrum. Assuming a pseudo-first order binding reaction between amiloride and the Na channel, the microscopic rate constants were determined from linear regression analysis of $2\pi f_c$ as a function of amiloride concentration as described for CDPC above. The estimated single channel current and channel density were 0.4 pA and 6.1 μm^{-2} respectively at 37°C. When these measurements were conducted at 27°C (to allow comparison of single channel properties with amphibian epithelia) the values of i and N were 0.1 pA and 3.2 μm^{-2} respectively. These estimates of i and N from rabbit colon agree within an order of magnitude with those reported for frog skin and toad urinary bladder. Thus the microscopic properties of Na channels in mammalian colon appear to be very similar to those found in amphibian epithelia.

In turtle colon, fluctuation analysis has been used to investigate the actions of carbachol on transepithelial Na transport using CDPC to induce fluctuations in the Isc.[53] This study showed that carbachol produces a reduction in Na current and channel number by 50% without any change in single channel current. These results imply that muscarinic regulation of Na absorption involves a reduction in the number of open channels in the apical membrane. This decrease could come about by (1) a decrease in open probability of the channel (2) an increase in the rate of channel inactivation or (3) a decrease in the rate of activation which would result in an accumulation of channels in the inactive pool. In general, it is not possible to distinguish between these possibilities using noise measurements. However, in some cases it has been possible to identify changes in open probability. Details of this analysis as applied to Na channels in frog skin can be found in Helman and Baxendale, 1990.[50]

Fluctuation analysis has also been used to examine characteristics of Na channels in hen coprodeum[52] using the amiloride analog triamterene. One of the methodological problems encountered in this study was that continuous oxygenation of the tissue was required to ensure viability but also produced extraneous noise of similar magnitude as those produced by triamterene. To overcome this problem short measurement times (20 sec) were used in which oxygenation of the tissue was eliminated. The low signal to noise ratio required the development of a new method for analyzing power density spectra based on integration of the power density spectrum to eliminate the influence of statistical variations in the difference spectrum. The details of this method can be found in Christensen and Bindslev, 1982.[52] The results of this study showed that the Na site density was 5.8 ± 1.0 μm^{-2} and the site conductance was 4 pS, similar to that reported for Na channels in frog skin.

Characterization of Basolateral K Channels

Fluctuation analysis has been used to investigate the properties of K channels located in the basolateral membrane of rabbit descending colon[20] and turtle colon.[54] In rabbit descending colon, nystatin was used to eliminate apical membrane resistance and as a result, produced a novel Lorentzian component to the power density spectrum. This Lorentzian component was blocked by 4 mM Ba^{2+}. The estimated single channel current was 0.01 pA and N was estimated to be 12 μm^{-2}. In turtle colon, studies with amphotericin treated tissues revealed the existence of a lidocaine sensitive K conductance that was induced in response to cell swelling. Previous single channel studies with lidocaine in turtle colon indicated that its effects were reversible and that it produced a flickery block of swelling induced K channels.[55] Lidocaine was subsequently used for fluctuation analysis experiments assuming a two state model that has been previously used to describe the blockade of Na channels by amiloride. Lidocaine was found to induce a Lorentzian component to the power density spectrum only under conditions where cell swelling was induced, consistent with its actions on the swelling induced K current. The single channel conductance for this channel using single channel recording techniques was 17 pS. Data obtained from fluctuation analysis estimated the conductance to be 20 pS and the number of channels/cm² = 29.7×10^{6}. Hence, the estimated single channel conductance from fluctuation analysis studies agreed well with single channel patch clamp measurements suggesting that the two state model reasonably described the interactions of lidocaine with the channel.

TRANSEPITHELIAL FLUX MEASUREMENTS

Radioisotopic flux studies have been important in establishing the ionic basis for the current changes that occur in response to transport inhibitors and various secretagogues.[11,12,56-64] They also provide a direct means of identifying electroneutral transport pathways that would not otherwise be detected from measurements of Isc.[56-59] Electroneutral processes can contribute significantly to the total solute flux across an epithelium and serve important roles in the regulation of cell volume and intracellular pH. By using flux measurements in combination with pharmacological agents and ion substitution maneuvers, it becomes possible to identify specific transport proteins responsible for the movement of a specific ion and to assess the relative contribution of multiple transport pathways to the total transport of electrolytes across the epithelium.[56-65]

EQUILIBRATION AND UNIDIRECTIONAL FLUX
MEASUREMENTS

Isotope Equilibration and Pairing of Tissues

Tissues can be prepared by either blunt dissection or by using the slide stripping procedure previously described. In general, flux measurements are performed under short circuit conditions with identical solutions on both sides of the tissue to eliminate the electrical and chemical driving forces for paracellular ion movements. Tissues should be allowed to stabilize for 30 minutes prior to the addition of radioisotopes to either the mucosal or serosal side of the tissue. For the measurement of Na or Cl fluxes, a 30-min incubation period is usually required to equilibrate the intracellular pools of these ions. For K (or Rb which in many cases can be substituted for K) this incubation period should be extended to 60 minutes or longer since the concentration of intracellular K is significantly higher than Na or Cl and more time is required to achieve complete equilibration.[60–63] If the intracellular pools are not completely equilibrated prior to the flux measurement, the unidirectional fluxes will underestimate the transcellular movement of isotope. Moreover, the unidirectional fluxes will not remain constant from one flux period to another. This can cause a significant problem in interpreting the effects of various blockers and secretagogues. To determine whether sufficient equilibration time has been allowed, two or three consecutive flux measurements can be made and compared with one another to see if there are any significant changes over time.

Another important issue when performing flux measurements is to be sure that tissues are adequately paired. Tissues are usually paired on the basis of conductance since this determines, to a large extent, the contribution of the paracellular pathway in the movement of isotope across the epithelium. This is most critical for so-called leaky epithelia where most of the isotope crosses the epithelium through the paracellular pathway.[65] In most cases, conductance should not vary by more than 25%. Ideally, this difference should be kept at a minimum to obtain the most accurate results.

Block Flux Measurements

In many situations, a block flux design is sufficient to examine the effects of blockers and regulatory substances on transepithelial ion transport. For these experiments, the first flux period usually serves as a control to establish the basal transport rates of the ion across the epithelium.[57–59] The tissue can then be treated with a hormone or transport inhibitor and a second flux measurement of equal duration performed. The duration of the flux period will depend on the duration of action of the substance under investigation. If the effect of a hormone for example is transient (e.g. < 5 min) it may be difficult to detect significant changes in transcellular isotope movement relative to paracellular ion movements. The net flux across the epithelium can be determined by subtracting the mucosa-to-serosa (M-S) and serosa-to-mucosa (S-M) unidirectional fluxes using paired tissues from the same animal. An example of this type of experiment is presented in Table 1 where the effects of carbachol on Na and Cl fluxes across the porcine distal colon are shown.[58] In this experiment Na and Cl fluxes were measured simultaneously following pretreatment with TTX to eliminate tonic neural activity and to prevent the release of other neurotransmitters by carbachol. This data shows that carbachol significantly decreases the M-S unidirectional fluxes of Na and Cl and increases the S-M unidirectional Cl flux. The net effect is stimulation of Cl secretion as well as increasing the residual flux. The residual flux is calculated from the equation below:

$$J^{Na} - J^{Cl} - I_{sc} = J^{R} \qquad (16)$$

Where J^{Na} and J^{Cl} represent the net fluxes for Na and Cl expressed as current and J^{R} is the residual flux. In this case, the residual flux is that component of the I_{sc} that cannot be accounted for by the net transporrt of Na and Cl. The increase in residual flux shown in table 1 could be explained by either an increase in anion absorption (presumably HCO_3) or by stimulation of cation (presumably K) secretion. Similar effects of carbachol in other intestinal epithelial preparations have been reported.[47,66]

TABLE 1

Effects of 10 μM Serosal Carbamylcholine on Transepithelial Na and Cl Fluxes in Isolated Porcine Distal Colon Under Short Circuit Conditions

					Na Flux			Cl Flux		
Control	n	Isc	J^R	G_t	ms	sm	net	ms	sm	net
Mean	11	0.6	0.0	14.4	9.6	6.0	3.6	11.5	8.5	3.0
±SE		0.2	0.9	1.8	0.8	0.6	1.2	0.4	0.4	0.5
Carbamylcholine										
Mean	11	1.7	2.3*	16.2	8.6*	7.2	1.4	9.9*	12.5*	−2.6*
±SE		0.2	1.1	1.5	0.8	0.8	1.1	0.4	0.9	0.8

Note: Tissues were paired on the basis of transepithelial conductance (Gt within 25%). Units for unidirectional and net fluxes, Isc and J^R are reported as mEq hr^{-1} cm^{-2} and G_t as mS cm^{-2}. All tissues were pretreated with 0.1 μM tetrodotoxin before the equilibration period. (*) signifies $p < 0.05$ compared to control values. Adapted from reference 58.

In some cases it may be useful to include a third or fourth flux period to investigate the effects of transport inhibitors following hormonal stimulation. An example of this type of experiment is shown in Table 2 where the effects of cAMP, norepinephrine and TEA on Rb secretion across the porcine gallbladder epithelium are presented.[65] In this experiment an initial control flux was measured followed by three treatment periods. Addition of 8-Br-cAMP produced an increase in the S-M unidirectional flux and in the net flux indicating stimulation of K secretion. Addition of NE did not significantly affect Rb fluxes but subsequent addition of TEA, a known inhibitor of K channels, to the mucosal solution produced a significant inhibition of

TABLE 2

Effects of cAMP, Norepinephrine (NE), Tetraethylammonium (TEA) on Transepithelial Rubidium (^{86}Rb) Fluxes across Isolated Gallbladder Epithelium (Fundus Region) Under Short-Circuit Conditions

			Rb Flux			
Control	n	ms	sm	net	Isc	G_t
Mean	5	0.24	1.38	−1.14	4.31	14
±SE		0.04	0.15	0.17	0.40	1
cAMP	n	ms	sm	net	Isc	G_t
Mean	5	0.28	2.39*	−2.12*	7.19*	16*
±SE		0.03	0.24	0.25	0.67	1
NE	n	ms	sm	net	Isc	G_t
Mean	5	0.23	2.04*	−1.18*	5.10	13
±SE		0.06	0.07	0.09	0.55	1
TEA	n	ms	sm	net	Isc	G_t
Mean	5	0.38*	1.83	−0.72*	5.44*	13
±SE		0.08	0.12	0.12	0.49	1

Note: Tissues were paired on the basis of conductance (G_t within 20%). Units for Isc and unidirectional and net fluxes are reported as mEq hr^{-1} cm^{-2}, G_t values are mS cm^{-2}. (*) signfies $p < 0.05$ compared to control values. Adapted from reference 65.

the S-M and net Rb flux compared to control levels. This experiment clearly demonstrates that cAMP induced Rb secretion is mediated by TEA sensitive pathways located in the apical membrane. It is worth noting that these flux experiments require statistical analysis involving multiple comparisons which is not true of two period flux experiments described above. This issue is addressed in the next section.

CONTROL STUDIES AND STATISTICAL ANALYSIS

Time Controls and Elimination of Tonic Regulatory Activity

Parallel time control flux measurements should be performed on paired tissues (for both 2 and 3 period flux experiments) to ensure that the basal transport rates do not spontaneously change over time. This is also important to ensure that complete equilibration of the tissue with isotope has occurred prior to flux measurements. To determine whether the actions of a regulatory substance or blocker is acting through submucosal nerves or through cyclooxygenase or lipoxygenase products, it is often useful to pretreat the tissue with TTX and indomethacin or 5,8,11,14-eicosatetraynoic acid (ETYA) to eliminate indirect effects. TTX, as mentioned earlier, is known to block nerve conduction and inhibit tonic and evoked release of neurotransmitters from submucosal nerves.[47,57–59] Indomethacin is known to block cyclooxygenase activity and thus inhibits prostaglandin synthesis. ETYA also effects arachidonic acid metabolism by inhibiting both cyclooxygenase and lipoxygenase activity.[58,59] Pretreatment of the tissue with these inhibitors will help to eliminate tonic release neurotransmitter substances or inflammatory mediators and in some cases provide a more consistent baseline for determining the direct actions of regulatory substances and transport inhibitors on the epithelium.

Statistical Analysis of Flux Data

A paired two-tailed "t" test is usually used for analysis of two period flux experiments. However, the "t" test is not sufficient for multiple comparisons required for analysis of a three period flux design. If the treatment periods of the flux are only compared with a common control measurement, then Dunnett's test is appropriate. However, if multiple comparisons are to be made between treatment conditions as well as the control condition, then Dunnett's test is not appropriate and Duncan's multiple range test should be used.[39,57,59,65] The level of significance for most studies is usually set at $p < 0.05$.

EXPERIMENTS WITH ISOLATED CRYPTS

Isolated crypts provide a useful preparation for characterizing the functional properties of different cell types that exist within intestinal epithelia. These structures retain their ability to transport solute and continue to proliferate under culture conditions. By using microelectrode and fluorescence imaging techniques, it is possible to resolve differences in the responsiveness of various cells types to inhibitors of transport proteins and to regulatory compounds.

ISOLATION OF SINGLE CRYPTS

Micro-Dissection

Individual crypts can be isolated from stripped colonic mucosa by micro-dissection using fine forceps and a fine dissecting needle.[67] The submucosal muscle layers are stripped from the epithelium using a glass microscope slide. Then, with the aid of a dissecting microscope, the mucosa is cut into small pieces using a fine dissecting needle. As the tissue is pulled apart, individual crypts become visible and partially isolated from the surrounding tissue. Using a fine pair of forceps it is possible to free the crypt from the remaining tissue and transfer the isolated crypt into a collecting dish using a pasture pipette. To avoid adhesion of the crypt to dissecting instruments or pipette glass, it is helpful to dip the instruments and pipette in Ringer solution containing 5% bovine serum albumin. To facilitate adherence of the crypts to the culture dish, the dishes can be coated with ether poly-L-lysine (5mg/ml) or with a thin coat of Matrigel. In general, the crypts maintain their crypt-like appearance in culture for approximately 24–36 hours. Crypts isolated from porcine distal colon attach to Matrigel coated dishes for microelectrode experiments within 12–15 hours while still retaining their crypt-like structure. After this time, the cells migrate away from the blind end of the crypt and begin to form a monolayer (Figure 5). In most cases a complete monolayer is not formed and the cells detach from the plate in about 4–6 days.

Mucosa Vibration

Intact crypts can also be isolated from colonic mucosa using a modification of the intestinal cell isolation procedure described by Bjerknes and Cheng.[9] Initially, the epithelium is stripped from the submucosa using a glass microscope slide as described above. The mucosa is then fixed onto a plastic holder using tissue adhesive (histoacryl blue, Braun-Melsungen, Melsungen FRG), transferred into Ca^{2+}-free Ringer solution containing 0.1% bovine serum albumin and gassed with $95\%O_2/5\%CO_2$ ($37°C$). After a 15-min incubation period, the holder is then vibrated (Vibromixer El, Chemap AG, Switzerland) once for 30 seconds. This procedure results in the isolation of intact crypts which can then attach to poly-L-lysine (5 mg/ml) coated slides. This technique allows for the isolation of large numbers of intact crypts that can be used for biochemical studies or for electrophysiological experiments.

ELECTROPHYSIOLOGICAL AND FLUORESCENCE IMAGING STUDIES WITH ISOLATED CRYPTS

Conventional Microelectrode Studies

The crypt is known to be the site of intestinal electrolyte and fluid secretion.[68] Recently, conventional microelectrodes were used to investigate the effects of vasoactive intestinal peptide (VIP) and carbachol (CCH) on membrane potential of micro-dissected crypts from rabbit colon. Initial studies by Biagi et al.[69] showed that isolated crypts bathed in rabbit Ringer solution ($37°C$) have a mean basolateral membrane potential of -67 mV. Addition of either VIP (10^{-10} M) or aminophylline produced prolonged (> 5 minutes) depolarizations (approximately 40 mV) of the basolateral membrane. This effect was not altered by TTX. CCH produced no significant change in membrane potential when added alone to VIP responsive cells. In a subsequent study by Greenwald and Biagi,[70] treatment of crypts with CCH following addition of VIP resulted in a rapid hyperpolarization of the basolateral membrane. This effect is consistent with CCH dependent activation of basolateral K channels. Preliminary experiments with micro-dissected porcine colonic crypts also show large, prolonged depolarizations of the basolateral membrane produced by VIP (Figure 6).[71] Moreover, addition of CCH alone caused a transient decrease in membrane potential in the absence of VIP. This effect was inconsistent with the notion that CCH increases basolateral K permeability and may indicate a reduction in basolateral K conductance. These results suggest that there may be some important species differences with respect to the regulation of ion transport by various secretagogues.

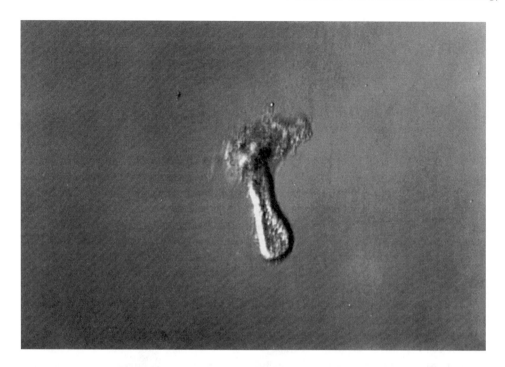

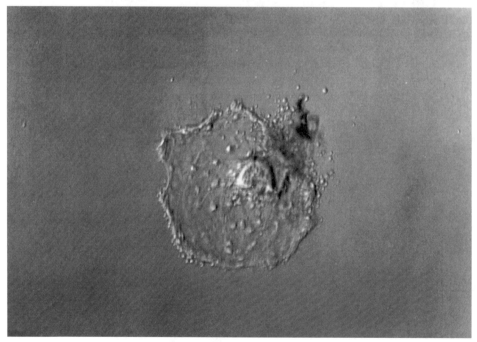

FIGURE 5   Isolated crypt from the porcine distal colon epithelium obtained by the micro-dissection technique (top). Following 24–48 hours in culture, the crypt cells migrate away from the initial point of attachment and begin to form a monolayer (bottom).

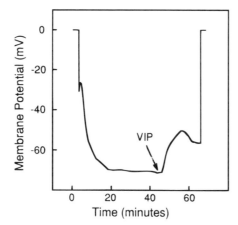

FIGURE 6 Effects of vasolactive intestinal peptide (VIP) on the basolateral membrane potential of a crypt cell following isolation of the intact colonic crypt. Note that VIP produces a prolonged depolarization of the membrane with a time course that is similar to its effects on Isc. This depolarization presumably results from activation of Cl channels located in the apical membrane.

Identification and Characterization of Cl Channels from Patch Clamp Experiments

The mucosal vibration technique has been previously used to prepare rat colonic crypts for study using single channel patch clamp recording techniques.[72] Following attachment to a poly-L-lysine coated slide, crypts were washed with Ringer solution containing 3 mM DTT to facilitate gigaohm seal formation to the basolateral membrane. The inside-out patch configuration was used to investigate the properties of Cl channels present in the basolateral membrane. From 28 patches, 5 contained Cl channels. These channels possessed linear current-voltage relationships with a slope conductance of 29 pS. They were blocked with anthracene-9-carboxylic acid and were not permeable to gluconate. The channels were similar to those found in the apical membrane of cells located near the surface of the crypt. This finding suggested the possibility that calcium removal may have sufficiently disrupted the tight junction during crypt isolation so that the apical channels may have migrated into the basolateral membrane of these cells. An alternative explanation is that Cl channels located in the basolateral membrane are physiologically important in transcellular Cl absorption or volume regulation.

Measurement of Secretagogue Induced Cl Permeability Changes in Isolated Crypts

Individual crypts, micro-dissected from the intact rabbit epithelium using the procedure outlined above, have been used to investigate the effects of PGE_2 and epinephrine on Cl permeability of crypt cells.[67] Following isolation, crypts were transferred to poly-lysine coated coverslips and placed into a perfusion chamber mounted onto the stage of an inverted microscope equipped for fluorescence imaging studies. They were then loaded with the halide sensitive dye 6-methoxy-N-[3-sulfopropylquinolinium] (SPQ) to determine intracellular Cl concentration and to assess changes in anion permeability across cell membranes. Hypotonic shock was used to load SPQ into crypt cells. This involved exposing the isolated crypts to a 5mM SPQ solution made using 50% NaCl Ringer solution for 5 minutes and then thoroughly washing away the excess dye. Experiments to investigate Cl permeability were performed after 10 minutes following return to standard NaCl Ringer solution. Images of the crypts included the lower three-quarters of the crypt since the neck region often curved out of the focal plane. Distinct cell boundaries were not observed presumably due to the narrow intercellular spaces. Flow of anions across the cell membrane prior to and following stimulation of secretion was assessed by replacement of Cl with Br, I or gluconate. PGE_2 and epinephrine produced transient decreases in cell [Cl] in approximately 50% of the crypt cells. Following stimulation with PGE_2 and epinephrine, Cl efflux and Br efflux were increased only in cells that that exhibited the decrease in cell [Cl] at the onset of stimulation. The fall in cell [Cl] is presumably due to the opening of Cl channels in response to secretagogue stimulation. The subsequent return of fluorescence intensity towards resting levels reflects an increase in Cl uptake presumably mediated by Na-K-2Cl cotransport activity and perhaps $Cl-HCO_3$ exchange. These results would suggest that activation of Cl secretion occurs sequentially where electrogenic Cl efflux precedes electroneutral uptake. The consequence of sequential activation of conductive and coupled transport mechanisms is an initial decrease in Cl concentration that will increase the driving force for Cl entry and reduce Cl exit from the cell. The results of this study also showed that the time course of fluorescence change induced by gluconate perfusion was different for PGE_2 and epinephrine. The prolonged increase in fluorescence during epinephrine stimulation suggested that the decrease in cell [Cl] was greater following epinephrine stimulation compared to PGE_2. This effect may result from the fact that PGE_2 stimulated Cl efflux across the apical membrane may be attenuated by accumulation of Cl in the lumen of the crypt, whereas epinephrine induced Cl efflux across the basolateral membrane is essentially unrestricted. It is also possible that a regulatory mechanism may exist that limits Cl efflux in response to PGE_2 stimulation. In summary, fluorescent imaging experiments with SPQ have shown that specific cell types within the crypt respond to secretagogue stimulation and that the time course of the fluorescence changes suggest sequential rather than simultaneous activation of Cl efflux and influx pathways.

SUMMARY AND CONCLUSIONS

The objective of this review was to discuss some of the *in vitro* techniques that have been used to investigate properties and regulation of electrolyte transport across intact epithelial preparations. These techniques have been important in establishing our present understanding of the mechanisms and control of epithelial transport function. They have demonstrated that epithelial tissues are remarkably complex, particularly in regard to the interactions that occur between different cell types (including submucosal nerves, enteroendocrine cells and associated immune cells). Knowledge of these interactions is essential for predicting the behavior of epithelial tissues under *in vivo* conditions. Moreover, results using these approaches should provide a useful context in which to interpret future data regarding molecular structure and detailed functional properties of specific transport proteins and receptor molecules involved in transepithelial electrolyte transport.

REFERENCES

1. **Altenberg, G., Copello, J., Cotton, C., Dawson, K., Segal, Y., Wehner, F. and Reuss, L.,** Electrophysiological methods for studying ion and water transport in Necturus gallbladder epithelium, *Methods in Enzymol.,* 192, 650, 1990.
2. **Reuss, L.,** Ion transport across gallbladder epithelium. *Physiol. Rev.,* 69, 503, 1989.
3. **Levis, R. A. and Rae, J. L.,** Constructing a patch clamp setup, *Methods in Enzymol.,* 207, 14, 1992.
4. **Rae, J. L. and Levis, R. A.,** Glass technology for patch clamp electrodes, *Methods in Enzymol.,* 207, 66, 1992.
5. **Koefoed-Johnson, V. and Ussing, H. H.,** The nature of the frog skin potential, *Acta Physiol. Scand.,* 42, 298, 1958.

6. **Dawson, D. C.,** Ion channels and colonic salt transport, *Annu. Rev. Physiol.,* 53, 321, 1991.
7. **Sullivan, S. K. and Field, M.,** Ion transport across mammalian small intestine, in *The Gastrointestinal System IV,* Schultz, S. G., Field, M. and Frizzell, R. A., Eds., American Physiological Society, New York, 287, 1991.
8. **Halm, D. R. and Frizzell, R. A.,** Ion transport across the large intestine, in *The Gastrointestinal System IV,* Schultz, S. G., Field, M. and Frizzell, R. A., Eds., American Physiological Society, New York, 257, 1991.
9. **Bjerknes, M. and Cheng, H.,** Methods for isolation of intact epithelium from the mouse intestine, *Anat. Rec.,* 199, 565, 1981.
10. **Bridges, R. J., Rack, M., Rummel, W. and Schreiner, J.,** Mucosal plexus and electrolyte transport across the rat colonic mucosa, *J. Physiol.,* 376, 531, 1986.
11. **Field, M., Fromm, D. and McColl, I.,** Ion transport in rabbit ileal mucosa: I. Na and Cl fluxes and short circuit current, *Am. J. Physiol.,* 220, 1388, 1971.
12. **Field, M.,** Ion transport in rabbit ileal mucosa II. Effects of cyclic 3′, 5′-AMP, *Am. J. Physiol.,* 221 992, 1971.
13. **Andres, H., Bock, R., Bridges, R. J., Rummel, W. and Schreiner, J.,** Submucosal plexus and electrolyte transport across rat colonic mucosa, *J. Physiol.,* 364, 301, 1985.
14. **Lewis, S. A., Ifshin, M. S., Loo, D. D. F. and Diamond, J. M.,** Studies of sodium channels in rabbit urinary bladder by noise analysis, *J. Memb. Biol.,* 80, 135, 1984.
15. **Zweibaum, A., Laburthe, M., Grasset, E. and Louvard, D.,** Use of cultured cell lines in studies of intestinal cell differentiation and function, in *The Gastrointestinal System IV,* Schultz, S. G., Field, M. and Frizzell, R. A., Eds., American Physiological Society, New York, 223, 1991.
16. **Dharmsathaphorn, K., Mandel, G., McRoberts, J. A., Tisdale, L. D. and Masui, H.,** A human colonic tumor cell line that maintains vectorial electrolyte transport. *Am. J. Physiol.,* 246, G204, 1984.
17. **Cereijido, M., Robbins, E. S., Dolan, W. J., Rotunno, C. A., Sabatini, D. D.,** Polarized monolayers formed by epithelial cells on a permeable and translucent support, *J. Cell Biol.,* 77, 853, 1978.
18. **Handler, J. S., Steele, R. E., Sahib, M. K., Wade, J. B., Preston, A. S., Laweson, N. L. and Johnson J. P.,** Toad urinary bladder epithelial cells in culture: Maintenance of epithelial structure, sodium transport and response to hormones, *Proc. Natl. Acad. Sci. USA,* 76, 4151, 1979.
19. **McCabe, R. D. and Dharmsathaphorn, K.,** Mechanism of VIP stimulated chloride secretion by intestinal epithelial cells, in *Vasoavtive Intestinal Peptides and Related Peptides.,* Said, S. I. and Mutt, V., Eds., New York Acad. Sci. 527, 326, 1988.
20. **Wills, N. K.,** Mechanisms of ion transport by the mammalian colon revealed by frequency domain analysis techniques, in *Current Topics in Membranes and Transport,* Wade, J. B. and Lewis, S. A. Eds., vol. 20, 61, 1984.
21. **Wills, N. J. and Biagi, B.,** Active potassium transport by rabbit descending colon epithelium, *J. Memb. Biol.,* 64, 195, 1982.
22. **Fuchs, W., Larsen, E. H. and Lindemann, B.,** Current-voltage curve of sodium channels and concentration dependence of sodium permeability in frog skin, *J. Physiol.,* 267, 137, 1977.
23. **Palmer, L. G., Edelman, I. S. and Lindemann B.,** Current-voltage analysis of apical Na transport in toad urinary bladder: Effects of inhibitors of transport and metabolism. *J. Memb. Biol.,* 57, 59, 1980.
24. **Palmer, L. G.,** Voltage-dependent block by amiloride and other monovalent cations of apical sodium channels in the toad urinary bladder, *J. Memb. Biol.,* 80, 153, 1984.
25. **Palmer, L. G., Lindemann B. and Edelman, I. S.,** Aldosterone control of the density of sodium channels in the toad urinary bladder, *J. Memb. Biol.,* 64, 91, 1982.
26. **Jack, H. Y., Palmer, L. G., Lindemann B. and Edelman, I. S.,** Role of sodium channel density in the natriferic response of the toad urinary bladder to an antidiuretic hormone, *J. Memb. Biol.,* 64, 77, 1982.
27. **Thompson S. M., Suzuki, Y., and Schultz, S. G.,** The electrophysiology of rabbit decending colon, *J. Memb. Biol.,* 66, 41, 1982.
28. **Wills, N. K. Lewis, S. A. and Eaton, D. C.,** Active and passive properties of rabbit descending colon: A microelectrode and nystatin study. *J. Memb. Biol.,* 45, 81, 1979.

29. **Taylor, A. and Windhager, E. E.,** Possible role of cytosolic calcium and Na-Ca exchange in regulation of transepithelial Na transport, *Am. J. Physiol.,* 236, F505, 1979.

30. **Palmer, L. G.,** Use of K depolarization to study apical transport properties in epithelia, in *Current Topics in Membranes and Transport,* Wade, J. B. and Lewis, S. A., Eds., vol. 20, 61, 1984.

31. **Clausen, C.,** Membrane area changes associated with proton secretion in turtle urinary bladder studied using imOpedence analysis techniques, in *Current Topics in Membranes and Transport,* Wade, J. B. and Lewis, S. A., Eds., vol. 20, 47, 1984.

32. **Clausen, C. and Wills, N. K.,** Impedence analysis in epithelia, in *Ion Transport by Epithelia: Recent Advances,* ed., Schultz, S. G., Raven Press, New York, 79, 1981.

33. **Weinstein, F. C., Posowski, J. J., Peterson, K., Delalic, Z. and Civan, M. M.,** Relationship of transient electrical properties to active Na transport by toad urinary bladder, *J. Memb. Biol.,* 52, 25, 1980.

34. **Lewis, S. A., Wills, N. K. and Eaton, D. C.,** Basolateral membrane potential of a tight epithelium: Ionic diffusion and electrogenic pumps, *J. Memb. Biol.,* 41, 81, 1979.

35. **Kirk, K. L., Halm, D. R. and Dawson, D. C.,** Active sodium transport by turtle colon via an electrogenic Na-K exchange pump, *Nature,* 287, 237, 1980.

36. **Halm, D. R., Dawson, D. C.,** Cation activation of the basolateral sodium-potassium pump in turtle colon, *J. Gen. Physiol.,* 82, 315, 1983.

37. **Hubel, K. A.,** The effects of electrical field stimulation and tetrodotoxin on ion transport bny the isolated rabbit ileum. *J. Clin Invest.,* 62, 1039, 1978.

38. **Hubel, K. A., and Shirazi, S.,** Human ileal ion transport *in vitro:* Changes with electrical field stimulation and tetrodotoxin, *Gastroenterology,* 83, 63, 1982.

39. **Hindebrand, K. R. and Brown, D. R.,** Intrinsic neuroregulation of ion transport in porcine distal jejunum, *J. Pharmacol. Exp. Ther.,* 255, 285, 1990.

40. **Bartfai T., Inverfeldt, K. and Fisone, G.,** Regulation of the release of coexisting neurotransmitters, *Ann. Rev. Pharmacol. Toxicol.,* 28, 285, 1988.

41. **Carey, H. V., Cooke, H. J. and Zafirova, M.,** Mucosal responses evoked by stimulation of ganglion cell somas in the submucosal plexus of the guinea pig ileum, *J. Physiol.,* 364, 69, 1985.

42. **Cooke, H. J.,** Influence of enteric cholinergic neurons on mucosal transport in guinea pig ileum, *Am. J. Physiol.,* 246, G263, 1984.

43. **Feldman, D. H., Olivera, B. M. and Yoshikami, D.,** Omega Conus geographus toxin: a peptide that blocks calcium channels, *FEBS Lett.,* 214, 295, 1987.

44. **Allescher, H. D., Willis, S., Schusdziarra, V. and Classen, M.,** Omega conotoxin GVIA speciffically blocks neuronal mechanisms in rat ileum, *Neuropeptides,* 13, 253, 1989.

45. **Perdue, M. H. and Davison, J. S.,** Response of jejunal mucosa to electrical transmural stimulation and two neurotoxins, *Am. J. Physiol.,* 251, G642, 1986.

46. **Diener, M., Knobloch, S. F., Bridges, R. J., Keilmann, T, and Rummel, W.,** Cholinergic-mediated secretion in the rat colon: neuronal and epithelial muscarinic responses, *Eur. J. Pharmacol.,* 168, 219, 1989.

47. **Zimmermann, T. W. and Binder, H. J.,** Effect of tetrodotoxin on cholinergic agonist-mediated colonic electrolyte transport, *Am. J. Physiol.,* 244, G386, 1983.

48. **Lindemann, B.,** Fluctuation analysis of sodium channels in epithelia, *Ann. Rev. Physiol.,* 46, 497, 1984.

49. **Hoshiko, T.,** Fluctuation analysis of apical sodium transport, in *Current Topics in Membranes and Transport,* Wade, J. B. and Lewis, S. A., Eds., vol. 20, 3, 1984.

50. **Helman, S. I. and Baxendale, L. M.,** Blocker related changes of channel density: analysis of a 3-state model for apical Na channels of frog skin, *J. Gen. Physiol.,* 95, 647, 1990.

51. **Els, W. J. and Helman, S. I.,** Activation of epithelial Na channels by hormonal and autoregulatory mechanisms of actions, *J. Gen. Physiol.,* 98, 1197, 1991.

52. **Christensen, O. and Bindslev, N.,** Fluctuation analysis of short-circuit current in a warm-blooded sodium-retaining epithelium: site current, density, and interaction with triamterine, *J. Memb. Biol.,* 65, 19, 1982.

53. **Wilkinson, D. J. and Dawson, D. C.,** Cholinergic modulation of apical Na channels in turtle colon: analysis of CDPC-induced fluctuations, *Am. J. Physiol.,* 259, C668, 1990.

54. **Dawson, D. C., Van Driessche, W. and Helman, S. I.,** Osmotically induced basolateral K conductance in turtle colon: lidocaine-induced K channel noise, *Am J. Physiol.,* 254, C165, 1988.
55. **Germann, W. J., Lowy, M. E., Ernst, S. A. and Dawson, D. C.,** Differentiation of two distinct K conductances in the basolateral membrane of turtle colon, *J. Gen. Physiol.,* 88, 237, 1986.
56. **Binder, H. J. and Foster, E. S., Budinger, M. E. and Hayslett, M. S.,** Mechanism of electroneutral sodium chloride absorption in distal colon of the rat, *Gastroenterology,* 93, 441, 1987.
57. **Traynor, T. R. and O'Grady, S. M.,** Mechanisms of Na and Cl absorption across the distal colon epithelium of the pig, *J. Comp. Physiol.,* 162, 47, 1992.
58. **Traynor, T. R., Brown, D. R. and O'Grady, S. M.,** Regulation of ion transport in porcine distal colon: effects of putative neurotransmitters, *Gastroenterology,* 100, 703, 1991.
59. **Traynor, T. R. and O'Grady, S. M.,** Brain natriuretic peptide stimulates K and Cl secretion across the porcine distal colon epithelium, *Am. J. Physiol.,* 260, C750, 1991.
60. **McCabe, R. D. and Smith, P. L. and Sullivan, L. P.,** Ion transport by rabbit descending colon: mechanisms of transepithelial K transport, *Am. J. Physiol.* 246, G594, 1984.
61. **Smith, P. L. and McCabe, R. D.,** Potassium secretion by rabbit descending colon: effects of adrenergic stimuli, *Am. J. Physiol.,* 250, G432, 1986.
62. **Halm, D. R. and Frizzell, R. A.,** Active K transport across rabbit distal colon: relation to Na absorption and Cl secretion, *Am. J. Physiol.,* 251, C252, 1986.
63. **McCabe, R. D. and Smith, P. L.,** Colonic potassium and chloride secretion: role of cAMP and calcium, *Am. J. Physiol.,* 248, G103, 1985.
64. **Sullivan, S. K. and Smith, P. L.,** Active potassium secretion by rabbit proximal colon, *Am. J. Physiol.,* 250, G475, 1986.
65. **DuVall, M. D. and O'Grady, S. M.,** Regulation of K secretion across the porcine gallbladder epithelium, *Am. J. Physiol.,* 264, C1542, 1993.
66. **Brown, D. R. and Miller, R. J.,** Neurohumoral control of fluid and electrolyte transport by the intestinal mucosa, in *The Gastrointestinal System IV,* Schultz, S. G., Field, M. and Frizzell, R. A., Eds., American Physiological Society, New York, 527, 1991.
67. **Halm, D. R., Kirk, K. L. and Sathiakumar, K. C.,** Stimulation of Cl permeability in colonic crypts of Lieberkuhn measured with a fluorescent indicator, *Am. J. Physiol.,* 265, G1, 1993.
68. **Welsh, M. J., Smith, P. L., Fromm, M. and Frizzell, R. A.,** Crypts are the site of intestinal fluid and electrolyte secretion, *Science,* 218, 1219, 1982.
69. **Biagi, B. A., Wang, Y. Z. and Cooke, H. J.,** Effects of tetrodotoxin on chloide secretion in rabbit distal colon: tissue and cellular studies, *Am. J. Physiol.,* 258, G223, 1990.
70. **Greenwald, L. and Biagi, B. A.,** Interaction between charbachol and vasoactive intestinal peptide in cells of isolated colonic crypts, *Am. J. Physiol.,* 262, G940, 1992.
71. **Traynor, T. R. and O'Grady, S. M.,** Control of electrolyte secretion in isolated crypts from porcine colon, *FASEB J.,* 7, 579, 1993.
72. **Diener, M., Rummel, W., Mestres, P. and Lindemann, B.,** Single chloride channels in colon mucosa and isolated colonic enterocytes of the rat, *J. Memb. Biol.,* 108, 21, 1989.

6 Criteria for Defining Enteric Neurotransmitters

Charles H. V. Hoyle and Geoffrey Burnstock

INTRODUCTION

Following the development of the theory of chemical transmission from concept to fact, it became necessary to lay down some ground rules for defining chemical neurotransmitters, and these evolved into the criteria for chemical transmission, including that in the myenteric plexus. In an early review, Werman[1] emphasized that the fundamental criterion for identification of a neurotransmitter is: the identity of action criterion. In other words, in an experimental situation, application of a putative transmitter substance should produce the same effect as the physiological transmitter. He also warned against the production of barriers to understanding due to the blithe acceptance of a set of rules, and a too narrow interpretation of them.

The criteria that have become widely accepted, and minor variations of which are most often quoted,[2–4] are based on those set out by Paton[5] in 1958, and a few years later by Eccles:[6] 1) the presynaptic neuron synthesizes and stores the transmitter; 2) the transmitter is released in a calcium-dependent manner; 3) there should be a mechanism for terminating the activity of the transmitter, either by enzymatic degradation or by cellular uptake; 4) local exogenous application of the transmitter substance should mimic its endogenous activity; 5) agents that block or potentiate the endogenous activity of the transmitter should also affect its exogenous application in the same way.

Some have found these criteria too restrictive for practical purposes,[7–10] and aside from adenosine-5′-triphosphate (ATP) and 5-hydroxytryptamine (5-HT, serotonin) they tend not to have been applied rigorously to non-classical transmitter candidates.[4]

Before going on to consider the classical criteria of neurotransmitters in more detail, it is necessary to discuss two developments in the field of neuroscience that will come to bear on the definition of a transmitter, namely cotransmission and neuromodulation. The phenomenon of cotransmission,[8–15] whereby a neuron utilizes a plurality of transmitters, is extant in both the peripheral and central nervous systems. In nearly all the cases examined, where it has been established that a population of neurons uses more than one transmitter substance, the transmitters involved have distinct temporal and frequency-dependent characteristics.[15] For example, in the sympathetic supply to the vas deferens ATP and noradrenaline act as cotransmitters, with ATP being responsible for an initial transient contraction, and noradrenaline causing a more latent, and more sustained contraction.[16–19] Furthermore, at low frequencies of stimulation the contractile responses may be purely purinergic, while at high frequencies of stimulation the adrenergic component predominates. The situation is similar in many other sympathetically innervated organs, such as blood vessels and seminal vesicles,[13,14,20–29] and cotransmission with other combinations of transmitter substances occurs in other autonomically innervated organs,[8,10–13,15] and also in the peripheral terminals of sensorimotor neurons.[8,10,12,30] In all divisions of the peripheral nervous system; in the enteric nervous system *par excellence;* fibers and cell bodies

0-8493-8304-8/96/$0.00+$.50

have been shown to contain several neuropeptides, which are putative transmitters.[12,15,31,32] In many cases the term "putative" still applies because the functions of the coexisting substances have not been identified. In some cases a coexisting neuropeptide functions as a neuromodulator as opposed to being a true transmitter; there is an important distinction to be made between the two.

In general terms, in line with the Identity of Action Criterion,[1] a neurotransmitter has an observable action, causing a direct effect on a postsynaptic or postjunctional cell whereas a neuromodulator is a substance that modulates the action of a primary transmitter. This action could occur at a presynaptic site, where it could cause an increase or decrease in the amount of transmitter released, or at a postsynaptic site, where it can enhance or diminish the effect of the transmitter, perhaps by altering the affinity of the postsynaptic transmitter-receptor, or by interfering with the transmitter clearance or degradation mechanisms.

Neuromodulators can be humoral agents, such as circulating hormones, or they can be neural agents, themselves released from nerve terminals. It is in this latter case that there is an important distinction to be made between a neurosecretion being a primary transmitter, which obeys all the neurotransmitter criteria, and a modulator, which may also appear to fulfil the neurotransmitter criteria, except that *its action is only manifest when there is a process of primary neurotransmission occurring.* For example, in some blood vessels neuropeptide Y (NPY) is found in sympathetic nerves that utilize ATP and noradrenaline as cotransmitters: exogenous NPY, on its own, has no observable effect on the tone of the vascular wall, but it potentiates the vasoconstrictor responses to exogenous noradrenaline, and to the adrenergic component of sympathetic nerve stimulation.[33–38] As another example, in the vas deferens, where NPY is also contained in sympathetic nerve terminals that utilize ATP and noradrenaline, the effects of NPY are concentration-dependent: application of low concentrations potentiate exogenous noradrenaline and the adrenergic component of neural stimulation; application of higher concentrations that do not have a direct effect on the smooth muscle itself cause a prejunctional inhibition of adrenergic transmission.[39–41] Thus, in these examples, although NPY is released from nerve terminals, and in other respects may fulfil the transmitter criteria, its lack of direct action prevents it from being classified as a primary transmitter. Instead it should be classified as a neuromodulator. However, the term "neuromodulator" encompasses a broad spectrum of compounds that are not necessarily released from nerves; it is important to pay attention to the context, or to use a qualifying term, thus: a *neuromodulatory transmitter* is a substance, released from neurons whose action is only manifest when another process of neurotransmission is occurring; a *humoral neuromodulator* is a substance that arises from a site remote from the site of neurotransmission that it modulates. In this chapter the term "transmitter" in the absence of any specific context or qualification will be taken to mean either a primary neurotransmitter or a neuromodulator transmitter. Also, the terms "synapse" and "synaptic" will be used in a general sense, and unless otherwise stated can be taken to mean "junction" and "junctional" as well.

In addition to releasing neurotransmitters, neurons may also release trophic factors. The essential difference between a trophic factor and a neurotransmitter is the time-course of their action. Whereas neurotransmission is a rapid process, in which a response may last for a number of milliseconds, seconds, or in more extreme cases, minutes; trophic responses may well be unobservable in the short term, requiring hours or days to become manifest. There is comparatively little information about the synthesis, storage and release of trophic factors from enteric neurones; thus trophic factors will not be considered in this chapter. However, the subject of growth factors in the enteric nervous system has recently been reviewed.[42]

Two further advances in neuroscience (both detailed below) that also call for a re-examination of the classic neurotransmitter criteria are, firstly, the realization that physiological or pathophysiological release of neurotransmitter is not necessarily calcium-dependent (reviews[43,44]), and secondly, the discovery that chemicals like the free radical of nitric oxide (NO) (reviews[45–51]) or perhaps even carbon monoxide (CO)[52,53] can function as neurotransmitters in many divisions of the nervous system, including the enteric nervous system.

The aims of this chapter are to examine the classical criteria of a neurotransmitter in a contemporaneous context, and to discuss whether or not they are still applicable given the advances in our understanding of chemical transmission processes. At the end of this chapter we present our revised definitions of them. Because neurotransmission is such a general principle, although the enteric nervous system and techniques relevant to its study are emphasized, models of transmission in regions outside the gastrointestinal tract are also presented.

SYNTHESIS AND STORAGE OF NEUROTRANSMITTERS

One of the original classical criteria was that a neuron must synthesize its transmitter,[5] and implicit in this is that the synthetic enzymes must be present in the neuron. Some authors who have addressed this question go as far to say that the transmitter must be contained within synaptic vesicles.[6,54] Taken at face value this would be an eminently suitable suggestion.

Synaptic vesicles (see review by Gabella[55]) have two main attributes: their size and their electron density. Small vesicles are up to 60–70 nm in diameter, those with greater diameters, but usually less than 120 nm, are called "large". Small agranular vesicles (with electron-lucent cores) are typically found in cholinergic nerve terminals, whether peripheral or central, autonomic or somatic, where they contain acetylcholine (ACh). Small granular vesicles (with electron-dense cores) are typically found in sympathetic nerve terminals and contain noradrenaline. Both adrenergic and cholinergic synaptic vesicles also contain ATP.[56–74] Small vesicles, granular or agranular, are possibly formed from recycled membranes of exocytosed large vesicles,[75–77] but the relationship between large and small granular vesicles in the same nerve fiber is not fully understood.

Large vesicles formed in the cell body, where they bud off from the Golgi apparatus, are transported down the axon on a microtubular system. Large adrenergic vesicles contain various neuropeptides[72,78] in addition to noradrenaline, but they also contain non-transmitter substances such as chromogranins,[79] which are involved in the packaging process, and dopamine β-hydroxylase (DBH) which converts dopamine to noradrenaline. Neuropeptides are not found in the small vesicles, only the large ones, and their range includes vasoactive intestinal polypeptide (VIP), NPY, enkephalins, endorphins and tachykinins.

The ultrastructural features of myenteric neurons (i.e. neurons in Auerbach's plexus), viewed electronmicroscopically, have been examined in detail, and several different populations of neurons, based on attributes such as cyton size and organelle distribution have been defined.[80] Based on attributes of the vesicles, including size, shape, electron density, and number, eight morphologically distinct types of axon have also been defined, along with two further types that were thought to represent different physiological conditions.[80] The fact that nerve terminals contain distinctive populations of transmitter vesicles, and that vesicles of several different shapes and sizes can be observed provides indications that neurons utilize several transmitters, and contain combinations of transmitters in various proportions. To date, nearly two dozen substances have been proposed to be neurotransmitters or neuromodulatory transmitters in the enteric nervous system (Table 1), approximately half of which have been shown to satisfy at least four of the classical criteria, with the remainder satisfying fewer than four of the criteria.[32,81–84]

Despite the fact that many neurotransmitters are stored within vesicles there are several questions that remain to be asked. Are all transmitter substances always stored within vesicles? Is it necessary for a transmitter to be stored within a vesicle in order to be released? Is it necessary for the transmitter to be synthesized within the neuron that releases it?

Not even classical transmitter substances are always packaged into vesicles. They may be present in the cytosol of nerve terminals, and be released from this cytosolic pool rather than

TABLE 1

Neurotransmitters and Neuromodulatory Transmitters in the Enteric Nervous System

* Acetylcholine (ACh)
* Adenosine 5′-triphosphate (ATP)
  Angiotensin
  Calcitonin gene-related peptide (CGRP)
  Carbon monoxide (CO)
  Dopamine
  Dynorphin
* Enkephalins
  Endorphins
  Galanin
* Gamma-aminobutyrate (GABA)
  Gastrin/cholecystokinin (CCK)
* 5-Hydroxytryptamine (5-HT, serotonin)
  Neurotensin
* Nitric oxide (NO)
* Noradrenaline (NA, norepinephrine)
  Pancreatic polypeptide
  Peptide histidine isoleucine (PHI)
  Somatostatin
* Substance P
* Vasoactive intestinal polypeptide (VIP)

Note: Substances flagged with an asterisk (*) have been shown to satisfy the transmitter criteria, and are generally accepted to be *bona fide* neurotransmitters or neuromodulatory transmitters. The remaining substances, have not yet been shown to satisfy all the criteria.

from vesicles.[43,44] Synaptic vesicles contain energy- and ion-dependent transporter proteins in their membranes[44,72,74,85,86] (see below), and these transporter proteins can become inserted into the presynaptic membrane of the nerve terminal, where they remain unless recycled into new synaptic vesicles. The orientation of these transporters is such that if, under normal operating conditions, they carried a transmitter into the vesicle, when inserted into the neurolemma they would carry the transmitter out of the nerve terminal,[44] and into the synaptic cleft.

Many transmitter substances such as ACh, noradrenaline, γ-aminobutyrate (GABA), glutamate and ATP exist at high concentrations in neuronal cytosol.[43,44,68,74,87–90] However, it should be borne in mind that while a vesicular storage system is specific for cells with a specialized secretory function, cytosolic "storage" is common to many types of cells, including glial, smooth muscle and endothelial cells.

The appreciation that neurons do not need to store transmitter substances within vesicles is exemplified by retinal horizontal cells. These cells are a type of interneuron, but in many species they do not contain synaptic vesicles: they synthesize their transmitter, GABA, and can accumulate it via a specific transporter protein, and can release it in a controlled fashion into the synaptic cleft, all without the aid of vesicular packaging.[44,88]

For some transmitter substances a vesicular storage mechanism is neither appropriate nor necessary. The synthetic enzyme of NO, NO-synthase (NOS) is constitutively present in neuronal cytosol in perikarya and neurites.[45,46,48,51,91–100] The enzyme is soluble and does not appear to be compartmentalized: it converts L-arginine to L-citrulline with the concomitant production of NO. NO readily diffuses through cell membranes, thus it could not be retained by a synaptic vesicle. Further, because of its transcellular mobility it does not require an exocytotic or a carrier-mediated release mechanism. Despite being atypical in this respect, it is synthesized and released by neurons, and is widely regarded as a neurotransmitter in the central (reviews[46,48,50,51,91,101–103]) and peripheral nervous system, including the enteric nervous system (reviews[47,103–105]).

Can a neuron utilize a substance as a transmitter that it has not synthesized or does not synthesize? It has been known for a long time that neurons can take up substances and incorporate them into synaptic vesicles or into a cytosolic pool, and ultimately release them in the manner of a neurotransmitter: so-called "false transmitters". False transmitters can develop as the result of certain therapeutic interventions, pathological or even physiological conditions.

In the condition of hepatic encephalopathy abnormal tyrosine metabolism results in excess production of octopamine, which can be handled by adrenergic nerves as if it were noradrenaline. Because octopamine is transported into synaptic vesicles in competition with, and at the expense of, noradrenaline, when adrenergic transmission is invoked it is not as effective as it should be, because, at the postsynaptic site, octopamine is neither as potent nor as efficacious as the noradrenaline that it has displaced.

In the gastrointestinal tract, 5-HT has been shown to be taken up and released as a function of nerve stimulation by the sympathetic innervation of the mesenteric arterial system.[106] In the normal isolated mesenteric vascular bed pressor responses evoked by periarterial nerve stimulation are predominantly (80–90%) adrenergic, the residual component is probably purinergic.[23,29,107] The uptake of [^{3}H]-5-HT into these sympathetic nerves is prevented by fluoxetine (a 5-HT uptake inhibitor) or cocaine (an amine uptake inhibitor), and its release is prevented by tetrodotoxin, guanethidine or calcium-free conditions.[106] In preparations where the pressor response has been reduced to its minimum by phentolamine, but in which the sympathetic nerves are otherwise functional, incubation with 5-HT causes a restoration of the pressor responses to nerve stimulation. These responses are reduced to control levels by 5-HT-receptor antagonists.[106] Fluoxetine and cocaine, both inhibiting 5-HT uptake, prevent this restorative action of 5-HT. Thus 5-HT can be taken up by these mesenteric sympathetic nerves, and can be effectively employed as a neurotransmitter; furthermore, it has also been suggested that it is utilized in this way physiologically to contribute to the maintenance of local vascular tone.[106]

CALCIUM-DEPENDENT RELEASE

Of all the criteria this is often the most easily tested, and may often be used as the only criterion. The basis of this criterion is that neurosecretory exocytosis, the mechanism by which transmitter vesicles empty their contents into the synaptic cleft, requires elevated levels of intracellular Ca^{2+}. This arises as a consequence of the opening of voltage-dependent Ca^{2+}-channels during the action potential as it invades the nerve terminal; the ensuing Ca^{2+}-entry initiates exocytosis, resulting in the fusion of transmitter vesicles with the neurolemma, and release of their contents into the extracellular space.[108–110] Functional and morphological studies indicate that release of transmitter from both small and large vesicles is Ca^{2+}-dependent.[76,111–113] There may be some functional differences between the mechanics of small and large vesicular exocytosis: small vesicles only seem to release their contents at specialized active zones of the nerve fiber, from terminals or terminal varicosities, whereas large vesicles may be able to fuse with any region of the neuronal membrane, be it dendrite, cell body, axon or terminal.[111–114] Furthermore, although elevation of cytosolic Ca^{2+} is essential for triggering release via exocytosis, the release mechanism can terminate even though intracellular Ca^{2+}-levels remain high.[115]

Although NO is not stored in nerve terminals its release is calcium-dependent, or rather its synthesis is. The constitutive NOS found in neurons needs to be bound to calmodulin to be fully active: the binding of calmodulin to NOS is reversible. Calmodulin itself is induced to bind NOS when it is activated by and bound to Ca^{2+}.[92,116,117] This occurs when the cytosolic levels of Ca^{2+} rise above 400 nM, such as during action potential discharge. Thus, although the release mechanism of NO is not controlled by action potential discharge and consequently Ca^{2+}, its synthesis, and therefore indirectly its release, is finely controlled in this way.

Considerable evidence has accumulated that transmitters can be released independently of an elevation of intracellular Ca^{2+}-levels (reviews[43,44]). Whether or not this is a truly physiological mechanism is still subject of investigation. The transmitters that are released in this way are "stored" free in the cytoplasm rather than in vesicles, and they are carried out of the cell by transporter proteins. These carriers are probably the same ones that are responsible for the transmitter uptake, and that can reverse their direction under certain conditions.[44] For example, GABA released from central neurons by a Ca^{2+}-dependent vesicular release mechanism has its action terminated by carrier mediated transport into glial cells and local neurons.[118,119] The energy for the uptake is derived from a chemiosmotic symport with Na^+ and Cl^-. The stoichiometry is $2Na^+:Cl^-:GABA$, thus the transport of GABA is electrogenic, carrying a net positive charge. The carrier can reverse its operation if there is an elevation in intracellular Na^+, or depolarization, and sufficient levels of cytosolic GABA.[74,120–124] In retinal horizontal cells that lack synaptic vesicles GABA release via this type of reversed uptake is very possibly physiological,[44] and the results from a study on rat forebrain growth cones also indicate that this is a physiological mechanism of GABA release.[125]

In the peripheral nervous system, noradrenaline has been shown to be released from a cytoplasmic compartment of cardiac sympathetic nerves during ischemic or cytotoxic hypoxia, in a calcium-independent manner.[126–130] The same compartment may be mobilized by cardiac glycosides such as digitalis.[131] Interestingly, NPY contained in large synaptic vesicles in adrenergic nerves does not appear to be able to be released by a non-exocytotic process.[132]

Synaptosomal preparations of the guinea-pig myenteric plexus, made by homogenizing isolated segments of small intestine that contain the myenteric plexus, followed by several steps of centrifugation to result in a pellet that essentially contains pinched-off nerve terminals together with their complement of synaptic vesicles, have been used to examine Ca^{2+}-dependent transmitter release. Many transmitter substances, including ACh, ATP, GABA and noradrenaline, have been shown to be released from such preparations.[133–138] However, evidence has been obtained from synaptosomes that transmitter release in the myenteric plexus may not always be Ca^{2+}-dependent. The release of ACh due to certain stimuli may, indeed, be independent of extracellular calcium ions.[139]

Using the more simple preparation of superfused isolated intestinal segments, in which the myenteric neurons can be electrically stimulated, and the superfusate subsequently analysed for putative transmitter content, Ca^{2+}-independent release of VIP has been demonstrated.[140] The actual release mechanism has not yet been determined, and questions such as whether or not VIP exists in a non-vesicular compartment, or whether there is a transporter for VIP remain to be answered. However, in some ways the release of VIP from enteric nerve terminals is known to be atypical, in that although it is released following neuronal activation[141–143] it does not appear to be released when neurons are depolarized by K^+.[140,144] Depolarization of nerve cells by applied K^+ is well known to evoke release of neurotransmitters.

There are several practical problems associated with the determination of transmitter release. One of these is in ensuring that the applied stimulus is effective, and a second one is whether the released transmitter is stable enough to allow it to be measured. The release of many transmitters is frequency-dependent or time-dependent (see reviews[15,32,73,133,145]), i.e. they may be released only at high frequencies of nerve stimulation, or after a relatively long time. In studies using intracellular microelectrodes to record membrane potential, in myenteric ganglia low stimulation frequencies (1 Hz) applied to presynaptic nerve terminals evoke only fast transient depolarizations, so-called fast excitatory synaptic potentials (f.e.p.s.ps), in the postsynaptic cell: this is due to released ACh acting on nicotinic receptors. At high frequencies

(10 Hz) there is also a latent, slow depolarization, the slow excitatory postsynaptic potential (s.e.p.s.p), which is due to a non-cholinergic transmitter. The release of this non-cholinergic transmitter is frequency-dependent since it is not manifest at low frequencies of stimulation.[146] Another example is the release of opioid peptides from the myenteric plexus, and this may only be evident following application of high stimulation frequencies, or when the stimulus has been applied for a long time.[147,148] Similarly, the release of substance P, which can be evoked by reflex activity or electrical stimulation, is dependent on its neurons firing at a relatively high frequency.[149–153]

Measuring the transmitter content of superfusates passed over isolated tissues, or of venous effluent from organs *in situ,* has proven to be useful in release studies of many substances (for example[32,73,81,140,154]). In some tissues and organs, if the rate of release is low and the rate of degradation or clearance is high, the transmitter substance may be undetectable in a sample of perfusate or venous outflow. Nevertheless, the transmitter may be shown to be functioning, and therefore released, by a pharmacological manipulation such as the application of a receptor antagonist causing a loss of response. Nitric oxide is a free radical with a very short biological half-life, of the order of seconds, making it difficult or impossible to identify its presence in a collected sample of perfusate. However, techniques have been developed that allow it to be determined, one of which is a bioassay.[155–158] An isolated section of donor tissue, in which NO is suspected to be a transmitter, is superfused in such a way that the effluent perfusate immediately passes over a segment of an isolated blood vessel (in particular, endothelium denuded rabbit aorta). In this cascade system electrical stimulation of the donor tissue evokes a response both in that tissue and in the recipient blood vessel. Because the effect of NO on the blood vessel has been defined, pharmacological manipulation of the responses (potentiation by L-arginine or superoxide dismutase; inhibition by hemoglobin) can confirm that NO is indeed being released in the donor tissue. This system works because of the proximity of the recipient to the donor tissue, allowing only a short period of time between NO release in the donor tissue and its potential activity in the recipient tissue, which is not long enough for too much of the NO to be inactivated. Using this assay method NO release has been shown in isolated strips of gastric fundus and ileocolonic sphincter.[155–158]

INACTIVATION OF NEUROTRANSMITTERS

As all physiological signal molecules or ions have some way of being inactivated, either by enzymic degradation, or by removal from the system by an active or a passive mechanism, should "transmitter inactivation" be given the status of a criterion?

This criterion that a transmitter must be degraded by extracellular enzymes, or taken up into either pre- or post-synaptic cells was established because the process of chemical neurotransmission needs to be actively terminated for it to be a finely controlled process. In essence this criterion is still upheld. Regardless of whether or not a transmitter is synthesized and stored in a neuron, and regardless of whether or not its release is calcium-dependent, a transmitter still needs to be inactivated.

This seems to be true for all transmitter substances, although in the case of many neuropeptides the inactivation mechanisms are not completely known. One slight exception is ATP, whose main degradation product is adenosine, which is still biologically active, but which can be removed rapidly from the synaptic region by uptake systems.

Acetylcholine is rendered inactive by acetylcholinesterase (AChE), found ubiquitously on the extracellular surface of many types of cell, and found within the cytosol of many types of nerves that are not necessarily cholinergic. AChE cleaves ACh into acetate and choline: the choline is recovered by an active uptake process into the nerve terminal, where it is re-synthesized into ACh by the enzyme choline acetyltransferase (ChAT); the acetate elutes into the blood stream. Noradrenaline and other amine transmitters such as glutamate, glycine, GABA and 5-HT are removed from the synaptic cleft by active transport processes mediated by fairly specific carriers. If taken up by neurons they can be re-utilized as transmitters, either being re-packaged into transmitter vesicles, or entering the cytosolic releasable pool. If taken up by non-neuronal cells such as glial or smooth muscle cells they may be catabolized by specific enzymes.

Neuropeptides are not known to be carried back into nerve terminals, but some may be internalized after binding to the receptor on the postsynaptic cell, and subsequently metabolized.[159–161] They are most likely hydrolysed into inactive components by non-specific peptidases or proteases such as endopeptidases, aminopeptidases or peptidyl peptidase (also known as angiotensin converting enzyme; ACE).[145]

For ATP the situation is different. Its sequential dephosphorylation be ectoenzymes yields ADP, AMP and adenosine. The conversion to adenosine is the rate limiting step, performed by $5'$-nucleotidase. Adenosine is transported via a nucleoside carrier into neurons and non-neuronal cells, where it may be catabolized by adenosine deaminase, or phosphorylated by the action of kinases to produce adenine nucleotides, preponderantly ATP.

The rapid hydrolysis of ATP often makes it difficult to determine whether it is acting *per se* or whether its activity is due to the formation of adenosine.[73,162] There are few unequivocal examples of adenosine being derived from neurally released ATP having a physiological action. In the rabbit pulmonary artery ATP is a cotransmitter with noradrenaline from sympathetic nerves.[163] In this vessel adenosine acts on theophylline-sensitive presynaptic P_1-purinoceptors to cause inhibition of transmitter release. Theophylline alone enhances the transmitter release, indicating that there is an "adenosine tone" present, and it has been suggested that this adenosine is derived from the neuronally released ATP.[163]

Nitric oxide does not have any need of an uptake mechanism, but it is rendered inactive by interaction with superoxide radicals, resulting in the formation of nitrites and nitrates.

MIMICRY AND ANTAGONISM

The criteria that exogenous application of a transmitter substance should mimic the action of endogenous transmitter release, and that application of a drug that affects the response of the exogenous agent should affect the endogenous transmitter in the same way, are pharmacological rather than physiological. As such they are secondary rather than primary criteria, and although they are superficially straightforward, in practice they can often cause problems.

Firstly, some differences between exogenous and endogenous application need to be appreciated. In the normal process of transmission, a high concentration of transmitter is delivered to a restricted area in a very short period of time. When a substance is applied exogenously, it may be applied at a physiological concentration, but in many experimental situations it is difficult to apply it to an appropriately restricted area, and because it usually has to diffuse a far greater distance, maybe through several layers of tissue, the rate of increase in concentration at the transmitter receptors is not as great. Thus, very often application of the transmitter substance does not mimic neurotransmission.

As mentioned earlier with respect to determination of transmitter release, a similar problem with mimicry may be the presence of degrading enzymes, or of powerful uptake mechanisms, which may be present in cells remote from the site of transmission as well as at the site of transmission, allowing exogenously applied substances to reach their receptors only at very low concentrations. In the central nervous system it is often very difficult to mimic the effects of ACh unless AChE has been blocked. Similarly, in the central nervous system applied ATP is rapidly degraded by ectoenzymes to adenosine, and in very few places has applied ATP been shown to have an action mediated via it own receptors, rather than adenosine receptors.[162,164–166] The inherent instability of the transmitter substance can also be a problem: this is exemplified by NO, with its half-life of seconds in physiological solutions.

A second problem is that the physiological process may well be cotransmission involving more than one transmitter, or a transmitter coupled with a neuromodulatory transmitter: thus two (or more) substances would need to be applied in order to mimic the true physiological response. The behavior of the transmitter receptors can also mean that the response to exogenous application is not the same as that which occurs during transmission. Several types of receptors undergo rapid desensitization or tachyphylaxis. Their kinetics are such that the response to a relatively slow increase in transmitter concentration is not the same as the response to the relatively rapid increase that occurs during transmission. To some extent experimental techniques have been developed to overcome this problem, but in many tissues it may be insurmountable.

As far as antagonism goes, perhaps the greatest drawback is the lack of available antagonists. Obviously the discovery of putative transmitters precedes the development of their antagonists. For ACh, noradrenaline, 5-HT, glutamate, GABA, dopamine, and some of the neuropeptides useful antagonists that may be specific or selective for subtypes of their receptors have been available for a long time. For ATP the situation is improving with the recent discoveries of the antagonistic properties of suramin and pyridoxalphosphate-6-azophenyl-2',4'-disulphonic acid (PPADS).[73,167–170] However, for many of the neuropeptides the range of antagonists is extremely limited. The situation concerning NO is somewhat different because it has no extracellular receptor. However, there are some powerful pharmacological manipulations that can be used. The synthetic enzyme of NO, NOS requires L-arginine as a substrate, and analogs of L-arginine can compete with the substrate binding site, and inhibit NO production (reviews[46–48,50,51,91,101–105]). In its target cell NO binds to the heme moiety of soluble guanylate cyclase, resulting in the synthesis of cyclic GMP (cGMP). Compounds such as methylene blue, which inhibits guanylate cyclase, and phosphodiesterase antagonists, which block the enzyme that metabolizes cGMP, have been used to produce a parallel effect on applied NO and neural transmission.[104,171–174] Further, because it is a free radical, agents such as hemoglobin and hydroquinone, which can inactivate free radicals, have also been used to produce a simultaneous inhibition of response to applied NO and the neurotransmission process.[175–179]

Nature, in her wisdom, lays down many principles, but she also provides many variations: although the original transmitter criteria were well founded on scientific principles, the many variations make them difficult to accept wholly. We have seen that neurotransmitters are not necessarily synthesized in neurons (e.g. 5-HT), nor are they necessarily stored in synaptic vesicles (e.g. glutamate in retinal horizontal cells), nor even stored at all (NO), nor is their release necessarily calcium-dependent (e.g. carrier-mediated release). The criterion of inactivation still holds good, although it is worth pointing out that all transmitter-like substances have a termination mechanism of some sort: in order to contextualize inactivation within the process of neurotransmission, it would be necessary to state that the inactivation mechanism has to be local to the site of transmission. The pharmacological manipulations of mimicry and antagonism cannot be regarded as criteria that define a neurotransmitter, they are criteria that can be applied in the experimental investigation of transmitters substances. Nevertheless, they are still valid, given the limitations that may be imposed by the experimental technique itself, the method of application of the transmitter substance, or the quality of the pharmacological tools.

Neurotransmission is a finely controlled process wherever it occurs: for classical transmission and for transmission by NO intracellular Ca^{2+} is the physiological regulator, entering the cell during action potential discharge. For physiological carrier-mediated transmission the mechanism that causes the depolarization that stimulates the export of transmitter is controlled, but in pathophysiological conditions this process may be initiated, but it is essentially unregulated.

CONCLUSIONS AND REVISED CRITERIA

In conclusion, based on the arguments provided above the transmitter criteria can be divided into primary and secondary groups. The primary criteria (1–3 below) relate to the physiological attributes of the transmitter substance, and the secondary criteria (4 and 5 below) relate to the pharmacological attributes.

REVISED CRITERIA FOR MYENTERIC NEUROTRANSMITTERS

1. The neuron must synthesize the transmitter. Synthesis can occur in the cell body, or in the nerve cell processes, or in the nerve terminals. Storage may be transient, synthesis being initiated with activity. It could be argued that false transmitters, i.e. those taken up and released for physiological actions can be included, even though they are not synthesized in the neuron from which they are released.
2. A transmitter must be released from the nerve. Transmitter release is usually, but not always, calcium-dependent.
3. Mechanisms for terminating transmitter activity, either enzymatically or by uptake, or by a combination of both, must be present locally.
4. Local application of the transmitter should mimic the nerve-mediated response, but some variations due to neuromodulatory mechanisms or receptor distribution need to be taken into account. Specialized extracellular receptors and specific intracellular sites of action are both acceptable.
5. Parallel effects of drugs that block or potentiate the response to nerve stimulation, by acting at a postsynaptic site, and exogenous application of the transmitter substance must occur.

ACKNOWLEDGMENTS

Dr. Jill Lincoln, Department of Anatomy, UCL, is thanked for her helpful discussion during the preparation of this article.

REFERENCES

1. **Werman, R.,** Criteria for identification of a central nervous system transmitter, *Comparative Biochemistry and Physiology,* 18, 745, 1966.
2. **McLennan, H.,** *Synaptic Transmission,* 2nd Ed., W. B. Saunders, Philadelphia, 1970.
3. **Mountcastle, V. B. and Sastre, A.,** Synaptic transmission, in *Medical Physiology,* 14th Edition, Mountcastle, V. B., Ed., CV Mosby, St. Louis, 1980, 184.
4. **Burnstock, G.,** Neurotransmitters and trophic factors in the autonomic nervous system, *Journal of Physiology,* 313, 1, 1981.
5. **Paton, W. D. M.,** Central and synaptic transmission in the nervous system (pharmacological aspects), *Annual Reviews of Physiology,* 20, 431, 1958.
6. **Eccles, J. C.,** *The Physiology of Synapses,* Academic Press, New York, 1964,
7. **Potter, D. D., Furshpan, E. J., and Landis, S. C.,** Multiple-transmitter status and "Dale's principle," *Neuroscience Comment,* 1, 1, 1981.
8. **Campbell, G.,** Cotransmission, *Annual Reviews of Pharmacology and Toxicology,* 27, 51, 1987.
9. **Furness, J. B., Morris, J. L., Gibbins, I. L., and Costa, M.,** Chemical coding of neurons and plurichemical transmission, *Annual Reviews of Pharmacology and Toxicology,* 29, 289, 1989.
10. **Kupfermann, I.,** Functional studies of cotransmission, *Physiological Reviews,* 71, 683, 1991.
11. **Burnstock, G.,** Do some nerve cells release more than one transmitter? *Neuroscience,* 1, 239, 1976.
12. **Burnstock, G.,** Innervation of bladder and bowel, *Ciba. Found. Symp.,* 151, 2, 1990.
13. **Burnstock, G.,** Co-Transmission: the fifth Heyman's memorial lecture, *Arch. Int. Pharmacodyn. Ther.,* 304, 7, 1990.

14. **Burnstock, G.,** Noradrenaline and ATP as cotransmitters in sympathetic nerves, *Neurochemistry International,* 17, 357, 1990.

15. **Morris, J. L. and Gibbins, I. L.,** Co-transmission and neuromodulation, in *Autonomic Neuroeffector Mechanisms,* Burnstock, G. and Hoyle, C. H. V., Eds., Harwood Academic Publishers, Chur, 1992, 33.

16. **Fedan, J. S., Hogaboom, G. K., O'Donnell, J. P., Coloby, J., and Westfall, D. P.,** Contribution by purines to the neurogenic response of the vas deferens of the guinea-pig, *Eur. J. Pharmacol.,* 69, 41, 1981.

17. **Sneddon, P. and Westfall, D. P.,** Pharmacological evidence that adenosine triphosphate and noradrenaline are co-transmitters in the guinea-pig vas deferens, *Journal of Physiology,* 347, 561, 1984.

18. **Allcorn, R. J., Cunnane, T. C., and Kirkpatrick, K.,** Actions of α, β-methylene ATP and 6-hydroxydopamine on the sympathetic neurotransmission in the vas deferens of the guinea-pig, rat and mouse: support for co-transmission, *British Journal of Pharmacology,* 89, 647, 1985.

19. **Kirkpatrick, K. and Burnstock, G.,** Sympathetic nerve-mediated release of ATP from the guinea-pig vas deferens is unaffected by reserpine, *Eur. J. Pharmacol.,* 138, 207, 1987.

20. **Nakanishi, H. and Takeda, H.,** The possible role of adenosine triphosphate in chemical transmission between the hypogastric nerve terminal and seminal vesicle in the guinea-pig, *Japanese Journal of Physiology,* 23, 479, 1973.

21. **Cheung, D. W.,** Two components in the cellular response of rat tail arteries to nerve stimulation, *Journal of Physiology,* 328, 461, 1981.

22. **Muramatsu, I., Fujiwara, M., Miura, A., and Sakakibara, Y.,** Possible involvement of adenine nucleotides in sympathetic neuroeffector mechanisms of dog basilar artery, *J. Pharmacol. Exp. Ther.,* 216, 401, 1981.

23. **Kügelgen, I. V. and Starke, K.,** Noradrenaline and adenosine triphosphate as co-transmitters of neurogenic vasoconstriction in rabbit mesenteric artery, *Journal of Physiology,* 367, 435, 1985.

24. **Meldrum, L. A. and Burnstock, G.,** Evidence that ATP is involved as a co-transmitter in the hypogastric nerve supplying the seminal vesicle of the guinea-pig, *European Journal of Pharmacology,* 110, 363, 1985.

25. **Sneddon, P. and Burnstock, G.,** ATP as a co-transmitter in rat tail artery, *European Journal of Pharmacology,* 106, 149, 1985.

26. **Cheung, D. W. and Fujioka, M.,** Inhibition of the excitatory junction potential in the guinea-pig saphenous artery by ANAPP$_3$, *British Journal of Pharmacology,* 89, 3, 1986.

27. **Muramatsu, I. and Kigoshi, S.,** Purinergic and non-purinergic innervation in the cerebral arteries of the dog, *British Journal of Pharmacology,* 92, 901, 1987.

28. **Warland, J. J. I. and Burnstock, G.,** Effects of reserpine and 6-hydroxydopamine on the adrenergic and purinergic components of the sympathetic nerve responses of the rabbit saphenous artery, *British Journal of Pharmacology,* 92, 871, 1987.

29. **Nagao, T. and Suzuki, H.,** Effects of α, β-methylene ATP on electrical responses produced by ATP and nerve stimulation in smooth muscle cells of the guinea-pig mesenteric artery, *General Pharmacology,* 19, 799, 1988.

30. **Maggi, C. A.,** The dual, sensory and "efferent" function of the capsaicin-sensitive primary sensory neurons in the urinary bladder and urethra, in *Nervous Control of the Urogenital System,* Maggi, C. A., Ed., Harwood Academic Publishers, Chur, 1993, 383.

31. **Furness, J. B. and Costa, M.,** *The Enteric Nervous System,* Churchill Livingstone, Edinburgh, 1987.

32. **Furness, J. B. and Costa, M.,** Identification of transmitters of functionally defined enteric neruons, in *Handbook of Physiology, Section 6: The Gastrointestinal System, Vol. 1,* Wood, J. D., Ed., American Physiological Society, Bethesda, 1989, 387.

33. **Dahlof, C., Dahlof, P., and Lundberg, J. M.,** Neuropeptide Y (NPY)-enhancement of blood pressure increase upon α-adrenoceptor activation and direct pressor effects in pithed rats, *European Journal of Pharmacology,* 109, 289, 1985.

34. **Abel, P. W. and Han, C.,** Effects of neuropeptide Y on contraction, relaxation, and membrane potential of rabbit cerebral arteries, *Journal of Cardiovascular Pharmacology,* 13, 52, 1989.

35. **Andriantsitohaina, R. and Stoclet, J. C.,** Potentiation by neuropeptide Y of vasoconstriction in rat resistance arteries, *British Journal of Pharmacology,* 95, 419, 1988.

36. **Revington, M. and McCloskey, D. I.,** Neuropeptide Y and control of vascular resistance in skeletal muscle, *Regulatory Peptides,* 23, 331, 1988.

37. **Nield, T. O.,** Actions of neuropeptide Y on innervated and denervated rat tail arteries, *Journal of Physiology,* 386, 19, 1987.

38. **Saville, V. L., Maynard, K. I., and Burnstock, G.,** Neuropeptide Y potentiates purinergic as well as adrenergic responses of the rabbit ear artery, *European Journal of Pharmacology,* 176, 117, 1990.

39. **Lundberg, J. M, Terenius, L., Hökfelt, T., Martling, C. R., Tatemoto, K., Mutt, V., Polak, J., Bloom, S. R., and Goldstein, M.,** Neuropeptide Y (NPY)-like immunoreactivity in peripheral noradrenergic neurons and effects of NPY on sympathetic function, *Acta Physiologica Scandinavica,* 116, 477, 1982.

40. **Lundberg, J. M. and Stjarne, L.,** Neuropeptide Y (NPY) depresses the secretion of ^{3}H-noradrenaline and the contractile responses evoked by field stimulation, in the rat vas deferens, *Acta Physiologica Scandinavica,* 120, 477, 1984.

41. **Stjarne, L., Lundberg, J. M., and Astrand, P.,** Neuropeptide Y—a co-transmitter with noradrenaline and adenosine 5'-triphosphate in the sympathetic nerves of the mouse vas deferens? A biochemical, pharmacological and electropharmacological study, *Neuroscience,* 18, 151, 1986.

42. **Saffrey, M. J. and Burnstock, G.,** Growth factors and the development and plasticity of the enteric nervous system, *Journal of the Autonomic Nervous System,* 49, 183, 1994.

43. **Adam-Vizi, V.,** External Ca^{2+}-independent release of neurotransmitters, *J. Neurochem.,* 58, 395, 1992.

44. **Attwell, D., Barbour, B., and Szatkowski, M.,** Nonvesicular release of neurotransmitter, *Neuron,* 11, 401, 1993.

45. **Moncada, S., Palmer, R. M. J., and Higgs, E. A.,** Nitric oxide: physiology, pathophysiology, and pharmacology, *Physiological Reviews,* 43, 109, 1991.

46. **Lowenstein, C. J. and Snyder, S. H.,** Nitric oxide, a novel biological messenger, *Cell,* 70, 705, 1992.

47. **Sanders, K. M. and Ward, S. M.,** Nitric oxide as a mediator of nonadrenergic noncholinergic neurotransmission, *American Journal of Physiology,* 262, G379, 1992.

48. **Snyder, S. H.,** Nitric oxide: first in a new class of neurotransmitters? *Science,* 257, 494, 1992.

49. **Vincent, S. R. and Hope, B. T.,** Neurons that say NO, *Trends in Neuroscience,* 15, 108, 1992.

50. **Garthwaite, J.,** Nitric oxide signalling in the nervous system, *Seminars in Neuroscience,* 5, 171, 1993.

51. **Lowenstein, C. J., Dinerman, J. L., and Snyder, S. H.,** Nitric oxide: a physiologic messenger, *Annals of Internal Medicine,* 120, 227, 1994.

52. **Rattan, S. and Chakder, S.,** Inhibitory effect of CO on internal anal sphincter: heme oxygenase inhibitor inhibits NANC relaxation, *American Journal of Physiology,* 265, G799, 1993.

53. **Verma, A., Hirsch, D. J., Glatt, C. E., Ronnett, G. V., and Snyder, S. H.,** Carbon monoxide: a putative neural messenger, *Science,* 259, 381, 1993.

54. **Orrego, F.,** Criteria for the identification of central neurotransmitters, and their application to studies with some nerve tissue preparations in vitro, *Neuroscience,* 4, 1037, 1979.

55. **Gabella, G.,** Fine strucure of post-ganglionic nerve fibres and autonomic neuro-effector junctions, in *Autonomic Neuroeffector Mechanisms,* Burnstock, G. and Hoyle, C. H. V., Eds., Harwood Academic Publishers, Chur, 1992, 1.

56. **Dowdall, M., Boyne, A. F., and Whittaker, V. P.,** Adenosine triphosphate: a constituent of cholinergic synaptic vesicles, *Biochemical Journal,* 140, 1, 1974.

57. **Lagercrantz, H., Fried, G., and Dahlin, I.,** An attempt to estimate the *in vivo* concentrations of noradrenaline and ATP in sympathetic large dense core nerve vesicles, *Acta Physiologica Scandinavica,* 94, 136, 1975.

58. **Boyne, A. F.,** Isolation of synaptic vesicles from *Narcine brasiliensis* electric organ—some influences on release of vesicular acetylcholine and ATP, *Brain Research,* 114, 481, 1976.

59. **Lagercrantz, H.,** On the composition and function of large dense cored vesicles in sympathetic nerves, *Neuroscience,* 1, 81, 1976.

60. **Fried, G., Lagercrantz, H., and Hökfelt, T.,** Improved isolation of small noradrenergic vesicles from rat seminal ducts following castration. A density gradient and morphological study, *Neuroscience,* 3, 1271, 1978.

61. **Zimmermann, H.,** Turnover of adenine nucleotides in cholinergic synaptic vesicles of the *Torpedo* electric organ, *Neuroscience,* 3, 827, 1978.

62. **Aberer, W., Stitzel, R., Winkler, H., and Huber, E.,** Accumulation of ^{3}H-ATP in small dense core vesicles of superfused vasa deferentia, *J. Neurochem.,* 33, 797, 1979.

63. **Zimmermann, H.,** Co-existence of adenosine 5'-triphosphate and acetylcholine in the electromotor synapse, in *Co-transmission,* Cuello, A. C., Ed., MacMillan, London, 1982, 243.

64. **Fried, G.,** Small noradrenergic stroage vesicles isolated from rat vas deferens—biochemical and morphological characterization, *Acta Physiologica Scandinavica,* Suppl.493, 111, 1, 1980.

65. **Israel, M., Dunant, Y., Lesbats, B., Manaranche, R., Marsal, J., and Meunier, F.,** Rapid acetylcholine and adenosine triphosphate oscillations triggered by stimulation of the *Torpedo* electric organ, *Journal of Experimental Biology,* 81, 63, 1979.

66. **Fredholm, B. B., Fried, G., and Hedqvist, P.,** Origin of adenosine released from rat vas deferens by nerve stimulation, *European Journal of Pharmacology,* 79, 233, 1982.

67. **Klein, R. L.,** Chemical composition of the large noradrenergic vesicles, in *Neurotransmitter Vesicles,* Klein, R. L., Lagercrantz, H. and Zimmermann, H., Eds., Academic Press, New York, 1982, 133.

68. **Fukuda, J., Fujita, Y., and Ohsawa, K.,** ATP content in isolated mammalian nerve cells assayed by a modified luciferin-luciferase method, *Journal of Neuroscience Methods,* 8, 295, 1983.

69. **Fried, G., Terenius, L., Hökfelt, T., and Goldstein, M.,** Evidence for differential localization of noradrenaline and neuropeptide Y in neuronal storage vesicles isolated from rat vas deferens, *J. Neurosci.,* 5, 450, 1985.

70. **Payne, C. M.,** Phylogenetic considerations of neurosecretory granule contents: role of nucleotides and basic hormone/transmitter packaging mechanisms, *Arch. Histol. Cytol.,* 52 Suppl, 277, 1989.

71. **Fu, W. M. and Poo, M. M.,** ATP potentiates spontaneous transmitter release at developing neuromuscular synapses, *Neuron,* 6, 837, 1991.

72. **Fillenz, M.,** Transmission: noradrenaline, in *Autonomic Neuroeffector Mechanisms,* Burnstock, G. and Hoyle, C. H. V., Eds., Harwood Academic Publishers, Chur, 1992, 323.

73. **Hoyle, C. H. V.,** Transmission: purines, in *Autonomic Neuroeffector Mechanisms,* Burnstock, G. and Hoyle, C. H. V., Eds., Harwood Academic Publishers, Chur, 1992, 367.

74. **Parsons, S. M., Prior, C., and Marshall, I. G.,** Acetylcholine transport, storage, and release, *International Reviews of Neurobiology,* 35, 279, 1993.

75. **Haggendal, J.,** Noradrenaline and dopamine-beta-hydroxylase levels in rat salivary glands after preganglionic nerve stimulation: evidence for re-use of amine storage granules in transmitter release, *J. Neural Transm.,* 53, 147, 1982.

76. **Buckley, K. M. and Landis, S. G.,** Morphological studies of neurotransmitter release and membrane recycling in sympathetic nerve terminals in culture, *J. Neurocytol.,* 12, 93, 1983.

77. **Boarder, M. R.,** Presynaptic aspects of cotransmission: relationship between vesicles and neurotransmitters, *J. Neurochem.,* 53, 1, 1989.

78. **Bastiaensen, E., Miserez, B., and De Potter, W.,** Subcellular fractionation of bovine ganglion stellatum: co-storage of noradrenaline, Met-enkephalin and neuropeptide Y in large 'dense-cored' vesicles, *Brain Research,* 442, 124, 1988.

79. **Hagn, C., Klein, R. L., Fischer-Colbrie, R., Douglas, B. H., and Winkler, H.,** An immunological characterization of five common antigens of chromaffin granules and of large dense-cored vesicles of sympathetic nerve, *Neuroscience Letters,* 67, 295, 1986.

80. **Cook, R. D. and Burnstock, G.,** The ultrastructures of Auerbach's plexus in the guinea-pig. I. Neuronal elements, *J. Neurocytol.,* 5, 171, 1976.

81. **Hoyle, C. H. V. and Burnstock, G.,** Neuromuscular transmission in the gastrointestinal tract, in *Handbook of Physiology, Section 6: The Gastrointestinal System, Vol. 1,* Wood, J. D., Ed., American Physiological Society, Bethesda, 1989, 435.

82. **Burnstock, G.,** Neuromuscular transmission and neuromodulation in the gastrointestinal tract, in *Gastrointestinal Dysmotility: Focus on Cisapride,* Heading, R. C. and Wood, J. D., Eds., Raven Press, New York, 1992, 41.

83. **Gershon, M. D., Mawe, G. M., and Branchek, T. A.,** 5-HT and enteric neurones, in *The Peripheral Actions of 5-HT,* Fozard, J. R., Ed., Oxford University Press, Oxford, 1989, 247.

84. **Milner, P. and Burnstock, G.,** Neurotransmitters in the gut, in *Constipation and Related Disorders: Pathophysiology and Management in Adults and Children,* Kamm, M. A. and Lennard-Jones, J. E., Eds., Wrightson Biomedical Publishing, Petersfield, 1994, 41.

85. **Sanchez-Armass, S. and Orrego, F.,** A major role for chloride in ^{3}H-noradrenaline transport by rat heart adrenergic nerves, *Life Sciences,* 20, 1829, 1977.
86. **Kuhar, M. J. and Zarbin, M. A.,** Synaptosomal transport: a chloride dependence for choline, GABA, glycine, and several other compounds, *J. Neurochem.,* 31, 251, 1978.
87. **Hertz, L.,** Functional interaction between neurons and astrocytes. 1. Turnover and metabolism of putative amino acid transmitters, *Progress in Neurobiology,* 13, 277, 1979.
88. **Radian, R. and Kanner, B. I.,** Stoichiometry of sodium- and chloride-coupled gamma-amino butyric acid transport by synaptic plasma membrane vesicles isolated from rat brain, *Biochemistry,* 22, 1236, 1983.
89. **Aragon, M. C., Gimenez, C., and Mayor, F.,** Stoichiometry of sodium- and chloride-coupled glycine transport in synaptic plasma membrane vesicles derived from rat brain, *FEBS Letters,* 212, 87, 1987.
90. **Kanner, B. I. and Schuldiner, S.,** Mechanism of transport and storage of neurotransmitters, *CRC Critical Reviews in Biochemistry,* 22, 1, 1987.
91. **Dawson, T. M., Bredt, D. S., Fotuhi, M., Hwang, P. M., and Snyder, S. H.,** Nitric oxide synthase and neuronal NADPH diaphorase are identical in brain and peripheral tissues, *Proceedings of the National Academy of Sciences, U. S. A.,* 88, 7797, 1991.
92. **Nathan, C.,** Nitric oxide as a secretory product of mammalian cells, *FASEB Journal,* 6, 3051, 1992.
93. **Moncada, S.,** The 1991 Ulf von Euler Lecture: The L-arginine:nitric oxide pathway, *Acta Physiologica Scandinavica,* 145, 201, 1992.
94. **Afework, M., Tomlinson, A., Belai, A., and Burnstock, G.,** Colocalization of nitric oxide synthase and NADPH-diaphorase in rat adrenal gland, *Neuroreport,* 3, 893, 1992.
95. **Belai, A., Schmidt, H. H. H. W., Hoyle, C. H. V., Hassall, C. J. S., Saffrey, M. J., Moss, J., Foerstermann, U., Murad, F., and Burnstock, G.,** Colocalisation of nitric oxide synthase and NADPH-diaphorase in the myenteric plexus of the rat gut, *Neuroscience Letters,* 143, 60, 1922.
96. **Hassall, C. J. S, Saffrey, M. J., Belai, A., Hoyle, C. H. V., Moules, E. W., Moss, J., Schmidt, H. H. H. W., Foerstermann, U., and Burnstock, G.,** Nitric oxide synthase immunoreactivity and NADPH-diaphorase activity in a subpopulation of intrinsic neurones of the guinea-pig heart, *Neuroscience Letters,* 143, 65, 1992.
97. **Bredt, D. S., Glatt, C. E., Hwang, P. M., Fotuhi, M., Dawson, T. M., and Snyder, S. H.,** Nitric oxide synthase protein and mRNA are discretely localized in neuronal populations of the mammalian CNS together with NADPH diaphorase, *Neuron,* 7, 615, 1991.
98. **Saffrey, M. J., Hassall, C. J. S., Hoyle, C. H. V., Belai, A., Moss, J., Schmidt, H. H. H. W., Foerstermann, U., Murad, F., and Burnstock, G.,** Nitric oxide synthase and NADPH diaphorase activity in cultured myenteric neurones, *Neuroreport,* 3, 333, 1992.
99. **Schmidt, H. H. H. W., Gagne, G. D., Nakane, M., Pollock, J. S., Miller, M. F., and Murad, F.,** Mapping of neural nitric oxide synthase in the rat suggests frequent co-localization with NADPH diaphorase but not with soluble guanylate cyclase, and novel paraneural functions for nitrinergic signal transduction, *Journal of Histochemistry and Cytochemistry,* 40, 1439, 1992.
100. **Schmidt, H. H. H. W., Lohman, S. M., and Walter, U.,** The nitric oxide and cGMP signal transduction system: regulation and mechanism of action, *Biochimica et Biophysica Acta,* 1178, 153, 1993.
101. **Snyder, S. H.,** Nitric oxide and neurons, *Current Opinions in Neurobiology,* 2, 323, 1992.
102. **Snyder, S. H. and Bredt, D. S.,** Biological roles of nitric oxide, *Scientific American,* May, 28, 1992.
103. **Schuman, E. M. and Madison, D. V.,** Nitric oxide and synaptic function, *Annual Reviews in Neuroscience,* 17, 153, 1994.
104. **Sneddon, P. and Graham, A.,** Role of nitric oxide in the autonomic innervation of smooth muscle, *Journal of Autonomic Pharmacology,* 12, 445, 1992.
105. **Sanders, K. M., Ward, S. M., Thornbury, K. D., Dalziel, H. H., Westfall, D. P., and Carl, A.,** Nitric oxide as a non-adrenergic, non-cholinergic neurotransmitter in the gastrointestinal tract, *Japanese Journal of Pharmacology,* 58 Suppl. 2, 220P, 1992.
106. **Kawasaki, H. and Takasaki, K.,** Vasoconstrictor response induced by 5-hydroxytryptamine released from vascular adrenergic nerves by periarterial nerve stimulation, *J. Pharmacol. Exp. Ther.,* 229, 816, 1984.
107. **Ramme, D., Regenold, J. T., Starke, K., Russe, R., and Illes, P.,** Identification of the neuroeffector transmitter in jejunal branches of the rabbit mesenteric artery, *Naunyn Schmiedebergs Archives of Pharmacology,* 336, 267, 1987.

108. **Katz, B.,** *Nerve, Muscle and Synapse,* McGraw-Hill, New York, 1966.

109. **Katz, B.,** *The Release of Neural Transmitter Substances,* Liverpool University Press, Liverpool, 1969.

110. **Jessell, T. M. and Kandell, E. R.,** Synaptic transmission: a bidirectional and self-modifiable form of cell-cell communication, *Cell,* 72/Neuron 10 (Suppl), 1, 1993.

111. **Thureson-Klein, A.,** Exocytosis from large and small dense cored vesicles in noradrenergic nerve terminals, *Neuroscience,* 10, 245, 1983.

112. **Pow, D. V and Morris, J. F.,** Dendrites of hypothalamic magnocellular neurons release neurohypophysial peptide by excocytosis, *Neuroscience,* 32, 435, 1989.

113. **Sudhof, T. C. and Jahn, R.,** Proteins of synaptic vesicles involved in exocytosois and membrane recycling, *Neuron,* 6, 665, 1991.

114. **Thureson-Klein, A., Klein, R. L., and Zhu, P. C.,** Exocytosis from large dense cored vesicles as a mechanism for neuropeptide release in the peripheral and central nervous system, *Scan. Electron Microsc.,* 179, 1986.

115. **Parnas, I. and Parnas, H.,** The "Ca-voltage" hypothesis for neurotransmitter release, *Biophysical Chemistry,* 29, 85, 1988.

116. **Knowles, R. G., Palacios, M., Palmer, R. M. J., and Moncada, S.,** Formation of nitric oxide from L-arginine in the central nervous system: a transduction mechanism for stimulation of the soluble guanylate cyclase, *Proceedings of the National Academy of Sciences, U. S. A.,* 86, 5159, 1989.

117. **Schmidt, H. H. H. W., Pollock, J. S., Nakane, M., Foerstermann, U., and Murad, F.,** $Ca^{2+}/$ Calmodulin-regulated nitric oxide synthases, *Cell Calcium,* 13, 427, 1992.

118. **Thompson, S. M. and Gahwiler, B. H.,** Effects of GABA uptake inhibitor tiagabine on inhibitory synaptic potentials in rat hippocampal slice cultures, *Journal of Neurophysiology,* 67, 1698, 1992.

119. **Isaacson, J. S., Solis, J. M., and Nicoll, R. A.,** Local and diffuse synaptic actions of GABA in the hippocampus, *Neuron,* 10, 165, 1993.

120. **Schwartz, E. A.,** Calcium-independent release of GABA from isolated horizontal cells of the toad retina, *J. Physiol. Lond.,* 323, 211, 1982.

121. **Bernath, S. and Zigmond, M. J.,** Characterization of GABA release from striatal slices: evidence for a calcium-independent process via the GABA uptake system, *Neuroscience,* 27, 563, 1988.

122. **Cunningham, J. R., Neal, M. J., Stone, S., and Witkovsky, P.,** GABA release from Xenopus retina does not correlate with horizontal cell membrane potential, *Neuroscience,* 24, 39, 1988.

123. **Dunlop, J., Grieve, A., Schousboe, A., and Griffiths, R.,** Stimulation of gamma-[3H]aminobutyric acid release from cultured mouse cerebral cortex neurons by sulphur-containing excitatory amino acid transmitter candidates: receptor activation mediates two distinct mechanisms of release, *J. Neurochem.,* 57, 1388, 1991.

124. **Bernath, S.,** Calcium-independent release of amino acid neurotransmitters: fact or artifact? *Progress in Neurobiology,* 38, 57, 1992.

125. **Taylor, J. and Gordon Weeks, P. R.,** Calcium-independent gamma-aminobutyric acid release from growth cones: role of gamma-aminobutyric acid transport, *J. Neurochem.,* 56, 273, 1991.

126. **Schomig, A., Dart, A. M., Dietz, R., Mayer, E., and Kubler, W.,** Release of endogenous catecholamines in the ischemic myocardium of the rat. Part A: Locally mediated release, *Circulation Research,* 55, 689, 1984.

127. **Carlsson, L., Graefe, K. H., and Trendelenburg, U.,** Early intraneuronal mobilization and deamination of noradrenaline during global ischemia in the isolated perfused rat heart, *Naunyn Schmiedebergs Archives of Pharmacology,* 336, 508, 1987.

128. **Schomig, A., Fischer, S., Kurz, T., Richardt, G., and Schomig, E.,** Nonexocytotic release of endogenous noradrenaline in the ischemic and anoxic rat heart: mechanism and metabolic requirements, *Circulation Research,* 60, 194, 1987.

129. **Kurz, T. and Schomig, A.,** Extracellular sodium and chloride depletion enhances nonexocytotic noradrenaline release induced by energy deficiency in rat heart, *Naunyn Schmiedebergs Archives of Pharmacology,* 340, 265, 1989.

130. **Richardt, G., Haass, M., and Schomig, A.,** Calcium antagonists and cardiac noradrenaline release in ischemia, *J. Mol. Cell Cardiol.,* 23, 269, 1991.

131. **Kranzhofer, R., Haass, M., Kurz, T., Richardt, G., and Schomig, A.,** Effect of digitalis glycosides on norepinephrine release in the heart. Dual mechanism of action, *Circulation Research,* 68, 1628, 1991.

132. **Haass, M., Hock, M., Richardt, G., and Schomig, A.,** Neuropeptide Y differentiates between exocytotic and nonexocytotic noradrenaline release in guinea-pig heart, *Naunyn Schmiedebergs Archives of Pharmacology,* 340, 509, 1989.

133. **Yau, W. M.,** Neurotransmitter release in the enteric nervous system, in *Handbook of Physiology, Section 6: The Gastrointestinal System, Vol. 1,* Wood, J. D., Ed., American Physiological Society, Bethesda, 1989, 403.

134. **Dowe, G. H. C., Kilbinger, H., and Whittaker, V. P.,** Isolation of cholinergic synaptic vesicles from the myenteric plexus of guinea-pig small intestine, *J. Neurochem.,* 35, 993, 1980.

135. **Yau, W. M., Youther, M. L., and Verdun, P. R.,** A presynaptic site of action of substance P and vasoactive intestinal polypeptide on myenteric neurons, *Brain Research,* 330, 382, 1985.

136. **Yau, W. M. and Verdun, P. R.,** Release of gamma-aminobutyric acid from guinea-pig myenteric plexus synaptosomes, *Brain Research,* 278, 271, 1983.

137. **Al-Humayyd, M. and White, T. D.,** Adrenergic and possible nonadrenergic sources of adenosine $5'$-triphosphate release from nerve varicosities isolated from ileal myenteric plexus, *J. Pharmacol. Exp. Ther.,* 233, 796, 1985.

138. **White, T. D. and Leslie, R. A.,** Depolarization-induced release of adenosine $5'$-triphosphate from isolated varicosities derived from the myenteric plexus of the guinea-pig small intestine, *J. Neurosci.,* 2, 206, 1982.

139. **Reese, J. H. and Cooper, J. R.,** Modulation of release of acetylcholine from ileal synaptosomes by adenosine and adenosine $5'$-triphosphate, *J. Pharmacol. Exp. Ther.,* 223, 612, 1982.

140. **Belai, A., Ralevic, V., and Burnstock, G.,** VIP release from enteric nerves is independent of extracellular calcium, *Regulatory Peptides,* 19, 79, 1987.

141. **Fahrenkrug, J., Gelbo, H., Holst, J. J., and Schaffalitzky de Muckadell, O. B.,** Influence of the autonomic nervous system on the release of vasoactive intestinal polypeptide from the porcine gastrointestinal tract, *Journal of Physiology,* 180, 405, 1978.

142. **Fahrenkrug, J., Haglund, U., Jodal, M., Lundgren, O., Olbe, L., and Schaffalitzky de Mucka-dell, O. B.,** Nervous release of vasoactive intestinal polypeptide in the gastrointestinal tract of cats: possible physiological implication, *Journal of Physiology,* 284, 291, 1978.

143. **Gaginella, T. S., O'Driscoll, T. M., and Hubel, K. A.,** Release of vasoactive intestinal polypeptide by electrical field stimulation of the rabbit ileum, *Regulatory Peptides,* 2, 165, 1981.

144. **Besson, J., Rostene, W., Lhiaubet, A-M., Pousin, B., and Rosselin, G.,** Release in vitro. Effect of various depolarizing agents, *Experientia,* 39, 732, 1983.

145. **Dockray, G. J.,** Transmission: peptides, in *Autonomic Neuroeffector Mechanisms,* Burnstock, G. and Hoyle, C. H. V., Eds., Harwood Academic Publishers, Chur, 1992, 409.

146. **Willard, A. L. and Nishi, R.,** Neurons dissociated from rat myenteric plexus retain differentiated properties when grown in cell culture. III. Synaptic interactions and modulatory effects of neuro-transmitter candidates, *Neuroscience,* 16, 213, 1985.

147. **Puig, M. M., Gascon, P., Craviso, G. L., and Musacchio, J. M.,** Endogenous opiate receptor ligand: electrically induced release in the guinea-pig ileum, *Science,* 195, 419, 1977.

148. **Schultz, R., Wuster, M., Simantov, R., Snyder, S., and Hertz, A.,** Electrically stimulated release of opiate-like material from the myenteric plexus of the guinea-pig ileum, *European Journal of Pharmacology,* 41, 347, 1977.

149. **Donnerer, J., Bartho, L., Holzer, P., and Lembeck, F.,** Intestinal peristalsis associated with release of immunoreactive substance P, *Neuroscience,* 11, 913, 1984.

150. **Donnerer, J., Holzer, P., and Lembeck, F.,** Release of dynorphin, somatostatin and substance P from the vascularly perfused small intestine of the guinea-pig small intestine during peristalsis, *British Journal of Pharmacology,* 83, 919, 1984.

151. **Baron, S. A., Jaffe, B. M., and Gintzler, A. R.,** Release of substance P from the enteric nervous system: direct quantification and characterization. *J. Pharmacol. Exp. Ther.,* 227, 365, 1983.

152. **Angel, F., Go, V. L. W., and Szurszewski, J. H.,** Innervation of the muscularis mucosae of canine proximal colon, *Journal of Physiology,* 357, 93, 1984.

153. **Holzer, P.,** Characterization of the stimulus-induced release of immunoreactive substance P from the myenteric plexus of the guinea-pig ileum, *Brain Research,* 297, 127, 1984.

154. **Belai, A. and Burnstock, G.,** Release of calcitonin gene-related peptide from rat enteric nerves is Ca^{2+}-dependent but is not induced by K^+ depolarization, *Regulatory Peptides,* 23, 227, 1988.

155. **Boeckxstaens, G. E., Pelckmans, P. A., Ruytjens, I. F., Bult, H., De Man, J. G., Herman, A. G., and van Maercke, Y. M.,** Bioassay of nitric oxide released upon stimulation of non-adrenergic non-cholinergic nerves in the canine ileocolonic junction, *British Journal of Pharmacology,* 103, 1085, 1991.

156. **Boeckxstaens, G. E., Pelckmans, P. A., Bult, H., De Man, J. G., Herman, A. G., and van Maercke, Y. M.,** Non-adrenergic non-cholinergic relaxation mediated by nitric oxide in the canine ileocolonic junction, *Eur. J. Pharmacol.,* 190, 239, 1990.

157. **Bult, H., Boeckxstaens, G. E., Pelckmans, P. A., Jordaens, F. H., van Maercke, Y. M., and Herman, A. G.,** Nitric oxide as an inhibitory non-adrenergic non-cholinergic neurotransmitter, *Nature,* 345, 346, 1990.

158. **Boeckxstaens, G. E., Pelckmans, P. A., Bogers, J. J., Bult, H., De Man, J. G., Oosterbosch, L., Herman, A. G., and Van Maercke, Y.,** Release of nitric oxide upon stimulation of nonadrenergic noncholinergic nerves in the rat gastric fundus, *J. Pharmacol. Exp. Ther.,* 256, 441, 1991.

159. **Misbin, R. I., Wolfe, M. M., Morris, P., Buynitzky, S. J., and McGuigan, J. E.,** Uptake of vasoactive intestinal polypeptide by rat liver, *American Journal of Physiology,* 243, G103, 1982.

160. **Nau, R., Ballmann, M., and Conlon, J. M.,** Binding of vasoactive intestinal polypeptide to dispersed enterocytes results in rapid removal of the NH_2-terminal histidyl residue, *Molecular Endocrinology,* 52, 97, 1987.

161. **Svoboda, M., De Neef, P., Tastenoy, M., and Christophe, J.,** Molecular characteristics and evidence for internalization of vasoactive intestinal polypeptide (VIP) receptors in the tumoral rat pancreatic acinar cell line, *European Journal of Biochemistry,* 176, 707, 1988.

162. **Hoyle, C. H. V. and Burnstock, G.,** ATP receptors and their physiological roles, in *Adenosine in the Nervous System,* Stone, T. W., Ed., Academic Press, London, 1991, 43.

163. **Katsuragi, T. and Su, C.,** Augmentation by theophylline of [^{3}H]purine release from vascular adrenergic nerves: evidence for presynaptic autoinhibition, *J. Pharmacol. Exp. Ther.,* 220, 152, 1982.

164. **Edwards, F. A., Gibb, A. J., and Colquhoun, D.,** ATP receptor-mediated synaptic currents in the central nervous system, *Nature,* 359, 144, 1993.

165. **Evans, R. J., Derkach, V., and Surprenant, A.,** ATP mediates fast synaptic transmission in mammalian neurones, *Nature,* 357, 503, 1993.

166. **Benham, C. D.,** ATP joins the fast lane, *Nature,* 359, 103, 1992.

167. **Ziganshin, A. U., Hoyle, C. H. V., Lambrecht, G., Mutschler, E., Baeumert, H. G., and Burnstock, G.,** Selective antagonism by PPADS at P_{2X}-purinoceptors in rabbit isolated blood vessels, *British Journal of Pharmacology,* 111, 923, 1994.

168. **Ziganshin, A. U., Hoyle, C. H. V., Bo, X., Lambrecht, G., Mutschler, E., Baeumert, H. G., and Burnstock, G.,** PPADS selectively antagonizes P_{2X}-purinoceptor-mediated responses in the rabbit urinary bladder, *British Journal of Pharmacology,* 110, 1491, 1993.

169. **Lambrecht, G., Friebe, T., Grimm, U., Windscheif, U., Bungardt, E., Hildebrandt, C., Baeumert, H. G., Spatz-Kuembel, G., and Mutschler, E.,** PPADS, a novel functionally selective antagonist of P_2-purinoceptor-mediated responses, *European Journal of Pharmacology,* 217, 217, 1992.

170. **Hoyle, C. H. V., Knight, G. E., and Burnstock, G.,** Suramin antagonizes response to P_2-purinoceptor agonists and purinergic nerve stimulation in the guinea-pig urinary bladder and taenia coli, *British Journal of Pharmacology,* 99, 617, 1990.

171. **Andersson, K. E., Garcia Pascual, A., Persson, K., Forman, A., and Tottrup, A.,** Electrically-induced, nerve-mediated relaxation of rabbit urethra involves nitric oxide, *J. Urol.,* 147, 253, 1992.

172. **Dokita, S., Morgan, W. R., Wheeler, M. A., Yoshida, M., Latifpour, J., and Weiss, R. M.,** N^G-nitro-L-arginine inhibits non-adrenergic, non-cholinergic relaxation in rabbit urethral smooth muscle, *Life Sciences,* 48, 2429, 1991.

173. **Trigo-Rocha, F., Aronson, W. J., Hohenfellner, M., Ignarro, L. J., Rajfer, J., and Lue, T. F.,** Nitric oxide and cGMP: mediators of pelvic nerve-stimulated erection in dogs, *American Journal of Physiology,* 264, H419, 1993.

174. **Rajfer, J., Aronson, W. J., Bush, P. A., Dorey, F. J., and Ignarro, L. J.,** Nitric oxide as a mediator of relaxation of the corpus cavernosum in response to nonadrenergic, noncholinergic neurotransmission, *New England Journal of Medicine,* 326, 90, 1992.

175. **Boeckxstaens, G. E., Pelckmans, P. A., Bogers, J. J., Bult, H., De Man, J. G., and Oosterbosch, L.,** Release of nitric oxide upon stimulation of nonadrenergic noncholinergic nerves in the rat gastric fundus, *J. Pharmacol. Exp. Ther.,* 256, 441, 1991.

176. **Toda, N., Baba, H., Tanobe, Y., and Okamura, T.,** Mechanisms of relaxation induced by K^+ and nicotine in dog duodenal longitudinal muscle, *J. Pharmacol. Exp. Ther.,* 260, 697, 1992.

177. **Toda, N., Tanobe, Y., and Baba, H.,** Suppression by N^G-nitro-L-arginine of relaxations induced by non-adrenergic, non-cholinergic nerve stimulation in dog duodenal longitudinal muscle, *Japanese Journal of Pharmacology,* 57, 527, 1991.

178. **Gillespie, J. S. and Sheng, H.,** The effects of pyrogallol and hydroquinone on the response to NANC nerve stimulation in the rat anococcygeus and the bovine retractor penis muscles, *British Journal of Pharmacology,* 99, 194, 1990.

179. **Gillespie, J. S. and Sheng, H.,** A comparison of haemoglobin and erythrocytes as inhibitors of smooth muscle relaxation by the NANC transmitter in the BRP and rat anococcygeus and by EDRF in the rabbit aortic strip, *British Journal of Pharmacology,* 98, 445, 1989.

7 Enteric Neurotransmitters and Hormone Receptors

David R. Brown

INTRODUCTION

The digestive system serves to process and assimilate consumed nutrients and defend the host organism against ingested pathogens and other noxious materials. Moreover, cells within this system are subject to continuous renewal in order to optimize digestive function. To accomplish its various tasks, the gastrointestinal tract manufactures a wide variety of chemical messenger molecules which are secreted into the extracellular milieu and participate in inter- and intracellular communication through their interactions with membrane-bound receptor proteins. The nature, organization, and complexity of this ornate tapestry of cells, chemical messengers and receptors have evolved differently among animal species as they adapted to particular ecological niches and food sources.

Due to their abundance and variety of receptors, gastrointestinal tissues have been widely used in pharmacological studies even before the formulation of the drug-receptor concept in the early twentieth century. Bayliss and Starling, for example, examined the actions of atropine in gut preparations.[1] Many early pharmacological experiments were in fact conducted to assess the effects of drugs on gastrointestinal motility and secretion. Perhaps the most popular model to be employed in *in vitro* experiments on drug action has been the cecal end of the guinea pig ileum. It was utilized in early pharmacological experiments as an *in vitro* tissue model for the analysis of drug action on smooth muscle contractility because it exhibits a relatively steady baseline in contrast to the high amplitude spontaneous activity which is often observed in isolated intestinal smooth muscle segments from other species.[2] Many of the classical studies of drug antagonism, "spare receptors" and partial agonism by Schild, Stephenson, Nickerson and others were performed using the isolated guinea pig ileum.[3–5] A field-stimulated preparation of guinea pig ileum which was utilized by Kosterlitz as a bioassay for opiate activity, played a key role in the identification of endogenous opioid peptides from brain, pituitary and gut extracts and in the discovery of opiate receptor heterogeneity.[6] Smooth muscle preparations from other regions of the digestive system or from other species also became important models for pharmacological studies. For example, the longitudinally-oriented taenia caeci from the guinea pig large intestine was employed by Burnstock and his colleagues in early studies of purinergic neurotransmission and the rat stomach fundus was used in investigations by Vane on 5-hydroxytryptamine receptors.[7,8]

Although isolated segments of gastrointestinal smooth muscle continue to hold an important place in pharmacological investigations, these have been supplemented by the use of both *in vivo* models of motor function and isolated smooth muscle cells. Over the past three decades, functional studies have extended beyond smooth muscle preparations to encompass the wide variety of other excitable and non-excitable cells in the gastrointestinal tract. These include investigations of receptors mediating gastric acid secretion, ion transport and growth in intestinal epithelial cells and host defense by the gut immune system. Moreover, several classes of receptors have been characterized that regulate aspects of neuronal activity in the enteric ganglionated plexuses or the release of hormones from gastrointestinal endocrine cells.

It is not the author's intention to undertake an exhaustive review of receptor characterization in any one cell type or system present in the digestive tract. Rather the objective of this chapter will be to provide some general concepts and guidelines for the design and execution of future experiments involving gastrointestinal neurotransmitter receptors. Due to space limitations, he apologizes in advance for the exclusion of many important papers in this dynamic field of investigation.

PHARMACODYNAMICS OF LIGAND-RECEPTOR INTERACTIONS

The selective interaction between a membrane receptor and its cognate ligands is a fundamental process in cell-to-cell communication. A majority of known receptor systems consist of an agonist recognition site which is coupled through a signal transduction mechanism to one or more effector molecules.[9] These effectors determine the nature of the ultimate cellular response to the initial agonist-receptor interaction (Table 1). The functional quantitation of ligand-receptor interactions is fundamentally based on the Law of Mass Action. In early receptor theory, the

---

TABLE 1
Receptor-Effector Systems

Representative Receptor Classes	Transduction Mechanism	Initial Effector(s)
A. Ion Channel-coupled Receptors		
Nicotinic cholinergic	Intrinsic conformational change in	Intrinsic cation channel
Ionotropic glutamatergic	multisubunit receptor protein	Intrinsic cation channel
$GABA_A$		Intrinsic chloride channel
Glycine		Intrinsic chloride channel
Serotonin (5-HT_3)	Intrinsic conformational change	Intrinsic cation channel
Purine receptors (P_{2X}, P_{2Z}, P_{2T})		Intrinsic cation channel
B. Receptors with Intrinsic Enzymatic Activity		
Atrial natriuretic factor	Intrinsic cytoplasmic guanylate	Cyclic GMP
Guanylin	cyclase activity	
Growth factors	Intrinsic tyrosine kinase activity	Various substrates
CD45	Intrinsic protein tyrosine	Various substrates
	phosphatase activity	
TGF-β	Intrinsic serine-threonine	Various substrates
	phosphatase activity	
C. Receptors Coupled to Heterotrimeric GTP-Binding (G) Proteins		
Adrenergic	G proteins (α, β, γ subunits)	Various substrates (adenylate
Muscarinic cholinergic		cyclase; inositol trisphosphate/
Serotonin		diacylglycerol; ion channels)
(5-HT_1, 5-HT_2, 5-HT_4 types)		
Neuropeptide		
Neurokinin		
Secretin		

cellular response in a biological system was thought to be directly proportional to the amount of agonist ligand that bound to a fixed number of receptors. Thus, occupation of the total receptor population by an agonist should yield a maximum effect. It was soon realized however that agonist efficacy exists as a continuum, i.e. that minor structural changes in ligand molecules produced full agonists, partial agonists or even antagonists. In subsequent modifications of classical theory, the cellular response in a given system was postulated to be a function of ligand-dependent and -independent variables.[10] Ligand-dependent variables include the efficacy of the ligand and its affinity in binding to the receptor. Properties of the biological system independent of the ligand include receptor density and the ability of the cell to convert ligand binding to a final cellular response. In the case of receptors coupled to guanine nucleotide-binding (G) proteins, proximal factors underlying cellular coupling efficiency might include the affinity of particular G proteins for cytoplasmic binding domains on the receptor, the relative amount of G protein in proximity to the receptor, and number of different G proteins capable of binding to and being activated by the receptor (i.e. the so-called "promiscuous" receptor).[11]

Full agonists may occupy a small fraction of receptors to achieve maximal effects, whereas partial agonists can bind to the entire population of active receptors and produce submaximal effects. Antagonists, which by definition lack efficacy, can block agonist binding sites in a competitive or non-competitive fashion. The actions of non-competitive antagonists cannot be surmounted by agonists and result from persistent blockade or modifications to the agonist binding domain or from interruptions in signalling pathways that contribute to the final cellular response but are inaccessible to agonists. The continuum of ligand efficacy can be powerfully exploited in the functional characterization of receptors and in the analysis of drug actions in the alimentary tract. It should be noted that there is not yet a unitary theory of ligand-receptor interactions; this area is undergoing some modification with the advent of new information on the structure and function of receptors. This is highlighted by pharmacological analyses of ligand-gated ion channels which, given the quantal nature of ionic fluxes as well as drug-induced changes in single channel conductances and open channel probabilities measured by current electrophysiological techniques, have theoretical foundations that diverge from classical receptor theory.[12] The reader is referred to several recent books for a more extensive discussion of receptor theories or on the design and interpretation of pharmacological experiments.[10,13–15]

CHARACTERIZATION OF RECEPTORS

GENERAL CONSIDERATIONS

Complexity of the Experimental Preparation

Functional experiments in gastrointestinal pharmacology have been designed using biological preparations possessing different levels of complexity. In whole animals, the integrated response to a drug may be measured, the influence of the circulating hormones might be determined or communication between the gut and other organ systems may be defined. Tissues, such as mucosal sheets or smooth muscle strips, provide a lower level of complexity that can be exploited in more precisely defining organ responses or signalling networks. A further reduction in complexity is represented by isolated primary cells or cultured cell lines as well as cell membranes or subcellular components. These provide information about the cellular or molecular mechanisms underlying drug effects or receptor mechanisms, but do not necessarily predict drug effects at the organismal level. Each level of complexity presents problems or has limitations, and a careful investigator will not attempt to overinterpret experimental results obtained in any one system.

Three general sets of factors influence the quantity of the ligand reaching a specific receptor compartment: 1) obstacles to ligand permeation, 2) mechanisms to reduce the effects of ligand interactions at the receptor, and 3) ligand removal processes. The more complex the system, the more these variables must be accounted for in evaluating ligand-receptor interactions. In tissue preparations, for example, the receptor compartment may be embedded within the substance of the tissue. A ligand would have to diffuse through the tissue bathing medium, penetrate the unstirred water layer surrounding the tissue, and diffuse through the tissue substance at a rate dependent upon the surface area, thickness, and morphology of the tissue. An agonist ligand, upon binding to receptors, may rapidly induce the desensitization or internalization of a portion of the receptor pool, a process which serves to limit agonist activity. Removal of the ligand from the receptor compartment might involve ligand internalization into cells, active ligand uptake through neurotransmitter transporters, and biotransformation or degradation. These various factors, together with the unique chemical characteristics of the ligand, impede equilibration between the ligand and receptor and affect the determination of relative pharmacological activities among a class of ligands.

In cellularly-heterogeneous preparations, ligand delivery is usually not discretely localized to the particular subset of cells in which pharmacological activity is being determined. Thus, the effect(s) observed are often the net result of a combination of influences impinging upon the measured cellular response that were brought into play by ligand administration. In preparations of gut tissue in which biological responses are often measured over short time scales (seconds to minutes), it is quite common to encounter the question of whether a particular substance, added to the tissue bathing medium, acts directly on target cells or indirectly modifies target cell function through its ability to alter the release of neurotransmitters, hormones, or paracrine/autocrine factors.

Moreover, the reader should bear in mind that such preparations, with a moderate to high degree of complexity, may possess multiple receptors on different cell types that are capable of interacting with the experimental substance. These situations complicate the determination of the sites at which an endogenous substance under investigation may normally act. The target sites for the endogenous substance may be discretely localized and be in close proximity to the substance's release sites under physiological conditions. Added to a tissue bath even at "physiologically-relevant" concentrations however, the sites of action for the same substance may appear to be widely-dispersed and numerous. For example, the antral hormone gastrin may elicit contractions in isolated smooth muscle cell preparations in concentrations as low as one femtomolar, but concentrations of the hormone that are some 5 to 7 orders of magnitude higher are necessary to contract muscle strips; it is likely that activation of cells other than the target serve to modify gastrin action measured in the more complex preparation.[16] It is essential to relate the results of studies conducted on preparations of high complexity with those of lower complexity before definitive conclusions can be made concerning the sites of drug action and the functional role of endogenous substances.

Drug Selectivity

Numerous drugs have been employed to characterize receptors, ion channels and transporters or other proteins in the gastrointestinal tract. Many of these have been employed as "selective" agonists or blockers to define the mechanisms underlying a tissue function or drug effect. Often they have been employed at a single arbitrary concentration and the results thus did not provide useful quantitative information about ligand-receptor interactions that could be extrapolated to other studies. Moreover, "selective" drugs may not adequately elucidate the basic mechanisms involved, especially at high concentrations. What has not been appreciated in many studies is the fact that even the most "selective" drug maintains its specificity over a narrow range of concentrations. A few examples drawn from different classes of drugs appear in Table 2 to underscore this point. Furthermore, the mechanisms by which an endogenous substance produces an effect may change with concentration. For example, the gut hormone cholecystokinin (CCK)

TABLE 2
Non-selective Effects of Drugs

Drug	Selective Action	Non-selective Effects
DIDS†	Anion-exchange inhibitor	Inhibits P-type ATPases[16]; activates α_2-adrenergic receptors[17,18]
Procaine	Local anesthetic	Blocks muscarinic cholinergic receptors[19]
Verapamil	Ca^{2+} channel blocker	Blocks Na^+ and K^+ channels; blocks α-adrenergic, muscarinic cholinergic and opiate receptors[20,21]
Yohimbine	α_2-Adrenergic antagonist	Blocks Na^+ channels; blocks α_1-adrenergic and 5-HT$_2$ receptors; inhibits monoamine oxidase and cholinesterase activity[22]

†4,4′-Diisothiocyanatostilbene-2,2′-disulfonic acid.

may elicit contractions of gallbladder smooth muscle by stimulating cholinergic neurons at low concentrations and by directly interacting with CCK_A receptors on smooth muscle cells at higher concentrations.[24]

Species and Individual Variations in Drug Response

There is a large species-related variability in drug activity in intestinal preparations. This is due in part to species differences in gut morphology and signaling circuitry in the gastrointestinal tract. In comparing the distribution of receptors regulating ion transport within the small intestine in several species, for example, differences in the cellular occurrence of some receptors emerge (Table 3). Recent molecular biological studies of cloned receptor cDNAs have demonstrated that substitutions in certain amino acids important in ligand binding and signal transduction can occur among species and impede receptor classification using selective agonists and antagonists.[57] Species and individual variations in drug biotransformation processes are well recognized and can influence pharmacological studies, especially at the *in vivo* level.[58] Recently, genetic polymorphisms in receptor structure within an individual have been recognized that may give rise to individual variability in drug effects. A rare polymorphism (Thr[164] → Ile) in the proposed ligand binding pocket of the human β_2-adrenergic receptor, for example, has been associated with decreases in agonist and antagonist affinities and impaired G protein activation.[59]

Regional Differences

Drug effects may vary with the region of the intestinal tract under study because the digestive system exhibits a high degree of regional specialization. Reports of regional variations in drug activity abound in the literature. For example, norepinephrine interacts with α_2-adrenergic receptors in the submucosal plexus of the porcine ileum to promote chloride absorption, but produces chloride secretion in porcine colon by activating α_1-adrenergic receptors present on epithelial cells.[32,60] In the porcine gallbladder, α_2-adrenergic receptors regulate salt absorption differently in the neck and fundus; in addition, β_2-adrenergic receptors which likely mediate chloride secretion are present only in the fundic epithelium.[61] In the guinea pig intestine, histamine acting on H_1-histamine receptors elicits contractions in longitudinal smooth muscle with greater potency in the ileum than in colon; this appears to result from regional differences in receptor reserve.[62] Regional variations in drug action have also been observed in three regions of the muscularis mucosae from rabbit colon.[63] The cellular and molecular mechanisms underlying such regional variations remain to be explored in greater detail.

TABLE 3

Species Differences in the Cellular Occurrence of Some Receptors Mediating Small Intestinal Ion Transport

Receptor Type	Animal Species	Cellular Location	
		Submucosal Neurons	Epithelial Cells
α_2-Adrenergic	Rabbit[25–27]	Probably	Yes
	Guinea pig[28]	Yes	Undefined
	Rat[29,30]	Probably	Yes
	Dog[31]	Yes	Undefined
	Pig[32,33]	Yes	No
	Human[34]	Undefined	Yes
Muscarinic cholinergic	Guinea pig[35–38]	Yes	Yes
	Rat[39,40]	Undefined	Yes
	Pig[33,41,42]	Yes	Yes
Neuropeptide Y	Rabbit[43]	Undefined	Yes
	Mouse[44]	Yes	No
	Rat[45–47]	Undefined	Yes
	Pig[48]	Yes	No
Opiate	Rabbit[49]	Probably	No
	Mouse[50]	Probably	No
	Guinea pig[28,51,52]	Yes	Undefined
	Rat[53,54]	Undefined	No
	Dog[31]	Yes	Undefined
	Pig[55,56]	Yes	No†

†Low-affinity μ-like binding sites detected autoradiographically in mucosa, but these may not function in transport regulation.

Drug Removal Processes

Estimates of drug potency and efficacy can be altered by the presence of removal processes in the assay preparation. These processes vary for different substances and could include degrading enzymes such as acetylcholinesterase or peptidases as well as neurotransmitter re-uptake mechanisms. Although they normally function to limit the effects of naturally-occurring agonist neurotransmitters and neuromodulators, these processes may act to differentially remove synthetic compounds, including antagonists. A few examples are presented to emphasize the importance of drug removal processes in the gut. Denervation of the rat jejunum is associated with a supersensitivity in the contractile actions of direct and indirect-acting cholinergic agonists; this effect has been attributed to a decrease in cholinesterase activity in the preparation.[64] The amount of cholinesterase activity may vary with the tissue preparation. The cholinesterase inhibitor neostigmine increases the secretory potency and efficacy of acetylcholine in isolated sheets of the rat colonic mucosa, but has no effect on acetylcholine activity in the porcine jejunal mucosa.[41,65]

Neuropeptides are catabolized by a variety of peptidases which lack specificity for any particular peptide class.[66] As is the case with many gut peptides, the biologically-active C-terminus of substance P is rapidly degraded by the cell surface enzyme endopeptidase 24.11. In organ bath preparations of the guinea pig taenia caeci or vas deferens, the half-life of substance P is about 2.5 minutes. The $t_{1/2}$ is increased by nearly 3-fold in the presence of phosphoramidon, a naturally-occurring endopeptidase inhibitor.[67] Phosphoramidon greatly increases the magnitude and duration of substance P-induced contractions in several smooth muscle preparations.[67,68]

Some non-homologous peptides, such as calcitonin gene-related peptide, when given in combination with substance P can serve as substrates for the peptidase and thus augment the activity of substance P by delaying its breakdown.[69]

Neurotransmitter transport proteins reside on the membranes of nerve terminals and other cell types and function to selectively remove neurotransmitters (eg. biogenic amines and amino acids) from the extracellular space by a sodium-dependent active transport mechanism.[70] Re-uptake mechanisms that avidly remove norepinephrine released from submucosal neurons reside in the rat colonic mucosa.[71] In sheets of the porcine ileal mucosa mounted in Ussing chambers, blockade of norepinephrine uptake with desipramine increases the effectiveness of the catecholamine to alter ion transport at low concentrations as manifested by a 1000-fold sinistral shift in the lower portion of the norepinephrine concentration-effect relationship.[32] Higher concentrations of the catecholamine apparently saturate the re-uptake mechanism. The numerous factors influencing the concentrations of drugs in the receptor compartment are discussed extensively elsewhere.[10] The possible influence of removal processes on drug action deserves important consideration in the design of experiments, particularly in comparisons of drug action.

Other Variables Affecting Drug Action

There are numerous other variables that can potentially affect ligand-receptor interactions in the gastrointestinal tract. The animal's strain, age, gender, reproductive condition, feeding habits and diet may influence drug action, as can certain preexisting disease states (eg. inflammation, diabetes). These various factors should be taken into account when designing experiments and interpreting results.

RECEPTOR CLASSIFICATION

Functional Approaches

Receptors are characterized primarily by their affinities for a series of selective agonists and competitive antagonists. Purely competitive antagonists are considered to be more useful than agonists in classifying receptors because they lack the complicating variable of intrinsic efficacy and their requirements for binding to receptor sites are not as limited as agonists (i.e. they need only to produce a competitive block of agonist binding). Hence, they are more capable of detecting structural differences in a class of receptor proteins.

Agonist and Antagonist Affinities

Functional determinations of agonist affinity can be executed if a state in which there is a linear relationship between receptor occupancy and agonist response exists. In the case of full agonists, this usually involves limiting agonist responses through the application of functional antagonists or by eliminating of a portion of the total receptor population through irreversible alkylation (as in the partial alkylation method of Furchtgott).[72,73] The first approach suffers from present theoretical limitations and the second depends upon the availability of receptor-selective alkylating agents and assumptions implicit in classical receptor theory (i.e. the existence of a linear relation between agonist-receptor occupancy and agonist effect). The affinity of partial agonists possessing relatively low efficacy can be estimated with fewer problems than is the case with full agonists. These methods involve comparisons of the efficacy of the partial agonist with that of a full agonist at equiactive concentrations or assessments of the ability of a partial agonist to shift the concentration-response relationship of a full agonist.[10] The method of partial irreversible receptor blockade noted above can also be employed with partial agonists.[14]

Assessment of antagonist potency is perhaps the most powerful means of classifying receptors. The degree to which varying concentrations of a given competitive and reversible antagonist shift the concentration-effect curves of an agonist in a rightward direction can be calculated on the basis of dose-ratios (i.e. the ratio between agonist EC_{50} values in the presence and absence of antagonist at a fixed concentration). This model assumes that equiactive concentrations of agonist occupy the same number of receptors in the absence and presence of antagonist.[74] By determining agonist potency in the presence of antagonist at a number of concentrations, one can obtain a number of dose-ratios which can be analyzed by linear regression procedures. A Schild regression on these data can provide information on the equilibrium dissociation constant (K_B) of the competitive antagonist and deviations from unity in the slope of the regression can be useful for detecting conditions which prevent the establishment of drug-receptor equilibrium (such as the presence of drug removal processes, multiple drug actions or multiple receptors).[10] Of course, this method of estimating antagonist potency has its limitations, notably in the requirement that many concentration-effect curves must be constructed. Thus, within a tissue preparation agonist concentration-effect curves must be determined in the absence and presence of antagonist at a fixed concentration. Moreover, much rests on the agonist concentration-effect curve in the control condition since dose-ratio values are based on it.

Alternative methods exist for estimating antagonist potency under the limitations of the experimental preparation or particular properties of the antagonist. A method for determining antagonist potency has been proposed for preparations in which only single concentration-effect curves can be determined. By analysis in a Clark plot, all of the data points in agonist control and antagonist-shifted concentration-effect curves are compared for estimation of the antagonist K_B.[75] Pharmacological resultant analysis can be employed for determining the affinity of an antagonist having more than one action through the addition of a second antagonist capable of competing for a common receptor site.[76] These and other procedures are described in more detail elsewhere.[10,77]

In the context of antagonism, the reader should be aware that antagonists have been employed when available as useful pharmacological tools to selectively interrupt endogenous neurohormonal pathways in the digestive system. Against exogenous agonists which can be experimentally applied at high concentrations, many of these drugs produce a *competitive* antagonism as evidenced by a parallel dextral shift in the agonist concentration-effect curve. When used to block endogenous pathways however, such competitive antagonists appear to produce an *insurmountable* receptor blockade because they reduce the maximal effectiveess of an transmitter-releasing stimulus or indirectly-acting agonist. The antagonism appears to be non-competitive due to *finite* tissue concentrations of endogenous agonist which limit the ability of the agonist to surmount antagonist occupancy at its cognate receptor. In studies of the suppressive effects of norepinephrine on neurally-mediated ileal ion transport, for example, it was observed that the α-adrenoceptor blocker phentolamine produced a decrease in norepinephrine potency but not efficacy. In contrast, it greatly reduced the efficacy of tyramine, a drug which evokes the release of norepinephrine from its endogenous stores.[32]

Receptor Desensitization or Protection Experiments

Two general techniques have been used to study receptors involved in mediating the actions of enteric hormones or neurotransmitters. With the lack of available antagonists for some receptor systems, selective desensitization of the receptor by treatment with an agonist has been employed in many studies. Continuous agonist exposure of both ion channel-linked and G protein-coupled receptors produces desensitization; in the case of the latter receptor class, the mechanisms underlying this phenomenon include a receptor down-regulation, which may result in a reduction in receptor density (i.e. a loss of receptors), and in receptor-effector uncoupling. These effects are dependent upon the concentration and efficacy of the agonist employed and vary with the duration of agonist exposure and the cell types affected. Comparisons of subsequent agonist actions after desensitization must be made using agonists with equivalent efficacies; in general, the effects of low efficacy agonists will be blunted by desensitization more than those produced by agonists of higher efficacy. Furthermore, the investigator should be cognizant that desensitization induced in one receptor type may extend to other unrelated receptor types through the activation of common intracellular signalling pathways (heterologous desensitization).[13]

Receptor protection experiments involve a general alkylation of receptor populations with a non-specific alkylating agent such as N-ethylmaleimide or somewhat more selective agents such as phenoxybenzamine or N-ethoxycarbonyl-2-ethoxy-1,2-dihydroquinoline (EEDQ). To ascertain a role for a particular receptor in an aspect of gut function, an ligand selective for that receptor is present at the time of alkylation and "protects" the receptor from inactivation. Using this method to examine the receptors involved in neurally-mediated relaxation of gastric fundus smooth muscle, Grider demonstrated that relaxation was preserved following protection of VIP receptors, but not ATP receptors. These results implicated VIP as the major inhibitory transmitter released by electrical field stimulation of this tissue.[78] There are several obvious limitations to this technique. The degree to which a receptor population is eliminated is dependent upon the concentration of and duration of exposure to the alkylating agent which produces, in effect, an irreversible antagonism. This is an important issue as most full agonists (and their endogenous counterparts) require only a small fraction of the entire receptor population to produce a cellular response, i.e. there are a great number of spare receptors. Alkylation must proceed to the point where unprotected receptors are effectively lost to full agonists. Moreover, the use of agonists to protect receptors by rendering them inaccessible to the alkylating agent may be accompanied by undesirable down-regulation (and thus loss) of "protected" receptors. Agonists that are used to protect a receptor should be selective for it. Finally, the alkylating agents may have non-specific effects on cell function and viability which can complicate the results of these experiments.

Immunoneutralization

Enteric peptides have been the subject of many investigations designed to determine their actions in the digestive system. As our knowledge of peptide receptors often lags behind the isolation and chemical synthesis of peptides, suitable antagonists that are both specific for peptide receptor subtypes and lacking in partial agonist activity may not be available to block chemical signaling. For this reason, passive immunoneutralization of endogenous peptides with peptide antibodies has been employed to reduce the amount of physiologically-released peptides at their site(s) of action. Antisera against vasoactive intestinal peptide (VIP) have been used in this way to confirm a role for VIP as a myorelaxant and pro-secretory transmitter in the intestine.[79, 80] By binding to an agonist, the high molecular weight antibody may restrict access of the agonist to its cognate receptors. To the extent that this happens, immunoneutralization will act similar to a natural and selective agonist removal process (such as re-uptake, see below) by producing a downward shift in the agonist concentration-effect relationship at low agonist concentrations. Moreover, the process should be saturated and thus be surmounted by the agonist at high concentrations. The kinetics of antibody-agonist complex formation are often slow relative to agonist-receptor interactions and thus immunoneutralization may not be a useful strategy for investigating rapid signalling events.[81] Obviously, the issue of selectivity comes into consideration when working with antisera as they will bind to any endogenous substance possessing the epitopic domain.

RADIOLIGAND BINDING ASSAYS

Radioligand binding assays determine the characteristics of receptor occupancy by a drug or endogenous substance. Therefore, like functional assays binding assays provide information on the affinities of agonists and antagonists in binding to a particular receptor population as well as provide information on the density of binding sites. Because they do not measure agonist efficacy or the nature of signal transduction processes which are coupled to the receptor, binding studies cannot discriminate between a receptor and other cellular proteins which manifest selective affinity for the ligand. Thus binding studies define "binding sites", but cannot by themselves define a "receptor", which by pharmacological criteria must be linked to a cellular response (Table 4).

With the major exception of biological activity, many receptor criteria could in fact apply equally well to other "acceptor" sites which may exhibit binding features resembling that of a receptor, i.e. displacement of radioligand with structurally-related drugs; stereospecificity, saturability, and reversibility of ligand binding; and regional distribution of sites.[82,83] Regionally-distributed uptake sites, which normally function to remove biogenic amines (i.e. norepinephrine, dopamine, serotonin, histamine) or amino acid (i.e. glutamate, taurine, aspartate) transmitters from the extracellular space and thus terminate their participation in intercellular signalling, represent one class of "acceptor" molecules. Although their affinity for binding these substances is usually lower than that of receptors, they can display specific ligand binding which is reversible, saturable, and displaced by chemically-related substances including antagonists. In some cases, the nature of the acceptor molecules can be quite unexpected. Some ligands selective for α_2-adrenergic receptors such as clonidine, UK-14,304 and idazoxan also bind saturably and selectively, but with lower affinity, to non-adrenergic imidazoline sites.[84] The muscarinic cholinergic antagonist [^{3}H]quinuclidinyl benzilate can bind to intestinal mucus with relatively low affinity, its binding is displaced by atropine which exhibits an IC_{50} value which is within an order of magnitude of that determined for displacement at mucosal cholinergic receptors (210 nM vs. 14 nM).[85] Hepatic membranes can contain degrading enzymes which may possess a pattern of ligand specificity similar to that of a receptor. Even talc can exhibit saturable binding to hormonal ligands![86] The presence of specific acceptor sites and non-specific binding sites represent potential artifacts which can complicate the results of binding assays. Radioligand binding studies should be accompanied by functional determinations of ligand affinity and selectivity.

There are numerous reviews and monographs dealing with the execution and interpretation of radioligand binding assays and the reader is referred to these for further information (cf. for example, refs.[13,87–90]). Essentially, receptor binding assays involve three different approaches. *Saturation experiments* examine the binding of varying concentrations of radioligand to a fixed concentration of receptors. They provide estimates of the radioligand dissociation constant (K_d, a measure of affinity) and of receptor density (B_{max}). By varying the time of radioligand-receptor interactions but keeping receptor and ligand concentrations constant, *kinetic experiments* can be performed which measure the rate of ligand-receptor interactions and permit the calculation

---

TABLE 4
Receptor Criteria

Concept	Experimental Validation
Receptor number is finite	Binding is saturable
Bind site represents a receptor	The order of ligand affinities at the binding site should correlate well with functional estimates of ligand affinity; selective drugs should display a similar degree of specificity in binding and in biological activity
Receptor occupancy obeys Langmuir binding isotherm model	Dissociation constants determined from kinetic and saturation experiments should agree
Receptor has steric requirements	Ligand binding should be stereospecific

of association and dissociation rate constants. Finally, *inhibition experiments* involve the addition of competing non-radioactive ligands at varying concentrations to the radioligand-receptor complex and provide estimates of affinity (K_i) for the competing cold ligand.

In designing binding assays, major factors that one must consider include (a) *the characteristics of the receptor preparation* (intact cells, cell membranes, crude homogenates, highly-purified membranes?), (b) the *type of tracer* to be employed (^{125}I has >30,000-fold higher specific activity than ^{14}C, but a shorter half-life) and (c) the *method used to separate free radioligand from receptor-bound radioligand* (typically rapid filtration or centrifugation). Preparations for binding assays may have various advantages and disadvantages. The procedures used to prepare tissues, dispersed cells or cell membrane fragments may alter the binding kinetics of the receptor. In some preparations, such as cell membranes or solubilized tissue, the biological activities linked to receptor activation may be difficult to measure or actually be eliminated. Moreover, the receptor is not in its normal environment (for example, it does not remain in contact with cytosolic proteins). On the other hand, these systems are thus easy to prepare and store. Cell preparations offer several advantages: 1) the ease of processing large numbers of samples; 2) receptors are present in their natural milieu; 3) binding and functional properties of receptors can be examined; and 4) aspects of receptor regulation can be studied. They also present disadvantages which include difficulties in controlling ligand and cell concentrations in mono-layer preparations and the possibility that changes in receptor characteristics may occur as the result of regulatory processes (such as receptor-effector uncoupling or receptor down-regula-tion).[87] An exact correlation between biochemically- and functionally-determined ligand affinit-ies may be difficult to achieve in cellularly-heterogenous tissues. Moreover, in isolated cells or tissues, the radioligand may be internalized or sequestered and thus alter the measurement of binding kinetics. Indeed, different levels of complexity in preparations employed in binding assays will be associated with varying amounts of non-specific binding. The reader should bear in mind that specific binding of 50% or less is not considered adequate for radioligand binding assays.[87] The actions of degrading enzymes, internalization processes or other removal mecha-nisms resulting in loss or non-specific binding of the radioligand should be controlled.

In addition to the critical selection of a ligand based on its selectivity and high affinity for a particular binding site or class of sites, the process of radiolabeling a ligand should not interfere with the its native biological activity. This point should be confirmed as one chooses a particular radioligand for use in binding assays. It is very important to verify the identity of bound radioactivity. The density of receptors may be low in some preparations, a factor necessitating the use of radioiodinated ligands with high specific activity. Ligands modified by radiolabeling should be examined for retention of biological activity. Radiodination of a peptide, for example, may result in the oxidation of key methionyl or cystinyl residues which can destroy biological activity and alter the binding affinity of the molecule.[91] Moreover, the relatively large iodine molecule may physically interfere with receptor binding.[92] In the case of tritiated peptides, storage at low temperatures ($< -20°$ C) will lessen destruction of these radioligands by β emissions.[93] Peptides in general represent a class of receptor ligands that pose many problems which require careful design of binding experiments. Some variables affecting the results of peptide binding assays (but which should be considered for other classes of ligands as well) are listed in Table 5. The reader should also keep in mind that the use of agonists as ligands may be accompanied by some degree of receptor down-regulation or complicated by changes in affinity due to receptor coupling and uncoupling to effectors. Unfortunately, suitable antagonist ligands may be non-existent or not readily available for some classes of receptors.

Separation of free from bound radioligand is a critical step which must be executed rapidly in order to prevent dissociation of ligand-receptor complexes. Rapid filtration assays are preferred for their relative rapidity and technical ease in measurements of high-affinity binding, but non-specific binding to glass fiber filters may constitute a disadvantage. Centrifugation assays are most useful for measuring ligand binding to receptors at lower affinities (>10 nM) and in

TABLE 5
Some Variables Affecting Peptide Binding Assays

Problem	Possible Solutions
Poor chemical stability of ligand	Reduce oxidation of critical amino acid residues by avoiding vigorous mixing; store peptide under inert gases and low temperatures; add antioxidants to ligand aliquots
Poor biological stability of ligand	Reduce degradation of ligands with peptidase inhibitors and lower incubation temperatures
Artificially low ligand affinity and binding site density; artifactual heterogeneity of binding sites	Check purity of ligands
Peptide adsorption to surfaces; high non-specific binding to filters	Treat glassware or filters with silicone, polylysine, polyethyleneimine or albumin; reduce incubation temperature; change receptor binding preparation; avoid use of polystyrene containers.

Information summarized from references 92 and 93.

situations where high specific binding or rapid ligand-receptor dissociation is a problem. Other separation methods, such as equilibrium dialysis or gel chromatographic approaches, are employed less frequently and are described in more detail elsewhere.[89]

Molecular Strategies

There is no question that the application of molecular biology techniques in pharmacology has revolutionized our thinking about the fundamental nature of receptors, including the many receptors present in the gastrointestinal tract. Taking the superfamily of G protein-coupled receptors as an example to illustrate the power of these approaches, it should be noted that since the cloning of a β-adrenergic receptor in 1986 over 200 receptors have been cloned to date.[94] Recent investigations with particular receptors have focused on the critical structural elements that influence ligand binding and signal transduction, important aspects of receptor regulation, and the link between mutations in receptor structure or defects in receptor regulation and the occurrence of disease.

The principles of receptor cloning have been the subject of recent reviews and the reader is referred to these sources for further information.[94,95] The amino acid sequences of receptors can be rapidly deduced after cloning and sequencing complementary DNAs (cDNAs) obtained after reverse transcription of messenger RNAs (mRNAs) encoding these proteins (Figure 1).

The sequence of a receptor in a particular cell type can be determined after isolation of cellular RNA and its reverse transcription (RT) to cDNA, which is then amplified by the polymerase chain reaction (PCR). This RT-PCR approach requires oligonucleotide primers that hybridize to particular sequences of receptor cDNA and are employed in cDNA amplification. The primers are usually based on consensus sequence motifs specific for a family of receptors which have been previously determined. Products from the RT-PCR reaction can be subcloned into an appropriate vector and sequenced; their sequence homologies to cloned receptor subtypes can then be evaluated. This strategy can be useful not only in confirming that a particular receptor mRNA of interest is expressed in cells, but provides probes for further analysis of receptor mRNA expression under different experimental conditions or for screening genomic or cDNA libraries in the isolation and analysis of receptor genes or gene transcripts. The RT-PCR strategy has recently been used, for example, as a highly sensitive means of detecting mRNAs encoding different adrenergic receptor subtypes in a variety of peripheral tissues includ-

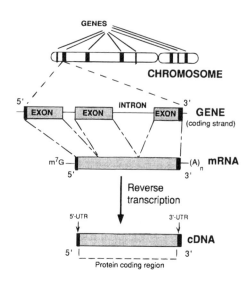

FIGURE 1 Relationship between chromosomes, receptor genes, messenger RNA (mRNA) and complementary DNA (cDNA). UTR, untranslated region; m^7G, 7-methylguanosine cap; $(A)_n$, polyadenylated tail. Shaded areas represent nucleic acid sequences that code for receptor protein.

ing the gut.[97,98] It has also been employed to examine the differential localization of neurokinin and histamine receptors in the canine colonic epithelium.[99]

The size and amount of receptor mRNAs, which are in relatively low abundance within cells, can be quantitatively detected through Northern hybridization analysis using labeled oligonucleotide, cDNA or cRNA receptor probes. For example, poly(A^+) RNA encoding the α_{2A}-adrenergic receptor was detected in the porcine ileal submucosa with this technique.[33] Other, more sensitive RNA quantitation techniques which also provide some information on RNA structure include S1 nuclease analysis and the primer extension and ribonuclease protection assays which require the use of highly specific, single-stranded probes.[100,101] The ribonuclease protection assay has been used in a recent study to compare α_{2A}-adrenergic receptor mRNA expression in crypt and villous cells of the human proximal colon.[34] These DNA-excess solution hybridization techniques are more sensitive than Northern hybridizations in measuring low abundance receptor mRNAs.[102] It should be emphasized that the detection or quantitation of receptor mRNAs through RT-PCR, Northern hybridization analysis or other techniques does not represent a measurement of receptor *protein* which is generated after extensive post-translational processing of mRNA. For example, mRNA encoding a subunit of the NMDA subtype of the ionotropic glutamate receptor could be detected by Northern hybridization in PC12 cells but no functional receptors could be found.[103] The results obtained from analyses of receptor mRNA cannot be directly and quantitatively related to those obtained in radioligand binding or functional assays. The specificity of these assays is dependent upon a number of factors including the nature and size of the probe, the structural characteristics of the region of RNA to be probed, and the hybridization and wash conditions.

The cDNA sequence of a receptor mRNA provides important information predictive of the amino acid sequence and structure of the receptor as well as its homologies to related proteins. It is critical that a cloned receptor cDNA be expressed and characterized functionally in cells in order to confirm its identity. Receptor cDNAs should be transfected into cultured cell lines that do not express the receptor endogenously, but nevertheless have the necessary cellular machinery to produce normal receptor protein. An orphan G protein-coupled receptor (LCR1), cloned from a bovine cDNA library, was found to selectively bind ^{125}I-neuropeptide Y (NPY) with high affinity after its transfection and expression in COS and CHO cells. Based on this evidence, it was proposed to represent a third subtype of NPY receptor.[104] However, subsequent experiments with LCR1 and its human homolog revealed that COS and CHO cells transfected with cDNAs for these receptors failed to express a functional NPY receptor; endogenous NPY binding sites on these cells constituted an artifact for radioligand binding assays.[105]

Receptors expressed on transfected cells can be used for functional, cell biological, and radioligand binding studies. Whenever possible, the pharmacological properties of the transfected receptor should be compared with those of the naturally-occurring receptor. Many cell lines express endogenous peptide receptors, for example, and these can be employed for functional comparisons of receptors transfected and expressed in another cell line. This is important as posttranslational processing of receptor proteins and the coupling of these receptors to effectors may vary in different cell lines and create alterations in receptor function. Point mutations or cassette mutations in the cDNA sequence prior to transfection can be made experimentally to alter the coding of single or multiple amino acid residues respectively; deletion mutations eliminate key amino acids.[106] Such manipulations of receptor sequence at the genetic level have yielded valuable insights into receptor function and regulation.

The sequence of the receptor gene yields information on genomic organization such as the presence and location of putative transcriptional regulatory motifs and promoter regions, the arrangement of protein-coding exons and the non-coding introns which interrupt them, the characteristics of the 5'- and 3'-untranslated regions and aspects of secondary DNA structure. Moreover, genomic DNA can be used for chromosomal mapping of receptor genes.[107] Comparisons of genomic DNA and cDNA sequences can also yield information on the post-transcriptional processing of the receptor, such as the existence of alternatively-spliced RNA variants (as in the case of CCK_B or somatostatin-2 receptors), species variations in receptor genes (e.g. the rat serotonin$_{1B}$ and human serotonin$_{1D\beta}$ receptors) or differently-sized RNA transcripts (e.g. the δ-opiate receptor).[108–111] Knowledge of the genomic sequence is essential for the analysis of receptor gene expression.[112]

LOCALIZATION OF RECEPTORS

RECEPTOR PROTEIN

Functional Localization and Sorting of Cells

The methods described in the preceding sections for the analysis of receptor protein and mRNA have been extended in procedures designed to localize receptors on specific cell populations or in particular anatomical regions. Cells bearing a particular class of receptors can be isolated or visualized on the basis of receptor-mediated signal transduction. For example, dissociated PC12 cells and enteroendocrine cells loaded with the calcium-indicating fluorescent dye indo-1 have been isolated through the activation of their respective M_4-muscarinic or CCK monitor peptide receptors (which are coupled to intracellular calcium elevations) and purified by fluorescence-activated cell sorting.[113,114] Subpopulations of enteric neurons responsive to nitric oxide (NO) have been visualized in the guinea pig intestine through immunohistochemically-detected elevations in cyclic GMP occurring in response to the NO donor, sodium nitroprusside.[115] These functional approaches for identifying cells bearing particular classes of receptors are quite powerful, providing that the specificity of the agonists used, possible paracrine interactions between responsive and "silent" cells, and other factors including those discussed above are taken into account.

Quantitative Receptor Autoradiography

Quantitative receptor autoradiography represents an extension of the radioligand binding assay and is quite useful for the visualization and quantitation of binding sites in complex tissues at low to moderate cellular resolution (usually in the micron range) by light microscopy. This receptor mapping technique has been the subject of many books and book chapters; the reader is referred to some of these for more details.[116–119] *In vivo* autoradiography involves the injection of a radioligand having high specific activity and affinity for the receptor in question into an animal and regional distribution of the radioligand in tissues is assessed over time. The procedure is relatively easy to execute, but adequate receptor characterization is a difficult process.[119] *In vitro* autoradiography, on the other hand, involves direct radioligand binding to tissue sections so that it is possible to better control conditions under which binding is measured and binding sites can be characterized through saturation, kinetic, and inhibition experiments. Other advantages of this latter approach when compared to *in vivo* autoradiography include the lower cost of experiments, better control of metabolic processes in tissue sections, and the ability to study different types of receptors in consecutive tissue sections.[116] In both procedures, radiolabeled tissue sections are mounted on emulsion-coated coverslips or slides and the density of exposed silver grains in the autoradiogram can be quantified against standards for accurate measurements of grain density or optical density. Many classes of receptors present in the intestinal tract have been studied by quantitative receptor autoradiography; these include binding sites for acetylcholine (muscarinic), atrial natriuretic factor, bombesin/gastrin-releasing peptide, neurokinins, neurotensin, norepinephrine, opiates and serotonin.

Receptor Immunohistochemistry

Receptor immunohistochemistry with antireceptor antibodies or anti-idiotypic antibodies to receptor ligands represents another approach to visualizing and mapping receptor proteins with a higher resolution than can be achieved with receptor autoradiographic procedures. Immunohistochemical techniques can be combined with electron microscopy, tract tracing, autoradiographic or *in situ* hybridization procedures to examine the localization and dynamics of receptors on cell subpopulations in a complex tissue preparation. Moreover, the availability of receptor antisera is useful for the co-detection of receptor proteins and effector molecules on Western blots. Although the results of immunohistochemical experiments provide information on the cellular and subcellular densities of receptor proteins, they do not yield information on the pharmacological properties of the receptor. In addition, suitable controls to assess the specificity of antibodies for particular receptors may not be available and different proteins bearing a similar antigenic determinant may be detected. This problem can be circumvented through the use of several antisera directed to different portions of the receptor which yield identical patterns of staining. The use of antireceptor antibodies for the localization of receptors in the gastrointestinal tract is in its beginning stages.[120]

RECEPTOR MESSENGER RNA

In Situ Hybridization Histochemistry

In situ hybridization histochemistry has been employed in mapping particular mRNAs in tissue sections.[121,122] As with the molecular methods discussed in the preceding sections, this reaction involves the hydrogen bonding between complementary nucleotides of two single-stranded nucleic acid molecules. One of these nucleic acids functions as a probe for the complementary RNA strand under investigation and therefore is labeled with a radioisotope or other detectable molecule. The characteristics of the nucleic acid probe are critical as they determine the stability of the nucleic acid hybrids formed and hence the success of the procedure. Double-stranded cDNA probes are easily to label, often to high specific activities, but must be denatured to separate the strands. Once denatured, only half the strands which are complementary to mRNA participate in the mixed-phase hybridization to mRNA; the other cDNA strand can reanneal to the probe and limit the availability of probe for RNA hybridization. Oligonucleotide probes can be easily synthesized and their shorter length facilitates tissue penetration. Because the sequence of oligonucleotides can be specified by the experimenter, probes can be constructed that possess a high specificity for a region of mRNA. The major disadvantage of relatively short probes is that they form less stable hybrids due to hybridization and wash conditions of relaxed stringency. Riboprobes, which are single-stranded RNA copies of cDNA (cRNA), form highly stable RNA-RNA hybrids. Moreover, they are single-stranded and do not reanneal like cDNA probes. They can be labeled to high specific activity through double nucleotide-labeling and other techniques. They are more labile than cDNA or oligonucleotides and have a greater propensity for non-specific hybridization, a factor which requires posthybridization ribonuclease treatment to reduce background labeling.[122] Proper controls must be executed to establish that probe hybridization is specific. In addition to posthybridization ribonuclease treatments, these include a demonstration of competition between labeled and unlabeled forms of the probe for target mRNA, the respective use of homologous and heterologous probes to demonstrate convergence and divergence in the pattern of target mRNA labeling, and the measurement of the thermal stability of hybrids by melting point analysis.[122] Of course, hybridization histochemistry should be combined, whenever possible, with immunocytochemistry or other methods designed to measure receptor protein concomitantly with receptor mRNA.

Although it has been used successfully in mapping receptor RNAs within the central nervous system, *in situ* hybridization histochemistry has not yet been utilized extensively in gastrointestinal tissues. However, in one recent study, mRNA encoding the M_3-muscarinic cholinergic receptor was found to be expressed in villous, but not crypt cells of the rat jejunal epithelium using this approach.[123]

SUMMARY AND CONCLUSIONS

The twentieth century has witnessed both the formulation of the receptor concept and the present golden era of receptor biology. Functional studies of receptors using highly selective agonists and antagonists have been conducted over much of this time period (i.e., the prerecombinant era) and the results of these experiments have been reproduced and extended by biochemical and molecular biological investigations. A complete understanding of receptor function can only be achieved through the proper application and amalgamation of old and new pharmacological techniques. The modern investigator must be acutely aware of their advantages and limitations as he or she unravels the complexities of receptor-mediated signal transduction in the digestive system.

REFERENCES

1. **Bayliss, W. M. and Starling, E. H.,** The movements and innervation of the small intestine, *J. Physiol. (London),* 24, 99, 1899.
2. **Daniel, E. E.,** Pharmacology of adrenergic, cholinergic, and drugs acting on other receptors in gastrointestinal muscle, in *Mediators and Drugs in Gastrointestinal Motility II [Handbk. Exp. Pharmacol.,* vol. 59/2), Bertaccini, G., Ed., Springer-Verlag, Heidelberg, 193, chap. 5.
3. **Schild, H. O.,** pA, a new scale for the measurement of drug antagonism, *Brit. J. Pharmacol.,* 2, 189, 1947.

4. **Nickerson, M.,** Receptor occupancy and tissue response, *Nature,* 178, 697, 1956.

5. **Stephenson, R. P.,** A modification of receptor theory, *Brit. J. Pharmacol.,* 11, 379, 1956.

6. **Lord, J. A. H., Waterfield, A. A., Hughes, J. and Kosterlitz, H. W.,** Endogenous opioid peptides: multiple agonists and receptors, *Nature,* 267, 495, 1977.

7. **Burnstock, G., Campbell, G. and Rand, M. J.,** The inhibitory innervation of the taenia of the guinea-pig caecum, *J. Physiol. (London),* 182, 504, 1966.

8. **Vane, J. R.,** A sensitive method for the assay of 5-hydroxytryptamine, *Brit. J. Pharmacol.,* 12, 344, 1957.

9. **Hollenberg, M. D.,** Structure-activity relationships for transmembrane signaling: the receptor's turn, *FASEB J.,* 5, 178, 1991.

10. **Kenakin, T. P.,** *Pharmacological Analysis of Drug-Receptor Interaction,* second ed., Raven Press, New York, 1993.

11. **Kenakin, T. P.,** Are receptors promiscuous? Intrinsic efficacy as a transduction phenomenon, *Life Sci.,* 43, 1095, 1988.

12. **Pallotta, B. S.,** Single ion channel's view of classical receptor theory, *FASEB J.,* 5, 2035, 1991.

13. **Limbird, L. E.,** *Cell Surface Receptors: A Short Course on Theory and Methods,* Martinus Nijhoff Publ., Boston, 1986.

14. **Tallarida, R. J., Raffa, R. B. and McGonigle, P.,** *Principles in General Pharmacology,* Springer-Verlag, New York, 1988.

15. **Pratt, W. B. and Taylor, P.,** *Principles of Drug Action: The Basis of Pharmacology,* third ed., Churchill Livingstone, New York, 1990.

16. **Vega, F. V., Cabero, J. L. and Mardh, S.,** Inhibition of H,K-ATPase and Na, K-ATPase by DIDS, a disulphonic stilbene derivative, *Acta Physiol. Scand.,* 134, 543, 1988.

17. **Periyasamy, S. M. and Somani, P.,** Sodium regulation of α_2-adrenoreceptors of human platelets: inactivation by 4,4′-diisothiocyano-2,2′-stilbene disulfonic acid (DIDS), *Biochem. Biophys. Res. Comm.,* 141, 222, 1986.

18. **Nieuwland, R., Van Willigen, G. and Akkerman, J.-W. N.,** 4,4′-Di-isothiocyanatostilbene-2,2′-disulphonic acid ('DIDS') activates protein kinase C and Na^+/H^+ exchange in human platelets via α_{2A}-adrenergic receptors, *Biochem. J.,* 293, 523, 1993.

19. **Ikei, N., Busik, J., Habara, Y. and Kanno, T.,** Competitive inhibition by procaine of carbachol-induced stimulus-secretion coupling in rat pancreatic acini, *Brit. J. Pharmacol.,* 110, 603, 1993.

20. **Janis, R. A. and Triggle, D. J.,** New developments in Ca^{2+} channel antagonists, *J. Med. Chem.,* 26, 775, 1983.

21. **Homaidan, F. R., Donowitz, M., Wicks, J., Cusolito, S., El Sabban, M. E., Weiland, G. A. and Sharp, G. W. G.,** Ca^{2+} channel blockers interact with α_2-adrenergic receptors in rabbit ileum, *Am. J. Physiol.,* 254, G586, 1988.

22. **Goldberg, M. R. and Robertson, D.,** Yohimbine: a pharmacological probe for study of the α_2-adrenoreceptor, *Pharmacol. Rev.,* 35, 143, 1983.

23. **Fox, J. E. T.,** Control of gastrointestinal motility by peptides. Old peptides, new tricks—new peptides, old tricks, in *Motility Disorders* [*Gastroenterology Clinics of North America, vol. 18*], Ouyang, A., Ed., W.B. Saunders, Philadelphia, 1989, p. 163.

24. **Grider, J. R.,** Peptidergic regulation of smooth muscle contractility, in *Gastrointestinal Regulatory Peptides* [*Handbk. Exp. Pharmacol.,* vol. 106], Brown, D. R., Ed., Springer-Verlag, Heidelberg, 1993, chap. 9.

25. **Chang, E. B., Field, M. and Miller, R. J.,** α_2-Adrenergic receptor regulation of ion transport in rabbit ileum, *Am. J. Physiol.,* 242, G237, 1982.

26. **Chang, E. B., Field, M. and Miller, R. J.,** Enterocyte α_2-adrenergic receptors: yohimbine and *p*-aminoclonidine binding relative to ion transport, *Am. J. Physiol.,* 244, G76, 1983.

27. **Hubel, K. A., Renquist, K. S. and Varley, G.,** Noradrenergic influence on epithelial responses of rabbit ileum to secretagogues, *Am. J. Physiol.,* 256, G919, 1989.

28. **Surprenant, A., Shen, K.-Z., North, R. A. and Tatsumi, H.,** Inhibition of calcium currents by noradrenaline, somatostatin, and opioids in guinea-pig submucosal neurones, *J. Physiol. (London),* 431, 585, 1990.

29. **Nakaki, T., Nakadate, T., Yamamoto, S. and Kato, R.,** *Alpha$_2$*-adrenergic receptor in intestinal epithelial cells. Identification with [^{3}H]yohimbine and failure to inhibit cAMP accumulation, *Mol. Pharmacol.,* 23, 228, 1983.

30. **Paris, H., Voisin, T., Remaury, A., Rouyer-Fessard, C., Daviaud, D., Langin, D. and Laburthe, M.,** *Alpha-2* adrenoceptor in rat jejunum epithelial cells: characterization with [^{3}H]RX821002 and distribution along the villus-crypt axis, *J. Pharmacol. Exp. Ther.,* 254, 888, 1990.

31. **Ahmad, S., Allescher, H. D., Manaka, H., Manaka, Y. and Daniel, E. E.,** Biochemical studies on opioid and α_2-adrenergic receptors in canine submucosal neurons, *Am. J. Physiol.,* 256, G957, 1989.

32. **Hildebrand, K. R. and Brown, D. R.,** Norepinephrine and *alpha*-2 adrenoceptors modulate active ion transport in porcine small intestine, *J. Pharmacol. Exp. Ther.,* 263, 510, 1992.

33. **Hildebrand, K. R., Lin, G., Murtaugh, M. P. and Brown, D. R.,** Molecular characterization of α_2-adrenergic receptors regulating intestinal electrolyte transport, *Mol. Pharmacol.,* 43, 23, 1993.

34. **Valet, P., Senard, J.-M., Devedijan, J.-C., Planat, V., Salomon, R., Voisin, T., Drean, G., Couvineau, A., Daviaud, D., Denis, C., Laburthe, M. and Paris, H.,** Characterization and distribution of α_2-adrenergic receptors in the human intestinal mucosa, *J. Clin. Invest.,* 91, 2049, 1993.

35. **Buckley, N. and Burnstock, G.,** Autoradiographic localisation of muscarinic receptors in guinea-pig intestine: distribution of high and low affinity agonist binding sites, *Brain Research,* 294, 15, 1984.

36. **North, R. A., Slack, B. E. and Surprenant, A.,** Muscarinic M$_1$ and M$_2$ receptors mediate depolarization and presynaptic inhibition in guinea-pig enteric nervous system, *J. Physiol. (London),* 368, 435, 1985.

37. **Carey, H. V., Tien, X.-Y., Wallace, L. J. and Cooke, H. J.,** Muscarinic receptor subtypes mediating the mucosal response to neural stimulation of guinea pig ileum, *Am. J. Physiol.,* 253, G323, 1987.

38. **Kachur, J. F., Sturm, B. L., Gaginella, T. S. and Noronha-Blob, L.,** Regulation of guinea pig ileal electrolyte transport by M3-muscarinic acetylcholine receptors *in vitro, Mol. Pharmacol.,* 38, 836, 1990.

39. **Wahawisan, R., Wallace, L. J. and Gaginella, T. S.,** Muscarinic receptors on rat ileal villus and crypt cells, *J. Pharm. Pharmacol.,* 38, 150, 1986.

40. **Stewart, C. P. and Turnberg, L. A.,** A microelectrode study of responses to secretagogues by epithelial cells on villus and crypt of rat small intestine, *Am. J. Physiol.,* 257, G334, 1989.

41. **Chandan, R., Megarry, B. H., O'Grady, S. M., Seybold, V. S. and Brown, D. R.,** Muscarinic cholinergic regulation of electrogenic chloride secretion in porcine proximal jejunum, *J. Pharmacol. Exp. Ther.,* 257, 908, 1991.

42. **Chandan, R., Hildebrand, K. R., Seybold, V. S., Soldani, G. and Brown, D. R.,** Cholinergic neurons and muscarinic receptors regulate anion secretion in pig distal jejunum, *Eur. J. Pharmacol.,* 193, 265, 1993.

43. **Hubel, K. A. and Renquist, K. S.,** Effect of neuropeptide Y on ion transport by the rabbit ileum, *J. Pharmacol. Exp. Ther.,* 238, 167, 1986.

44. **Rivière, P. J. M., Rao, R. K., Pascaud, X., Junien, J. L. and Porreca, F.,** Effects of neuropeptide Y, peptide YY and *sigma* ligands on ion transport in mouse jejunum, *J. Pharmacol. Exp. Ther.,* 264, 1268, 1993.

45. **Laburthe, M., Chenut, B., Rouyer-Fessard, C., Tatemoto, K., Couvineau, A., Servin, A. and Amiranoff, B.,** Interaction of peptide YY with rat intestinal epithelial plasma membranes: binding of the radioiodinated peptide, *Endocrinology,* 118, 1910, 1986.

46. **Cox, H. M., Cuthbert, A. W., Hakanson, R. and Wahlestedt, C.,** The effect of neuropeptide Y and peptide YY on electrogenic ion transport in rat intestinal epithelia, *J. Physiol. (London),* 398, 65, 1988.

47. **Nguyen, T. D., Heintz, G. G., Kaiser, L. M., Staley, C. A. and Taylor, I. L.,** Neuropeptide Y. Differential binding to rat intestinal laterobasal membranes, *J. Biol. Chem.,* 265, 6416, 1990.

48. **Brown, D. R., Boster, S. L., Overend, M. F., Parsons, A. M. and Treder, B. G.,** Actions of neuropeptide Y on basal, cyclic AMP-induced, and neurally evoked ion transport in porcine distal jejunum, *Regul. Peptides,* 29, 31, 1990.

49. **Binder, H. J., Laurenson, J. P. and Dobbins, J. W.,** Role of opiate receptors in regulation of enkephalin stimulation of active sodium and chloride absorption, *Am. J. Physiol.,* 247, G432, 1984.

50. **Sheldon, R. J., Rivière, P. J. M., Malarchik, M. E., Mosberg, H. I., Burks, T. F. and Porreca, F.,** Opioid regulation of mucosal ion transport in the mouse isolated jejunum, *J. Pharmacol. Exp. Ther.,* 253, 144, 1990.

51. **Mihara, S. and North, R. A.,** Opioids increase potassium conductance in submucous neurones of guinea-pig caecum by activating δ-receptors, *Brit. J. Pharmacol.,* 88, 315, 1986.

52. **Kachur, J. F. and Miller, R. J.,** Characterization of the opiate receptor in the guinea-pig ileal mucosa, *Eur. J. Pharmacol.,* 81, 177, 1982.

53. **Hardcastle, J., Hardcastle, P. T. and Redfern, J. S.,** Morphine has no direct effect on PGE_2-stimulated cyclic AMP production by rat isolated enterocytes, *J. Pharm. Pharmacol.,* 34, 68, 1982.

54. **Gaginella, T. S., Rimele, T. J. and Wietecha, M.,** Studies on rat intestinal epithelial cell receptors for serotonin and opiates, *J. Physiol. (London),* 335, 101, 1983.

55. **Quito, F. L. and Brown, D. R.,** Neurohormonal regulation of ion transport in the porcine distal jejunum. Enhancement of sodium and chloride absorption by submucosal opiate receptors, *J. Pharmacol. Exp. Ther.,* 256, 833, 1991.

56. **Quito, F. L., Seybold, V. S. and Brown, D. R.,** Opiate binding sites in mucosa of pig small intestine, *Life Sci.,* 49, PL219, 1991.

57. **Hall, J. M., Caulfield, M. P., Watson, S. P. and Guard, S.,** Receptor subtypes or species homologues: relevance to drug discovery, *Trends Pharmacol. Sci.,* 14, 376, 1993.

58. **Baggot, J. D.,** *Principles of Drug Disposition in Domestic Animals: The Basis of Veterinary Clinical Pharmacology,* W. B. Saunders, Philadelphia, 1977, chap. 4.

59. **Green, S. A., Cole, G., Jacinto, M., Innis, M. and Liggett, S. B.,** A polymorphism of the human β_2-adrenergic receptor within the fourth transmembrane domain alters ligand binding and functional properties of the receptor, *J. Biol. Chem.,* 268, 23116, 1993.

60. **Traynor, T. R., Brown, D. R. and O'Grady, S. M.,** Regulation of ion transport in porcine distal colon: effects of putative neurotransmitters, *Gastroenterology,* 100, 703, 1991.

61. **Duvall, M. D. and O'Grady, S. M.,** Regional adrenergic regulation of ion transport across the isolated porcine gallbladder, *Am. J. Physiol.,* 264, R703, 1993.

62. **Barker, L. A.,** Regional variation in the sensitivity of longitudinal smooth muscle to histamine at H_1-receptors in guinea-pig ileum and colon, *Brit. J. Pharmacol.,* 85, 377, 1985.

63. **Percy, W. H., Rose, K. and Burton, M. B.,** Pharmacologic characterization of the muscularis mucosae in three regions of the rabbit colon, *J. Pharmacol. Exp. Ther.,* 261, 1136, 1992.

64. **Osinski, M. A. and Bass, P.,** Chronic denervation of rat jejunum results in cholinergic supersensitivity due to reduction of cholinesterase activity, *J. Pharmacol. Exp. Ther.,* 266, 1684, 1993.

65. **Browning, J. G., Hardcastle, J., Hardcastle, P. T. and Sanford, P. A.,** The role of acetylcholine in the regulation of ion transport by rat colon mucosa, *J. Physiol. (London),* 272, 737, 1977.

66. **Conlon, J. M.,** Proteolytic inactivation of neurohormonal peptides in the gastrointestinal tract, in *Gastrointestinal Regulatory Peptides* [*Handbk. Exp. Pharmacol., vol. 106*], Brown, D.R., Ed., Springer-Verlag, Heidelberg, 1993, chap. 6.

67. **Hall, J. M., Fox, A. J. and Morton, I. K. M.,** Peptidase activity as a determinant of agonist potencies in some smooth muscle preparations, *Eur. J. Pharmacol.,* 176, 127, 1990.

68. **Rouissi, N., Nantel, F., Drapeau, G., Rhaleb, N-E., Dion, S. and Regoli, D.,** Inhibitors of peptidases: how they influence the biological activities of substance P, neurokinins, bradykinin and angiotensin in guinea pig, hamster and rat urinary bladders, *Pharmacology,* 40, 196, 1990.

69. **Nyberg, F., Le Grevés, P. and Terenius, L.,** Modulation of endopeptidase activity by calcitonin gene related peptide: a mechanism affecting substance P action?, *Biochimie,* 70, 65, 1988.

70. **Amara, S. G. and Kuhar, M. J.,** Neurotransmitter transporters: recent progress, *Ann. Rev. Neurosci.,* 16, 1993.

71. **Wu, Z. C. and Gaginella, T. S.,** Functional properties of noradrenergic nervous system in rat colonic mucosa: uptake of [^{3}H]norepinephrine, *Am. J. Physiol.,* 241, G137, 1981.

72. **Leff, P., Martin, G. R. and Morse, J. M.,** Application of the operational model of agonism to establish conditions when functional antagonism may be used to estimate agonist dissociation constants, *Brit. J. Pharmacol.,* 85, 655, 1985.

73. **Furchtgott, R. F.,** The use of β-haloalkylamines in the differentiation of receptors and in the determination of dissociation constants of receptor-agonist complexes, in *Advances in Drug Research, vol. 3,* Harper, N.J. and Simmonds, A.B., Eds., Academic Press, New York, 1993, p. 21.

74. **Arunlakshana, O. and Schild, H. O.,** Some quantitative uses of drug antagonists, *Brit. J. Pharmacol.,* 14, 48, 1959.

75. **Stone, M. and Angus, J. A.,** Developments of computer-based estimation of pA_2 values and associated analysis, *J. Pharmacol. Exp. Ther.,* 207, 705, 1978.

76. **Black, J. W., Gerskowitz, V. P., Leff, P., and Shankley, N. P.,** Analysis of competitive antagonism when this property occurs as part of a pharmacological resultant, *Brit. J. Pharmacol.,* 89, 547, 1986.
77. **Ott, L., Weiner, D., Cheng, H. and Woodward, J.,** Estimating pA_2 values for different designs, *J. Pharmacol. Meth.,* 5, 75, 1981.
78. **Grider, J. R.,** Identification of neurotransmitters by selective protection of postjunctional receptors, *Am. J. Physiol.,* 258:G103, 1990.
79. **Grider, J. R. and Makhlouf, G. M.,** Colonic peristaltic reflex: identification of vasoactive intestinal peptide as a mediator of descending relaxation, *Am. J. Physiol.,* 251, G40, 1986.
80. **Cooke, H. J., Zafirova, M., Carey, H. V., Walsh, J. H. and Grider, J.,** Vasoactive intestinal polypeptide actions on the guinea pig intestinal mucosa during neural stimulation, *Gastroenterology,* 92, 361, 1987.
81. **van Oers, J. W. A. M., van Bree, C., White, A. and Tilders, F. J. H.,** Antibodies to neuropeptides as alternatives for peptide receptor antagonists in studies on the physiological actions of neuropeptides, in *Progress in Brain Research,* vol. 92, Joosse, J., Buijs, R.M. and Tilders, F.J.H., Eds., Elsevier, Amsterdam, 225, 1992, chap. 19.
82. **Laduron, P. M.,** Criteria for receptor sites in binding studies, *Biochem. Pharmacol.,* 33, 833, 1984.
83. **Laduron, P. M.,** Stereospecificity in binding studies. A useful criterion though insufficient to prove the presence of receptors, *Biochem. Pharmacol.,* 37, 37, 1988.
84. **Kilpatrick, A., Brown, C. C. and Mackinnon, A. C.,** Non-α_2-adrenoceptor idazoxan binding sites: a new target for drug development, *Transact. Biochem. Soc.,* 20, 113, 1992.
85. **Rimele, T. J. and Gaginella, T. S.,** Binding of [^{3}H]quinuclidinyl benzilate to intestinal mucus. An artifact in identification of epithelial cell muscarinic receptors, *Biochem. Pharmacol.,* 31, 515, 1982.
86. **Cuatrecasas, P. and Hollenberg, M. D.,** Binding of insulin and other hormones to non-receptor materials: saturability, specificity and apparent "negative cooperativity", *Biochem. Biophys. Res. Comm.,* 62, 31, 1975.
87. **Bylund, D. B. and Toews, M. L.,** Radioligand binding methods: practical guide and tips, *Am. J. Physiol.,* 265, L421, 1993.
88. **Gardner, J. D.,** Receptors for gastrointestinal hormones, *Gastroenterology,* 76, 202, 1979.
89. **Yamamura, H. I., Enna, S. J. and Kuhar, M. J., Eds.,** *Neurotransmitter Receptor Binding,* second ed., Raven Press, New York, 1985.
90. **Yamamura, H. I., Enna, S. J. and Kuhar, M. J., Eds.,** *Methods in Neurotransmitter Receptor Analysis,* Raven Press, New York, 1990.
91. **Heward, C. B., Yang, Y. C. S., Sawyer, T. K., Bregman, M. D., Fuller, B. B., Hruby, V. J. and Hadley, M. E.,** Iodination associated inactivation of β-melanocyte stimulating hormone, *Biochem. Biophys. Res. Comm.,* 88, 266, 1979.
92. **Quirion, R. and Gaudreau, P.,** Strategies in neuropeptide binding research, *Neurosci. Biobehav. Rev.,* 9, 413, 1985.
93. **Hanley, M.,** Peptide binding assays, in *Neurotransmitter Receptor Binding,* second ed., Yamamura, H.I., Enna, S.J. and Kuhar, M.J., Eds., Raven Press, New York, 1985, chap. 4.
94. **Dixon, R. A. F., Kobilka, B. K., Strader, D. J., Benovic, J. L., Dohlman, H. G., Frielle, T., Bolanowski, M. A., Bennett, C. D., Rands, E., Diehl, R. E., Mumford, R. A., Slater, E. E., Sigal, I. S., Caron, M. G., Lefkowitz, R. J. and Strader, C. D.,** Cloning of the gene and cDNA for mammalian β-adrenergic receptor and homology with rhodopsin, *Nature,* 321, 75, 1986.
95. **Eva, C. and Sprengel, R.,** Cloning of G protein-coupled receptors, in *Receptors: Molecular Biology, Receptor Subclasses, Localization, and Ligand Design,* Conn, P.M., Ed., Academic Press, New York, 1993, chap. 2.
96. **Laburthe, M., Kitabgi, P., Couvineau, A. and Amiranoff, B.,** Peptide receptors and signal transduction in the digestive tract, in *Gastrointestinal Regulatory Peptides* [*Handbk. Exp. Pharmacol., vol. 106*], Brown, D.R., Ed., Springer-Verlag, Heidelberg, 1993, chap. 5.
97. **Thomas, R. F. and Liggett, S. B.,** Lack of β$_3$-adrenergic receptor mRNA expression in adipose and other metabolic tissues in the adult human, *Mol. Pharmacol.,* 43, 343, 1993.
98. **Eason, M. G. and Liggett, S. B.,** Human α_2-adrenergic receptor subtype distribution: widespread and subtype-selective expression of α_2C10, α_2C4, and α_2C2 mRNA in multiple tissues, *Mol. Pharmacol.,* 44, 70, 1993.

99. **Khan, I., LaPierre, N. and Rangachari, P. K.,** Messenger RNAs for neurokinin and histamine receptor subtypes in isolated canine colonic crypts, *J. Pharmacol. Exp. Ther.,* 272, 1285, 1995.

100. **Wiesner, R. J. and Zak, R.,** Quantitative approaches for studying gene expression, *Am. J. Physiol.,* 260, L179, 1991.

101. **Farrell, R. E., Jr.,** *RNA Methodologies: A Laboratory Guide for Isolation and Characterization,* Academic Press, New York, 1993.

102. **Hadcock, J. R., Williams, D. L. and Malbon, C. C.,** Physiological regulation at the level of mRNA: analysis of steady-state levels of specific mRNAs by DNA-excess solution hybridization, *Am. J. Physiol.,* 256, C457, 1989.

103. **Sucher, N. J., Brose, N., Deitcher, D. L., Awobuluyi, M., Gasic, G. P., Bading, H., Cepko, C. L., Greenberg, M. E., Jahn, R., Heinemann, S. F. and Lipton, S. A.,** Expression of endogenous NMDARI transcripts without receptor protein suggests post-transcriptional control in PC12 cells, *J. Biol. Chem.,* 268, 22299, 1993.

104. **Rimland, J., Xin, W., Sweetnam, P., Saijoh, K., Nestler, E. J. and Duman, R. S.,** Sequence and expression of a neuropeptide Y receptor cDNA, *Mol. Pharmacol.,* 40, 869, 1991.

105. **Jazin, E. E., Yoo, H., Blomqvist, A. G., Yee, F., Weng, G., Walker, M. W., Salon, J., Larhammar, D. and Wahlestedt, C.,** A proposed bovine neuropeptide Y (NPY) receptor cDNA clone, or its human homologue, confers neither NPY binding sites nor NPY responsiveness on transfected cells, *Regul. Peptides,* 47, 247, 1993.

106. **Buckley, N. J., Hulme, E. C. and Birdsall, N. J. M.,** Use of clonal cell lines in the analysis of neurotransmitter receptor mechanisms and function, *Biochim. Biophys. Acta,* 1055, 43, 1990.

107. **Wilkie, T. M., Chen, Y., Gilbert, D. J., Moore, K. J., Yu, L., Simon, M. I., Copeland, N. G. and Jenkins, N. A.,** Identification, chromosomal location, and genome organization of mammalian G protein-coupled receptors, *Genomics,* 18, 175, 1993.

108. **Vanetti, M., Kouba, M., Wang, X., Vogt, G. and Höllt, V.,** Cloning and expression of a novel mouse somatostatin receptor, *FEBS Lett.,* 311, 290, 1992.

109. **Song, I., Brown, D. R., Wiltshire, R. N., Gantz, I., Trent, J. M. and Yamada, T.,** The human gastrin/cholecystokinin type B receptor gene: alternative splice donor site in exon 4 generates two variant mRNAs, *Proc. Natl. Acad. Sci. U.S.A.,* 90, 9085, 1993.

110. **Adham, N., Romanienko, P., Hartig, P., Weinshank, R. L. and Branchek, T.,** The rat 5-hydroxytryptamine$_{1B}$ receptor is the species homologue of the human 5-hydroxytryptamine$_{1D\beta}$ receptor, *Mol. Pharmacol.,* 41, 1, 1992.

111. **Bzdega, T., Chin, H., Kim, H., Jung, H. H., Kozak, C. A. and Klee, W. A.,** Regional expression and chromosomal localization of the δ-opiate receptor gene, *Proc. Natl. Acad. Sci. U.S.A.,* 90, 9305, 1993.

112. **Harrington, C. A. and Buckley, N. J.,** Methods for studying the control of receptor gene expression: promoter mapping and analysis of transcription regulation, in *Receptors: Molecular Biology, Receptor Subclasses, Localization, and Ligand Design,* Conn, P.M., Ed., Academic Press, New York, 1993, chap. 1.

113. **Ransom, J. T., Cherwinski, H. M., Delmendo, R. E., Sharif, N. A. and Eglen, R.,** Characterization of the m4 muscarinic receptor Ca^{2+} response in a subclone of PC-12 cells by single cell flow cytometry. Inhibition of the response by bradykinin, *J. Biol. Chem.,* 266, 11738, 1991.

114. **Liddle, R. A., Misukonis, M. A., Pacy, L. and Balber, A. E.,** Cholecystokinin cells purified by fluorescence-activated cell sorting respond to monitor peptide with an increase in intracellular calcium, *Proc. Natl. Acad. Sci. U.S.A.,* 89, 5147, 1992.

115. **Young, H. M., McConalogue, K., Furness, J. B. and De Vente, J.,** Nitric oxide targets in the guinea-pig intestine identified by induction of cyclic GMP immunoreactivity, *Neuroscience,* 55, 583, 1993.

116. **Kuhar, M. J.,** Receptor localization with the microscope, in *Neurotransmitter Receptor Binding,* second ed., Yamamura, H.I., Enna, S.J. and Kuhar, M.J., Eds., Raven Press, New York, 1985, chap. 7.

117. **Boast, C. A., Snowhill, E. W. and Altar, C. A.,** Eds., *Quantitative Receptor Autoradiography,* Alan R. Liss, New York, 1986.

118. **Leslie, F. M. and Altar, C. A.,** Eds., *Receptor Localization: Ligand Autoradiography,* Alan R. Liss, New York, 1988.

119. **Kuhar, M. J. and Unnerstall, J. T.,** Receptor autoradiography, in *Methods in Neurotransmitter Receptor Analysis,* Yamamura, H.I., Enna, S.J. and Kuhar, M.J., Eds., Raven Press, New York, 1990. chap. 7.

120. **Vigna, S. R., Bowden, J. J., McDonald, D. M., Fisher, J., Okamoto, A., McVey, D. C., Payan, D. G., and Bunnett, N. W.,** Characterization of antibodies to the rat substance P (NK-1) receptor and to a chimeric substance P receptor expressed in mammalian cells, *J. Neuroscience,* 14, 834, 1994.

121. **Penschow, J. D., Haralambidis, J., Darling, P. E., Darby, I. A., Wintour, E. M., Tregear, G.W. and Coghlan, J.P.,** Hybridization histochemistry, *Experentia,* 43, 741, 1987.

122. **Tecott, L. H., Eberwine, J. H., Barchas, J. D. and Valentino, K. L.,** Methodological considerations in the utilization of *in situ* hybridization, in *In Situ Hybridization: Applications to Neurobiology.* Valentino, K.L., Eberwine, J.H. and Barchas, J.D., Eds., Oxford University Press, New York, 1987, chap. 1.

123. **Przyborski, S. A. and Levin, R. J.,** Enterocytes on rat jejunal villi but not in the crypts possess m3 mRNA for the M_3 muscarinic receptor localized by *in situ* hybridization, *Exp. Physiol.,* 78, 109, 1993.

8 *In Vivo* Motility Techniques

Norman W. Weisbrodt and Paul Bass

INTRODUCTION

GENERAL APPROACH TO THE STUDY OF MOTILITY

The choice of techniques used to study gastrointestinal motility depends upon the question(s) being addressed. Oftentimes the question involves the motility response as it relates to the activities of multiple tissues and/or organs. In such cases, the choice may be to use *in vivo* techniques. Studies of gastrointestinal motility that utilize *in vivo* techniques can be divided roughly into categories—those in which the organ of interest is isolated as much as possible so that its response to various agents can be tested in the absence of influence from other organs, and those in which measurements are made with minimal intervention so that the effects on "normal" motility can be deduced. Although studies of the first type seem close to those conducted *in vitro,* they offer the advantage that the influence of extrinsic nerves and hormones can be determined. Also, normal blood flow is intact to better insure proper oxygenation of the relatively thick-walled organs comprising the gut. Studies of the second type may be conducted by surgically implanting monitoring devices that can be used while the animal is fully conscious and minimally restrained, or by using totally non-invasive techniques such as fluoroscopy. One can also use hybrids of the two types of studies. For example, 1 or 2 cannulas can be implanted chronically in various areas of the tract. These may be used to place luminal recording devices or even add inert markers for monitoring activity. Yet another common technique is to place a silicon tube into the stomach and upper small intestine. These tubes deliver a marker for measuring either gastric emptying or intestinal transit. Within each category of studies, many techniques have been devised. This chapter will discuss how one decides which technique is best to test the hypothesis that has been formulated.

Although the most important point in the choice of technique(s) is consideration of the hypothesis being tested, an equally important point is to clearly define what one means by "motility" prior to choosing a method to test an hypothesis. General statements that "motility is either increased or decreased" usually are meaningless. For example, just because the number and/or force of contractions are increased does not mean that emptying and/or transit is enhanced. In several species, morphine will enhance force and frequency of intestinal muscle contractions, yet decrease gastric emptying and prolong intestinal transit at the same time. An explanation for this delaying effect is given below.

We view motility as measured *in vivo* as falling into 3 categories: 1) phasic activity associated with or without tonal changes due to either or both circular and longitudinal muscle, 2) transit through part or the entire gut and 3) volume or tonal changes of the various organs of the gut. The above 3 categories can emphasize local activity as well as overall patterns of activity on or between organs. Obviously, many methods are applicable only to animal studies. However, hypotheses based on *in vivo* data from animals have had excellent extrapolation to humans. For example, muscle contractile patterns associated with interdigestive and digestive states in the dog have a direct extrapolation to humans.

HISTORICAL PERSPECTIVE

Direct observations of the various gastrointestinal tract organs have provided insight into their function. Accidents to individuals have yielded human models who have been studied by various physicians and scientists. An example of such an individual was Alexis St. Martin, a French-Canadian, who had a chronic gastrocutaneous fistula inflicted on him by an accidental gunshot wound. His attending physician William Beaumont successfully studied gastric physiology of St. Martin primarily between the years 1825–1833. Much of Beaumont's "laboratory" was an old log hospital in Prairie du Chien, Wisconsin, a site currently honored in a modern museum that contains several remnants from that time. Beaumont's diaries contain writings that confirmed and clarified many physiological principles. These include the movement of the body and antrum of the stomach. Beaumont recognized that various foods were ground and mixed with gastric contents. He also had insight into the antrum's ability to sieve particles when he observed that chyme entered the duodenum while crude food particles were retained in the stomach. Other ideas in physiology confirmed by Beaumont were that the stomach produced hydrochloric acid and that there was a CNS influence on gastric secretions. As a point of interest, Mr. St. Martin outlived Beaumont by over 30 years. St. Martin is buried north of Montreal, Canada. He was honored by the Canadian Physiology Society in 1962 with a graveyard plaque that reads in both English and French, "Through his affliction, he serves all humanity." More recently, a Mayo surgeon (M. G. Sarr) and one of us (P. B.) editorialized why the fistula did not heal.[1] Since Beaumont's observations, various types of fistulae and pouches in both people and animals have been described mainly for secretions but also for muscle movement. In more recent times, Harold Wolff and Stewart Wolf made several key observations, especially on psychological factors that influence the fistulated stomach of their subject Tom. These and several other observational type of studies are summarized in a chapter by W. C. Alvarez.[2]

Direct observation as described above allows for long-term study and for descriptions; however, quantification is difficult. Roentgen's discovery in 1897 lead to the introduction of various X-ray opaque materials that permitted the visualization of the lumen of the gastrointestinal tract. Cannon used this technique around the turn of the century to depict and describe the patterns of movement of bismuth within the intestine of conscious cats.[3] Many of the terms and descriptions from his classic paper still are in use today. Over the years, other technologies have been combine with radiography to produce, for example, X-ray cinematography. The latter is the forerunner of ultrasound techniques and even nuclear magnetic resonance (NMR) imaging. X-ray technology also has been used to identify opaque materials, as for example lead shot, placed under the serosa. Several of these techniques clearly outline the shortening of the circular and longitudinal muscle. An example of such a technique is described by Steggerda and Giantarco.[4] They injected X-ray contrast media (thorotrast) into the submucosal area of the bowel. With this method they could demonstrate the movement of various parts of the muscle wall. In another example, specific points along the esophagus of the cat were marked by implanting small tantalum markers and cineroentgenography was used to correlate constrictions and shortening of the esophageal wall with intraluminal pressure changes.[5]

Methods for measuring contractions of the gastrointestinal tract in anesthetized animals were also introduced in the late nineteenth century. The technique of passing a balloon into the lumen to record contractions was described by Bayliss and Starling.[6] Such measurements were quantitative and yielded permanent records. Also, various modifications of the technique allowed for measurements at more than one site and from unanesthetized animals, including humans.

One popular modification in use today is to employ small catheters with openings through which fluid is perfused. If the system has a low compliance, accurate determinations of intraluminal pressure around the openings can be obtained.

More recently, methods have been developed to monitor contractions of the musculature by placing sensors on the serosal surface of the gut. Both myoelectrical and mechanical activities have been recorded. Alvarez and Mahoney recorded electrical activity from the musculature of the gut as early as 1922.[7] However, it was not until the introduction of improved electronic recorders that interest in the method blossomed.[8]

Transplanted segments of bowel have been used for studying motility by placing balloons or open-tipped catheters into their lumen. An example is a Thiry-Vella loop in which a segment of bowel is freed and the two ends brought to the abdominal wall. We have also used "suitcase handles" in which a loop of bowel is placed into a tube of skin. Such a chronic preparation, referred to as a Beible loop, permits the recording of electric and motor activity from well-trained unanesthetized dogs. This preparation was used to initiate studies on the electric events of the canine small intestine at the Mayo Foundation.[8] This was the first of a long series of studies that climaxed in the characterization of the migrating myoelectric complex.[9]

Transit of material through the GI tract has been studied at all levels of sophistication. At one extreme, markers such as charcoal are taken orally and their appearance in the stool then noted. At the other, markers are placed within a specific organ and their emptying from or transit along that organ is followed from moment to moment.

Practically all of the methods discussed in this chapter have been derived from those described above. Various modifications have been made to combine two or more methods, to make a method less invasive and less likely to alter the motility pattern being monitored, and/or to increase the reliability and duration of data acquisition. In all cases, the need for modifications has been driven by the results of previous investigations.

ASSESSMENTS OF MOTILITY—SOME DEFINITIONS

The methods described in this chapter are used almost exclusively in unanesthetized animals. It must have been obvious to Walter B. Cannon that the patterns of gut contractions were different between the anesthetized and unanesthetized state because he was careful to study various GI parameters in unanesthetized animals. From 1889 to 1914, Cannon studied the passage of X-ray opaque substances through a variety of organs ranging from the esophagus of the goose to small bowel and colon activity in various mammals. Cannon was the first to characterize typical fed patterns of muscle activity initiated in animals. He mixed bismuth subnitrate with canned salmon and fed it to conscious cats that were trained to lie quietly on his lap. The type of gut transit and muscle activities described by Cannon could not be seen or recorded in anesthetized preparations. Then as now, anesthetics and narcotic analgesics profoundly affect transit as well as muscle contractions.

Before deciding what methodology to utilize, a decision must be made about what aspect of motility needs to be monitored in order to test the hypothesis being proposed. Each of the methods most commonly utilized provides information about one or more of four parameters—transit, wall motion, muscle contraction, and intraluminal pressure. Transit (sometimes designated as propulsion) refers to the linear displacement of a marker within the lumen of the gut. Wall motion refers to the physical displacement of the wall in response to contraction of the muscle comprising the wall or to stresses on the wall developed by lumenal contents. Muscle contraction refers to the active stress that is developed within the muscle comprising the wall. It is important to note that contraction may or may not result in wall motion. Intraluminal pressure refers to the hydrostatic pressure detected by a sensor placed in the lumen. Determination of the genesis of the pressure depends upon characteristics of the sensor and of the muscle contractions and wall motions producing the pressure.

GASTROINTESTINAL TRANSIT

The movement of material within and through organs of the gastrointestinal tract (i.e. Transit) must be coordinated and regulated so that digestion and absorption can take place in an orderly fashion. This is the function accomplished by contractions of the gut smooth muscle. So one can argue that if transit is the end point, the best assessment of overall motility is transit itself. Once transit is characterized, then the contractile patterns responsible for the transit and the regulatory pathways controlling the contractile patterns responsible for transit can be elucidated.

All methods that evaluate transit involve collection or detection of measurable material at one or more points of the gastrointestinal tract after its administration at another, usually orad, point. In order to be quantitative, it is best if the material being monitored is neither absorbed nor secreted within the organ through which transit is being assessed. This is especially relevant if transit through the small intestine is being evaluated due to the marked digestion and absorption that takes place in this organ. On the other hand, using inert markers may provide information only on the movement of the marker itself and not the movement of the digestible material the marker is incorporated into.

Although the force and frequency of contractions of the circular muscle markedly influence gastrointestinal transit of digestive and nondigestive substances, one cannot assume that the rate of transit will increase as force and frequency increase. This has been well documented using drugs. Narcotics that stimulate circular muscle contractions prolong transit time;[10,11] laxatives that inhibit muscle activity shorten transit time.[12] The apparent paradox is easily understood if one visualizes a circular muscle contraction as obliterating the bowel lumen and increasing the resistance to flow. Similarly, minimizing or reducing circular muscle activity enhances transit. Thus, contractile patterns of motility as influenced by interdigestive or digestive states, diseases, or drugs may be more important than force and frequency in determining the rate and spread of substances through various organs of the gastrointestinal tract. In this section, we will address the various ways of evaluating transit through the entire as well as the separate organs of the GI tract.

Non-Invasive Techniques

Stool Frequency

Frequency of defecation is an overall indication that transit and gut function is normal. Connell et al.[13] defined normal bowel habits as easily passed formed stools at a rate not greater than twice per day nor less than once every 2 days. Based on the above normal patterns, the FDA adapted the definition of constipation as less than 3 bowel movements per week.[14] Based on this definition, stool frequency and stool characteristics are parameters that are used to assess laxatives. Studies on quantifying stools from normal and constipated individuals have been reported.[15,16] A similar study in evaluating fecal output in rats for evaluating antidiarrheal and laxative drugs has also been described.[17]

Total Transit

Techniques are available to monitor mouth-to-anus or total transit time. Total transit information is helpful in assessing prokinetic and antidiarrheal drugs as well as normal and pathophysiological conditions. Total transit also may be helpful for demonstrating the residence time of various sustained release medications. For example, an oral sustained release preparation of several beta blocking drugs has been evaluated for gradual release from an osmotic pressure-sensitive device marketed under the trade name Oros®. Oral ingestion of Oros® by humans resulted in a total transit time ranging from 5 to 58 hours (Figure 1). Note that this wide range could result in marked differences in the absorption of nutrients and drugs from one individual to another.

The substance used for total transit studies should be solid, nonabsorbable, and of reasonably small particle size to assess transit at all levels of the GI tract. It has been shown that the stomach empties liquids, digestible solids, and indigestible solids in a differential manner.[19] In humans, several substances like dyes, barium, glass beads, and radioactive chromium salts may be taken orally and then the stool collected and the substance identified in the stool. A popular method for measuring total transit time was reported by Hinton et al.[20] The test is easy to do, noninvasive, inexpensive, and avoids radiation exposure. Hinton used 25 rings of barium impregnated polyethylene catheters (3 mm outside diameter). He simply sectioned radiopaque cardiac catheters into small rings and placed them into a gelatin capsule which quickly dissolved in the stomach. The capsule is taken orally, the stool collected, flattened, placed under a regular X-ray tube, and the number of rings per stool counted. From such studies, it has been demonstrated that the first rings may appear in the stool as early as 18 hours after ingestion. Approximately 80% of the rings are present on average in most people by around 60 hours. The Hinton method was modified to assess transit by a single stool analysis.[21] This was made practical by administering 3 different shaped markers on three consecutive days and identifying which of the markers were present in the stool on day 4 after the initiation of the study.

There are several markers whose location in the gastrointestinal tract can be monitored by devices external to the body. Radiopaque substances, such as barium, can be imaged using x-rays. Advantages of this technique are that barium preparations are simple and cheap and standard x-ray machines are widely available. Also, by using image intensifiers and videocameras, continuous and permanent visualizations can be obtained. A major disadvantage is that significant levels of radiation are encountered if prolonged measurements are made. Also, most radiopaque substances are relatively dense and may not transit the gut like normal gut contents. A second technique, called scintigraphy,[22,23,24] avoids some of the complications encountered when using x-rays. Scintigraphy uses various gamma ray emitting isotopes. These isotopes are used to label both solid and liquid components of a meal. Then, movement of the label is detected by gamma cameras. By using proper placements of the cameras and appropriate considerations, the method can yield quantitative results. Also, if more than one isotope is used,

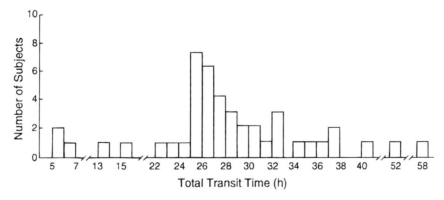

FIGURE 1 Histogram of the individual total gastrointestinal transit times for an ingested drug delivery system. Total transit times is shown on the abscissa and the number of subjects with the indicated transit times is shown on the ordinate. (Modified from reference 18.)

differential movement of labeled solids and labeled liquids can be followed. Major disadvantages are that gamma cameras are not found as commonly in research laboratories and isotopes still are involved. Also, isotope may be released from the carrier and may not necessarily follow the substance of interest that is being transported or absorbed. Other considerations of scintigraphy have been discussed by Sandefer and Digenis.[25] A more recent technique that avoids the use of radiation is ultrasonography.[26,27,28] Used in the proper mode, both flow and the direction of flow can be monitored.

All of the techniques described above can provide important information; innovations and improvements in equipment are making them more and more valuable. However, there are limitations. The major one is that transit cannot be followed in all regions of the GI tract. In order to be useful, the region of the GI tract being monitored must be delineated. This is relatively easy if the esophagus and stomach are the organs of interest. Also, information about transit through the colon can be surmised. On the other hand, it is difficult to follow movement of material through regions of the small intestine due to the overlapping of intestinal loops. With ultrasound, only small regions can be monitored for flow. Finally, all of these methods require that the subjects remain still during monitoring. This often is not possible in animal experiments unless restraint is used, a procedure that could itself alter transit.

Oral-Cecal Transit

A novel technique for measuring mouth-to-cecum transit was introduced by Bond and Levitt in 1975 (Figure 2). This technique takes advantage of the fact that certain carbohydrates such as lactulose are not digested by enzymes produced in the mammalian small intestine; however, they are metabolized by intestinal bacteria found in the colon. One product of this metabolism is hydrogen that is absorbed from the lower gut and excreted via the lungs. Thus, if lactulose is ingested, the time of appearance of increased hydrogen in the breath can be taken as an indication of the time of transit to the cecum and proximal colon.[30] Recently, one of us (PB) has employed this technique in the rat.[31] Advantages of this technique are that it is non invasive and does not employ radiation. Breath hydrogen detectors are relatively inexpensive and easy to use. On the other hand, the method does not distinguish between gastric emptying and intestinal transit unless the lactulose is placed directly into the intestine. Also, the test is less valid if there is bacterial overgrowth of the small intestine for any reason. Other potential problems have been discussed by Summers and Soffer.[32]

Labeled carbon can also be used to monitor transit in the gut. One technique utilizes ^{14}C or ^{13}C-octanoic acid bound to egg yolk to monitor the gastric emptying of food made with the egg.[33] As the octanoic acid empties from the stomach, it is readily absorbed in the proximal

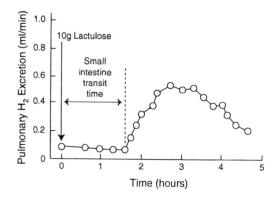

FIGURE 2 Pulmonary hydrogen excretion as a function of time after ingestion of lactulose. (Modified from reference 29.)

small intestine and delivered to the liver where it undergoes metabolism with labeled CO_2 as one of the products. The labeled CO_2 collected serves as an index of gastric emptying.

Invasive Techniques

There are two major problems involved in determining transit in and through specific areas of the gastrointestinal tract. One is the rapid placement of the marker at the starting point. Unless esophageal transit or gastric emptying is being studied, this cannot be accomplished without cannulation. Even for studies of gastric emptying, cannulation can be avoided only if the subject can cooperate by voluntarily and quickly ingesting the material. The second major problem is in collecting or quantitatively monitoring the marker within and at the end of the organ through which transit is being evaluated. This also often involves cannulation or sacrifice of the animal.

The most common and perhaps least invasive of the techniques involves placing intraluminal catheters. In studies of gastric emptying, the stomach can be intubated via the mouth or via a cannula placed in the esophagus or body of the stomach. The test meal that contains a marker can be gavaged into the stomach and the catheter removed during the period of gastric emptying. Then the catheter can be reinserted and the gastric contents recovered. From knowing the amount of marker instilled and the amount recovered, gastric emptying can be determined. Such a technique was used by Hunt and co-workers to elucidate much of what we know about the regulation of gastric emptying in humans.[34] We and others have adapted this technique to the study of gastric emptying in dogs.[35,36] The data in Figure 3 clearly show that liquid meals of varying composition empty at different rates.[35] These different rates of emptying were correlated with different patterns of contraction of the stomach and proximal small intestine which were monitored with serosal strain gage transducers (See figure in reference 35). A major limitation of using catheters to deliver test meals is that it is difficult to study the emptying of solids which have been shown to empty in a pattern differing from that of liquids.[19]

Placement of catheters also has been used to study transit through short segments of intestine. Dillard et al.[37] have described a multi-lumen catheter that allows for the simultaneous measurement of flow rate, mean transit time, and intestinal segment volume. The catheter is passed to the desired location and a "steady state" is created by the infusion of isotonic electrolyte solution through the most proximal catheter. Marker is then injected as a bolus through this catheter. Ten cm distal to this catheter, a second catheter is used to sample the marker that has

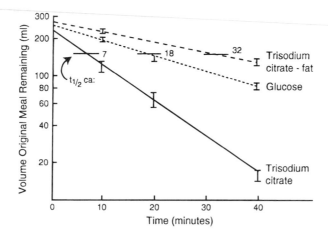

FIGURE 3 Gastric emptying of three equiosmolar liquid test meals. The addition of fat to the citrate meal increases its half-emptying time from 7 to 32 min. The emptying of glucose ($t^{1/2} = 18$ min) is faster than oleate. (Modified from reference 35.)

mixed with the perfusion fluid. A third catheter, 20–40 cm distally is used to take an additional sample. From the pattern of change in marker between the two sampling sites, mean transit time, flow rate, and volume of the intestine can be determined. The major limitations of this method are that the catheters and the infusion of fluid themselves may alter transit.

For studies in animals, permanent fistulas can be prepared to lessen the need for catheterization. Cooke and co-workers implanted gastric cannulas so that contents could be added to and drained from the stomach without orally intubating the dogs they studied.[38] They, as well as Meyer and co-workers, implanted cannulas in the proximal duodenum so that contents emptying from the stomach of dogs could be collected directly.[39] By allowing the animals to eat various meals, they were able to study the emptying of solids as well as liquids. Construction of permanent duodenal cannulas suitable for such studies has been described by Rubinstein et al.[40] In addition to allowing study of gastric emptying, the quantity and quality of effluent from cannulas of this type can be used to monitor the phases of the interdigestive cycle.[41] The major limitation with this modification is that the cannulas have the potential to distort the movement of the organ in question and could thus alter the parameter being monitored.

Placement of permanent cannulas also has been used to monitor intestinal transit and to perfuse materials into the intestine in order to study their effect on other motility parameters such as gastric emptying. The major advantage of the use of cannulas is that repeated measurements can be made with minimal disturbance of the animals. An ingenious method to obtain the same measurements but without the use of a cannula was reported by Summers and co-workers.[42] They prepared, in dogs, a Beible loop of intestine and placed a Geiger tube next to it. Isotope placed in the proximal intestine then could be detected as it passed through the loop.

A limitation of the above-mentioned techniques to monitor intestinal transit is that they provide information only on the appearance of material at the collection sites. They do not provide information on the distribution of the material within the intestine at any given instant in time. Also, the techniques are difficult to use in small animals such as rats. In 1976, Summers and co-workers reported on a method in which rats were given a radioactive marker and then killed at various times.[43] The entire intestine was removed and a Geiger tube was passed along the intestine so that the distribution of marker could be determined. Over the years, we and others have modified this technique. One modification has been to implant catheters into the duodenum so that the marker could be instantaneously placed in the small bowel, thus avoiding the complication of gastric emptying.[44,45] Other modifications have been to divide the intestine into ten segments to make statistical comparisons easier (Figure 4), and to employ fluorescent markers to avoid the use of isotopes.[46,47] Although this technique is very reproducible, fast, and relatively easy, it does require the use of groups of animals to obtain single data points.

Special Transit Techniques for the Colon

Two early studies using bismuth subnitrate as a contrast medium or a pea-flour water gruel, respectively, clearly demonstrated that colon transit is at different rates in different segments of the colon.[3,48] These early transit studies showed that the cecum and sigmoid colon are major areas of delay in the lower bowel.

Original distribution of markers in the whole colon over time has been estimated by Metcalf et al.[49] Markers are ingested for several consecutive days followed by an abdominal X-ray 4 days after the initial ingestion.

Scintigraphy of the colon is used to assess total and regional distribution of different substances with relatively short isotopic half-lives. The use of scintigraphy has been utilized extensively for clinical studies by various researchers at the Mayo Clinic. Details of several methods for measuring transit have been reviewed and presented by van der Ohe and Camilleri.[50] A brief description of two methods of monitoring colonic transit time is in humans presented below.

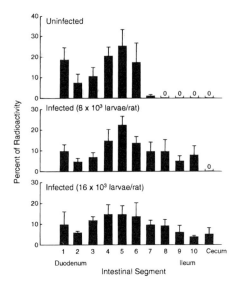

FIGURE 4   Distribution of marker (^{51}Cr) along the length of intestine in uninfected rats and rats infected with *T. spiralis*. The small intestine was divided into 10 segments of equal length. (Modified from reference 45.)

Delayed Release Capsule

Proano et al.[51] used polystyrene amberlite cation exchange resin pellets which measured 0.5–1.8 mm in diameter and were radiolabeled with ^{111}In. Approximately 1000 of the labeled pellets were placed in a 00 gelatin capsule and coated with various layers of methacrylate (Eudragit S-100). Methacrylate is sensitive to pH, disrupting at approximately pH 7. Thus the pellets in the gelatin capsule are not released till a pH of approximately 7.2. The coated capsule transits the stomach and most of the small bowel. It is most likely to disintegrate in the terminal ileum, delivering the labeled pellets into the colon.

Oral-Cecal Tube

The second approach was to place an oral-cecal tube into volunteers. In this study, a liquid radioisotope, ^{111}In-diethylenetriamine penta-acetic acid is placed into the cecal area of the bowel. This permits the measurement of liquid marker through various regions of the colon. The method obviously has the disadvantage of intubation.

WALL MOTION

As described under Historical Perspective, the earliest studies of wall motion were made by injecting contrast medium into the wall of an organ and by attaching radiopaque markers to the serosa. Marker movement then was determined radiographically. The major advantage of this technique is that it is about the only way to obtain information on changes in distance between two points along the length of the gut. Disadvantages are that markers must be surgically implanted and that radiography is required.

Measurements of wall motion can provide information about changes in diameter and length of the organ monitored. On the other hand, they do not necessarily provide information about contractions of the muscle. For example, an increase in diameter of a region of the small intestine can result from both a relaxation of the circular muscle and from the propulsion of contents into that region from another region.

Induction coils as a method to monitor wall motion were introduced by Brody and Quigley in 1944[52] and have been used mostly to monitor the diameter of the pylorus.[53] The technique involves placing two coils on the serosal surface directly opposite each other. Electric current passed through one of the coils sets up an electric field that is sensed by the other coil. The strength of the field depends in part upon the distance between the coils. Advantages of this technique are that once the coils are implanted, animals can be studied over long periods of time and that permanent records of moment-to-moment changes in diameter can be obtained. Disadvantages are that absolute calibration is difficult due to changes in local environment and in circumferential movement of the coils. Ehrlein and co-workers have combined output from coils placed on the pylorus with strain gage transducer measurements of antral and duodenal contractions and with radiography to carefully evaluate the mechanisms of gastric emptying (Figure 5).

In addition to monitoring flow, ultrasound also can be used to follow wall movements. The advantage of this technique is that sound waves are reflected in a manner dependent upon the density of the material. Because the wall has a density different from that of the contents in the lumen, lumen diameter can be assessed. By determining diameter at several locations and by making assumptions about the shape of the stomach, investigators have calculated changes in volume of the stomach and thus gastric emptying.[28,55]

MUSCLE CONTRACTION

The major limitations with observing the transit of lumenal content and/or wall motion is that one can speculate about, but not quantify, the relationship of the event to the responsible muscle contractions. The shortcomings of acute, anesthetized preparations in which contractions could be monitored directly, and the lack of muscle information from transit studies performed *in vivo* prompted many investigators after the Second World War (post 1945), to document intraluminal pressure events from the gastrointestinal tract during normal states. This involved studies performed on friendly unanesthetized animals to determine muscle activities during either digestive or interdigestive states. The desire to characterize the contractile patterns of the muscle during these states drove the development of additional muscle recording devices. In this review, we have divided these sensors of GI muscle activity into either intraluminal or extraluminal (i.e., serosal or even abdominal) recordings.

Electric Activity

As stated in several reviews,[56,57] the use of intact animals and recording of serosal surface potentials have several advantages: (a) the preparation can be physiological; (b) multiple tests

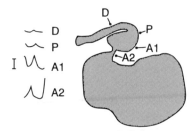

FIGURE 5 Stomach outline obtained via radiography, pyloric diameter (P) obtained via induction coils, and contractile force of the antrum (A1 and A2) and duodenum (D) obtained via strain gage transducers. From the permanent records obtained with these methods, correlations among the activities could be made. (Modified from reference 54.)

can be made on the same animal under a variety of conditions over a prolonged period; (c) several areas of the tract from the same preparation are easily explored simultaneously; (d) activity is recorded from a localized area; (e) the recording unit does not obstruct the bowel lumen or act as an abnormal stimulus to the mucosal reflexes; (f) the electric event is a more sensitive parameter than intraluminal pressure for monitoring motor activity. *In vivo*, bioelectric phenomena can supplement data obtained from manometry, radiology and other methods of motility evaluation.

Serosal Electrodes

The characteristics and properties of the *in vivo* electric activity of the small bowel was reviewed by one of us (P.B.).[56] Similar reviews on the electric activity of the stomach and colon have also been presented. The development of various electric sensing devices was established by the late 1960s. More recent reviews of electric activity contain the results of using serosal recordings in various, unanesthetized preparations. The construction of electrodes for chronic implants were made and reported by McCoy and Bass.[58]

The motivation for the electric development was to measure accurately an electric signal from minimally distorted normal bowel. It was also desirable to work with intact bowel rather than extrapolate information from partial organ systems. The signals, named electrogastro- or electroenterograms are the surface potentials or voltages detected with external electrodes from the surface of tissue, the extracellular fluid of the organ, or both. These extracellular gut electric signals are similar in nature to the electrocardiograms or electroencephalograms.

In the antrum of the stomach and most of the small bowel, the electric signal consists of two types of potentials that bear a close relationship to each other (Figure 6). One having a cyclic periodicity has many names; slow waves, action currents, electric control activity (ECA), slow potential and several others. The author (P. B.) prefers the term basic electric rhythm (BER). BER was first used by C. F. Code who first characterized the maximal frequency of the small intestinal mechanical contractile frequency of the dog as recorded by intraluminal devices to be 18 contractions per minute. This was described in the 1950's as basic rhythm, the most fundamental maximal rate of contractions observed at the time of recording. It was an easy extrapolation for Dr. Code to add the word "electric" to this concept. The name BER is purely descriptive of an omnipresent cyclic phenomena. The term "rhythm" denotes periodicity, "electric" describes the type of phenomena, "basic" indicates the persistent or fundamental nature of the event. Certain factors can alter the BER, but in the intact, undisturbed stomach or small intestine of most species studied, it is omnipresent. In contrast, the other popular terms like slow waves or ECA have a time or function connotation that is not supported by experimental data.

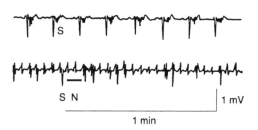

FIGURE 6   Postprandial myoelectric antral, upper electromyogram, and duodenal, lower electromyogram, activity. The BER frequencies of the antrum and duodenum are approximately 4.8 and 18 cpm, respectively. S marks the spike potentials of the antrum and duodenum. N denotes the nonspiking interval on the duodenal electromyogram. Note that the mechanical counterpart to the spike potentials are muscle contractions. (Modified from reference 59.)

The second form of electric activity consists of single or multiple oscillations that represent the electric event that precedes actual muscle contractions. The most common term used is again descriptive, "spike potentials". Other terms are fast activity, action potentials, and electric response activity (ERA).

Both BER and spike potentials can be recorded on magnetic tape or by polygraphs that detect a response from essentially d-c to about 50 cycles per second. Frequently, a shorter time constant is used that eliminates the BER and permits continuous recording of only the spike potentials. This can give a 24-hour record of gut activity that readily lends itself to frequency or pattern analysis. Instruments for recording such high frequency response were not available until the 1950s. Thus, early electric studies of the gastrointestinal tract lacked spike potentials and were not properly interpreted.[56]

The construction of electrodes has been detailed.[58] Briefly, an electrode may be made from silver or platinum. The electrode may be a few mm long, needle-like, or a flat surface. Both will record similar signals. The electrode is soldered to a conducting wire and the solder junction carefully waterproofed with an epoxy. This water proofing insures that only a few mm of bare, conducting tip is in contact with the serosa of the gut. Multiple electrodes can be sewn onto the bowel and led to a common electric plug. The wire at the electric plug must be waterproofed to prevent shorting. The waterproofed plug is frequently housed in an aluminum holder that is mounted to the abdomen of or between the scapulae of an animal. Following surgery, such animals may be used for several months. It is the author's experience that rats prepared with such electrodes are useful for 3–4 weeks. Dog and cat preparations may be used for 4–5 months. The clarity of the signal eventually deteriorates; the amplitude becomes less. This may be due to the presence of the platinum or silver causing a slight necrosis and damage to the tissue where it is in contact with the metal.

Modifications of the electrodes have been made by two separate groups.[60,61] These changes facilitated the recording from the rat gut. In the latter, a silicone tube is used as a "mold". A 4 mm piece of silver wire is bent at 90°, soldered to a length of 36 gauge silver-copper wire that is Teflon insulated. The silver tip of the electrode is pierced through a silicone tube. The tube is then filled with an epoxy resin injected from a syringe. After drying, the silastic tube is cut away, the silver electrode shaped and filed, the epoxy notched and the finished electrode is ready for assembly into a plug. A large silver coiled wire may be used as a reference electrode. Alternatively, 2 electrodes may be made in a single silastic tube and used as a bipolar recorder. Another type of wire electrode was developed by Ruckebusch and co-workers[62] who used 60 μ diameter insulated nichrome wire. They burned away the insulation from approximately 4 mm from the tip of the wire. These investigators then inserted a size 27 needle through the serosa and muscle at the site of the bowel to be implanted, placed the bared wire into the needle and pulled the unit out, thus implanting the wire into the muscle of the bowel. The wire is then twisted so as to have a portion of the bared end under or in close contact with the muscle. The authors achieved bipolar recording by fixing 2 wires less than 2 mm apart. The method has been useful for recording from the intestine of lambs in utero[63] as well as parts of the GI tract in the rat.

An electrode may be used in a single monopolar configuration,[64] or 2 electrodes close together as a bipolar system.[65] The use of a monopolar electrode involves placing a recording electrode on or in the gut muscle while a reference or indifferent electrode is placed in a nonintestinal area, frequently subcutaneously in the thigh area. Bipolar recordings measure potentials between two electrodes in the same tissue.

Mucosal Electrodes

In humans, electric activity has also been recorded from the mucosal surface.[66] Christensen et al. were successful in using intraluminal electrodes in normal subjects and patients with various diseases.[67] Clinically, electric events have been recorded from patients with ileostomies by placing a recording electrode into the exteriorized portion of bowel.[68,69] Electric events have also been recorded from thiry fistulas of unanesthetized dogs. However, isolated segments of bowel generate patterns that differ from the signals of intact gastrointestinal tract.

Abdominal Electrodes

As early as 1922, Alvarez was using non-invasive electrodes placed on the abdomen to record electric signals from the gastrointestinal tract. He reported in people a distinctive 3 per minute cyclic wave. Several laboratories throughout the world have duplicated the ability to record the 3 per minute signal from the antrum of humans.[70,71] A clear description of electrodes and recording instruments has been reported by one of us (P. B.).[72] We not only confirmed the presence of 3 per minute signal but also reported on the presence of a DC potential. We used 16 standard pediatric electrodes on the abdomen of several volunteers. This large electrode array on the abdomen enabled us to precisely locate the optimal gastric signal which was essentially just above the antrum. We also correlated a recording from a mucosal suctional electrode with the abdominal electrodes that verified that the 3 cycles per minute from the abdomen corresponded in frequency to the BER signal obtainable from either the mucosa or serosa.[73] The abdominal signal is approximately 100 microvolts, much lower than the usual 3 millivolts signal obtained directly from the serosal surface. The attenuation factor of 30 is caused by both increased distance from the signal source, the antrum, and out of phase potentials from other areas of the stomach. The low volt signal obtained by abdominal recording methods requires great care and minimal body movement to record the signal without noise.

Mechanical Activity

When muscle contracts, force develops parallel to the long axis of the myofilaments. The consequence of this force depends upon the orientation of the muscle cell. For cells oriented along the longitudinal axis of the GI tract, contraction may result in changes in organ length. For cells oriented circumferentially, contraction may result in changes in organ diameter. The degree of changes in length and diameter produced by a contraction depends upon the forces opposing the contraction. Often contraction results in visible wall displacement. On the other hand, contraction may result in no change in muscle cell length or organ size. That is the contraction may be isometric. This can occur when the forces opposing contraction are equal to or greater than those developed by muscle contraction. Contraction also may or may not correlate with intraluminal pressure development. If a contraction does not result in occlusion of the lumen or compression of the contents under the contraction, there may be no measurable change in pressure in the region of contraction. On the other hand, a remote contraction can cause an increase in a region that is not contracting if the two regions are connected by a "common cavity." Finally, the forces imparted upon intraluminal contents depend not only on contractions occurring at a single point, but on the coordinated contractions that occur at multiple adjacent points. Thus, the technique that one chooses to record mechanical properties has a major influence on what conclusions can be drawn about muscle contractions.

Strain Gage Transducers

Transducers monitor the stress applied by muscle contraction. When sewn onto the serosal surface, the transducer detects unidirectional, isometric muscle contraction. The development of the strain gage transducer as applied to the gastrointestinal tract is an interesting demonstration of collaboration between two groups of pharmacologists in academics and industry. As indicated in Jacoby et al.,[74] the idea of measuring muscle stress in the walls of hollow organs *in vivo* led Walton and Brody to develop a transducer that was applicable for acute recording of myocardial contractions. Dr. Donald Bennet, a pharmacologist at the University of Michigan, and one of us (P. B.), employed at Parke, Davis and Company, speculated that the cardiac recording unit could be refined for chronic recording of gut muscle. Henry Jacoby, then a graduate student, was the first to explore this idea by evaluating various strain gages, waterproofing materials and bonding agents. Technical assistance was provided by W. T. Bean, a consulting aeronautical engineer in Detroit, MI, regarding the properties of strain gages, and by people at Dow Corning in Midland, MI, on silicone technology. The initial transducer implants were a success—they lasted 8 days! Refinements by Rienke et al. produced a transducer with longer life. This increased working time allowed him to describe several physiological events such as the interdigestive and digestive states. Another example of information obtainable using such units is the series of studies on the effects of nicotine on the colon of the dog by the two of us.[76] A detailed description of the construction of the transducer currently used in the dog and other animals is given in Bass and Wiley.[77] The miniaturization of transducers for use on the gi tract of the rat and other small animals is described in Pascaud et al.[78] Such miniature transducers also have been adapted to record muscle activity from the Ussing Chamber.[79] From 1971 on, Ruth Bass, University of Wisconsin, taught construction techniques to investigators and later provided a commercial outlet for the serosal strain gage transducer (Figure 7). Whether constructed by individuals or purchased, investigators, using these transducers, have been able to define many aspects of gut physiology and pharmacology.

Strain gage transducers have been used to record sustained contractions or relaxations (changes in tone) as well as circular and longitudinal muscle phasic activity. When sewn in the transverse axis of the bowel, transducers record phasic contractions which may be superimposed on tonal changes of circular muscle activity. Because circular muscle contraction usually is concentric, circular muscle under the transducer contracts at the same time as the muscle at the ends of the transducer. Thus, transducer compression occurs. Strain gage transducers can also reproduce tonic contractions or relaxations; phenomena less dynamic than phasic contractions and more difficult to quantify. For example, relaxations of gastric fundic and gallbladder muscle have been detected during filling of the stomach[80,81] (Figure 8) and gallbladder. Contractions of the longitudinal muscle have not been studied extensively. Muscle cells located beneath the transducer may not contract synchronously so that stretch as well as compression of the transducer may occur. Thus, results from transducers placed in the longitudinal axis are more difficult to interpret; the transducers may generate upward and downward wave forms that indicate phasic muscle relaxation or contraction activity.

Strain gage transducers offer several advantages over other methods of recording GI motility: 1) The units directly record the contractile activity of the smooth muscle. 2) They are sewn on the serosal surface of the GI tract. Thus, their use avoids any interference with flow of intraluminal

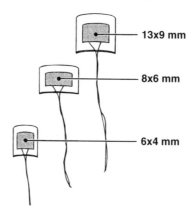

FIGURE 7   The three sizes and configurations of strain gage transducers currently available.

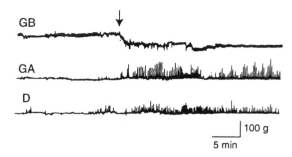

FIGURE 8   Contractile response to feeding in a conscious dog as measured by strain gage transducers. Transducers were placed to monitor circular muscle activity on the gastric body (GB), gastric antrum (GA), and duodenum (D). (Modified from reference 81.)

contents and avoids stimulation of mucosal receptors. Since they are permanently fixed in position, the same site can be monitored repeatedly without using elaborate procedures to place the sensors in the desired position. 3) The units can be used in combination to monitor multiple sites of the gastrointestinal tract. 4) They can be used to monitor separately the activity of the circular and longitudinal muscle layers of the intestines. 5) There is no need to prepare fistulae or isolated loops of bowel. Conversely, there are some disadvantages: 1) An electrical connection is needed between the animal and the recording unit. This necessity removes the animal from its normal environment and could influence the motor patterns. 2) Only contractions of the muscle and not the physiological function of the contractions are monitored. Thus, it is difficult to determine if a given sequence of contractions results in mixing or propulsion of intraluminal contents. 3) It is difficult to adapt the units for use in humans.

Mercury Strain Gages

These gages operate on the principle that the electrical resistance offered by a column of mercury enclosed in a segment of silicone rubber tubing will increase as it becomes longer and narrower. Once sewn on the serosal surface of an organ, they provide information about the circumference of that organ. Theoretically, these units should be especially useful in monitoring activity of those regions of the gut such as the stomach that undergo changes in tone and volume. However, they have not be utilized widely.[83]

Impedance Planimetry

This method makes use of the principle that the impedance of a saline solution inside a distensible balloon is proportional to the cross-sectional area of the balloon. As developed by Gregersen and co-workers,[84] the device consists of two pairs of electrodes mounted on a segment of catheter that is located inside a balloon (Figure 9). A constant alternating current is passed between the outer electrodes. The signal detected by the inner electrodes will depend upon the cross-sectional area of the balloon which is determined by the volume of saline injected into it. If a pressure sensor also is included, the device can be used to estimate compliance and wall stress in hollow, distensible organs such as those found in the GI tract. The balloon is placed in the organ and inflated and deflated by stepwise infusing and withdrawing saline that is at body temperature. At each volume, cross-sectional area and intraballoon pressure is determined. If the balloon is such that it offers little resistance to stretch at the volumes used, properties of the organ wall and not of the balloon are determined.

The advantage of this device is that it is the only way in which certain biomechanical properties, such as wall stress, of GI organs can be obtained *in vivo.*[85] It may prove particularly useful in monitoring "compliance" and "parallel elastic" properties of the gut wall. It is too early to determine precise advantages and disadvantages of this relatively new method.

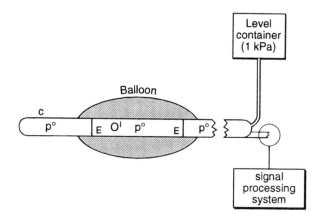

FIGURE 9 Schematic representation of the sensor system for making impedance estimates of cross-sectional area. C, probe; E, electrode; O^I, infusion channel; p°, side hole for pressure measurement. (Modified from reference 85.)

Measurement of Volume

Changes in volume of the body of the stomach, proximal colon, as well as other areas of the gut are of interest. Increases in volume occur in the stomach with ingestion of liquids or food and in the proximal colon when ileal effluent is discharged. The smooth muscle properties of the body of the stomach and proximal colon, shared with the urinary bladder and gallbladder, permits expansion of these various organs while maintaining a low intra-organ pressure. Volume changes may be objectively measured by a technique developed by Malagelada and coworkers[86] (Figure 10). The instrument for measuring organ volume change is referred to as a barostat which actually documents the isotonic muscle changes of a given organ. The barostat consists of a balloon that is introduced into the organ. The pressure in the balloon is maintained constant; the volume changes are recorded. The balloon is connected to a pump capable of moving air in and out of the unit in response to changes of volume in the organ. Volume balloon sizes are available to accommodate human as well as dog stomach, and colon. The documented measurement is usually referred to as organ tone. A recent instrument developed by a French company

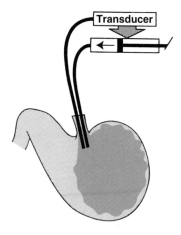

FIGURE 10 Schematic representation of the gastric barostat. A constant pressure is maintained within the intragastric bag. When the stomach relaxes, the system injects air; when the stomach contracts, air is aspirated. From the volume of air injected and aspirated, and the set pressure, changes in gastric volume can be deduced. (Modified from reference 86.)

is described by Bradette et al.[87] The thin walled (40 μm) balloon has a 700 ml air compliance without affecting pressure. This was more than adequate for measuring colonic tone in humans.

The limitations of the barostat relate to the device only being useful in an empty organ, the balloon may interfere with the flow of organ content and the properties of the balloon may contribute to limits of recording distensibilities.

INTRALUMINAL PRESSURE

Techniques that monitor intraluminal pressure take advantage of the fact that in many areas of the gastrointestinal tract, localized contractions of the muscularis externa will increase the pressure locally within the lumen. In particular, intraluminal devices are most useful in monitoring sphincteric regions where tonic contractions of the musculature maintain localized closure of the lumen. Intraluminal devices can detect resting pressures as well as changes that represent both relaxation and contraction of sphincters. Such information is difficult if not impossible to obtain with other methods. Intraluminal devices offer the advantages that they can be passed into place through the mouth or anus or through fistulae placed in any organ of the gut. Also, long-term recordings can be obtained in fully conscious animals as well as humans. Improvements over the years have resulted in units that can be passed to just about any region of the GI tract with minimal discomfort so that recordings can be made from multiple sites at the same time. The size of the units also has been reduced so that they probably have minimal influence upon the activity being recorded.[88] On the other hand, intraluminal devices always have the potential of stimulating mucosal receptors to alter motility. Also, the bowel does have a tendency to slip or "telescope" over the catheter so that the exact location of the activity being monitored can be called into question.[89] Finally, there are regions of the GI tract such as the gastric fundus where measurements of intraluminal pressure do not always reflect contractile activity of the wall.

Perfused Catheters

This method probably is the most widely used today. It was developed and refined between the early '50s and middle '70s. Prior to their use, small balloons and non-infused open-tipped, water-filled catheters were placed in the lumen. These catheters were then connected to pressure transducers external to the subject. Although these devices yielded approximation of the pressures being generated, design limitations limited their usefulness, especially for areas of the GI tract in which pressures changes were phasic and rapid. Detailed studies begun by Pope and Horton[90] and continued by Dodds and co-workers[91] demonstrated that the slow infusion of saline utilizing a high-pressure, low-compliance system would provide very accurate pressure recordings, even in regions, such as the esophagus, that contract rapidly. Improvements and modifications over the years have been made so that very low rates of infusion are needed.[92] Also, catheters and infusion pumps now are commercially available so that one no longer has to fashion his/her own systems. Perfused catheters were first most heavily used to study the esophagus, a relatively accessible organ of moderate length and possessing a relatively limited repertoire of contractile patterns and functions. They currently are used to monitor activity in just about every region of the alimentary canal including the colon and biliary tract.[93]

Solid-State Transducers

These devices are similar to perfused catheters in the activities they monitor.[94] Thus, they offer no theoretical advantages. On the other hand, they do offer the advantages that neither a column of fluid nor perfusion is required. Also, the pressure sensors are located right in the regions of the GI tract being monitored. Thus, there is no need to have external pressure transducers nor to ensure that the transducers are placed at the right height so that hydrostatic pressures do not develop. Outputs from the pressure sensors can be recorded directly on a small recorder that is portable. Thus, they have been used to obtain 24-hour ambulatory recordings. Major disadvantages of this technique are that the units are relatively expensive and are not as durable as perfused catheters. One interesting modification of this method is the "radiopill".[95,96] This device contains a pressure transducer and a transmitter in the shape of a capsule. Once this capsule is swallowed, its general location within the GI tract can be followed and the intraluminal pressures surrounding it can be monitored. Thus, an indication of both transit and pressure can be obtained. However, the device has not been characterized enough to determine its usefulness.

Sleeve Catheter

One of the problems with open-tipped catheters or solid-state transducers is that they monitor pressures localized to a small region. Thus, as the organ slips over the catheter, activity at different adjacent sites will be monitored. This is especially bothersome in sphincteric regions such as the lower esophageal sphincter. Placement of a catheter tip within a sphincteric region at rest will indicate a pressure above that either orally or aborally. If the pressure suddenly falls, one cannot be certain if it fell because the sphincter relaxed or because the sphincter region moved orally or aborally to the tip. One way to obviate this problem is to place multiple catheters with closely-spaced tips in the region. Another way was developed by Dent[97] (Figure 11). This technique utilizes a sleeve placed over one of the catheter holes such that the sleeve is sealed immediately orad to the catheter hole and is open at the aborad end. If fluid is perfused through the system, compression of the sleeve anywhere along its length will reflect a similar pressure. Thus, it does not matter if the gut wall moves in relation to the hole in the catheter. This device has been used extensively to study the lower esophageal sphincter. It appears to be ideally suited to this region because resting activity is minimal both orad in the esophageal body and aborad in the gastric fundus. It also is being used in other regions such as the pylorus; however, the extensive contractile activity of the antrum, the duodenum, and even the two muscle rings separating the antrum from the duodenum[98] may complicate the measurements.

Balloon catheters have also been used. Except for specialized devices such as the barostat, intraluminal balloons currently are not popular.

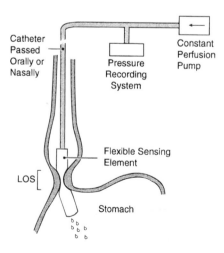

FIGURE 11 Schematic of the sleeve element in place at the lower esophageal sphincter (LOS). A constant flow infusion is maintained so that changes in resistance to outflow caused by contraction of the sphincteric muscle results in changes in the pressure recorded. (From Dent, J., measurement and control of lower esophageal sphincter pressure, Thesis, 1978.)

COMBINATION OF RECORDING DEVICES

In evaluating a hypothesis, one may occasionally combine recording devices to verify that two phenomena are related. Combinations of sensors also evaluate the respective sensitivities of the detecting units. The demonstration that spike potentials correlate with intraluminal pressure or circular muscle contractions was clearly shown by combining an electrode with an intraluminal pressure recorder or a transducer.[8,11,99] A 3-way sensor comparison was recorded from Daniel's laboratory.[100,101] They compared two intraluminal devices, a perfused catheter, and an intraluminal tube mounted strain gage with a serosal strain gage transducer (Figure 12). The intraluminal pressure probe and serosal transducer responded in parallel to various smooth muscle stimuli. The intraluminal strain gage device response was unpredictable with polarity responses exhibiting both positive and negative deflections. The authors conclude, using the serosal transducer as the standard, that perfusion manometry from the colon of the anesthetized dog "albeit imperfect, is a superior technique for the measurement of colonic contractile events" when compared with a novel intraluminal device.[100]

A biased, questionable conclusion is also possible when comparing two sensors. Edelbroek et al.[102] compared an intraluminal sleeve sensor to a serosal strain gage transducer that was supposedly sewn on the terminal antrum of the dog. In this case, a fixed 8×1.4 cm transducer on the serosa is compared to a 4.8 cm long sleeve sensor placed in the lumen of the antrum and duodenum. Intraluminal pressures with catheters and serosal electrode electric activity were also recorded. The muscle sampling areas of the sleeve and serosal transducer are clearly different. Also, though the authors claim the serosal transducer was sewn onto the "distal pyloric muscle loop," the myograms in their Figures 2 and 3 suggest otherwise. It is well established that the entire stomach, including the distal pyloric loop has cyclic electric frequency (BER) of 4.5 cycles/minute. This electric cyclical phenomena mandates the highest frequency of contractions. The authors' figures contains contractile frequency as recorded by the serosal transducers well in excess of 4.5 cycles/minute. The obvious conclusion from the data is that

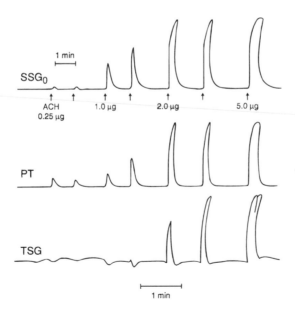

FIGURE 12 Changes in colonic motor activity induced by acetylcholine. Recordings were obtained by strain gage transducers mounted on the serosa (SSG), perfused tubes (PT), and tube-mounted strain gages (TSG). Note that the polarity of events recorded by TSG often differed from that obtained with the other two methods. (Modified from reference 100.)

the serosal "pyloric" transducer is recording some duodenal contractible activity. Interpretation of results may lead to opposite conclusions suggested in the published literature.

SENSORS WITH POTENTIAL FOR USE ON THE GASTROINTESTINAL TRACT

A microminiature (1.6 mm $\times$ 0.4 mm) force transducer was developed for recording hollow organ activity by Thomas Nelsen at Stanford University.[103,104] The units were successfully implanted on a rabbit oviduct which measures 1 mm in diameter. The units achieved an average life of 60 days, and were stable in monitoring muscle tension. The transducer was designed and produced by James Angell of the Electrical Engineering Department and supported by an NIH contract. Unfortunately, no GI studies have been reported with this device. In the hands of one of us (P. B.) the units were found to be too fragile for implantation on the stomach or small intestine of the dog. Thus the preliminary attempt for G. I. application was not successful.

Semi-conductor elements have been used for constructing serosal transducers used on the gut[105] as well as on the rabbit oviduct.[106] Extraluminal displacement transducers have also been described for simultaneous recording of mechanical activities of the circular and longitudinal muscle.[107] An independent construction of a displacement transducer has also been described by Kingma et al.[108]

Sensors for recording other organs have been reported. The technology may be applicable to the gut. One example is the description of a pressure probe for recording contractions of the teat sphincter in bovines.[109]

A miniature intraluminal transducer 1–1.2 mm diameter has been described for implantation into the oviduct of a rabbit.[110] Impedance measurements for documenting the diameter of the fallopian tube of the rabbit have been obtained.[111] In the miscellaneous category, a unique housing unit for long-term monitoring of rat intestinal electric and strain gage transducer activity has been reported.[112]

ORGAN SPECIFIC STUDIES

The above portions of the review emphasize the various methods for monitoring essentially three parameters: transit, wall motion, and muscle activity. Each organ in the gastrointestinal tract has physiological functions, pathological changes and pharmacological responses that may best be monitored by different methods or a combination of methods. Below are itemized a few approaches that we favor for monitoring different areas of the gastrointestinal tract.

Esophagus

This organ is most commonly studied with devices that register intraluminal pressure in the body as well as in the sphincters. The two most common devices are perfused catheters and sleeve catheters. Transit is usually noted with scintigraphy or with radiographic opaque substances.

Stomach

The stomach is really two organs, the body and antrum separated from the duodenum by a 2-ring muscle complex.[98] Contractions and relaxations of the body of the stomach can best be studied using the barostat as described under measurement of tone. Antral activity is best monitored in animals with serosal transducers or electrodes. In humans catheters or more recently ultra-sonography reveal antral activity. Transit and stomach emptying can be monitored with both liquid and solid test meals. Actual gastric aspiration and/or duodenal collection of contents via tubes or cannulas are commonly used in human and animal studies respectively. Scintigraphy currently appears to be the most common method used in humans. The antral-duodenal area is most difficult to objectively study and understand.

Small Bowel

Mixing and transit in this organ are two areas under active evaluation. Animals are studied with serosal electrodes and transducers. In humans, inaccessibility and intestinal loop overlap are major challenges to objective measurements. Various methods used in the esophagus and stomach are applicable to the small intestine.

Colon and Anal Canal

Methods that permit measurement of mixing, transit, tonal evaluation and evacuation are used on these segments of the gastrointestinal tract.

REFERENCES

1. Editorial: "The famous gastrocutaneous fistula of Alexis St. Martin. Why didn't it close? Or should we refer to it as a gastric stoma?" M. G. Sarr, P. Bass, E. Woodward. *Dig. Dis. Sci.* 36, 1345, 1991.
2. **Alvarez, W. C.,** Early studies of the movements of the stomach and bowel, in *Handbook of Physiology,* Vol. 4, Code, C. F., Ed., Williams & Wilkins, Baltimore, 1968, 1573.
3. **Cannon, W. B.,** The movements of the intestines studied by means of the roentgen rays, *Am. J. Physiol.,* 6, 251, 1902.
4. **Steggerda, F. R. and C. Giantarco,** A method for visualizing different organs in the normal unanesthetized animal, *Anat. Rec.* 67, 405, 1937.
5. **Dodds, W. J. and E. T. Stewart,** Evaluation of esophageal movement using intramural tantalum wire markers, in *Proceedings 4th International Symposium of Gastrointestinal Motility,* Mitchell Press Ltd., Vancouver, Canada, 1974, 313.
6. **Bayliss, W. M. and Starling, E. H.,** The movements and innervation of the small intestine, *J. Physiol.* (Lond.), 24:99, 1899.
7. **Alvarez, W. C. and Mahoney, L. J.,** Action currents in stomach and intestine, *Am. J. Physiol.,* 58, 476, 1922.
8. **Bass, P., Code C. F. and Lambert, E. H.,** Motor and electric activity of the duodenum, *Am. J. Physiol.* 201, 287, 1961.
9. **Code, C. F. and Marlett, J. A.,** The interdigestive myoelectric complex of the stomach and small bowel of *J. Physiol. (Lond.),* 246, 289, 1975.
10. **Plant, O. H. and Miller, G. H.,** Effects of morphine and some other opium alkaloids on the muscular activity of the alimentary canal, *J. Pharmacol. Exp. Ther.* 27, 361, 1926.
11. **Bass, P. and Wiley J. N.,** Effects of Ligation and Morphine on Electric and Motor Activity of the Duodenum of Dog, *Am. J. Physiol.* 208, 908, 1965.
12. **Stewart, J. J. and Bass P.,** Effects of Ricinoleic and Oleic Acids on the Digestive Contractile Activity of the Canine Small and Large Bowel, *Gastroenterology,* 70, 371, 1976.
13. **Connell, A. M., Hilton, C., Irvine, G., Leonnard-Jones J. E., and Misiewicz, J. J.,** Variation of bowel habit in two population samples, *Br. Med.* J. 2, 1095, 1965.
14. FED REG. Laxative Drug Products for Over-the-Counter Human Use: Tentative Final Monograph 50, 2124, 1985.
15. **Bass, P. and Dennis, S.,** The laxative effects of lactulose in normal and constipated subjects, *J. Clin. Gastroenterol.* 3 (Suppl 1), 23, 1981.
16. **Marlett, J. A., Li, B. U. K., Patrow, C. J., and Bass, P.,** Comparative laxation of psyllium with and without senna in an ambulatory constipated population, *Am. J. Gastroenterol.* 87, 333, 1987.

17. **Bass, P., Kennedy, J., and Wiley, J. N,.** Measurement of fecal output in rats, *Am. J. Dig. Dis.* 17, 925, 1972.
18. **John, V. A., Shotton, P. A., Moppert, J., and Theobald, W.,** Gastrointestinal transit of Oros drug delivery systems in healthy volunteers: a short report, *Br. J. Clin. Pharmac.,* 19, 203S, 1985.
19. **Camilleri, M., Malagelada, J-R., Brown, M. L., Becker, G., and Zinsmeister, A. R.,** Relation between antral motility and gastric emptying of solids and liquids in humans, *Am. J. Physiol.,* 249, G580, 1985.
20. **Hinton, J. M., Leonnard-Jones, J. E., and Young, A. C.,** A new method for studying gut transit times using radiopaque markers, *Gut,* 10, 842, 1969.
21. **Cummings, J. H. and Wiggins, H. S.,** Transit through the gut measured by analysis of a single stool, *Gut,* 17, 219, 1976.
22. **Caride, V. J., Prokop, E. K., Troncale, F. J., Buddoura, W., Winchenbach, K., and McCallum, R. W.,** Scintigraphic determination of small intestinal transit time: Comparison with the hydrogen breath technique, *Gastroenterology,* 86, 714, 1984.
23. **Jacobs, F., Akkermanns, L. M. A., Yoe, O. H., Hoekstra, A., and Wittebol, P.,** A radioisotope method to quantify the function of fundus, antrum, and their contractile activity in gastric emptying of a semi solid and solid meal, in *Motility of the Digestive Tract,* Wienbeck, M., Ed., Raven Press, 233, 1981.
24. **Tolin, R. D., Malmud, L. S., Reilley, J., and Fisher, R. S.,** Esophageal scintigraphy to quantitate esophageal transit (quantitation of esophageal transit), *Gastroenterology,* 76, 1402, 1979.
25. **Sandefer, E. P. and Digenis, G. A.,** Techniques in monitoring functions relevant to drug delivery in the gastrointestinal tract, in *Current Status on Targeted Drug Delivery to the Gastrointestinal Tract,* Capsugel Americas, Greenwood, S.C., U.S.A., 191, 1993.
26. **Ricci, R., Bontempo, I., Corazziari, E., LaBella, A., and Torsoli, A.,** Ultrasonic sizing of antrum as an indicator of gastric emptying, *Gut,* 34, 173, 1993.
27. **Kawagishi, T., Nishizawa, Y., Okuno, Y., Shimada, H., Inaba, M., Konishi, T., and Morii, H.,** Antroduodenal motility and transpyloric fluid movement in patients with diabetes studied using duplex sonography, *Gastroenterology,* 107, 403, 1994.
28. **Brown, B. P., Schulze-Delrieu, K., Schrier, J. E., and Abu-Yousef, M. M.,** The configuration of the human gastroduodenal junction in the separate emptying of liquids and solids, *Gastroenterology,* 105, 433, 1993.
29. **Bond, J. H., and Levitt, M. P.,** Investigation of small bowel transit time in man utilizing pulmonary hydrogen (H_2) measurements, *J. Lab. Clin. Med.,* 85, 546–555, 1975.
30. **Corbett, C. L., Thomas, S., Read, N. W., Hobson, N., Bergman, I., and Holdsworth, C. D.,** Electrochemical detector for breath hydrogen determination: Measurement of small bowel transit time in normal subjects and patients with the irritable bowel syndrome, *Gut,* 22, 836, 1981.
31. **Luck, M. S., White, J. C., and Bass, P.,** Gastrointestinal transit is not impaired by regional loss of myenteric neurons in rat jejunum, *Am. J. Physiol.,* 265, G654, 1993.
32. **Summers, R. W., and Soffer, E. E.,** Evaluation of intestinal motility, in *Motility Disorders of the Gastrointestinal Tract,* Anuras, S., Ed., Raven Press, New York, 1992, 89.
33. **Maes, B., Ghoos, Y., Hiele, M., Vantrappen, G., and Rutgeerts, P.,** Breath tests in gastric emptying and transit studies: clinical aspects, in *Progress in Understanding and Management of Gastrointestinal Motility Disorders,* Janssens, J., Ed., Department of Medicine, Division of Gastroenterology, K. U. Leuven, Leuven, 1993, 181.
34. **Hunt, J. N., and Knox, M. T.,** Regulation of gastric emptying, in *Handbook of Physiology,* Vol.4, Code, D. F., Ed., Williams & Wilkins, Baltimore, 1968, 1917.
35. **Weisbrodt, N. W., Overholt, B. F., Wiley, J. N., and Bass, P.,** A relation between gastrointestinal muscle contractions and gastric emptying, *Gut,* 10, 543, 1969.
36. **Russell, J. and Bass, P.,** Method for the quantitation of gastric emptying time of viscous test meals. *Am J Clin Nutr.,* 40, 647, 1984.
37. **Dillard, R. L., Eastman, H., and Fordtran, J. S.,** Volume-flow relationship during the transport of fluid through the human small intestine, *Gastroenterology,* 49, 58, 1965.
38. **Cooke, A. R., Chvasta, T. E., and Weisbrodt, N. W.,** Effect of pentagastrin on emptying and electrical and motor activity of the dog stomach, *Am. J. Physiol.,* 223, 934, 1972.
39. **Meyer, J. H., Thomson, J. B., Cohen, M. B., Shadchehr, A., and Mandiola, S. A.,** Sieving of solid food by the canine stomach and sieving after gastric surgery, *Gastroenterology,* 76, 804, 1979.

40. **Rubinstein, A., Li, V. H. K., Gruber, P., Bass, P., and Robinson, J. R.,** Improved intestinal cannula for drug delivery studies in the dog, *J. Pharmacol. Meth.,* 19, 213, 1988.

41. **Gruber, P., Rubinstein, A., Li, V. H. K., Bass, P., and Robinson, J. R.,** Gastric emptying of nondigestible solids in the fasted dog, *J. Pharm. Sci.,* 76, 117, 1987.

42. **Summers, R. W., Helm, J., and Christensen, J.,** Intestinal propulsion in the dog, *Gastroenterology,* 70, 753, 1976.

43. **Summers, R. W., Kent, T. H., and Osborn, J. W.,** Effects of drugs, ileal obstruction, and irradiation on rat gastrointestinal propulsion, *Gastroenterology,* 70, 753, 1976.

44. **Castro, U. A., Badial-Aceves, F., Smith, J. W., Dudrick, S. J., and Weisbrodt, N. W.,** Altered small bowel propulsion associated with parasitism, *Gastroenterology,* 71, 620, 1976.

45. **Weisbrodt, N. W., Badial-Aceves, F., Copeland, E. M., Dudrick, S. J., and Castro, G. A.,** Small-intestinal transit during total parenteral nutrition in the rat, *Am. J. Dig. Dis.,* 23, 363, 1978.

46. **Miller, M. S., Galligan, J. J., and Burks, T. F.,** Accurate measurement of intestinal transit, *J. Pharmacol. Methods,* 6, 211, 1981.

47. **Runkel, N. S. F., Moody, F. G., Smith, G. S., Rodriguez, L. F., Chen, Y., LaRocco, M. T., and Miller, T. A.,** Alterations in rat intestinal transit by morphine promote bacterial translocation, *Dig. Dis. Sci.,* 38, 1530, 1993.

48. **Elliot, T. R., and Barclay-Smith, E.,** Antiperistalsis and other muscular activities of the colon, *J. Physiol. (Lond),* 31, 272–304, 1904.

49. **Metcalf, A. M., Phillips, S. F., Zinsmeister, A. R., MacCarthy, R. L., Beart, R. W., and Wolff, B. G.,** Simplified assessment of segmental colonic transit, *Gastroenterology* 92, 40–47, 1987.

50. **von der Ohe, M. R. and Camilleri, M.,** Measurement of small bowel and colonic transit: indications and methods, *Mayo Clin. Proc.* 67, 1169, 1992.

51. **Proano, M., Camilleri, M., Phillips, S. F., Brown, M. L., and Thomforde, G. M.,** Transit of solids through the human colon: regional quantification in the unprepared bowel, *Am. J. Physiol: Gastrointest. Liver Physiol.,* 258, G856, 1990.

52. **Brody, D. A., and Quigley, J. P.,** Application of the inductograph to the registration of movements of body structures such as the pyloric sphincter, *J. Lab. Clin. Med.,* 29, 863, 1944.

53. **Louckes, H. S., Quigley, J. P., and Kersay, J.,** Inductograph method of recording muscle activity especially pyloric sphincter physiology, *Am. J. Physiol.,* 199, 301, 1960.

54. **Prove, J., and Ehrlein, H-J.,** Motor function of gastric antrum and pylorus for evacuation of low and high viscosity meals in dogs, *Gut,* 23, 150, 1982.

55. **Holt, S., Cervantes, J., Wilkinson, A. A., and Wallace, J. H. K.,** Measurement of gastric emptying rate in humans by real-time ultrasound, *Gastroenterology,* 90, 918, 1986.

56. **Bass, P.,** In vivo electrical activity of the small bowel, in *Handbook of Physiology,* Vol. 4, Code, C. F, Ed, American Physiological Society, Washington, D. C., 1968, 2051

57. **Weisbrodt, N. W.,** Motility of the small intestine, in *Physiology of the gastrointestinal tract, 2nd ed.,* Johnson, L. R., Ed., Raven Press, New York, 1987, 631.

58. **McCoy, E. J. and Bass, P.,** Chronic electric activity of gastric duodenal area: Effects of food in certain catecholamines, *Am. J. Physiol.* 205, 439, 1963.

59. **Russell, J., Bass, P., Shimizu, M., Miyauchi, A., and Go, V. L. W.,** Canine intestinal ulcer: myoelectric components and the effect of chronic hypergastrinemia, *Gastroenterology,* 82, 746, 1982.

60. **Ruckebusch, M., and Fioramonti, J.,** Electrical spiking activity and propulsion in small intestine in fed and fasted rats, *Gastroenterology,* 68, 1500, 1975.

61. **Sussman, S. E., Stewart, J. J., Burks, T. F., and Weisbrodt, N. W.,** Effects of morphine sulfate on motility of the small intestine, *J. Pharmacol. Exp. Ther.,* 214, 333, 1980.

62. **Grivel, M. L., and Ruckebusch, Y.,** The propagation of segmental contractions along the small intestine, *J. Physiol.,* 227, 611, 1972.

63. **Ruckebusch, Y., and Grivel, M. L.,** A technique for long-term studies of the electrical activity of the gut in the foetal and neonate, in *Proceedings 4th International Symposium of Gastrointestinal Motility,* Daniel, E. E., Ed., Mitchell Press Ltd., Vancouver, Canada, 1974, 427.

64. **Fox, D. and Bass, P.,** Selective myenteric neuronal denervation of the rat jejunum; differential control of the propagation of migrating myoelectric complex and basic electric rhythm, *Gastroenterology,* 87, 572, 1984.

65. **Dwinell, M. B., Bass, P., and Oaks, J. A.,** Intestinal myoelectric alterations in rats chronically infected with the tapeworm *Hymenolepis diminuta, Am. J. Physiol.: Gartrointest. Liver Physiol.,* 267, G851, 1994.

66. **Fleckenstein, P., and Oigaard, A.,** Electrical spike activity in the human small intestine, *Am. J. Dig. Dis.,* 23, 776, 1978.

67. **Christensen, J., Schedl, H. P., and Clifton, J. A.,** The basic electrical rhythm of the duodenum in normal human subjects and in patients with thyroid disease, *J. Clin. Invest.,* 43, 1659, 1964.

68. **Daniel, E. E., Honour, A. J., and Bogoch, A.,** Antagonism of serotonin-induced contraction and electrical activity in the ileum, *Gastroenterology,* 39, 62, 1960.

69. **Forster, F. M., Helm, J. D. Jr., and Ingelfinger, F. J.,** The electric potentials of the human small intestine, *Am. J. Physiol.* 139, 433, 1943.

70. **Geldof, H., van der Schee, E. J., Smout, A. J. P. M., and Grashuis, J. L.,** Electrogastrography, in *Gastric and Gastroduodenal Motility,* Akkermanns, L. M. A., Johnson, A. G., and Read, N. W., Eds, Praeger, New York, 1984, 163.

71. **Chen, J. D. Z., Schirmer, B. D., and McCallum, R. W.,** Serosal and cutaneous recordings of gastric myoelectrical activity in patients with gastroparesis, *Am. J. Physiol.,* 266, G90, 1994.

72. **Myers, T. J., Bass, P., Webster, J. G., Fontaine, A. B., and Miyauchi, A.,** Human surface electrogastrograms: AC and DC measurements, *Journal Am. Biomed. Eng.* 12, 319, 1984.

73. **Hamilton, W., Bellahsene, B. E., Reichelderfer, M., Webster, J. D., and Bass, P.,** Human electrogastrograms comparison of surface and mucosal recordings, *Dig. Dis. Sci.,* 31, 33, 1986.

74. **Jacoby, H. I., Bass, P., and Bennet, D. R.,** In vivo extraluminal contractile force transducer for gastrointestinal muscle, *J. Appl. Physiol.,* 18, 658, 1963.

75. **Reinke, D. A., Rosenbaum, A. H., and Bennet, D. R.,** Patterns of dog gastrointestinal contractile activity monitored in vivo with extraluminal force transducers, *Am. J. Dig. Dis.,* 12, 113, 1967.

76. **Weisbrodt, N. W., Hug, C. C. Jr., Schmiege, S. K., and Bass, P.,** Effects of nicotine and tyramine on contractile activity of the colon, *European J. Pharmacol.,* 12, 310, 1970.

77. **Bass, P. and Wiley, J. N.,** Contractile force transducer for recording muscle activity in unanesthetized animals, *J. Appl. Physiol.,* 32, 567, 1972.

78. **Pascaud, X. B, Genton, M. J. H., and Bass, P.,** A miniature transducer for recording intestinal motility in unrestrained chronic rats, *Am. J. Physiol.* 235:E532, 1978.

79. **Li, Y. F., Weisbrodt, N. W., Harari, Y., and Moody, F. G.,** Use of a modified Ussing chamber to monitor intestinal epithelial and smooth muscle functions, *Am. J. Physiol.* 261, G166, 1991.

80. **Itoh, Z., Takeuchi, S., Aizawa, I., and Takayanagi, R.,** Characteristic motor activity of the gastrointestinal tract in fasted conscious dogs measured by implanted force transducers, *Digestive Diseases,* 23, 229, 1978.

81. **Itoh, Z.,** Hormones, peptides, opioids and prostaglandins in normal gastric contractions, in *Gastric and Gastroduodenal Motility,* Akkermans, L. M. A., Johnson, A. G., and Read, N. W., Eds., Praeger, New York, 1984, 41.

82. **Itoh, Z. and Takahashi, I.,** Periodic contractions of the canine gallbladder during the interdigestive state, *Am. J. Physiol.,* 240, G183, 1981.

83. **Kelly, M. and Kennedy, T.,** Motility changes in the antrum after proximal gastric vagotomy, *Br. J. Surg.,* 62, 215, 1975.

84. **Gregersen, H., Kraglund, K., and Djurhuus, J. C.,** Variations in duodenal cross-sectional area during the interdigestive migrating motility complex, *Am. J. Physiol.: Gastrointest. Liver Physiol.,* 259, G26, 1990.

85. **Orvar, K. B., Gregersen, H., and Christensen, J.,** Biomechanical characteristics of the human esophagus, *Dig. Dis. Sci.,* 38, 197, 1993.

86. **Azpiroz, F. and Malagelada, J. R.,** Physiological variations in canine gastric tone measured by an electronic barostat, *Am. J. Physiol.,* 248, G229, 1985.

87. **Bradette, M., Delvaux, M., Staumont, G., Fioramonti, J., Bueno, L., and Frexinos, J.,** Evaluation of colonic sensory thresholds in IBS patients using a barostat: definition of optimal conditions and comparison with healthy subjects, *Dig. Dis. and Sci.,* 39, 449, 1994.

88. **Lydon, S. B., Dodds, W. J., Hogan, W. J., and Arndorfer, R. C.,** The effect of manometric assembly diameter on intraluminal esophageal pressure recording, *Dig. Dis.,* 20, 968, 1975.

89. **Hirsch, J., Ahrens, E. H., and Blankendom, D. H.,** Measurement of the human intestinal length *in vivo* and some causes of variation, *Gastroenterology,* 31, 274, 1956.

90. **Pope II, C. E. and Horton, P. F.,** Intraluminal force transducer measurements of human oesophageal peristalsis, *Gut,* 13, 464, 1972.

91. **Dodds, W. J., Stef, J. A., and Hogan, W. J.,** Factors determining pressure measurement accuracy by intraluminal esophageal manometry, *Gastroenterology,* 70, 117, 1976.

92. **Berseth, C. L.,** Gestational evolution of small intestinal motility in preterm and term infants, *J. Pediatr.,* 115, 646, 1989.

93. **Dodds, W. J., Hogan, W. J., and Geenen, J. E.,** Motility of the biliary system, in *Handbook of Physiology, sect 6; the gastrointestinal system,* Schultz, S. J., Wood, J. D., and Rauner, B. B., Eds., American Physiological Society, Bethesda, 1989, 1055.

94. **Mathias, J. R., Sninsky, C. A., and Millar, H. D.,** Clench, M. H., and Davis, R. H., Development of an improved multi-pressure-sensor probe for recording muscle contraction in human intestine, *Dig. Dis. Sci.,* 30, 119, 1985.

95. **Browning, C., Valori, R. M., and Wingate, D. L.,** A new pressure-sensitive ingestible radiotelemetric capsule, *Lancet,* 2, 504, 1981.

96. **Evans, D. F., Foster, G. E., and Hardcastle, J. D.,** The motility of the human antrum and jejunum during the day and during sleep: an investigation using a radiotelemetry system, in *Motility of the Digestive Tract,* Wienbeck, M., Ed., Raven Press, New York, 1982, 185.

97. **Dent, J.,** A new technique for continuous sphincter pressure measurement, *Gastroenterology,* 71, 263, 1976.

98. **Torgersen, J.,** Muscular build and movement of the stomach and duodenum, *Acta. Radiol. Suppl.,* 45, 3, 1942.

99. **Bass, P. and Wiley, J. N.,** Electrical and extraluminal contractile-force activity of the duodenum of the dog., *Am. J. Dig. Dis.,* 10, 183, 1965.

100. **Cook, I. J., Reddy, S. N., Collins, S. M., and Daniel, E. E.,** Influence of recording techniques on measurement of canine colonic motility, *Dig. Dis. Sci.,* 33, 999, 1988.

101. **Valori, R. M., Collins, S. M., Daniel, E. E., Reddy, S. N., Shannon, S., and Jury, J,** Comparison of methodologies for the measurement of antroduodenal motor activity on the dog, *Gastroenterology,* 61, 546, 1986.

102. **Edelbroek, M., Schuurkes, J., De Ridder, W., Horowitz, M., Dent, J., and Akkermans, L.,** Pyloric motility: sleeve sensor versus strain gauge transducer, *Dig. Dis. Sci.,* 39, 577, 1994.

103. **Muller, H. H. and Nelsen, T. S.,** Rabbit oviduct isthmus contraction patterns in estrus and after human chorionic gonadotropin and progesterone treatment, *Biology of Reproduction,* 21, 563, 1979.

104. **Nelsen, T. S., Nunn, T. A., and Angell, J. B.,** Microminiature transducers for oviductal motor function, in *Ovum Transport and Fertility Regulation,* Harper, M. J. K., Pauerstein, C. J., Adams, C. E., Coutinho, E. M., Croxatto, H. B., and Paton, D. M., Eds., Scriptor, Copenhagen, 75.

105. **Hubel, K. A. and Follick, M.,** A small strain gage for measuring intestinal motility in rats, *Am. J. Dig. Dis.,* 21, 1075, 1976.

106. **Jeutter, D. C. and Fromm, E.,** Silicon force transducer for extraluminal measurement of oviduct contractile activity, *IEEE Transactions on Biomedical Engineering,* BME-24, 226, 1977.

107. **Lambert, A., Eloy, R., and Grenier, J. F.,** Transducer for recording electrical and mechanical chronic intestinal activity, *J. Appl. Physiol.,* 41, 942, 1976.

108. **Kingma, Y. J., Bowes, K. L., Kocylowski, M. S. K., and Szmidt, J.,** Inductive displacement gauge, *Am. J. Physiol.,* 239, G128, 1980.

109. **Lefcourt, A. M.,** Rhythmic contractions of the teat sphincter in bovines: an expulsion mechanism, *Am. J. Physiol.,* 242, R181, 1982.

110. **Blair, W. D., Gilliland, B. E., and Sauer, B. W.,** An intraluminal transducer/telemetry system for oviductal motility studies, *J. Appl. Physiol.,* 40, 999, 1976.

111. **Guha, S. K., Anand, S., and Talwar, G. P.,** *In vivo* motility of the unobstructed fallopian tube, *J. Appl. Physiol.,* 40, 114, 1976.

112. **Wright, J. W., Healy, T. E. J., Balfour, T. W., and Hardcastle, J. D.,** A method for long-term recording of intestinal mechanical and electrical activity in the unrestrained rat, *J. Pharmac. Methods,* 6, 233, 1981.

9 *In Vitro* Techniques for the Study of Gastrointestinal Motility

William H. Percy

CRITERIA FOR PERFORMING *IN VITRO* EXPERIMENTS

Meaningful *in vitro* studies of intestinal smooth muscle function date back to the now legendary works of Magnus[1–6] at the turn of the century. Although these studies were not original in their use of isolated intestinal smooth muscle,[7,8] they represent the first serious attempts to relate structure to function and to characterize the mechanisms underlying such phenomena as spontaneous contractile activity. While many of Magnus' original conclusions about intestinal muscle function have now been superseded through the use of more sophisticated technology, his contribution to the area must be acknowledged as the point of origin for even the most complex present day experiments.

The *in vitro* methods that will be discussed in this section are based largely on techniques which, although borrowing from Magnus' ideas, begin with Trendelenburg's work on the peristaltic reflex of the guinea pig ileum in 1917.[9] This seminal study was followed by the classic works of Finkleman, 1930,[10] Garry and Gillespie, 1954, 1955[11,12] and Paton, 1955.[13] Although there is now an expansive literature on the *in vitro* physiological and pharmacological properties of the muscles which comprise the gut, each in some way owes its origins to these earlier works.

The primary aim of an *in vitro* experiment involving intestinal muscle is to be able to study a selected aspect of muscle function under conditions where the influence of external factors (e.g. circulating hormones) is removed, but the muscle itself performs in a manner analogous to its *in vivo* capacity. In order to ensure that this is possible, a number of important questions must be answered before beginning any experimental protocol; these questions include:

1. What is the most appropriate physiological solution with which to maintain the tissue?
2. Can tissue be stored or should it be used immediately and does the ambient temperature affect its performance?
3. Is isometric recording preferable to isotonic recording?
4. What load should be placed on the muscle so that its mechanical performance is optimal?
5. Should concentration-related phenomena be studied and how are such data best presented and analyzed?
6. What techniques are available for the study of intrinsic and extrinsic nerves, different muscle types and different intestinal regions?

At a time when increasing emphasis is being placed upon events at the cellular and molecular level it is important to realize that most questions about *integrated intestinal function* cannot be answered utilizing such techniques. The *in vitro* methods discussed in this chapter offer investigators realistic tools with which to selectively assess the roles and interactions of the various components which comprise the gastrointestinal tract as a whole. However, the continuing contribution of these methods to our understanding of the physiology and pharmacology of the gut relies heavily upon an understanding of their applications and limitations. The following section is designed to address these concerns.

CHOICE OF PHYSIOLOGICAL SOLUTION

One of the first decisions that has to be made when beginning a series of *in vitro* experiments using gastrointestinal tissue is the appropriate physiological medium for the task in hand. The survival of a tissue and its ability to respond to mechanical, pharmacologic or electrical stimuli are critically dependent upon the medium in which it is maintained. The consequences of choosing an inappropriate solution may be fairly profound, but the fact that one generally does not routinely compare physiological solutions as an integral part of most experimental protocols may obscure this error.

For example, it has been noted that when using the guinea pig esophageal muscularis mucosae reducing the calcium ion concentration of the bathing medium between 3.6 mM and 0.9 mM increases the threshold and the EC_{50} values for acetylcholine by approximately one order of magnitude.[14] Conversely, in the same series of experiments it was found that the maximum response of this tissue to acetylcholine still occurs at the same concentration regardless of the available calcium unless none is present. In contrast to its esophageal muscularis mucosae, in the guinea pig ileum alterations in available calcium over the same concentration range have little or no effect on the longitudinal muscle responses to acetylcholine.[14] However, analysis of the amount of acetylcholine being released from the myenteric plexus of this preparation in response to low frequency electrical stimulation has shown that it initially rises as available calcium is reduced from 2.54 to 1.27 mM, but declines as the calcium ion concentration is further decreased.[15]

From these examples it may be concluded that the choice of physiological solution is crucial with respect to the question which the experimental protocol seeks to answer. Similarly, one cannot arbitrarily select a particular solution and expect that it will work equally well for all tissues.

It is generally assumed that the physiological bathing medium used in *in vitro* experiments involving gastrointestinal smooth muscle reproduces the extracellular environment *in vivo*. However, this is not entirely correct and from a comparison of Tables 1 and 2 it can be seen that both a typical Tyrode's solution[16] and a modified Krebs' solution[17] contain chloride at a higher concentration than would generally be found in the blood of a variety of species. Similarly, relative to the blood of the same species Tyrode's solution is low in potassium and bicarbonate while Krebs' solution and most of its modifications contain almost double the typical level of glucose. These observations are in keeping with Tyrode's original observation that the solution which he derived experimentally was more successful in prolonging tissue viability than solutions used by his contemporaries which mimicked the ionic composition of blood.[16]

When selecting a physiological medium for a particular series of experiments one should be aware of the calcium ion concentration which can reasonably be used with such bicarbonate buffered solutions. In general, solutions similar in composition to those described in Table 1 are capable of maintaining Ca^{2+} in solution in the range 0–5 mM, provided they are gassed with both O_2 and CO_2 in approximately a 95-5% ratio. If a particular experimental procedure calls for investigating the effects of elevating Ca^{2+} to concentrations such as 10 mM these solutions will not be adequate and an alternative buffer system such as HEPES or MOPS should be considered.

TABLE 1
Physiological Solutions

Salt	Molecular Weight	Tyrode Solution		Original Krebs[a]		Modified Krebs	
		g/l	mM	g/l	mM	g/l	mM
NaCl	58.44	8.00	136.89	5.54	94.79	6.925	118.50
KCl	74.56	0.20	2.68	0.35	4.69	0.354	4.75
CaCl$_2$	110.99[b]	0.20	1.80	0.28	2.52	0.282	2.54
NaH$_2$PO$_4$	155.99	0.05	0.32	—	—	0.186	1.19
KH$_2$PO$_4$	136.10[b]	—	—	0.16	1.17	—	—
MgSO$_4$.(7H$_2$O)	246.48	—	—	0.29	1.17	0.293	1.19
MgCl$_2$	95.21[b]	0.10	1.05	—	—	—	—
		GAS EACH OF THESE WITH 95% O$_2$ AND 5% CO$_2$[c]					
		BEFORE ADDING GLUCOSE AND SODIUM BICARBONATE					
Glucose	180.10	1.0	5.55	2.10	11.65	1.982	11.0
NaHCO$_3$	84.01	1.0	11.90	2.10	25.00	2.100	25.0

[a]The original Krebs' solution[17] also contained the sodium salts of pyruvic acid (4.88 mM), fumaric acid (10.81 mM) and glutamic acid (4.89 mM). Shown for comparison is a typical modified Krebs' solution used today.
[b]Refers to the molecular weight of the anhydrous form.
[c]It should be noted that Tyrode was fortunate in selecting a low Ca^{2+} ion concentration for his solution as he chose to gas it with O$_2$ alone.

As is found in the body, the ability of the bicarbonate buffer system to work effectively is a function of the amount of CO$_2$ available to interact with water to form carbonic acid. The dissociation of carbonic acid provides the necessary H$^+$ ions required to prevent the solution from becoming too alkaline. If CO$_2$ is not available for the continuous production of carbonic acid, this buffering capacity is lost because the H$^+$ ions are rapidly depleted. Thus, under conditions where a bicarbonate buffered physiological solution is not provided with sufficient CO$_2$, the pH increases and Ca^{2+} in combination with other anions will form a precipitate. When this happens the solution becomes cloudy, taking the appearance of having had a tablespoon of milk added. While in theory it is possible to reverse this by vigorous gassing with an O$_2$/CO$_2$ gas mixture or by the addition of measured amounts of HCl, in practical terms (i.e. time saved) it is more judicious to simply make a fresh solution.

TABLE 2
Ranges of Blood Concentrations (mM) of Principal Ions in Different Species

	Guinea pig	Rabbit	Rat	Cat	Dog	Human
Na$^+$	120–149	100–145[¥]	140–156	147–156	135–180	136–145[#]
K$^+$	3.8–7.9	3.6–6.9[¥]	5.4–7.0	4.0–6.0	3.5–6.7	3.5–5.0[§]
Ca^{2+} [a]	1.32–2.99	2.07–2.73	1.24–3.49	1.24–3.24	0.72–2.91	2.12–2.61[#]
Cl$^-$	90–115	95–120	100–110	110–123	99–121	100–106[#]
GLUCOSE	4.55–5.93	2.77–5.17[¥]	2.77–7.49	3.33–8.04	3.55–6.66	3.88–5.55[#]
HCO$_3$$^-$	13–30	16–32	13–32	14–27	15–29	22–26[§]

[a]Assumes that all calcium is present in the ionized form.
All values have been adapted from reference 18 except; [¥] from reference 19; [#] from reference 20; [§] from reference 21.

It is also important to consider the potential effects of the metabolic substrate which is to be utilized. While almost without exception glucose is selected, it has been known since 1912 that gastrointestinal smooth muscle can function with a variety of different substrates.[22] This phenomenon has recently been studied in detail using muscle from the opossum esophageal body and lower esophageal sphincter subjected to different pharmacologic stimuli. As a result of these experiments it was found that under certain conditions incubation with glucose was not always associated with the largest agonist-induced contractions.[23]

Thus, in summary, the correct choice of physiological solution is crucial to the success of the experiment to be performed. Determination of the appropriate solution should be made experimentally and should not be based solely on "previous experience," particularly if one is moving from one region of the gastrointestinal tract to another or if a different species is to be used.

STORAGE CONDITIONS AND THE EFFECTS OF AMBIENT TEMPERATURE

In addition to choosing the best physiological medium to sustain an isolated intestinal smooth muscle preparation the way in which it is treated prior to the start of the experiment and the temperature at which the experiment itself is performed will also influence the outcome.

The ability of intestinal smooth muscle to contract once removed from the body was described as long ago as 1854.[7] However, the conditions under which it could be stored and still perform this function were given only cursory consideration[8] until the studies of Gunn & Underhill in 1914.[24] These authors carried out a series of experiments in which the viability of rabbit and cat intestinal smooth muscle was assessed after storage for varying periods of time at different temperatures.

It was concluded from these studies that the muscle was still capable of producing rhythmic pendulum movements (spontaneous contractions) and responding to cholinergic and adrenergic stimulation after 5 days of storage at 3–7°C. As the storage temperature was increased the duration of tissue viability decreased, such that at 37°C the tissue was only considered to "live" for approximately 8 hours and then, only if oxygen was *not* made available. Based on the figures provided by the authors these conclusions must be qualified with the observations that the resting tone, spontaneous contractile amplitude and responses to agonists were all significantly attenuated with cold storage. Thus, one cannot accept at face value the authors' statement that as long as the muscle exhibits spontaneous contractions upon re-warming it continues to respond "normally" to pharmacologic stimuli.

More recent studies have demonstrated in a quantitative fashion that cold storage of gastrointestinal smooth muscle has profound effects upon both the nerves and muscle present in the tissue sample. Even moderate cooling (to 24°C) of the guinea pig ileum may result in an irreversible loss of the emptying phase of the peristaltic reflex, which requires both an intact myenteric plexus and a functional muscularis propria (the longitudinal and circular muscle layers).[25] This process occurs without a loss of muscle function,[25] providing evidence for the process now known as "cold denervation" as described by Filogamo.[26]

Although smooth muscle responses to agonists may appear normal following cold storage there is considerable evidence that even short term cooling causes profound mechanical and pharmacological changes to take place. For example, rat colonic longitudinal muscle stored at 4°C for periods of from 1–7 days shows a significant increase in stress relaxation (the decline in force per unit area that is seen when a smooth muscle is held under a fixed load) with a concurrent significant decrease in Young's modulus (the relationship between the load which is applied to the muscle and the resulting change in length).[27] These alterations alone will have a significant impact on any attempt to quantitate the length-tension characteristics of the muscle.

From an electrophysiological standpoint, cooling of gastrointestinal smooth muscle may be associated with membrane depolarization[28,29] and a reduction in both the number and amplitude of slow waves.[28] At room temperature ($\approx 22°C$) the duration of muscle hyperpolarization in response to intrinsic nerve stimulation may also be increased almost 100%.[29] In addition to these changes, cooling of the guinea pig ileum has been shown to elicit muscarinic receptor-mediated spontaneous contractions of the longitudinal muscle[30] and in rat esophageal muscularis mucosae 48 hours cold storage unmasks serotonin receptors that are not evident in freshly prepared tissue.[31]

An additional example which emphasizes the importance of temperature relates to the responses of the esophageal muscularis mucosae to electrical field stimulation. In 1969 Christensen and Lund[32] noted that at 36–38°C the esophageal muscularis mucosae of the North American opossum responded to electrical field stimulation with a monophasic "duration" contraction. This observation was subsequently confirmed and extended by Christensen and Percy in 1984 who demonstrated that this response was cholinergic in origin.[33] However, using the same tissue at 30°C Domoto et al.[34] observed a two phase response consisting of an initial cholinergic phasic component and a tonic component which they attributed to the release of substance P. It is known that both spontaneous and evoked acetylcholine release from enteric nerves are depressed as the ambient temperature is decreased.[35,36,37] Thus, because the tonic component of the esophageal muscularis mucosae response at 30°C was depressed by eserine and by carbachol,[34] it is likely that the substance P-evoked component was not evident at 37°C because it was being suppressed by the amount of endogenous acetylcholine being released upon stimulation.

Clearly, therefore, cooling, storage and ambient temperature have multiple and somewhat unpredictable effects on intestinal smooth muscle and its intrinsic innervation. Thus, unless one wishes to perform experiments that are directly related to one or other of these conditions, or if cooling is required as an aid to dissection,[12] fresh tissue should always be used and the ambient experimental temperature regulated to that of the body of the donor species. In circumstances where it is not practicable to use fresh tissue (e.g. with human tissue samples which may be difficult to acquire) control experiments relating to mechanics and pharmacology should be performed over the time frame involved to ensure that hour to hour or day to day differences are taken into consideration when evaluating the results of the experiment.

CHOICE OF TRANSDUCER

In the earliest experiments in which gastrointestinal smooth muscle contraction was studied *in vitro,* measurements were made under isotonic conditions (i.e. development of muscle tension was associated with a change in length). To achieve this, segments of whole intestine were attached to a lever system such that the muscle pulled against a load at one end of the lever and this same end marked a slowly rotating smoked drum, giving a measure of the amplitude of shortening and lengthening. However, a review of the current *in vitro* literature will quickly reveal that virtually all experiments involving gastrointestinal smooth muscle are now carried out using isometric transducers, where the muscle develops tension but does not change length. This is a curious development because, even a cursory glance into the abdominal cavity of an anesthetized (or recently euthanized) animal will demonstrate that, for the most part, gastrointestinal smooth muscle does not function isometrically but rather, contracts isotonically. The reasons underlying this apparent paradox between *in vitro* measurement and *in vivo* function relate to the mechanics of the different types of transducers and the information that can be obtained with either one.

The isometric transducer (Figure 1A) involves no muscle movement and, therefore, relies solely upon electronics to translate force into a measurable signal. In this instance the force

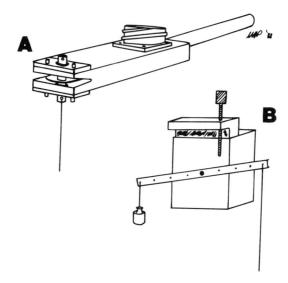

FIGURE 1   A. Type of transducer typically used for recording isometric tension. The load on the tissue is pre-set by elevating or lowering the transducer relative to the top of the preparation when it is anchored to the base of the organ bath. This transducer allows for actual force generated by the muscle to be quantitated but has the disadvantage that, as the preparation relaxes, the load on the tissue decreases and true isometric recording does not take place. (Note that this transducer type can be modified to perform in an isotonic fashion by the insertion of appropriate springs between the preparation and the transducer itself). B. Typical isotonic transducer. In this case the load on the tissue is the weight suspended from the transducer arm. With this system the tissue contracts and relaxes with a concurrent change in length during which the load remains constant. Using this type of transducer it is possible to measure actual muscle shortening or lengthening. However, this method has the disadvantage that one cannot measure the corresponding forces that are being generated.

applied to the transducer causes an alteration in one arm of a Wheatstone bridge circuit. This is seen as a voltage difference by the amplifier to which the transducer is attached. With this type of transducer the load applied to the tissue is the result of the transducer being moved away from the tissue, parallel to its long axis, thus stretching it by a measurable amount. Contraction of the tissue in response to a challenge is then measured based upon the force generated by the muscle pulling against the transducer.

The modern day isotonic transducer (Figure 1B) utilizes the same lever system as its predecessor, but movement of the lever is translated into a changing electrical signal by such methods as using movement of the spindle to which the center of the lever is attached to move a variable density filter between a light source and a photoelectric cell. The basic principle of the system remains unchanged in that the muscle is stretched by the load placed upon it and, when stimulated, develops tension by shortening and pulling against the load. One important feature of this system is that as the muscle changes length the load remains constant.

The types of information that can be obtained utilizing isometric and isotonic transducers are quite different. For example, under isometric conditions smooth muscle is capable of generating forces of a magnitude comparable to those produced by skeletal muscle preparations whereas, under isotonic conditions it can shorten to as little as 20% of is original length.[38] Thus, from a quantitative standpoint the most important difference between isometric and isotonic transducers is that with the former one can measure the amount of force being produced by a tissue sample but not the corresponding shortening; with the latter, one can measure change in length but not actual force. This may not appear to be significant because, if one normalizes concentration-response data to a tissue's maximum contraction to an agent such as acetylcholine, carbachol or potassium, expression of the data would always be relative to a known 100% and the method used to ascertain this would be immaterial. However, the differences between transducer types *is* important because, as has been shown in airway smooth muscle, maximum tension generation does not necessarily correspond to maximum shortening.[39] This is because shortening is limited by the volume of the muscle and, therefore, isotonically recorded contractions may be appear maximal at drug concentrations where force generation would still be increasing under isometric conditions. Thus, if one is interested in obtaining information from the linear portion of a concentration-response curve such a difference may not be critical, but if it is important to know what happens a tissue's maximum responses under a variety of conditions this may be more clearly seen under isometric recording conditions.

An important property of intestinal smooth muscle which is often not considered in the choice of transducer is its ability to relax. As noted above, under isotonic recording conditions the load on a tissue remains constant irrespective of its length. Contrary to expectations, under isometric recording conditions muscle relaxation *is* associated with an increase in length. This means that the effective distance between the top of the tissue and the transducer is reduced and, therefore, the load on the tissue is decreased in proportion. Thus, by definition, one cannot measure an "*isometric relaxation*". However, having made this statement, under most conditions it is possible to assess, at least qualitatively, whether or not a muscle relaxes in a concentration- or stimulus-dependent manner when attached to an isometric transducer. As a result of the load on the tissue decreasing as its length increases, isometric concentration-relaxation curves may appear quite shallow (*i.e.* they reach a maximum within a small concentration range). This may be further complicated if the tissue has a capacity to relax which exceeds the load placed upon it. This could occur if the optimal length for the generation of active tension (L_o) (see below) was reached at a tension equivalent to a 1 g load (9.8 mN) but, when stretched, the tissue is capable of relaxing by amount equivalent to 1.5 g (14.7 mN). This would mean that, at a particular concentration of the agent inducing the relaxation, the baseline on the chart recorder would return to zero and would be flat at all concentrations of the drug beyond this point. The end result of this is that a significant portion of the concentration-response relationship may be lost.

In contrast, under isotonic conditions the ability to measure relaxation is not complicated by variability of the load for any given muscle length. Thus, if an appropriate load is chosen (see below) it is possible to construct a complete concentration-response curve in which the maximum relaxation observed represents the true ability of the tissue to increase in length and does not merely reflect the limitations of the recording system.

Having outlined the differences between the two types of transducer it is important to note that certain muscle types may perform optimally with only one type of transducer. Thus, guinea pig ileum longitudinal muscle will contract and relax equally well under isometric or isotonic conditions.[13,15,40,41] The opossum lower esophageal sphincter on the other hand, has a high resting tone and does not relax and return to its original resting length particularly well under isotonic conditions (Percy, unpublished observations), but will do so for hours when attached to an isometric transducer.[42] Human distal colonic longitudinal and circular muscles give clearly defined isometric and isotonic contractile responses but exhibit significant relaxations (as opposed to a loss of spontaneous contractions) only under isotonic recording conditions[43] (Figure 2).

Thus, before embarking upon a series of experiments in which intestinal muscle responses are to be evaluated, it is a worthwhile exercise to consider whether an isometric or an isotonic transducer is the most appropriate choice to answer the questions that are being asked. In many instances it will be of value to the investigator to carry out preliminary experiments such that the correct selection is made based upon experimentally derived information.

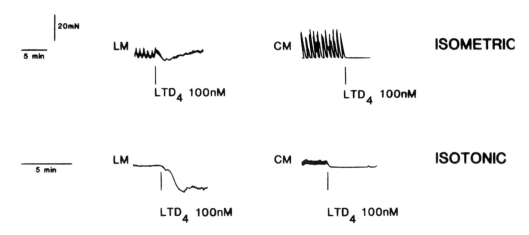

FIGURE 2 A comparison of the inhibitory responses of human distal colonic longitudinal muscle (LM) and circular muscle (CM) to leukotriene D4 under isometric (top) and isotonic (bottom) recording conditions. Tissues are from the same colon sample. Note that under isometric conditions only spontaneous contractions are lost whereas, under isotonic conditions there is a significant loss of tone. The vertical calibration is in milliNewtons (mN) for isometric recordings but, because force cannot be measured with an isotonic transducer there is no corresponding measurement for these traces. (From Percy, W. H. et al., *Gastroenterology* 99, 1324, 1990. With permission.)

DETERMINATION OF THE LOAD TO PLACE UPON THE TISSUE

Having decided upon a particular transducer type the next question that needs to be addressed is what load to place upon the tissue. In many cases an otherwise sound experimental protocol may be significantly weakened by a failure to apply a sufficient load to the muscle or, by overstretching it.

A common error is to assume that virtually any gastrointestinal smooth muscle preparation will respond optimally if it is attached to an isometric transducer and placed "under 1 gram of tension". For some muscles this will be far less than is required[e.g. 43,44,45,46] whereas, for others this would be 2–5 times the optimal load.[e.g. 14,47,48,49] Furthermore, it is important to note that although the expression "grams of tension" has been employed for some considerable time, it is incorrect because the gram is a unit of mass not force. In the more current literature force is correctly expressed in Newtons (N) or milliNewtons (mN). To convert from grams to Newtons is a relatively simple calculation based on the relationship between mass and gravitational acceleration (9.8 msec^{-2}):

$$1 \text{ g} = 980 \text{ dynes and } 1N = 100,000 \text{ dynes}$$
$$1 \text{ g} = 980/100,000 N$$
$$1 \text{ g} = 0.0098 N$$
$$\mathbf{1 \text{ g} = 9.8 \text{ mN or } 10 \text{ mN} = 1.02 \text{ g}}$$

Based on this, correct expressions to describe the amount of stretch placed on a preparation attached to an isometric transducer could be either "under 10 mN of tension" or "under a *tension equivalent to a* 1.02 g load". Clearly this problem does not arise with an isotonic transducer where the preparation is literally operating "under a 1g load".

To ascertain the appropriate load for a particular tissue it is necessary to construct a length-tension relationship. This involves placing the tissue under step-wise increases in tension, allowing an equilibration period and then measuring the contractile response to an agonist or a K^+ challenge. The following protocol would be appropriate for use with an isometric transducer but could, with difficulty, be carried out using an isotonic transducer. In almost all cases the optimal muscle load determined under isometric conditions can be used with the same muscle type connected to an isotonic transducer.

Ideally, to carry out this protocol a strip of mucosa-free muscle, 1–2 cm long by 2–4 mm wide, cut in the longitudinal or circular axis should be used. If one uses a segment of whole intestine the responses are complicated by several factors. First, the actions of the circular muscle layer, which is at 90° to the plane of recording, tend to oppose contraction in the longitudinal axis.[38] Second, unless the threads anchoring the preparation to the transducer and the base of the tissue bath are positioned at precisely corresponding locations on the oral and aboral circumference, the longitudinal muscle will tend to contract in a spiral fashion and true force measurements will not be obtained. Third, if one wishes to calculate the *stress* (force per unit of cross sectional area) produced by the muscle under study it is virtually impossible to do this for a whole segment. This is because the contractions that are measured are largely a function of the muscle fibers between the two anchoring points and the further one gets from this region in a circumferential direction the smaller the contribution of those muscle fibers to the overall response. However, because the calculation of *stress* is based on muscle mass this inherent error leads to an underestimate of the true force the muscle is capable of producing. Fourth, although it is generally ignored, a segment of whole intestine will almost certainly contain a longitudinally oriented muscularis mucosae which may make a significant contribution to the overall force which is recorded. This possibility is supported by the observation that in the rabbit distal colon, *on a mm²* basis, the muscularis mucosae is capable of producing between 150% and 200% of the *stress* produced by the corresponding region of longitudinal muscle (compare references 43 and 50). Fifth, in certain regions of the intestine such as the stomach, the mucosa constitutes the majority of the tissue mass and, as such, can significantly interfere with the ability of the muscularis propria to contract and relax.

Having produced an appropriate tissue sample first, suspend it in an organ bath at 37 ± 0.5°C and allow it to equilibrate for approximately 30 minutes, changing the bathing medium every 10 minutes. Next, raise the isometric transducer to a point where the tissue is held upright and rigid in the bath, but no tension is recorded by the system. Measure the length of the tissue (in centimeters) between the threads which anchor it to the base of the bath at the bottom and the transducer at the top. This is the initial muscle length, sometimes referred to as the resting length, denoted as L_i. Raise the transducer to increase the tissue length by the increment you have chosen to use throughout this procedure (1–2 mm would be a reasonable amount). When the tension produced by this load has reached a steady state note its magnitude above the baseline (which denotes zero tension). This represents the passive tension developed at this length. A contractile response should now be evoked using the pharmacologic agent of choice (one whose effects can be reversed within a short period of time is preferable). The difference between the zero baseline and the peak of the phasic component of this evoked response is the total tension developed at this length. The active tension (i.e. the component caused by the agonist) is then calculated as the total tension minus the passive tension.[51] As this process is repeated at each incremental increase in tissue length it will be noted that although passive tension continues to increase the active tension initially increases, reaches a maximum and, as the length continues to increase, begins to decline. The tissue length at which the active tension is maximal is known as the optimal length for the generation of active tension, and is referred to as L_o. Data obtained in such an experiment may be represented graphically with all values normalized with respect to either the maximum active tension[52] or the total tension[51] generated at L_o. The ratio of L_o to L_i varies between muscle types and values of 1.5 to 2.5 (*i.e.* L_o = 150% to 250% of L_i) are common.[42,43]

The size of this range means that the load stretching the muscle to L_o must be determined experimentally for each new muscle type to be studied. It cannot simply be assumed for example, that a value obtained using the longitudinal muscle of the guinea pig ileum would be appropriate for the same muscle in the distal colon. In fact, the mechanical properties of any one muscle layer in the intestine vary considerably in relation to factors such as, the age of the animal, duration of tissue storage or location along the length of an organ.[27] Significant differences have also been noted between the longitudinal and circular muscle layers in the same anatomical location.[43]

Having constructed a length-tension relationship for a particular muscle it is of value to calculate the maximum active, passive and total *stress* developed at L_o. From the equation density = mass/volume and from the assumption that the tissue sample is somewhere in shape between a cuboid and a cylinder with cross sectional area (A) and length (L) it follows that (A) is equal to the mass (g)/density (g/ml) × length (cm). The density of smooth muscle in Krebs' solution has previously been calculated[51] to be 1.056 gml^{-1} and the mass and length of the tissue are values that can be measured directly. (NOTE: If the tissue sample contains both longitudinal and circular muscle the mass of the muscle in the plane of recording must first be calculated by histologically determining what percentage of the total mass this represents.[43,53] This is critical because the ratio of longitudinal to circular muscle varies along the length of the intestine). Therefore, based upon calibration of the isometric transducer with a known weight in grams, *stress* can easily be determined by combining this information. It will also be evident that, should it be necessary, *stress* at every tissue length studied can also be computed by measuring the actual length of the tissue at each increment and then applying these equations.

Conducting 4 or 5 preliminary experiments should be sufficient to establish the load which stretches the muscle L_o. Provided that one does not make a significant change in the way in which future tissues are obtained (e.g. using older animals, moving to a different anatomical location within the same organ or cutting longer/shorter segments) this value may be used each time this particular preparation is studied.

CONSTRUCTING CONCENTRATION-RESPONSE CURVES

Perhaps the most useful but most mis-used analytical tool available for the study of gastrointestinal smooth muscle *in vitro* is the concentration-response curve. Although originally these were referred to as "dose-response curves," with the advent of expressing how much drug was being administered to the bathing medium in terms of "moles per liter" rather than "μg," "concentration-response curve" has become the accepted name.

It is not the aim of this section to describe the fundamental concepts upon which concentration-response relationships are based and the reader is referred to the excellent monograph by Tallarida and Jacob[54] for this information. What follows is designed to assist in experimental design and to help researchers avoid many of the common pitfalls that are associated with the use of this technique.

The first question to be addressed is: *Can valid information be obtained by the use of an agonist at one concentration or should an entire concentration-response curve be constructed?* The answer to this may be taken from the early literature where it was common practice to perform experiments in which drugs were almost always added at a single effective concentration. The rationale for choosing this concentration was generally not explained and the responses obtained were never quantified in terms of their amplitude relative to the smallest and largest effects the drug could produce. The absence of this important information often led investigators to draw erroneous conclusions based on their data. For example, in their studies on the effects of cold storage on intestinal muscle function, Gunn and Underhill[24] were of the impression that cold storage had little effect on the muscle itself because, unless it was "dead" it always responded in the same way to the one concentration of pilocarpine and epinephrine which they used. However, had they performed experiments in which concentration-related contractions and relaxations were studied their conclusion would have been quite different.

Similarly, if one compares drug effects on an isolated muscle preparation without examining minimum to maximum responses important information may be lost. For example, Gallacher et al.[55] studied the actions of both acetylcholine (10 μg/ml) and histamine (1 μg/ml) on the isolated rabbit distal colonic muscularis mucosae. While they observed that both could cause contractions, the subsequent work of Percy et al.[49] clearly demonstrated that the concentration-response curve for histamine lies somewhat to the left of that for acetylcholine and that, on an equimolar basis, at concentrations greater than 10^{-7} M histamine always produces larger responses than acetylcholine. This is important information with respect to the properties of these agents because, as one moves in an oral direction, this relationship changes to the extent that, on proximal colonic muscularis mucosae, histamine and acetylcholine are essentially equipotent.[49] This conclusion could not have been reached on the basis of studying only one concentration of each agonist.

A second important problem associated with the use of agonists at only one concentration is a failure to observe concentration-dependent biphasic responses. In the experiments of Boschov et al.[56] it was noted that low concentrations of bradykinin applied to the longitudinal muscle of the rat duodenum caused relaxations. However, as the concentration of bradykinin was increased these relaxations were followed by progressively larger contractions. On rabbit proximal colonic muscularis mucosae norepinephrine causes relaxations at low concentrations which, as the concentration is increased, are reduced in amplitude by concurrent contractions that eventually become the predominant response.[49] In each of these cases the true nature of the agonist effect could not have been accurately predicted if only one concentration had been studied. In the former case the contractile effects of bradykinin could have been overlooked and, in the latter, not only would contractile responses have been overlooked, but the ability of norepinephrine to cause inhibition would have been greatly underestimated.

It should be clear from these simple examples that one should always determine the entire concentration-response relationship at some stage in any experimental protocol, regardless of whether novel compounds are being studied or not. Ideally, a correctly constructed concentration-response curve will contain at least one and preferably two concentrations of the agonist that cause no response. These may be used as additional vehicle controls and, in addition, they allow the threshold concentration required to elicit a contraction or relaxation to be determined. The curve should also contain a minimum of four points in the linear portion and at least two points which are maximal, to ascertain that the top of the concentration-response curve has, in fact, been reached.

Having obtained this information there are several way in which it can be expressed and analyzed. While the method chosen will depend upon the type of question that the protocol is attempting to answer, some forms of data expression will always be preferable to others.

EXPRESSION OF DATA

One method of data expression is to designate the largest response to each agonist tested as 100% and to normalize the data by expressing responses to each concentration as a fraction of this value. The drawback to this method is that all drugs used on an individual tissue appear to produce maximum responses. Information presented in this fashion is of little value for anything other than qualitative analysis. No conclusions may be drawn regarding intrinsic activity or potency and EC_{50}/IC_{50} values have no meaning under these circumstances.

A more rigorous approach is to determine what constitutes a tissue maximum response using an agent such as carbachol or a high K^+ solution. The responses to different concentrations of the various drugs used are then expressed as a percentage of the tissue's 100% response. In this way the relative potencies and/or intrinsic activities of individual agonists can be quantitatively assessed. Furthermore, EC_{50} or IC_{50} values can be calculated for those agents that produce a 100% response. The drawback to this method of data expression is that if one wishes to compare control tissue with tissue that has undergone some manipulation (e.g. inflammation, denervation or hypertrophy) the relationships between agonists in terms of potency or intrinsic activity might appear to be unchanged even although the muscle itself is producing much smaller contractions or relaxations to each concentration of the drug. For examples which address these problems the reader is referred to reference 50.

A third method of data expression which circumvents the problems associated with the techniques described above is to measure the actual *stress* generated by the muscle in response to different concentrations of agonists. Provided one knows the maximum *stress* the tissue can produce, the intrinsic activities and potencies of the various agonists can be obtained and EC_{50}/IC_{50} can be calculated. In addition, this method allows for differences between control and "treated" tissues to be compared directly. However, as the determination of *stress* requires a not inconsiderable amount of additional experimentation and calculation (weighing, measuring etc.), employing this technique is only of value in this particular experimental design. This caveat may be explained by considering an experiment where only control tissue is used and, when expressed as a percentage, the maximum response to acetylcholine is found to be twice that produced to a different agent. Clearly, this ratio would be unchanged by expressing the same data in terms of *stress* and the effort expended in the extra computation will provide no additional information. Examples of data expression illustrating the above points are contained in the reference by Yagi et al.[57]

ANALYSIS OF DATA

A number of methods exist for the mathematical manipulation of concentration-response data to allow it to be analyzed and interpreted. Such techniques have been elegantly described by Tallarida and Jacob,[54] DeLean et al.,[58] Carpenter[59] and Meddings et al.[60] and are beyond the scope of this review. The following section is merely designed to illustrate some important reasons why log concentration-response data cannot be analyzed with simple statistical tests and why more sophisticated methods must be employed.

A common error when comparing two log concentration-response curves that each have means and standard errors from 5 or more replicates (such as, control and control + antagonist), is to assume that corresponding points on each curve can be compared with either a paired or a non-paired Students t-test. Unfortunately the t-test is not appropriate for this type of comparison. First, because repeated use of this test greatly increases the likelihood of incorrectly identifying means as being significantly different when they are not[61] (i.e. a Type I or "α" error). Second, it will be noted that the standard errors on data points on a log concentration-response curve tend to be larger in the linear portion than they are at either end. This is because small responses tend to be uniformly small and near maximal responses are always very large. The greatest variability occurs over the concentration range where responses are not at either extreme. The responses in this range cause problems in situations where one might wish to compare a control concentration-response curve with a second curve obtained after treatment with an antagonist. If the antagonist is present in sufficient concentration to shift the curve to the right, some agonist concentrations which originally produced near maximal responses will be found to cause effects that lie on the linear portion of the curve. Similarly, points on the lower end of the linear portion will have moved to the non-linear lower limb of the curve. Thus, corresponding concentrations on the two curves now produce responses whose means almost certainly have non-homogeneous standard errors.

The standard error (SE) is the standard deviation (SD) divided by the square root of the number of observations (n) (*i.e.* SE = SD/$\sqrt{n}$). The standard deviation is the square root of the variance (s^2) (*i.e.* SD = $\sqrt{s^2}$). From this arithmetic relationship, it may be deduced that means which have disparate standard errors may represent population samples that have significantly different variances. Statistical tests, such as the t-test, require that the population samples being compared have similar distributions about their respective means, i.e. they have similar variances.[61] Clearly, therefore, under certain conditions this criterion cannot be met even by parallel log concentration-response curves and using t-tests for comparisons would be inappropriate. Errors produced by this method of analysis of concentration-response data are highlighted in reference 59, Figure 6, where t-tests were applied to the same data which had been mathematically expressed in two different forms. In one case only two points were found to be significantly different whereas, in the second 9 of the 10 points appeared to be different.

However, having stated what are the wrong tests to use it should be noted that there is no single method which can be used to determine the correct statistical method to analyze the data which comprise two or more log concentration-response curves. In large part this is because the conditions under which such data are obtained can differ dramatically depending on the experimental protocol. Some concentration-response data may represent cumulative additions of an agonist, others may involve multiple antagonist concentrations and, in some circumstances, one curve may be from a control group of tissues while the second is from a separate group of animals that has received some pretreatment. Data obtained using each of these methods cannot be analyzed by the same statistical test. At the very least if one has produced several log concentration response curves the data should be analyzed using some form of analysis of variance (ANOVA). This test includes in the calculation a compensation for the fact that multiple comparisons are being made.[61] It may also be desirable to first mathematically transform the data and then use an even more rigorous test such as an analysis of covariance (ANCOVA).[62]

Valid statistical analysis is an important part of any experimental protocol. Ideally, therefore, the experimental design should be based on sound statistical practices, rather than the all too common alternative of trying to find an appropriate test to use once the experiment has been performed.

STIMULATION OF THE EXTRINSIC NERVES OF THE INTESTINE

THE SMALL INTESTINE

Although the extrinsic parasympathetic innervation of the stomach had previously been studied,[63] the first *in vitro* technique by which it was possible to investigate the role of postganglionic sympathetic nerves innervating the intestine was devised by Finkleman in 1930.[10] At the time of his experiments little was known about the sympathetic innervation of the gut, and it was generally assumed that these nerve fibers released epinephrine. The aim of Finkleman's study was to compare the effects of nerve stimulation with those of epinephrine to try to determine if, in fact, this was correct. Although he was very elegantly able to demonstrate the release of an inhibitory substance following splanchnic nerve stimulation (Figure 3), due to the lack of specific pharmacologic tools he was unable to show conclusively that epinephrine was not the neurotransmitter involved. It was not until several years later that the identity of this neurotransmitter was established as norepinephrine.[64,65]

In 1953 Munro[66] described a modification of the Finkleman preparation which, in theory, was capable of measuring intraluminal pressure as opposed to simple longitudinal muscle contraction. Although this technique was later developed and utilized by other workers e.g.[67] it has provided little additional information regarding sympathetic innervation of the small intestine. Despite technological advances such as the development of immersible electrodes,[68] or the use of this technique in different species,[66,67,69] there have been few significant modifications of Finkleman's original preparation in the sixty-five years since it was first published.

The Finkleman preparation provides a useful tool for the study of the relationship between sympathetic nerves and gastrointestinal smooth muscle. There are, however, some limitations with respect to the amount and type of information that it can be used to collect.

First, as noted by Finkleman,[10] the magnitude of the inhibitory responses evoked by sympathetic nerve stimulation is highly dependent upon the resting tone of the preparation. If resting tone is high, spontaneous contractions are inhibited and the preparation also loses tone. If, on the other hand resting tone is low, only spontaneous contractions are depressed. To a certain extent this makes quantitative inter-preparation comparisons somewhat difficult.

Second, sympathetic nerve-induced inhibitory responses generally do not recover rapidly, therefore, the preparation cannot be stimulated at frequent intervals over the course of a typical all day experiment. In addition, sympathetic nerve mediated inhibitory responses in the small intestine may, under certain physiological and pharmacological conditions, be complicated by the presence of cholinergic contractions.[67,70,71]

PREPARATION OF A SMALL INTESTINAL SEGMENT WITH ATTACHED MESENTERIC NERVES

In his original publication on this technique Finkleman[10] described the production of two preparations, one from the duodenum and another from the ileum. It is now known that this

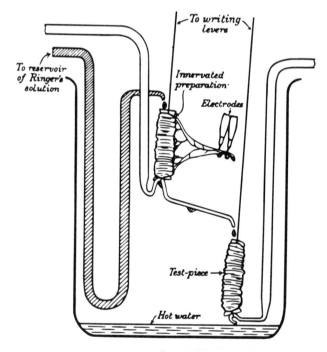

FIGURE 3 The Finkleman preparation as used in a bioassay system to measure the release of substances following stimulation of the extrinsic innervation. The tissues were kept moist by the hot water in the base of the beaker through which oxygen was bubbled. The upper, innervated intestinal segment was superfused with Ringer's solution and, via the glass rod, the superfusate then trickled over the lower test piece of tissue. Stimulation of the extrinsic nerves of the upper tissue resulted in a relaxation of the lower tissue following a lag time which, in part, would be determined by the rate of superfusion. Note that the electrode design does not allow for its immersion in a bathing medium. (From Finkleman, B., *J. Physiol. (Lond.)* 70, 145, 1930. With permission.)

method can be used with virtually any region of the small intestine and distal colon (see below) that has an adequate mesenteric attachment.

Rabbits (or any other species) to be utilized in this protocol should not be from the upper weight range of the species. This is because the deposition of large amounts of adipose tissue on the mesentery hampers its placement in an electrode and also provides a significant electrical resistance.

Once the abdomen has been opened the desired section of intestine can be excised with its mesentery attached and placed in a 7 inch Petri dish filled with warm (37°C) oxygenated (95% O_2/5/CO_2) physiological solution. The luminal contents should be flushed out from the oral end taking great care not to over-distend the segment or pull on its mesentery. The preparation should then be placed in clean, warm (37°C), oxygenated (O_2/CO_2) physiological solution and cut to appropriate lengths. The use of warm physiological solution ensures that the cut length will be very close to the length of the preparation in the tissue bath. If segments are cut in a room temperature solution they may increase to as much as double their original length when warmed and placed under tension. In his original paper Finkleman used 8–10 cm segments, but the technique will work with segments as short as 3cm provided that one is not relying upon the release of large quantities of mediators as part of a bioassay experiment.[10]

Appropriate lengths of 4-0 or 3-0 black, braided surgical thread should then be sutured through the anti-mesenteric wall of the preparation to be used in anchoring it to the base of the bath and connecting to the transducer. Based on the previous discussion of transducer types it may be deduced that this preparation will produce the most clearly defined inhibitory responses when recordings are made under isotonic conditions. Depending on the length of the preparation a load of 1-2.5 g would be appropriate. It should be noted that this method of suspending the tissue in the organ bath is somewhat different to the approach of Finkleman[10] who tied the ends of the segment shut to "prevent contamination of the Ringer's solution with intestinal contents". Flushing the lumen prior to mounting the tissue largely prevents this from taking place. In addition, having the lumen open allows for more complete oxygenation of the preparation and also prevents the accumulation of epithelial secretions which may reach sufficient volume to initiate peristalsis.

The mesenteric attachment which contains the blood vessels and postganglionic sympathetic nerves should next be placed in a bipolar electrode. Finkleman's original electrode design (see Figure 3) was such that a portion of the mesentery had to be lifted out of the bathing medium for extended periods of time to prevent current shunting through the ion rich solution in which the tissue was suspended. Since this has deleterious effects on the nerves under study it is desirable to use one of the many types of immersible electrodes[68] that are now available.

The optimal stimulus parameters to use depend somewhat on the phenomenon under study. Finkleman noted that inhibitory responses were obtained at stimulus frequencies of 20–40 Hz and, in fresh preparations, small excitatory responses were revealed at frequencies of 2–4 Hz. Pulse durations of 0.5 msec are appropriate[70] although values as high as 2.0 msec have been reported[72] and trains of stimuli up to 30 seconds in length have been used.[70,71,72]

THE LARGE INTESTINE

In 1953 Munro[66] took the next logical step with the Finkleman preparation and applied it to the distal colon of the guinea pig. He found that, as with the small intestine, the motor responses of the distal colon to sympathetic nerve stimulation were dependent upon the resting tone of the preparation. These observations went unchallenged until the works of Garry and Gillespie[11,12] who, in 1955, characterized the now famous "doubly innervated rabbit colon preparation" which allowed for the responses of the longitudinal muscle of the colon to both parasympathetic and sympathetic nerve stimulation be observed *in vitro*. This technique, represented a unique combination of the *in vitro* Finkleman preparation[10] and *in vivo* studies of the motor responses of the colon to extrinsic parasympathetic nerve stimulation.[73,74]

In contrast to previous observations in the small intestine, stimulation of the sympathetic nerves to the colon (the lumbar colonic nerves) was found to always produce a relaxation, regardless of the frequency of stimulation. Similarly, pelvic nerve stimulation always resulted in a contractile response. These conclusions were based on results obtained when studying a wide range of stimulus frequencies and voltages in preparations with high and low initial resting tone.[12] However, it should be noted that Varagic[75] has claimed that in the presence of tolazoline (an α-adrenoceptor antagonist) low frequency stimulation of the lumbar colonic nerves can produce a contractile response of this preparation prior to the onset of relaxation.

Over the years this technique has been successfully used to study both receptor-[46,76,77] and non receptor-mediated phenomena[41] associated with the extrinsic innervation of the colon in a variety of species. However, the original technique suffers from the limitation that only longitudinal muscle contractions and relaxations may be measured whereas, responses of the circular muscle layer must be qualitatively assessed by visual inspection. Furthermore, using this preparation one cannot determine if all neurons in the myenteric or submucosal plexus receive synaptic input from either or both of the lumbar colonic or pelvic nerves.

In addressing these problems certain modifications to the original technique have been made that have added significantly to the amount of information that can be obtained from this preparation. For example, Bianchi et al.,[77] using the guinea pig colon, combined the technique of Garry and Gillespie[11] with that of Paton.[13] This hybrid method revealed, through the use of transmural stimulation (20 Hz, 1 msec pulse duration for 30 seconds) the presence of non-adrenergic, non-cholinergic inhibitory nerves which did not receive preganglionic input from either the sympathetic or the parasympathetic extrinsic innervation. More recently, the Garry and Gillespie preparation for the rabbit colon has been modified to allow for the simultaneous recording of longitudinal and circular muscle activity along with transepithelial potential difference[78] (Figure 4). This has allowed the role of the extrinsic innervation in the control of colonic muscle and epithelial function to be simultaneously studied *in vitro* for the first time.

Thus, since its introduction in 1954 the Garry and Gillespie technique has developed into perhaps the most powerful and comprehensive tool available for the *in vitro* study of integrated neural control of colonic function.

PREPARATION OF A COLONIC SEGMENT WITH ATTACHED EXTRINSIC NERVES

As recommended by Garry and Gillespie in 1955,[12] rabbits to be used for this preparation should be at the lower end of the adult weight range (1.5–2.0 kg). This is because the presence of large amounts of fat around the extrinsic nerves will hinder the dissection procedure and will also present a significant barrier to the passage of electric current.

A question often raised at this point is: *Can one carry out this entire dissection in an anesthetized animal?* While it is practicable to do this in a species like the dog,[74] in the rabbit and guinea pig the highly vascular region around the bladder and distal colon and the relative fragility of these tissues make this an almost untenable proposition. Pooling and clotting of blood around the extrinsic nerves hastens their demise and, in addition, makes location of structures like the pelvic nerves virtually impossible. It is advisable, therefore, to follow the protocol described by Garry and Gillespie[11] (Figure 4) although, as an aid to locating the pelvic nerves it may be advisable to omit the exsanguination procedure.

The abdomen should be opened along the *linea alba* (mid line) and the cartilagenous joint of the *symphysis pubis* opened using a scalpel. The *symphysis pubis* can then be fully opened by forcing the hind legs apart. (If epithelial function is to be studied it will be necessary at this

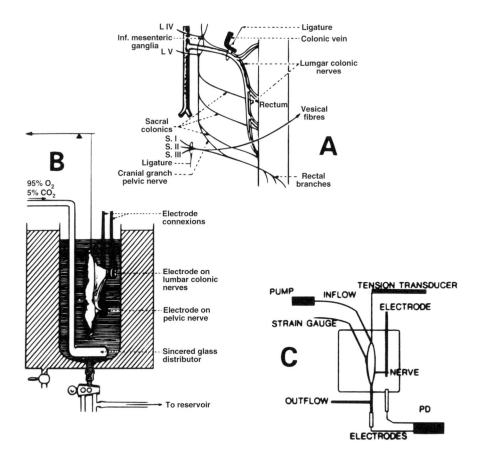

FIGURE 4   A. Schematic representation of the anatomical landmarks associated with the dissection procedures necessary to obtain a segment of colon with intact extrinsic sympathetic and parasympathetic innervation. (From Garry, R. C. and Gillespie, J. C., *J. Physiol. (Lond.)* 123, 60P, 1954. With permission). B. Appearance of the finished Garry and Gillespie doubly innervated rabbit colon preparation in the organ bath. Note that the electrodes are immersible such that the nerves do not have to be lifted out of the bathing medium for stimulation to take place. (From Garry, R. C. and Gillespie, J. C., *J. Physiol. (Lond.)* 128, 557, 1955. With permission). C. Schematic representation of a modified Garry & Gillespie preparation which allows for transepithelial potential difference to be measured in association with both longitudinal and circular muscle activity. The proximal end of the tissue is attached to an isometric transducer for measurement of longitudinal muscle contractions. A strain gauge is sewn to the serosal surface, oriented to the circular muscle layer, to measure mechanical activity in that plane. Potential difference (PD) is measured using two agar salt bridge electrodes, one in contact with the lumen and the other placed in the bathing solution. Krebs' solution is continuously perfused through the lumen, draining from the system via the outflow tube. (From Goldhill, J. M. and Percy, W. H., *Am. J. Physiol.* 265, G1064, 1993. With permission.)

time to introduce a perfusion catheter into the colon proximal to the area of interest, and to begin perfusing with cold, carboxygenated Krebs' or Tyrode's solution[78]). The bladder should be emptied and as much adipose tissue in the region as possible removed. To facilitate the latter procedure the entire area should be liberally moistened with ice cold Krebs' (or Tyrode's) solution. This has the dual effect of preserving tissue viability and facilitating the removal of fat. Throughout the following dissection procedures liberal application of chilled physiological solution should be continued.

The pelvic nerves (Figure 4A) can be located by first removing the lateral fat pads which are found under the part of the colon that lies beneath the *symphysis pubis*. If the animal has not been exsanguinated this will reveal one large circumferentially-oriented blood vessel on each side of the colon. The left and right pelvic nerves lie close to this vessel. Using a gentle blunt dissection technique free both pelvic nerves from adjacent connective tissue and follow their path to the point where they exit from the muscle covering the spine. The nerves should be ligated as far back from the colon as possible with Krebs'- (or Tyrode's-) soaked 5-0 to 7-0 black braided surgical suture, making sure that a sufficient length is used to allow placement of the nerves in the stimulating electrode. In some preparations when the pelvic nerves are ligated a wave of contraction may be seen to occur in the colonic region immediately proximal to the point where they appear to meet the wall of the colon. It is important to note that the pelvic nerves should not be cut out of the surrounding skeletal muscle at this time because, even in an "exsanguinated" animal, this can release significant quantities of blood.

The lumbar colonic sympathetic nerves can be isolated by tracing them through the mesocolon (mesenteric attachment) to their origin at the inferior mesenteric ganglion. This ganglion can be identified as two white/brown "lumps" in the mesentery close to the inferior mesenteric artery (Figure 4A). The mesentery, inferior mesenteric artery and vein can then be ligated at the inferior mesenteric ganglion. The mesenteric region containing the lumbar colonic nerves can now be isolated and dissected free from the surrounding tissues.

The bladder attachment to the colon should be severed and the pelvic nerves dissected free from the skeletal muscle layer in which they are partly embedded. A section of colon 4–5 cm long with each of these extrinsic nerve attachments is then removed and placed in a beaker of warm (37°C), carboxygenated Krebs' (or Tyrode's) solution. The use of a warm solution at this point facilitates the expulsion of fecal pellets by muscle action. This is preferable to the potential damage that could be done by attempting to clean the colonic lumen with forceps or a similar instrument.

Suitable lengths of 5-0 or 3-0 surgical suture should now be attached to the oral and aboral ends of the preparation. These will be used to connect it to the transducer and anchor it to the base of the bath respectively. Both pelvic nerves together can now be placed within the electrode of choice, which should be submersible[68] without leaking current to the bathing medium. The entire preparation is then mounted in an appropriately sized organ bath (approximately 50 ml) under a 2–3 g load and allowed to equilibrate for 30 minutes. A representation of the finished preparation is shown in Figure 4B.

The pelvic nerves can be stimulated at 10 Hz for periods of 10 seconds once per minute (0.017 Hz) with supramaximal pulses each having a duration of 0.5–1 msec.[12,41] When utilized in this fashion large contractile responses can be obtained for extended periods of time and the signal to noise ratio (amplitude of evoked contraction relative to spontaneous contractions) should be quite high. However, if the preparation has been dissected to include a significant amount of extreme distal colon/rectum, the signal to noise ratio will be much lower because the majority of fibers originating in the pelvic plexus enter ascending fiber bundles.[79,80] It may be noted that in some cases the response of the preparation to stimulation of the pelvic nerves will increase over the first 3–4 minutes and remain relatively stable thereafter. Thus, if one wishes to study the effect of a drug on this system 5–10 control periods of contraction should first be obtained.

In their original study Garry and Gillespie[12] found that lumbar colonic nerve stimulation for 30 seconds caused relaxation of the colon over a wide range of frequencies (10–1000 Hz) and that the optimal pulse duration was 1 msec. This inhibition persists for the duration of the stimulation and exhibits no decay or "escape phenomenon". For practical purposes it has subsequently been established that $\geq$ 90% inhibition occurs at a stimulus frequency of 50 Hz[46] and that this would be an appropriate frequency to use in studies of this system. However, in contrast to the rapid recovery of the colon from pelvic nerve stimulation, the inhibitory response to lumbar colonic nerve stimulation persists well beyond the end of the period of stimulation.

This means, therefore, that lumbar colonic nerve-evoked relaxations cannot be produced as often as pelvic nerve-evoked contractions.

STIMULATION OF THE INTRINSIC NERVES OF THE INTESTINE

The effect of passing an electrical current through a piece of intestine was described by Magnus in 1904.[3] Almost 50 years later Paton published his now classic *in vitro* method for electrically stimulating an intrinsically innervated segment of guinea pig ileum.[13] He described the resulting contractions as being "twitch-like" in nature at low frequencies of stimulation (0.1 Hz) and, in a subsequent paper, described "tetanus-like" contractions at higher frequencies of stimulation (≥ 5 Hz).[40] The development of this preparation represented a major breakthrough in studies of gastrointestinal neuroeffector transmission because it appeared that researchers now had the autonomic equivalent of a skeletal muscle preparation such as, for example, the phrenic nerve-hemidiaphragm. Such a tool was invaluable because, for the first time, the pre- and post-junctional (not "synaptic," because there is no anatomical modification of intestinal smooth muscle cells in the region of their innervation[81]) effects of a variety of agents on the intestine could be clearly distinguished. However, it has subsequently been established that nerve-muscle interactions within this tissue are more complex than events at the neuromuscular junction. For example, as the frequency of stimulation changes, contractile amplitude does not vary in proportion to the amount of acetylcholine being released[15] and other neurotransmitters such as substance P[82] are involved in the overall response. Furthermore, the actual amount of acetylcholine released with each stimulus pulse decreases as the stimulus frequency increases[15] while, in contrast, norepinephrine release per pulse is greatly increased under the same conditions.[83]

However, if one is prepared to accept such limitations, the electrically stimulated isolated guinea pig ileum can provide a useful assay system for the investigation of the pharmacologic properties of novel compounds. The principal reasons for this are:

1. When properly prepared the preparation has a very high signal to noise ratio *i.e.* the evoked responses are very large relative to any ongoing spontaneous mechanical activity.
2. The longitudinal muscle layer of the guinea pig ileum and its intrinsic innervation are exquisitely sensitive to pharmacologic agents and exhibit clearly defined responses over relatively low concentration ranges (e.g. 10^{-10}M–10^{-6}M for many excitatory and inhibitory drugs).
3. Unlike other intestinal smooth muscle preparations the isolated guinea pig ileum recovers rapidly from the excitatory and inhibitory effects of pharmacologic agents even when these are maximal. This is partly related to point #2 above because maximal responses are produced by relatively low concentrations of drugs. This has the advantage that concentration-response experiments can be completed within a relatively short time frame, thus minimizing concerns about significant changes in tissue viability between the beginning and the end of an experiment.
4. The motor responses of this tissue to low frequency electrical stimulation are not complicated by long duration non-adrenergic, non-cholinergic (NANC) relaxations.

PREPARATION OF THE COAXIALLY STIMULATED GUINEA PIG ILEUM

Ideally guinea pigs to be used for this technique should weigh 250–300 g. Following euthanasia open the abdomen along the midline and locate the ileum at its junction with the caecum. Move approximately 10 cm oral to this point because, as the ileum approaches the ileo-cecal sphincter, its pharmacologic properties change.[84,85] Cut through the ileum at this point, continuing a few millimeters into the mesenteric attachment. Take hold of the open end of the ileum (the bottom of the piece to be removed) using medium sized rats tooth forceps and, gently but firmly, pull the ileum out of the abdominal cavity. If the force applied is just sufficient to sever the mesenteric attachment the tissue will be undamaged by this procedure. If too much force is applied the muscle may function normally but the intrinsic innervation is likely to be damaged. Continue this process until a useful length of ileum has been freed (20–30cm). Cut through the ileum at the oral end of this segment marking it clearly with additional cuts so that it can subsequently be distinguished from the aboral end of the preparation (see below).

Place the entire length of the ileum in a 7 inch Petri dish filled with warm (37°C) oxygenated (O_2/CO_2) Krebs' solution. Gently place the end of a (37°C) Krebs'-filled narrow tip 1ml glass pipette in the marked oral end of the segment (if you do not know which is the oral end you may damage the segment by overfilling because you are trying to initiate peristalsis by a distension initiated at the aboral end). Raise the mouthpiece of the pipette 30–40 degrees above horizontal and allow Krebs' solution to flow slowly into the ileal lumen. Usually this will be sufficient to initiate a peristaltic wave and expel the luminal contents. If further Krebs' is required for complete emptying repeat this process. Always use a 1ml pipette as this will avoid the possibility of over-distending the ileum during the cleaning procedure.

Immediately upon expulsion of the luminal contents transfer the entire segment to a beaker containing 100–150 ml of warm (37°C) Krebs' solution and, by gentle agitation, clean any residual material from the serosal surface. Return the segment to a Petri dish again containing warm (37°C) oxygenated Krebs' solution. At this point it is necessary to cut the segment into lengths appropriate for the depth of bath in which they are being used, taking care to avoid Peyer's patches (5–10 mm diameter "spots" that are white/grey in color and are composed of epithelial lymphoid tissue). The use of warm Krebs' throughout each of these procedures means that the ileal longitudinal muscle is not contracted and the length cut in the Petri dish will be close to the ultimate length of the tissue in the organ bath. If cold Krebs' is used for the cleaning procedures, upon warming the tissue in the organ bath it will relax and may increase its length by as much as 100%.

Once again it is important to have identified which is the oral end of the segment that has now been cut. Carefully insert a 26 gauge platinum wire electrode through the lumen from the oral end. To avoid damage to the tissue the end of the electrode should be bent back upon itself so that one does not run the risk of pushing a potentially sharp pointed object through the gut wall. It is necessary for the electrode to be 1 or 2 cm longer than the preparation. The oral end of the electrode should be shielded with a plastic insulator (e.g. PVC tubing) glued to the wire. This insulator should extend 5 mm or so into the lumen.

With the electrode inserted as described, firmly tie the oral end in place using 4-0 or 3-0 black, braided surgical suture (not nylon or other "plastic" suture), leaving sufficient length to also secure this end of the preparation to the transducer. It is sometimes argued that the distensibility of a thread such as this might interfere with quantitative assessment of subsequent responses. However, in practice the elastic properties of the tissue and the magnitude of the forces it is capable of generating are small enough such that, for most experimental purposes, this is not an important consideration.

The aboral end of the preparation should now be tied firmly over the end of a "fluted" glass rod which runs through the stopper that fits in the base of the organ bath. The purpose of this tube is to allow any residual luminal contents and sloughed mucosa to drain out of the preparation so that it does not become distended during the time that it is in the organ bath. It is important, therefore, to ensure that the aboral end of the preparation corresponds to the aboral end of the ileum *in situ* so that if necessary, this process can be assisted by peristalsis. If the ileum is upside down in the bath, the luminal contents will be peristalsed to the top of the preparation causing an increasing distension which will produce an elevated motor activity as this reaches the threshold for peristalsis. Over time this will result in a significant decrease in the signal to noise ratio for any given experiment.

The preparation can now be mounted in the organ bath which should have a volume of between 10 and 20 ml. A second electrode is placed in the bathing medium so that electrical current can be passed across the wall of the ileum (*transmural stimulation*).

At this point the oral end of the preparation may be connected to either an isometric or an isotonic transducer and placed under an appropriate load (see sections on "choice of transducer" and "determination of load"). A properly prepared segment of ileum will exhibit no peristaltic activity once in the organ bath and the preparation will appear flat because the lumen is closed by the pressure exerted by the surrounding bathing medium.

Since the luminal electrode is insulated from the bathing medium whereas the other is contained within it, the passage of current is now almost exclusively a function of the resistance of the gut wall. Note that it is important to measure the current being passed through the system to ensure that constant stimulation is being utilized throughout the duration of the experiment. This can be achieved by the insertion of a 100Ω resistor in series with the cathode as shown in Figure 5. By measuring the voltage across the resistor with an oscilloscope, from Ohm's law ($V = IR$) if $R = 100\Omega$, every 10 V on the oscilloscope corresponds to a current of 0.1 A, i.e. 100 mA. For most *in vitro* experiments involving stimulation of intrinsic nerves in gastrointestinal tissues an appropriate supramaximal current would be in the range 100–120 mA. It will also be noted when performing this calculation that the voltage output from the stimulator may not be linearly related to the current being passed through the system, particularly at higher voltages (Figure 6). For this reason it is almost meaningless to describe stimulus parameters in terms of voltage alone; clearly, 50 V being passed through 5 ml of Krebs' solution would produce a significantly higher current than 50 V being passed through 50 ml of the same solution. Thus, to a certain extent expression of electrical stimulation in terms of current and not voltage may be thought of as analogous to the expression of concentration in molar rather than µg/ml.

An important question that it is necessary to address at this point is, how can one be certain

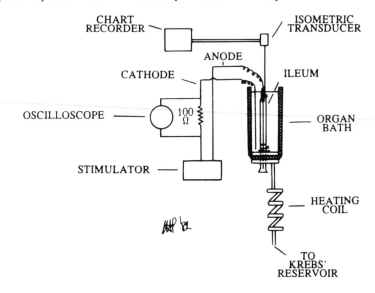

FIGURE 5 Schematic representation of a typical apparatus used for transmural (coaxial) electrical stimulation of a segment of isolated guinea pig ileum. The preparation, which is maintained at 37°C in a carboxygenated Krebs' solution, may be connected to either an isometric or an isotonic transducer. Insertion of a 100Ω resistor in series with the cathode allows for current in the system to be measured. Note that because of an insulator at the oral end of the anode this electrode does not make contact with the bathing medium.

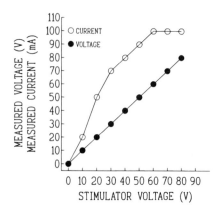

FIGURE 6 Comparison of the voltage output from a typical physiological stimulator passing current through 10 ml of Krebs' solution in a system similar to that in Figure 5. Note that there is a good agreement between the voltage that the stimulator is supposed to be producing and that actually measured at the output. On the other hand, the relationship between voltage read on the stimulator dial and current measured in the circuit is not linear.

that electrically-evoked responses are the result of nerve activation rather than direct stimulation of the muscle itself?

Extracellular electrophysiological investigation of the events surrounding myenteric plexus/ longitudinal muscle excitation following an applied current demonstrated that there are two components to the response. These consist of an early tetrodotoxin-sensitive action potential followed approximately 200 msec later by a Mn^{2+}-sensitive muscle action potential complex. When the relationship between the duration of the excitatory stimulus pulse and the nerve action potential was calculated it was found that the chronaxie (twice the threshold pulse duration required to initiate the action potential) was 0.1 msec. However, when a stimulus of this duration was applied in the presence of tetrodotoxin no muscle action potential complex could be elicited.[86] Thus, short duration pulses are ineffective in causing direct muscle excitation and, therefore, based on the pulse duration nerve and muscle excitation can be clearly separated. However, it should be noted that these values were calculated using a preparation consisting of only myenteric plexus and longitudinal muscle[87] and that, in practice, to pass a sufficient current across the entire thickness of the wall of the guinea pig ileum pulse durations of 0.3–0.5 msec are normally required. Furthermore, the stimulus parameters that are appropriate for the guinea pig ileum may be sub-effective in tissues from larger species where the connective tissue content is higher. For example, the use of pulse durations of 0.1 msec on the rabbit colonic muscularis mucosae produced barely discernable contractile responses in some, but not all preparations.[55] When the pulse duration was increased to 1 msec substantially larger responses were obtained and the number of preparations exhibiting these was increased.[49] Pulse durations in the region of 1 msec are still well below that necessary for direct muscle excitation, particularly if relatively low stimulus frequencies ($\leq$ 50 Hz) are employed.

It is also important to note that the above observations are equally valid for isolated tissue segments that are stimulated by placing them between electrodes that are both immersed in the bathing medium. This process is known as *electrical field stimulation* (EFS)[88] and differs from *transmural stimulation* in that the resistance between the electrodes is that of the bathing medium rather than of the tissue itself.

STUDIES ON THE PERISTALTIC REFLEX

The ability of an isolated segment of dog intestine to expel its luminal contents via circular-muscle activity was known almost a century ago.[8] In 1917 Trendelenburg,[9] drawing upon this knowledge described a method for the quantitative *in vitro* study of the peristaltic reflex of the small intestine. He noted that radial distension produced a two phase response which involved an initial shortening of the preparation *(preparatory phase)* followed by expulsion of the luminal contents via contraction of the circular muscle *(emptying phase)*. This technique in its original form (Figure 7A), proved to be invaluable in subsequent pharmacologic studies designed to investigate the basis of the peristaltic reflex in the small intestine.

From these early experiments it was found that, in the guinea pig ileum, longitudinal and circular muscle activity were not interdependent and that pharmacologic agents which depress the response of one layer do not necessarily affect the other. For example, Kosterlitz and Robinson[89] demonstrated that, following exposure to a high concentration of acetylcholine, the longitudinal muscle failed to contract upon luminal filling whereas, circular muscle responses were unaltered. Conversely, a low concentration of hexamethonium could abolish the circular muscle response to filling although longitudinal muscle contractions were unaltered.

Although studies such as these were instrumental in developing our understanding of the neural coordination of peristalsis in the guinea pig ileum, it was apparent to many researchers that the original Trendelenburg preparation had a number of important shortcomings. Perhaps the most important amongst these was the inability to determine the effects of luminally applied pharmacologic agents. This was a very germane concern because many orally ingested bioactive compounds pass through the gastrointestinal tract in a relatively high concentration. Thus, in 1958 Beleslin and Varagic[25] developed a modification of the Trendelenburg technique which allowed for drugs to be applied to the bathing medium and, in addition, through the lumen of the ileum. Using this method they were able to demonstrate that luminally applied 5-hydroxytryptamine could restore the peristaltic reflex when it had first been abolished by cooling the preparation.

In the same year Bülbring and Lin[90] independently described a more comprehensive modification of Trendelenburg's original apparatus (Figure 7B). This model allowed not only for drugs to be applied to the luminal surface, but also addressed a second shortcoming of the Trendelenburg preparation namely, the inability to measure flow through the intestinal segment under study. This was an important point because Trendelenburg's original technique measures movement of fluid that is introduced through the aboral end of the segment and undergoes a "regurgitation" process, moving in and out of the lumen as the muscle layers contract. This process is conducive to fatigue of the preparation and, in addition, gives no indication of the true relationship between muscle movement and the antegrade propulsion of the luminal contents.

Utilizing their novel method Bülbring and Lin[90] were able to demonstrate that intraluminal pressure and the amount of fluid moved through the segment underwent significant changes over time. In addition, they reported that 5-hydroxytryptamine applied to the lumen lowered the threshold for peristalsis whereas, application to the serosal side always caused inhibition. In contrast, low concentrations of acetylcholine caused stimulation whether applied to the mucosal or serosal surface while histamine caused muscle contraction when applied serosally but was without effect when applied to the lumen. Due to the versatility of this technique these authors were also able to demonstrate that 5-hydroxytryptamine was being released by the tissue into the luminal perfusate and that this release declined over time. This meant that, in theory, it was now possible to measure biological mediators being released by the mucosa and related structures and to correlate this with ongoing peristaltic activity.

Most recently the Trendelenburg preparation has been modified by Schulze-Delrieu[91] in such a way that the contractile activity of discrete areas of small intestine during peristalsis can be visualized (Figure 7C). This adaptation has allowed for important differences to be discerned between the mechanical responses of the duodenum and ileum to both luminal perfusion and bolus injections. Thus, it is now known that the volume of fluid accommodated by the ileum and its luminal diameter are both greater than the corresponding duodenal values under the same experimental conditions. Such observations have added an important new dimension to

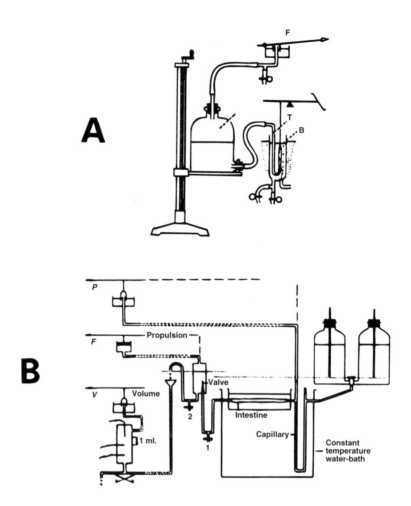

FIGURE 7   A. Schematic representation of a typical Trendelenburg apparatus. The segment of intestine is mounted on over a tube (T) which connects it to the reservoir (R) filled with physiological solution. When the fluid level in the reservoir is 1–2cm above that in the organ bath (B) peristalsis will be elicited by hydrostatic pressure. The ensuing contraction of the muscle layers of the ileal segment will then force fluid back into the reservoir. This displaces the air between the fluid and the float recorder (F) causing movement of the writing lever. Longitudinal muscle contractions are recorded via the lower writing lever. Note that the serosal bathing solution and that introduced into the lumen should both be at 37°C. (From, Staff, Department of Pharmacology, University of Edinburgh, *Pharmacological Experiments on Isolated Preparations,* 2nd ed. Churchill Livingstone, Edinburgh, 1970. With permission.) B. Trendelenburg preparation as modified by Bülbring and Lin. Note that in this instance fluid is introduced via the oral end of the segment and that measurements of pressure, propulsion and volume are based on the amount of liquid that actually passes through the preparation. By connecting the two reservoirs via a stopcock it is possible to perfuse the lumen with at least one solution containing a particular pharmacologic agent at a known concentration. (From Bülbring, E. and Lin, R. C. Y., *J. Physiol. (Lond.)* 140, 381, 1958. With permission.) C. (see next page) Trendelenburg preparation as modified by Schulze-Delrieu. Note that with this modification fluid entering the preparation from the reservoir is measured in terms of the weight decrease of the reservoir itself. Fluid can also be injected as a bolus from the syringe located between the reservoir and the intestine. The force generated by the intestinal segment in response to either stimulus is measured via the pressure transducer. These signals can then be integrated with that from the video camera which shows the physical configuration of the intestinal segment over time. (From Schulze-Delrieu, K., *J. Lab. Clin. Med.* 117, 44, 1991. With permission.)

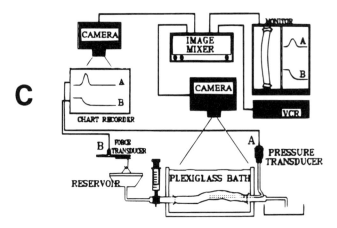

FIGURE 7 (continued).

studies of small intestinal peristalsis because the factors governing luminal transit can now be expanded to include wall compliance.

An important difference between the small and large intestine that was appreciated as early as 1900 by Bayliss and Starling[92] was the consistency of the luminal contents in different anatomical-locations. Thus, a final shortcoming of the Trendelenburg preparation which it was necessary to address is that although a fluid stimulus might be appropriate for certain regions of the small intestine (and can produce motor responses from the stomach[93] and colon[94,95]), the esophageal, gastric and colonic contents are often solid or semi-solid. Under these circumstances one might reasonably expect different behavior from the muscles which comprise these organs and that a measure of intraluminal pressure *per se* might not be an accurate representation of their motor activity in different regions.

In the isolated opossum esophagus Christensen and Lund[32] approached this problem by using a Trendelenburg-like apparatus in which the stimulus for esophageal peristalsis was balloon distension. In this system longitudinal muscle shortening was measured directly by connecting the oral end of the preparation to a transducer; the responses of the circular muscle layer were then measured manometrically. Using this technique it was possible to distinguish the "duration response" (a response which persists for the duration of the stimulus) of the longitudinal muscle, which occurred throughout the period of distension, from the "off response" (a response which occurs at some point after the stimulus has been switched off) of the circular muscle, which followed removal of the stimulus. Interestingly, use of this technique also revealed that the responses of the esophageal muscle layers to distension could be accurately reproduced by focal bipolar electrical stimulation. In a more recent modification of this technique Schulze-Delrieu et al.[96] opened the esophagus along its longitudinal axis, anchored one edge within the chamber and recorded circular muscle and lower esophageal sphincter activity via transducers connected to the free edge. While this preparation does not allow for the measurement of peristalsis *per se,* it did demonstrate for the first time that the circular muscle of the esophagus and the lower esophageal sphincter respond to electrical stimulation of both the stomach and esophagus. This observation shed new light on gastro-esophageal function, suggesting that information was transmitted both orally and aborally between the esophagus and stomach via the intrinsic nervous structures.

Studies of the responses of the stomach to luminal distension or to drugs have been somewhat fewer than in other regions of the intestinal tract. The intact, isolated stomach of the guinea pig has been utilized with a modification of the Trendelenburg apparatus.[93] However, the results obtained with this system are somewhat qualitative in that only total fluid movement can be assessed and this does not allow for any distinction to be made between the mechanical activities of the fundus, corpus and antrum.

To overcome such difficulties two methods of studying the isolated intact stomach were developed in the early 1970s. In 1972 Haffner and Stadaas[97] took the isolated rabbit stomach and inserted a balloon catheter through the stomach wall into each of the fundus, corpus and antrum. The sections containing the balloons were then partitioned from each other by placing sutures around the region. This method of recording was able to clearly distinguish different regional motor patterns following exposure to pharmacologic stimuli. For example, in response to serosally applied carbachol, the fundus exhibited a tonic contraction, the antrum developed a pattern of phasic contractions and the corpus produced a tonic contraction with superimposed phasic oscillations. The validity of this recording technique was subsequently established when it was utilized with guinea pig and rat stomachs[98] and striking similarities and differences between the three species were observed. Furthermore, these data were in good agreement with electrophysiological recordings from various regions in the isolated, perfused dog stomach.[99]

One major concern associated with the use of the isolated stomach is its susceptibility to oxygen starvation. The stomach from even a relatively small animal such as the rat or guinea pig, presents a significant barrier to the passage of oxygen if it is available only in the serosal bathing medium. Hypoxia has been shown to rapidly abolish myoelectric activity in the isolated stomach[99] and clearly, by extrapolation this would have deleterious effects on motor function. Thus, although at various times the isolated stomach has been perfused with physiological media for the purposes of *in vitro* study,[93,99] maintaining an adequate oxygenation is a valid concern.

To deal with this problem Kowalewski and Kolodej[100] developed a system whereby it was possible to perfuse the isolated stomach with the blood of a donor animal. This allowed for the perfusate to be constantly dialyzed and oxygenated as it circulated through the donor. Gastric motor function and myoelectric activity were then monitored via strain gauges and electrodes placed on the serosal surface. While this technique was very elegant and allowed for drugs to be administered directly into the perfusing arterial blood, it was not utilized to its full potential because responses to changes in intra-gastric pressure were not studied and, because the preparation does not sit in a bathing medium as such, serosal application of drugs could not be performed. It is worth noting at this point, therefore, that the addition of pharmacologic agents via the arterial tree may produce strikingly different results to those obtained by serosal application via the bathing medium.[101,102] Furthermore, in view of the complexity of the apparatus required and the additional surgery involved, it is not clear if this technique offers a worthwhile alternative to the isolated stomach perfused with a physiological medium. Thus, in terms of *in vitro* studies utilizing the whole stomach to investigate the movement of the gastric contents there is a relative paucity of information that may be attributed, in part, to the lack of a universally acceptable model system.

Studies of the movement of the colonic contents have been somewhat less problematic. Using the guinea pig and cat isolated colon and a modified Trendelenburg preparation, Frigo and Lecchini[103] measured persitaltic activity using a balloon distension stimulus. However, in addition to measuring circular muscle activity manometrically they also quantitated this parameter based upon photographic records of changes in luminal diameter in the guinea pig and with strain gauges in the cat. Through the use of this technique it was found that, in contrast to the ileum of the guinea pig, the longitudinal muscle of the colon of this species may undergo relaxation prior to aboral movement of the bolus. Furthermore, in the guinea pig ileum peristalsis measured using the traditional Trendelenburg apparatus reveals alternating periods of longitudinal and circular muscle contraction[40,89] whereas, in the colon, longitudinal muscle often exhibited an initial relaxation and aboral propulsion was found to be associated with a progressive tonic contraction of the longitudinal muscle layer.[103] Similar results were obtained using the cat colon but in addition, because its size facilitated the placement of circumferentially-oriented strain gauges, circular muscle contraction above and relaxation below the bolus were also observed.

In both species the balloon was moved through the colon with a maximal velocity of 1.0–1.5 mmsec^{-1} and, in order for movement to be achieved, an intact mucosa was required.

From these data it may be concluded that *in vitro* measurement of the peristaltic reflex can now be carried out at a very sophisticated level. Thus, in addition to measuring simple patterns of muscle contraction it is now possible to quantitate, luminal flow rate/speed of bolus movement, luminal diameter, wall compliance and substances being produced by the mucosa. However, it is important to stress that in order to produce meaningful data such experiments must be carried out using an appropriate stimulus and that this is more easily achieved in some regions than in others.

STUDIES ON THE INDIVIDUAL MUSCLE LAYERS OF THE INTESTINE

For many years it was an acceptable practice to study gastrointestinal smooth muscle function by suspending an appropriate segment of whole intestine in an organ bath and measuring longitudinal muscle contraction. However, such experiments do not provide all of the available information, particularly if one considers a system such as the esophagus where each muscle layer exhibits a totally different and characteristic response to stimulation of its intrinsic nerves.[32,42] In addition, when working with preparations from larger species, including human tissue, it is not practicable to adequately oxygenate a full thickness segment of intestine for the duration of a typical *in vitro* experiment e.g. 103. It is necessary, therefore, to have available alternative techniques with which it is possible to study smaller preparations of the individual muscle layers which comprise the organ in question. In this respect it is important to note that although one frequently hears reference to "both muscle layers of the intestine," with the exception of the stomach which has four, there are, in fact, three layers; longitudinal muscle, circular muscle and the muscularis mucosae (muscularis of the mucosa) which may itself be composed of two layers at 90 degrees to each other, depending on the species and anatomical location from which it is derived.[55,104–107] The following section describes techniques by which these layers can be studied and the advantages/disadvantages of using these.

THE MUSCULARIS PROPRIA

The idea of separating a strip of smooth muscle from the whole organ for *in vitro* study is far from new e.g.[63,87] and represents a mechanism whereby the properties of a particular muscle layer can essentially be evaluated in isolation. The advantages of this technique are that one can compare several strips from a single tissue sample, the influence of substances released from the mucosa on the muscularis propria is removed and the access of oxygen and pharmacologic agents is greatly enhanced. The disadvantages are first, that in utilizing an isolated muscle strip one makes the assumption that the whole organ is homogeneous and that each strip is representative of the entire muscle mass. Second, the magnitude of the responses from an isolated muscle strip may be so small that the gain on the amplifier has to be increased to clearly distinguish small contractions and/or relaxations; this generally equates with a decrease in the signal to noise ratio. Third, although it may seem trivial, this technique assumes that strips are cut parallel to the plane of the muscle they are supposed to represent. However, one rarely sees histological evidence which unequivocally establishes that this was the case for the muscle strip which was used in the actual experiment. Clearly, if the strip is cut at an angle to the actual orientation of the muscle fibers, the responses it produces will be less than optimal. With a mucosa-free, full thickness strip the further one goes from the plane of, for example, the longitudinal muscle, the more the circular muscle will influence the observed response.

Thus, although the use of a muscle strip might appear to be one of the simplest methods available for the study of gastrointestinal smooth muscle, these important points must be considered and addressed before performing the first experiment.

Methods for the preparation of muscle strips representing longitudinal or circular muscle can be typified by those used in the esophagus by Christensen et al.[32,42] In their original preparations the esophagus was opened longitudinally, the mucosa was removed and full thickness strips representing circular muscle were cut transversely while longitudinally-oriented sections were taken to represent the longitudinal muscle. Through the use of these differently oriented muscle preparations it was possible to distinguish the "duration response" of the longitudinal muscle from the "off response" of the circular layer. In later experiments the technique of cutting esophageal muscle strips was further refined in that an attempt was made to standardize the strip size by making cuts with a series of razor blades held in a clamp with measured spaces in between. This method of cutting muscle strips from the esophagus and esophagogastric region provided sufficient resolution for longitudinal muscle, circular muscle and lower esophageal sphincter muscle to be clearly distinguished from each other based upon their respective responses to electrical field stimulation.

However, it should not be assumed that cutting a muscle strip in the orientation of the muscle of interest was the first method employed for this purpose[87] or that it is practicable to do this in all intestinal regions in every species.[57] For example, in the mouse or the newborn rabbit[57] the colonic circumference may be so small that a circularly-oriented muscle strip cannot realistically be produced and/or used. Under these circumstances it would be necessary to consider an alternative technique such as that described by Harry in 1963.[47] In this protocol a segment of intestine is opened along its longitudinal axis and pinned out flat in a dish of oxygenated physiological solution. A series of cuts at 90 degrees to the long axis and extending about 75% of the width of the preparation are then made. These cuts are approximately 3 mm apart and each starts on the opposite side to the previous cut. When the preparation is stretched in an organ bath the cuts that have been made remove the influence of the longitudinal muscle and the contractions recorded are the result of circular muscle activity. This technique could, therefore, be used to substitute for cutting strips in the circular axis where this is not feasible. The resulting preparation has sufficient pharmacologic resolution that Harry[47] was able to make the now well known observation that the circular muscle of the guinea pig ileum is less responsive to acetylcholine that is the longitudinal muscle.

Thus, there are several techniques available for the study of the individual muscle layers which comprise the *muscularis propria.* Provided that one is cautious in their use and realizes the limitations of each, considerable useful information can be obtained from even a reasonably simple, but well conceived experiment.

THE MUSCULARIS MUCOSAE

Although it was demonstrated by Magnus in 1904[3] that the mucosa, submucosa and muscularis mucosae could be separated from the *muscularis propria,* no use was made of this information until the work of Gunn and Underhill in 1914.[24] These authors took a segment of cat small intestine and, by removing the external muscle layers (i.e. the *muscularis propria*) produced a cylinder composed entirely of muscularis mucosae. Through the use of this preparation they were able to demonstrate that, from a mechanical standpoint, the fibers of the muscularis mucosae in this region are not longitudinally-oriented but instead exhibit a spiral pattern. This they deduced from the observation that unless the threads anchoring the preparation to the transducer and to the base of the bath were placed on opposite sides of the circumference of the oral and aboral ends, the preparation was mechanically quiescent and did not respond well to stimulation by pharmacologic agents. What was unique about their observations was the relatively slow rate of spontaneous contractions exhibited by the muscle ($\approx$ 1 per minute) and the discovery that, in contrast to its effects on the *muscularis propria,* epinephrine caused a contraction of the muscularis mucosae. This latter result was subsequently confirmed *in situ* using dog small intestinal muscularis mucosae by King and Arnold.[104]

A further insight into the unique pharmacologic characteristics of the muscularis mucosae came from the *in vivo* experiments of King and Arnold[104] who demonstrated that in the dog small intestine stimulation of the vagus had only a minimal effect on duodenal and jejunal mucosal movement whereas, stimulation of the splanchnic nerves caused a widespread excitatory effect. Thus, at this point there was a good agreement between the behavior of the muscularis mucosae *in vitro* and *in vivo* in that in both cases it was excited by stimulation of adrenoceptors.

It is surprising to find, therefore, that in the period from 1922 to 1969 there were no significant advances in our understanding of muscularis mucosae function. Even the works of Walder,[108] Hughes[109,110] and Onori et al.[111] merely involved modifications of the Gunn and Underhill preparation applied to different anatomical locations.

It was not until 1969 that the intrinsic innervation of the muscularis mucosae was investigated using electrical field stimulation (20 Hz, 1 msec duration pulses) of tissue from the distal esophagus of the North American opossum.[32] This revealed that the muscularis mucosae and the longitudinal muscle both exhibited a "duration response." In contrast, when similar experiments were performed on the distal colonic muscularis mucosae of the rabbit (100 Hz, 0.1 msec duration pulses for 15–30 sec) by Gallacher et al.[55] this preparation was found to first contract and then relax, thus providing evidence for the presence of both excitatory and inhibitory innervation by intrinsic nerves. In 1979 Kamikawa and Shimo[112] further developed this technique for the guinea pig esophageal muscularis mucosae by removing the entire esophagus plus vagus nerves, dissecting most of the *muscularis propria* away from the submucosa thus leaving only that required to allow an intact vagal input to the preparation. Stimulation of the vagus nerve (10 Hz, 0.2 msec duration pulses for 6 sec) then revealed that it provides the submucosal plexus in this region with excitatory synaptic input.

Although each of the methods outlined above allows for information to be obtained about muscularis mucosae function in particular regions these methods are not applicable throughout the intestine in all species. For example, although cylinders of guinea pig esophageal[112] and rat colonic muscularis mucosae[113] may be studied *in vitro,* for larger species this is impractical because of the size of the tissue bath that would be necessary and the physical characteristics of a large, thin cylinder of tissue. Similarly, while strips of muscularis mucosae from dog stomach and colon[114] or opossum esophagus[33,34] function appropriately *in vitro* because of the relative rigidity of the mucosa, this is not the possible in all parts of the intestine because, in some cases the mucosa tends to wrap around the outside of the preparation, thus presenting a significant barrier to the diffusion of both oxygen[105] and pharmacologic agents.[115]

To circumvent the problems outlined above a novel technique was developed by Percy and Christensen in 1986[115] which, by ensuring that the mucosa was on the inner aspect of the preparation, allowed for strips of muscularis mucosae from different anatomical locations[49] to be studied. This method, as used with colonic tissue, is described below and is represented in Figure 8.

A 5 cm segment of colon is removed, opened along its mesenteric border and rinsed in warm Krebs solution to remove residual fecal material. The preparations is then pinned out mucosal surface down in a Sylgard® (Dow Corning)-coated 7 inch Petri dish in oxygenated Krebs' solution. Full thickness segments 3 cm $\times$ 3 mm in the longitudinal axis are excised. The *muscularis propria* can then be separated from the mucosa/muscularis mucosae/submucosa by sharp dissection. The isolated muscularis mucosae is known to be an extremely delicate tissue[116] thus, in the following procedures it should not be over-stretched or handled roughly.

The remaining strip of mucosa, muscularis mucosae and submucosa is then tied in the middle with 5-0 surgical thread and folded, mucosal surfaces inwards, to be half its original

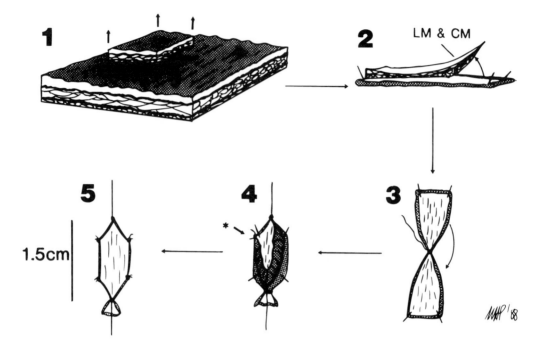

FIGURE 8 Schematic representation of the steps involved in preparing the colonic muscularis mucosae for measurement of its contractile properties. 1. A full thickness longitudinally-oriented segment of colonic tissue 3–5 cm × 0.5 cm is cut from the opened preparation. 2. The longitudinal (LM) and circular (CM) muscle layers (muscularis propria) are discarded. 3. With the mucosal surface underneath, a 4-0 suture line is tied around the middle of the preparation; the mucosal surfaces are then brought together (arrow). 4. The edges of the preparation are sutured (*) to prevent the mucosa (stippled area) from curling over the underlying muscle. 5. In the finished preparation the muscularis mucosae is fully exposed to the bathing medium and the mucosal surface is on the inner aspect. (Diagram based on Percy and Christensen, reference 115.)

length. The oral and aboral ends, now side by side, are tied together to form a loop. The vertical edges of the preparation are then sutured at four points with 7-0 surgical thread. This holds the preparation flat and ensures that the submucosa and muscularis mucosae are fully exposed to the bathing medium, but does not compromise its ability to contract. The finished preparation can then be connected to either an isotonic[115] or an isometric[49] transducer under an appropriate load.

Muscularis mucosae utilized in this fashion gives reproducible responses to drugs and to electrical field stimulation for several hours at a time. By using this technique it has been possible to show that the pharmacologic properties of the muscularis mucosae vary along the length of the colon,[49] that the muscularis mucosae is pharmacologically distinct from the corresponding region of longitudinal and circular muscle[49] and that in a rabbit model of inflammatory bowel disease the pharmacologic and mechanical properties of the muscularis mucosae are altered before any changes in the *muscularis propria* can be detected.[50]

Data obtained to date illustrate that the function of the muscularis mucosae is far from clearly understood. In addition, it seems likely that it will only be elucidated through the use of in vitro techniques such as those described above.

SUMMARY AND CONCLUSIONS

When instituting a series of *in vitro* experiments utilizing gastrointestinal smooth muscle the choice of physiological solution is critical as this provides the ions, oxygen and glucose upon which survival of the tissue is dependent. Commonly used physiological solutions such as Tyrode's or Krebs' are not exact representations of either blood or extracellular fluid. Thus, the choice of bathing medium cannot be based on a knowledge of the chemistry of these body fluids alone and the most appropriate solution should be determined experimentally. Whenever possible it is recommended that fresh tissue be used for any *in vitro* experiment. Storage, whether in a refrigerator, at room temperature or body temperature has unpredictable and deleterious effects on the properties of the nerves of the enteric nervous system and on the muscle itself. Similarly, unless the experimental protocol relates to the effects of cooling, the muscle under study should always be maintained at the "normal" body temperature of the species from which it was derived. Operating at lower temperatures has effects on both pharmacologic receptors, on the muscle itself and on the transmitters being released from the intrinsic innervation. Measurement of smooth muscle contraction may be made with either an isometric or an isotonic transducer. Isometric transducers are of particular value when it is necessary to measure force generation; isotonic transducers are most useful where relaxation responses are involved because they keep the load on the muscle constant. However, there is no hard and fast rule governing the choice of transducer the selection should be made based on experimental evidence. Regardless of which type of transducer is selected the load placed upon the tissue should be that which is determined to stretch the muscle to the length at which it produces the largest contractile responses to a pharmacological or electrical stimulus. Once a choice of transducer has been made the tissue should be exposed to the pharmacologic agents of choice over a wide concentration range. The data can then be expressed in one of a number of ways and presented as one or more log concentration-response curves. It is important to note that corresponding points on a series of such curves should not be statistically compared using Student's t-tests. Several preparations are available to study the role of the extrinsic sympathetic and parasympathetic nerves to the intestine. In the small intestine extrinsic sympathetic nerve function can easily be examined whereas, in the distal colon the effects of extrinsic sympathetic and parasympathetic nerves plus their interactions can be studied. Intestinal responses to the extrinsic nerves vary by region and the choice would be governed by the aim of the protocol. In smaller species such as the guinea pig or rabbit, intrinsic nerve function can be determined via the use of a whole segment of intestine and the technique of transmural stimulation. Where this is not practicable, representative strips of the appropriate muscle region can be subjected to electrical field stimulation by placing them between two electrodes immersed in the bathing medium. These techniques differ from extrinsic nerve stimulation in that all enteric nerves are activated when current is passed. All regions of the gastrointestinal tract exhibit some form of propulsive activity which might be termed peristalsis. A variety of methods exist whereby this can be studied in the esophagus, stomach, small and large intestine and measurement can be made of several parameters including, longitudinal and circular muscle contraction, flow, wall compliance, luminal diameter and velocity of propulsion. However, it is important to note that there may be significant regional variations within any one organ as to how peristaltic activity is accomplished. Furthermore, for the study of peristalsis it is of vital importance to ensure that the distending stimulus is appropriate, e.g. liquid in the small intestine but more solid in the colon. When it is necessary to study the individual muscle layers of the intestine rather than their combined responses, several methods are available which allow this to be achieved. Through the use of these various methods the innervation, pharmacologic and mechanical properties of each muscle type can be evaluated and compared. The various techniques available for the study of gastrointestinal smooth muscle *in vitro* continue to make an important contribution to our understanding of the integrated motor function of the gastrointestinal tract in health and in pathological states.

ACKNOWLEDGMENT

    The author wishes to thank Ms. Maureen Burton for having the presence of mind to document the pitfalls associated with several of these procedures while we were using them.

REFERENCES

1. **Magnus, R.:** Versuche am überlebenden Dünndarm von Säugethieren I. *Pflügers Arch.* **102:** 123, 1904.
2. **Magnus, R.:** Versuche am überlebenden Dünndarm von Säugethieren II. Die Beziehungen des Darmnervensystems zur automatischen Darmbewegung. *Pflügers Arch.* **102:** 349, 1904.
3. **Magnus, R.:** Versuche am überlebenden Dünndarm von Säugethieren III. Die Erregungsleitung. *Pflügers Arch.* **103:** 515, 1904.
4. **Magnus, R.:** Versuche am überlebenden Dünndarm von Säugethieren IV. Rhythmizitäre Periode. *Pflügers Arch.* **103:** 525, 1904.
5. **Magnus, R.:** Versuche am überlebenden Dünndarm von Säugethieren V. Wirkungsweise und Angriffspunkt einiger Gifte am Katzendarm. *Pflügers Arch.* **108:** 1, 1905.
6. **Magnus, R.:** Versuche am überlebenden Dünndarm von Säugethieren VI. *Pflügers Arch.* **106:** 152, 1906.
7. **Hafter, W.:** Neue Versuche über den Nervus splanchnicus major. *Zeitschr. f. rat. Med.* **4:** 322, 1854.
8. **Mall, F.:** A study of the intestinal contraction. *Johns Hopkins Hospital Reports.* **1:** 37, 1896.
9. **Trendelenburg, P.:** Physiologische und Pharmacologische Versuche über die Dünndarmperistaltic. *Arch. Exp. Pathol. Pharmacol.* **81:** 55, 1917.
10. **Finkleman, B.:** On the nature of inhibition in the intestine. *J. Physiol. (Lond.)* **70:** 145, 1930.
11. **Garry, R. C. and Gillespie, J. C.:** An *in vitro* preparation of the distal colon of the rabbit with orthosympathetic and parasympathetic innervation. *J. Physiol. (Lond.)* **123:** 60P, 1954.
12. **Garry, R. C. and Gillespie, J. C.:** The responses of the musculature of the colon of the rabbit to stimulation *in vitro* of the parasympathetic and sympathetic outflows. *J. Physiol. (Lond.)* **128:** 557, 1955.
13. **Paton, W. D. M.:** The responses of the guinea pig ileum to electrical stimulation by coaxial electrodes. *J. Physiol. (Lond.)* **127:** 40P, 1955.
14. **Kamikawa, Y., Uchida, K. and Shimo, Y.:** Heterogeneity of muscarinic receptors in the guinea pig esophageal muscularis mucosae and ileal longitudinal muscle. *Gastroenterology* **88:** 706, 1985.
15. **Cowie, A. L., Kosterlitz, H. W. and Waterfield, A. A.:** Factors influencing the release of acetylcholine from the myenteric plexus of the ileum of the guinea-pig and rabbit. *Br. J. Pharmacol.* **64:** 565, 1978.
16. **Tyrode, M. V.:** The mode of action of some purgative salts. *Arch. Int. Pharmacodyn.* **20:** 205, 1910.
17. **Krebs, H. A.:** Body size and tissue respiration. *Biochim. Biophys. Acta.* **4:** 249, 1950.
18. *Guide to the care and use of experimental animals.* Canadian Council on Animal Care, 79, 1984.
19. **Kozma, C., Macklin, W., Cummins, L. M. and Mauer, R.:** Anatomy, physiology and biochemistry of the rabbit. In, *The biology of the laboratory rabbit:* Weisbroth, S. H., Flatt, R. E. and Kraus, A. L. Eds. Academic Press, New York, 1974, 50.
20. **Ganong, W. F.:** *Review of medical physiology:* 6th ed., Lange Medical Publications, Los Altos, 1973, 579.
21. **Ratnoff, O. D.:** Blood components. *Physiology:* 3rd ed., Berne, R. M. and Levy, M. N. Eds. Mosby, St. Louis, 1993, 327.
22. **Neukirch, P. and Rona, P.:** Experimentelle Beiträge zur Physiologie des Darmes. *Pflügers Arch.* **144:** 555, 1912.
23. **Percy, W. H., Sutherland, J. and Christensen, J.:** Paradoxical relationship between substrates and agonist-induced contractions of opossum esophageal body and sphincter *in vitro. Dig. Dis. Sci.* **36:** 1057, 1991.
24. **Gunn, J. A. and Underhill, S. W. F.:** Experiments on the surviving mammalian intestine. *Q. J. Exp. Physiol.* **8:** 275–296, 1914.
25. **Beleslin, D. and Varagic, V.:** The effect of cooling and of 5-hydroxytryptamine on the peristaltic reflex of the isolated guinea-pig ileum. *Br. J. Pharmacol.* **13:** 266, 1958.
26. **Filogamo, G.:** Sulla denervazione dell'intestino a mezzo del freddo. *Boll. Soc. Ital. Biol. Sper.* **45:** 552, 1969.
27. **Watters, D. A. K., Smith, A. N., Eastwood, M. A., Anderson, K. C. and Elton, R. A.:** Mechanical properties of the rat colon: The effect of age, sex and different conditions of storage. *Q. J. Exp. Physiol.* **70:** 151, 1985.

28. **Barajas-Lopez, C., Chow, E., Den Hertog, A. and Huizinga, J. D.:** Role of the sodium pump in pacemaker generation in dog colonic smooth muscle. *J. Physiol. (Lond.)* **416**: 369, 1989.

29. **Kauvar, D., Crist, J. and Goyal, R. K.:** Effect of cold temperature on membrane potential responses in opossum esophageal circular muscle. *Am. J. Physiol.* **257**: G637, 1989.

30. **Tsai, C. S. and Ochillo, R. F.:** Low temperature and muscarinic receptor activities. *Cryobiol.* **26**: 485, 1989.

31. **Akbarali, H., Bieger, D. and Triggle, C. R.:** Effects of cold storage on relaxation responses in the rat oesophageal tunica muscularis mucosae. *Canad. J. Physiol. Pharmacol.* **65**: 23, 1987.

32. **Christensen, J. and Lund, G. F.:** Esophageal responses to distension and electrical stimulation. *J. Clin. Inv.* **48**: 408, 1969.

33. **Christensen, J. and Percy, W. H.:** A pharmacological study of oesophageal muscularis mucosae from the cat, dog and American opossum *(Didelphis virginiana). Br. J. Pharmacol.* **83**: 329, 1984.

34. **Domoto, T., Jury, J., Berezin, I., Fox, J. E. T. and Daniel, E. E.:** Does substance P comediate with acetylcholine in nerves of opossum esophageal muscularis mucosa?. *Am. J. Physiol.* **245**: G19, 1983.

35. **Harry, J.:** Effect of cooling, local anaesthetic compounds and botulinum toxin on the responses of and the acetylcholine output from the electrically transmurally stimulated isolated guinea-pig ileum. *Br. J. Pharmacol.* **19**: 42, 1962.

36. **Johnson, E. S.:** The origin of the acetylcholine released from the guinea-pig isolated ileum. *Br. J. Pharmacol.* **21**: 555, 1963.

37. **De La Lande, I. S. and Porter, R. B.:** Factors influencing the action of morphine on acetylcholine release in the guinea-pig intestine. *Br. J. Pharmacol.* **29**: 158, 1967.

38. **Gabella, G.:** Isometric contraction, isotonic contraction and passive contraction in smooth muscles. In, *Cells and tissues: A three dimensional approach by modern techniques in microscopy;* Proceedings of the VIII International symposium on Morphological Sciences, Rome, Italy, 1988. Pietro M. Motta Ed. Alan R. Liss, Inc. New York, 1989, 133.

39. **Armour, C. L., Diment, L. M. and Black, J. L.:** Relationship between smooth muscle volume and contractile response in airway tissue. Isometric versus isotonic measurement. *J. Pharmacol. Exp. Ther.* **245**: 687, 1988.

40. **Paton, W. D. M.:** The action of morphine and related substances on contraction and on acetylcholine output of co-axially stimulated guinea-pig ileum. *Br. J. Pharmacol.* **12**: 119, 1957.

41. **Lees, G. M. and Percy, W. H.:** Antibiotic associated colitis: An *in vitro* investigation of the effects of antibiotics on intestinal motility. *Br. J. Pharmacol.* **73**: 535, 1981.

42. **Christensen, J., Conklin, J. L. and Freeman, B. W.:** Physiologic specialization at esophagogastric junction in three species. *Am. J. Physiol.* **225**: 1265, 1973.

43. **Percy, W. H., Burton, M. B., Fallick, F. and Burakoff, R.:** A comparison *in vitro* of human and rabbit distal colonic muscle responses to inflammatory mediators. *Gastroenterology* **99**: 1324, 1990.

44. **Rand, M. J. and Ridehalgh, A.:** Actions of hemicholinium and triethylcholine on responses of guinea-pig colon to stimulation of autonomic nerves. *J. Pharm. Pharmacol.* **17**: 144, 1965.

45. **Del Tacca, M., Soldani, G., Selli, M. and Crema, A.:** Action of catecholamines on release of acetylcholine from human taenia coli. *Eur. J. Pharmacol.* **9**: 80, 1970.

46. **Gillespie, J. S. and Khoyi, M. A.:** The site and receptors responsible for the inhibition by sympathetic nerves of intestinal muscle and its parasympathetic motor nerves. *J. Physiol. (Lond.)* **267**: 767, 1977.

47. **Harry, J.:** The action of drugs on the circular muscle strip from the isolated guinea-pig ileum. *Br. J. Pharmacol.* **20**: 399, 1963.

48. **Herman, J. R. and Bass, P.:** Altered carbachol-induced contractile responses of rat jejunal smooth muscle following local myenteric plexus ablation. *Dig. Dis. Sci.* **35**: 1146, 1990.

49. **Percy, W. H., Rose, K. and Burton, M. B.:** Pharmacologic characterization of the muscularis mucosae in three regions of the rabbit colon. *J. Pharmacol. Exp. Ther.* **261**: 1136, 1992.

50. **Percy, W. H., Burton, M. B., Rose, K., Donovan, V. and Burakoff, R.:** *In vitro* changes in the properties of rabbit colonic muscularis mucosae in colitis. *Gastroenterology* **104**: 369, 1993.

51. **Gordon, A. R. and Siegman, M. J.:** Mechanical properties of smooth muscle. 1. Length-tension and force-velocity relations. *Am. J. Physiol.* **221**: 1243, 1971.

52. **Herlihy, J. T. and Murphy, R. A.:** Length-tension relationship of smooth muscle of the hog carotid artery. *Circ. Res.* **33:** 275, 1973.

53. **Percy, W. H., Burton, M. B., Fallick, F. and Burakoff, R.:** Rat colonic motor responses to inflammatory mediators *in vitro:* A poor model for the human colon. *J. Gastro. Motility* **3:** 229, 1991.

54. **Tallarida, R. J. and Jacob, L. S.:** *The dose-response relation in pharmacology.* Springer-Verlag, New York, 1979.

55. **Gallacher, M., MacKenna, B. R. and McKirdy, H. C.:** Effects of drugs and of electrical stimulation on the muscularis mucosae of rabbit large intestine. *Br. J. Pharmacol.* **47:** 760, 1973.

56. **Boschov, P., Paiva, A. C. M., Paiva, T. B. and Shimuta, S. I.:** Further evidence for the existence of two receptor sites for bradykinin responsible for the diphasic effect in the rat isolated duodenum. *Br. J. Pharmacol.* **83:** 591, 1984.

57. **Yagi, H., Snape, W. J. and Hyman, P. E.:** Perinatal changes in bombesin-stimulated muscle contraction in rabbit stomach and colon. *Gastroenterology* **100:** 980, 1991.

58. **DeLean, A., Munson, P. J. and Rodbard, D.:** Simultaneous analysis of families of sigmoidal curves: application to bioassay, radioligand assay, and physiological dose-response curves. *Am. J. Physiol.* **235:** E97, 1978.

59. **Carpenter, J. R.:** A method for presenting and comparing dose-response curves. *J. Pharmacol. Methods* **15:** 283, 1986.

60. **Meddings, J. B., Scott, R. B. and Fick, G. H.:** Analysis and comparison of sigmoidal curves: application to dose-response data. *Am. J. Physiol.* **257:** G982, 1989.

61. **Zivin, J. A. and Bartko, J. J.:** Statistics for disinterested scientists. *Life Sci.* **18:** 15, 1976.

62. **Pitts, D. K., Kelland, M. D., Shen, R-Y., Freeman, A. S. and Chiodo, L. A.:** Statistical analysis of dose-response curves in extracellular electrophysiological studies of single neurons. *Synapse* **5:** 281, 1990.

63. **McSwiney, B. A. and Robson, J. M.:** The response of smooth muscle to stimulation of the vagus nerve. *J. Physiol. (Lond.)* **68:** 124, 1929.

64. **Boura, A. L. A. and Green, A. F.:** The actions of bretylium: adrenergic neurone blocking and other effects. *Br. J. Pharmacol.* **14:** 536, 1959.

65. **Szerb, J. C.:** The effect of morphine on the adrenergic nerves of the isolated guinea-pig ileum. *Br. J. Pharmacol.* **16:** 23, 1961.

66. **Munro, A. F.:** Effect of autonomic drugs on the responses of isolated preparations from the guinea-pig intestine to electrical stimulation. *J. Physiol. (Lond.)* **120:** 41, 1953.

67. **Bentley, G. A.:** Studies on sympathetic mechanisms in isolated intestinal and vas deferens preparations. *Br. J. Pharmacol.* **19:** 85, 1962.

68. **Garry, R. C. and Wishart, M:** Fluid electrodes with a rubber diaphragm. *J. Physiol. (Lond.)* **115:** 61P, 1951.

69. **Van Harn, G. L.:** Responses of muscles of cat small intestine to autonomic nerve stimulation. *Am. J. Physiol.* **204:** 352, 1963.

70. **Day, M. D. and Rand, M. J.:** Effect of guanethidine in revealing cholinergic sympathetic fibres. *Br. J. Pharmacol.* **17:** 245, 1961.

71. **Boyd, G., Gillespie, J. S. and Mackenna, B. R.:** Origin of the cholinergic response of the rabbit intestine to stimulation of its extrinsic sympathetic nerves after exposure to sympathetic blocking agents. *Br. J. Pharmacol.* **19:** 258, 1962.

72. **Day, M. D.:** Effect of sympathomimetic amines on the blocking action of guanethidine, bretylium and xylocholine. *Br. J. Pharmacol.* **18:** 421, 1962.

73. **Langley, J. N. and Anderson, H. K.:** On the innervation of the pelvic and adjoining viscera. Part 1. Lower portion of the intestine. *J. Physiol. (Lond.)* **18:** 67, 1895.

74. **Wells, J. A., Mercer, T. H., Gray, J. S. and Ivy, A. C.:** The motor innervation of the colon. *Am. J. Physiol.* **138:** 88, 1942.

75. **Varagic, V.:** The effect of tolazoline and other substances on the response of the isolated colon of the rabbit to nerve stimulation. *Arch. Int. Pharmacodyn.* **106:** 141, 1956.

76. **Kennedy, C. and Krier, J.:** [Met[5]]enkephalin acts via δ-opioid receptors to inhibit pelvic nerve-evoked contractions of cat distal colon. *Br. J. Pharmacol.* **92:** 291, 1987.

77. **Bianchi, C., Beani, L., Frigo, G. M. and Crema, A.:** Further evidence for the presence of non-adrenergic inhibitory structures in the guinea-pig colon. *Eur. J. Pharmacol.* **4:** 51, 1968.

78. **Goldhill, J. M. and Percy, W. H.:** A novel *in vitro* technique to study extrinsic neural control of rabbit colonic muscle and epithelial function. *Am. J. Physiol.* **265:** G1064, 1993.

79. **Christensen, J., Stiles, M. J., Rick, G. A. and Sutherland, J.:** Comparative anatomy of the myenteric plexus of the distal colon in eight mammals. *Gastroenterology* **86:** 706, 1984.

80. **Christensen, J. and Rick, G. A.:** Distribution of myelinated nerves in ascending nerves and myenteric plexus of cat colon. *Am. J. Anat.* **178:** 250, 1987.

81. **Gabella, G.:** Innervation of the gastrointestinal tract. *Int. Rev. Cytol.* **59:** 129, 1979.

82. **Franco, R., Costa, M. and Furness, J. B.:** Evidence for the release of endogenous substance P from intestinal nerves. *Naunyn-Schmiedeberg's Arch. Pharmacol.* **306:** 195, 1979.

83. **Henderson, G, Hughes, J. and Kosterlitz, H. W.:** The effects of morphine on the release of noradrenaline from the cat isolated nictitating membrane and the guinea-pig ileum myenteric plexus-longitudinal muscle preparation. *Br. J. Pharmacol.* **53:** 505, 1975.

84. **Feldberg, W.:** Effects of ganglion blocking substances on the small intestine. *J. Physiol. (Lond.)* **113:** 483, 1951.

85. **Munro, A. F.:** The effects of adrenaline on the isolated guinea-pig intestine. *J. Physiol. (Lond.)* **112:** 84, 1951.

86. **Kosterlitz, H. W. and Lydon, R. J.:** Impulse transmission in the myenteric plexus-longitudinal muscle preparation of the guinea-pig ileum. *Br. J. Pharmacol.* **43:** 74, 1971.

87. **Ambache, N.:** Separation of the longitudinal muscle of the rabbit's ileum as a broad sheet. *J. Physiol. (Lond.)* **125:** 53P, 1954.

88. **Burn, J. H. and Rand, M. J.:** The relation of circulating noradrenaline to the effect of sympathetic stimulation. *J. Physiol. (Lond.)* **150:** 295, 1960.

89. **Kosterlitz, H. W. and Robinson, J. A.:** Inhibition of the peristaltic reflex of the isolated guinea-pig ileum. *J. Physiol. (Lond.)* **136:** 249, 1957.

90. **Bülbring, E. and Lin, R. C. Y.:** The effect of intraluminal application of 5-hydroxytryptamine and 5-hydroxytryptophan on peristalsis; the local production of 5-HT and its release in relation to intraluminal pressure and propulsive activity. *J. Physiol. (Lond.)* **140:** 381, 1958.

91. **Schulze-Delrieu, K.:** Intrinsic differences in the filling response of the guinea pig duodenum and ileum. *J. Lab. Clin. Med.* **117:** 44, 1991.

92. **Bayliss, W. M. and Starling, E. H.:** The movements and innervation of the large intestine. *J. Physiol. (Lond.)* **26:** 107: 1900.

93. **Spedding, M.:** A modified guinea-pig stomach preparation. *Br. J. Pharmacol.* **61:** 155P, 1977.

94. **McKirdy, H. C.:** Factors influencing tone in the rabbit large intestine. *Q. J. Exp. Physiol.* **63:** 111, 1978.

95. **Weems, W. A. and Weisbrodt, N. W.:** Comparison of colonic and ileal propulsive capabilities under conditions requiring hydrostatic work. *Am. J. Physiol.* **246:** G587, 1984.

96. **Schulze-Delrieu, K., Percy, W. H., Ren, J., Shirazi, S. S., and Von Derau, K.:** Evidence for inhibition of opossum LES through intrinsic gastric nerves. *Am. J. Physiol.* **256:** G198, 1989.

97. **Haffner, J. F. and Stadaas, J.:** Pressure responses to cholinergic and adrenergic agents in the fundus, corpus and antrum of isolated rabbit stomachs. *Acta Chir. Scand.* **138:** 713, 1972.

98. **Haffner, J. F. W.:** Pressure responses to cholinergic and adrenergic agents in the fundus corpus and antrum of isolated rat and guinea-pig stomachs. *Acta Chir. Scand.* **139:** 650, 1973.

99. **Green, W. E. R. and Hardcastle, J. D.:** The myoelectrical activity of the isolated perfused canine stomach. *J. Physiol. (Lond.)* **222:** 41P, 1972.

100. **Kowalewski, K. and Kolodej, A.:** Effect of prostaglandin E2 on myoelectrical and mechanical activity of totally isolated, *ex vivo*-perfused, canine stomach. *Pharmacol.* **13:** 325, 1975.

101. **Sakai, K.:** A pharmacological analysis of the contractile action of histamine upon the ileal region of the isolated, blood perfused small intestine of the rat. *Br. J. Pharmacol.* **67:** 587, 1979.

102. **Sakai, K., Akima, M., and Shiraki, Y.:** Comparative studies with 5-hydroxytryptamine and its derivatives in isolated, blood perfused small intestine and ileum strip of the rat. *Jap. J. Pharmacol.* **29:** 223, 1979.

103. **Frigo, G. M. and Lecchini, S.:** An improved method for studying the peristaltic reflex in the isolated colon. *Br. J. Pharmacol.* **39:** 346, 1970.

104. **King, C. E. and Arnold, L.:** The activities of the intestinal motor mechanism. *Am. J. Physiol.* **59:** 97, 1922.

105. **King, C. E., Glass, L. C., and Townsend, S E.:** The circular components of the muscularis mucosae of the small intestine of the dog. *Am. J. Physiol.* **148:** 667, 1947.

106. **Titkemeyer, C. W. and Calhoun, M. L.:** A comparative study of the small intestines of domestic animals. *Am. J. Vet. Res.* **16:** 152, 1955.

107. **Jamdar, M. N. and Ema, A. N.:** The submucosal glands and the orientation of the musculature in the oesophagus of the camel. *J. Anat.* **135:** 165, 1982.

108. **Walder, D. N.:** The muscularis mucosae of the human stomach. *J. Physiol. (Lond.)* **120:** 365, 1953.

109. **Hughes, F. B.:** The muscularis mucosae of the esophagus of the cat, rabbit and rat. *J. Physiol. (Lond.)* **130:** 123, 1955.

110. **Hughes, F. B.:** Drug responses of the human fetal esophagus. *Am. J. Physiol.* **191:** 37, 1957.

111. **Onori, L., Friedmann, C. A., Frigo, G. M., and Tonini, M.:** Effects of catecholamines, nicotine, acetylcholine and potassium on the mechanical activity of the colonic muscularis mucosae of the cat. *Dig. Dis. Sci.* **16:** 689, 1971.

112. **Kamikawa, Y. and Shimo, Y.:** Cholinergic and adrenergic innervations of the muscularis mucosae in guinea-pig esophagus. *Arch. Int. Pharmacodyn.* **238:** 220, 1979.

113. **Bailey, S. J. and Jordan, C. C.:** A study of [D-Pro^2,D-Phe^7,D-Trp^9]-substance P and [D-Trp^{7,9}]-substance P as tachykinin partial agonists in the rat colon. *Br. J. Pharmacol.* **82:** 441, 1984.

114. **Angel, F., Schmalz, P. F., Morgan, K. G., Go, V. L. W., and Szurszewski, J. H.:** Innervation of the muscularis mucosa in the canine stomach and colon. *Scand. J. Gastroenterol.* **17:** (Suppl. 71) 71, 1982.

115. **Percy, W. H. and Christensen, J.:** Pharmacological characterization of opossum distal colonic muscularis mucosae *in vitro*. *Am. J. Physiol.* **250:** G98, 1986.

116. **King, C. E. and Church, J. G.:** The motor reaction of the muscularis mucosae to some drugs. *Am. J. Physiol.* **66:** 428, 1923.

10 Isolated Smooth Muscle Cells

John R. Grider and K. S. Murthy

INTRODUCTION

The study of gut smooth muscle and its regulation by neurotransmitters and hormones is based on the use of a variety of preparations, each with distinct advantages and disadvantages. Isolated whole segments of gut and muscle strips retain all or some components of the enteric nervous system. In whole segments, physiological stimuli such as distension or mucosal contact can be used to activate enteric reflex pathways. Muscle strips can be prepared so as to include the myenteric or submucosal plexus of the enteric nervous system, and can be stimulated pharmacologically or electrically. The responses can be measured as a change in muscle tension or phasic contractile activity, or as a change in membrane potential.

The usefulness of intact smooth muscle tissue is limited by its heterogeneity which makes it difficult to determine the relationship between the mechanical response and various biochemical correlates of the response. Characterization of receptors by radioligand binding is limited by the presence of neural membranes in tissue homogenates; although neurons constitute only 1–2% of the muscle tissue mass, the density of receptors on them can be much higher than on smooth muscle cells. Furthermore, basal or induced transmitter release can complicate analysis of pharmacological responses making it difficult to distinguish direct action on smooth muscle cells from indirect, neurally-mediated actions. Release of transmitters by pharmacological agents can be eliminated by neural toxins, such as tetrodotoxin. The toxins, however, can introduce artifacts of their own: by eliminating all neural influences, including the dominant inhibitory influence, tetrodotoxin can unmask intrinsic myogenic phasic activity.[1,2] It should be noted that neural toxins which act by blocking axonal conduction may not eliminate transmitter release caused by presynaptic effects of pharmacological agents.

In contrast, suspensions of dispersed smooth muscle cells are devoid of neural elements and are, therefore, morphologically homogenous. This makes it possible to characterize receptors pharmacologically by measurement of mechanical response or a biochemical correlate of response (e.g., inositol 1,4,5-trisphosphate, cAMP, cGMP, $[Ca^{2+}]_i$, etc.) or immunochemically by measurement of radioligand binding. Single muscle cells can also be used to measure mechanical response as well as to characterize membrane events (e.g., membrane potential and ion channel activity). Intact and permeabilized single muscle cells and suspensions of cells can be used to examine various components of the signal transduction pathways initiated by the action of agonists, including GTP-binding proteins and effector enzymes.

CELL DISPERSION AND ISOLATION TECHNIQUE

Smooth muscle cells have been isolated from all regions of the gut including esophagus, lower esophageal sphincter, stomach, gallbladder and cystic duct, small intestine, large intestine,

0-8493-8304-8/96/$0.00+$.50
© 1996 by CRC Press, Inc.

225

and internal anal sphincter and from a variety of species including guinea pig, rat, rabbit, cat, dog, pig, and human (Table 1). The techniques of smooth muscle cell dispersion and isolation are based on the original method described by Bagby et al.[82] for preparation of muscle cells from the stomach of the amphibian Bufo marinus. The technique varies slightly with the species and the region of the gut from which smooth muscle cells are prepared. Gastric muscle cells are prepared following removal of the mucosa by blunt dissection and cutting the muscularis into 4 mm by 5 mm strips.[9,20,21] Intestinal muscle is first separated into circular and longitudinal muscle by gentle tangential stroking before cutting into strips. In species in which the muscularis is thick (e.g. rabbit, dog, and human) the tissue is sliced with a Stadie-Riggs slicer to facilitate digestion and improve cell yield.[9,10,13]

The muscle strips are digested by incubation at 31°C for two successive 40-minute periods in Ca^{2+}-free HEPES medium containing 1% collagenase (Type II) and 0.1% soybean trypsin inhibitor. The partially digested tissue is washed free of enzyme and the smooth muscle cells allowed to disperse spontaneously in collagenase-free HEPES medium. The cells are harvested by filtration through 500 μm Nitex mesh followed by three cycles of centrifugation at $100 \times$ g for 15 min and resuspension in HEPES medium containing 2 mM Ca^{2+}. Using this technique, 1 to 2 million cells can be obtained from guinea pig stomach and many more from larger animals.[9,10,20] This basic technique has been modified to include addition of other enzymes such

---

TABLE 1

Regions of the Gut and Species from which Smooth Muscle Cells have been Isolated

Region	Species	Reference
Esophagus	Cat	3,4
LES	Cat	3,5
Muscularis mucosa	Rabbit	6
Stomach	Human	7–10
	Dog	8,11–14
	Rabbit	8,15–18
	Guinea pig	7,9,19–31
Gallbladder	Human	32–35
	Dog	36–38
	Guinea pig	22,39,40
Cystic duct	Dog	37
Small Intestine	Human	7,8,41–45
	Dog	8,46,47
	Pig	47–49
	Rabbit	47,50,51
	Rat	8,47,52
	Guinea pig	7,41,43,47,53–59
Large intestine		
Colon	Human	60
	Dog	61–64, 123
	Cat	65
	Rabbit	60,66–70
	Rat	71–73
	Guinea pig	73–74
Tenia coli	Guinea pig	75–80
Internal Anal Sphincter	Human	60
	Rabbit	60,81

as trypsin, pronase and papain.[13,14,44,49,62,77] The absence of neural membranes in suspensions of smooth muscle cells has been confirmed by the absence of [^{3}H]saxitoxin binding.[15] Saxitoxin binds specifically to neuronal sodium channels and has been used as a marker for neural membranes in muscle tissue homogenates.[83]

The viability of the smooth muscle cells prepared by this technique is evident from their ability to 1) exclude trypan blue (98%),[20,64] 2) contract and relax in response to appropriate agonists, 3) maintain normal metabolism, incorporating labeled amino acids and rubidium and producing normal amounts of lactate,[84,85] 4) express normal ion channels and produce action potentials in response to electrical stimulation,[4,6,39,45,86] and 5) demonstrate initial velocities of shortening and generate force per crossectional area similar to that of intact muscle strips.[85]

CONTRACTION AND RELAXATION OF ISOLATED MUSCLE CELLS

MEASUREMENT OF MECHANICAL RESPONSE

Measurements of the mechanical responses to contractile and relaxant agonists have been made using suspensions of muscle cells as well as single muscle cells attached to a coverslip. Measurements in suspensions involve comparison of mean cell length in a control suspension to which no agonist has been added and mean cell length in a suspension to which a contractile agonist has been added.[10,20] An aliquot of cells ($\sim$10^4 cells/ml) is incubated with a test agent and the reaction terminated at intervals, usually 30 seconds, by addition of acrolein to a final concentration of 1%.

Cell measurement is usually made by image scanning micrometry.[10,20] The technique involves the direct measurement of cell lengths by eyepiece micrometer, image-scanning micrometer or computerized image analysis. The lengths of the first 50 randomly encountered cells in separate slides prepared from control and stimulant-treated suspensions are measured and compared. Contraction is expressed as the absolute decrease in mean cell length (μm) or percent decrease from control. Measurements using this technique have been validated by photomicrometry.

Control muscle cells do not undergo further relaxation; accordingly, relaxation is measured in cells exposed to a maximal concentration of a contractile agonist (e.g., 1 μM acetylcholine or 1 nM cholecystokinin octapeptide).[10,19] The cells are preincubated with the relaxant agonist for 60 seconds and together with the contractile agonist for another 30 seconds, after which the reaction is terminated with acrolein. Relaxation is determined from the change in mean length of contracted cells and expressed as percent inhibition of contraction.

Contraction and relaxation can also be measured in individual cells.[21,22,43] Because of their negative surface charge, the cells can be electrostatically anchored to a positively charged coverslip (coated with poly-L-lysine or similar agent) that forms the ceiling of a minichamber (0.1 ml in volume). The cells can be viewed continuously by phase-contrast microscopy and perfused at a rate of 1 ml/min with media containing contractile and relaxant agonists and antagonists. The length of single cells within the microscopic field can be measured at 10-second intervals by scanning micrometry and the change in length monitored continuously. The time course (Figure 1) and stoichiometry (Figure 2) of contraction of individual cells mimics closely those determined in cell suspensions.[21,43]

Other techniques have also been used for measurement of contraction. Singer and Fay[87] have use automated cell counting techniques to measure changes in cell length or width. Pulses induced by the passage of 10,000 cells through an orifice are collated into histograms in which pulse duration is equivalent to cell length and pulse height is equivalent with cell width. Contraction is measured as the lateral shift in the histogram in response to a contractile agonist.

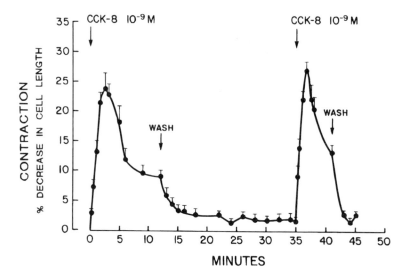

FIGURE 1   Kinetics of the contraction elicited by a maximal concentration of cholecystokinin (CCK-8) in single muscle cells from guinea pig stomach. The initial rapid maximal contraction was followed by a lower sustained plateau. The response was reversible upon washing and was repeatable by restimulation with CCK-8. (From *Am. J. Physiol.,* 250, G357, 1986, Figure 2. With permission.)

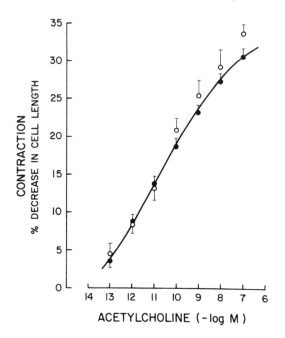

FIGURE 2   Concentration-response curves for the effect of acetylcholine on suspensions (open circles) and single (closed circles) muscle cells isolated from guinea pig stomach. (From *Am. J. Physiol.,* 250, G357, 1986, Figure 6. With permission.)

CHARACTERISTICS OF CONTRACTION AND RELAXATION

A large number of peptide and non-peptide agonists have been examined for their ability to cause contraction or relaxation of isolated smooth muscle cells from all regions of the gut

(Tables 2 and 3). With few exceptions, all of these agonists elicit responses in cells from all species in all regions of the gut.

Upon exposure to a contractile agonist, cells begin to contract immediately, attain an initial peak of contraction within 30 seconds independently of the agonist used. Peak contraction is followed by a more gradual decline to a plateau approximately 40% of peak response. Peak and plateau contraction is concentration-dependent with a maximal contraction corresponding to between 25 and 35% decrease in cell length. Maximal responses induced by full agonists are not significantly different from each other. Concentration-response curves are characteristically wide-spanned and with responses obtained at concentrations as low as 10 fM with some agonists. The reason for the exquisite sensitivity of dispersed muscle cells is not known. Wide-spanned concentration-response curves suggest the existence of receptor heterogeneity.

In many, perhaps most instances, the response reflects the net effect mediated by various receptor subtypes, such as histamine H_1 and H_2, adenosine A_1 and A_2, and 5-HT_2 and 5-HT_4. The histamine H_1 receptor mediates contraction and its effect predominates over that of the H_2 receptor which mediates relaxation. The effect of H_2 receptors is evident in the presence of H_2 antagonists which shift the concentration-response curve to the left.[89]

TABLE 2
Receptors on Isolated Muscle Cells for Peptides

	Pharmacological Response	Radioligand Binding	Messenger	References
CCK-A	C	NT	Ca ↑	22,90,91
CCK-B/gastrin	C	NT	Ca ↑	
BB/GRP	C	+	Ca ↑	23,26,42,60
NMB	C	+	Ca ↑	
NK-1	C	+	Ca ↑	52,53
NK-2	C	+	Ca ↑	
NK-3	C	NT	Ca ↑	
Opioid μ	C	+	Ca ↑/cAMP ↓	41,51,92,93
δ	C	+	Ca ↑/cAMP ↓	
κ	C	+	Ca ↑/cAMP ↓	
NPY_1	Nil	NT	cAMP ↓	94
NPY_2	C	NT	Ca ↑/cAMP ↓	
Motilin	C	+	Ca ↑	56,68,69
CGRP	R	+	cAMP ↑	25,28,31
VIP/PACAPII	R	+	cAMP ↑/cGMP ↑	16,79,80,95,96
PHI	R	+	cAMP ↑	
PACAP (Ap)	R	NT	G_k	
Somatostatin	Nil	+	cAMP ↓	7,97
Galanin	R	+	cAMP ↑	47,98
Endothelin A	C	+	Ca ↑	57,99
B	C	+	Ca ↑	

C = contraction, R = relaxation, Nil = no response, NT = not tested, (Ap) = apamin sensitive receptor

TABLE 3
Receptors on Isolated Muscle Cells for Nonpeptides

	Pharmacological Response	Radioligand Binding	Messenger	Reference
Muscarinic M2	C	+	cAMP $\downarrow$	27,43,59,63,66
M3	C	+	Ca $\uparrow$/cAMP $\uparrow$	77,88,100,106
Adrenergic α2	C	+	Ca $\uparrow$/cAMP $\downarrow$	64
β2	R	+	cAMP $\uparrow$	30,65
Dopamine 1	R	NT	cAMP $\uparrow$	24
5-HT$_2$	R	+	Ca $\uparrow$	55,101
5-HT$_4$	C	+	cAMP $\uparrow$	
Histamine H$_1$	C	NT	Ca $\uparrow$	89
H$_2$	R	NT	cAMP $\uparrow$	
Adenosine A$_1$	C	NT	Ca $\uparrow$	102,103
A$_2$	R	NT	cAMP $\uparrow$	
Leukotriene C4	C	NT	Ca $\uparrow$	104
D4/E4	C	NT	Ca $\uparrow$	

C = contraction, R = relaxation, NT = not tested

CHARACTERIZATION OF RECEPTORS ON SMOOTH MUSCLE CELLS

PHARMACOLOGICAL CHARACTERIZATION OF RECEPTORS

Pharmacological characterization of receptors involves measurement of cell response (contraction, relaxation, changes in levels of intracellular messengers, etc.) in the presence or absence of specific antagonists. As for muscle strips, the measurements yield estimates of EC$_{50}$, IC$_{50}$, and inhibitory dissociation constants (K$_i$) by Schild analysis. The co-existence of receptor subtypes mediating opposite actions (see above) can complicate analysis unless the effect of one subtype is suppressed by the use of a subtype-specific antagonist. An alternative approach involves the use of agonists that are highly selective for a given receptor subtype. This approach has been effectively used to identify the presence of receptor subtypes for neurokinins (NK-1, NK-2 and NK-3),[52] cholecystokinin (CCK-A),[22,90,91] gastrin (CCK-B), pituitary adenylate cyclase activating peptide (PACAP) and VIP receptors (VIP/PACAP-II),[16,80,95,96,] opioid receptors (μ, κ, and δ),[41,92,93] neuropeptide Y (NPY-Y$_1$ and NPY$_2$),[94] acetylcholine (muscarinic M$_2$ and M$_3$),[43,86,88] serotonin (5-HT$_2$ and 5-HT$_4$),[55] histamine (H$_1$ and H$_2$),[89] and adenosine (A$_1$ and A$_2$).[102,103]

The same complements of receptors are present in smooth muscle cells from various regions of the gut. The main exceptions are the absence of opioid and NPY receptors from longitudinal muscle cells of the intestine in humans and animals.[41,51] Relatively minor species differences in receptor subtypes have been reported. Muscle cells from rat and hamster intestine possess NK-2b receptors whereas muscle cells from human, rabbit and guinea pig possess NK-2a receptors.[52,105] The distinction has been facilitated by the availability of species-specific selective neurokinin antagonists.

The absence of a contractile or relaxant response to an agonist need not imply the absence of receptor. Some agonists which have no contractile or relaxant effects can nonetheless act as modulatory agents that augment or inhibit the response to other agonists. Thus, somatostatin which has no direct contractile or relaxant effect on gastric muscle cells can inhibit relaxation induced by VIP or β-adrenergic agonists.[7,97] The effect reflects the ability of somatostatin to interact with a receptor negatively coupled to adenylate cyclase via an inhibitory G protein sensitive to pertussis toxin. Neuropeptide Y (NPY) is another example of a substance which can act as a neuromodulatory peptide.[94] Accordingly, measurements of mechanical response should be complemented by other cellular measurements and by radioligand binding.

CHARACTERIZATION OF RECEPTORS BY RADIOLIGAND BINDING

Receptors for a variety of transmitters and hormones have also been demonstrated on isolated smooth muscle cells by the technique of radioligand binding as indicated in Tables 2 and 3. This technique is similar to that described for binding of radioligands to membranes except that suspensions of smooth muscle cells are used. Briefly, a radioligand is added to a suspension of smooth muscle cells for a defined period, after which the radioligand bound to cells is separated from unbound radioligand by rapid centrifugation or filtration. Specific binding is determined from the difference between total and nonspecific binding; the latter is defined as binding in the presence of an excess of unlabeled ligand. Time course and temperature dependence are determined and saturation and competition curves constructed as for membranes.

The characterization of receptors by radioligand binding in isolated cells offers several advantages over pharmacological characterization of receptors, allowing direct analysis of the interaction of the ligand with the receptor and calculation of association and dissociation rate constants, affinity constants, the number of binding sites and the existence of high and low affinity states. Furthermore, radioligand binding can reveal the existence of receptors for modulatory ligands that do not elicit detectable pharmacological responses by themselves. Compared to pharmacological studies, radioligand binding studies require large numbers of cells ($1\text{--}3 \times 10^5$ cells per sample). While this is not a limiting factor in large animals, it precludes the use of isolated cells for measurement of binding in some locations, for example, sphincteric regions of small animals. In these regions, however, autoradiographic techniques have proved to be an alternative quantitative approach.[106]

Radioligand binding has also been used to characterize receptors in crude or purified tissue homogenates from smooth muscle.[107,108] Although neural membranes represent only a small percentage of the total mass of tissue, the density of receptors on neural membranes is higher than it is on smooth muscle membranes and can therefore contribute substantially to binding in crude homogenates. The use of differential centrifugation and density gradients can yield partially purified membrane preparations enriched in smooth muscle or nerve membranes, using 5′-nucleotidase activity and [^{3}H] saxitoxin as markers of smooth muscle and neural membranes.[83,109] Preparations enriched with neural membranes have been used to characterize neural receptors. It should be emphasized, however, that these membranes retain a substantial contaminant of muscle membranes as defined by the presence of 5′-nucleotidase activity. In contrast, muscle cell suspensions can be obtained that are entirely free of neural elements as determined by absence of saxitoxin binding and can be used to identify specifically receptors on smooth muscle cells.

The characteristics of receptors as determined by radioligand binding in suspensions of intact muscle cells more closely parallels the biological response of the cells. Binding to cells is maximal within the first 5–15 minutes and achieves near maximal binding within the first few minutes.[27,28,51,77,96,98,101] This is more consistent with the rapid biochemical and mechanical events which occur upon addition of agonists to tissues. In contrast, the kinetics of binding to membrane preparations requires 60–90 minutes to achieve a steady state.

The number of receptors for peptides on muscle cells is low by comparison with the number of receptors for non-peptides. Based on the binding of [^{3}H]quinuclidinyl benzilate or [^{3}H]-N-methylscapolamine, the number of muscarinic receptors in the stomach[27,110] and intestine[67] of various species ranges from 250,000 to 600,000 receptors per cell. Similar estimates have been obtained for the number of β-adrenergic receptors.[30] In contrast, the number of receptors for peptide transmitters and hormones is usually a 100-fold lower (1,000 receptors/cell for VIP,[16] ~5,000 receptors/cell for motilin,[68] and ~20,000 receptors/cell for galanin[98]).

Radioligand binding studies have confirmed the presence of opioid receptor subtypes on circular muscle of the intestine and their absence from longitudinal muscle.[51] Using selective synthetic ligands of each opioid receptor, the number of receptors for each subtype were 480 for δ receptors, 830 for μ receptors and 1120 for κ receptors. It is worth noting in this context that the original binding studies that identified the existence of opioid receptors utilized homogenates prepared from strips of longitudinal muscle with adherent myenteric plexus. Given the absence of receptors on longitudinal muscle, binding to the crude homogenates reflected exclusively binding to neural membranes, from cholinergic and noncholinergic neurons.

CHARACTERIZATION OF RECEPTORS BY SELECTIVE RECEPTOR PROTECTION

A technique of selective receptor protection, whereby smooth muscle cells can be enriched in a single receptor type has been used to facilitate receptor characterization in isolated muscle cells.[92] Muscle cells are incubated with a selective agonist or antagonist which interacts with and thus protects the receptor during the subsequent incubation with the alkylating agent, N-ethylmaleimide (NEM). After washing, cells treated in this manner respond only to agonists of the protected receptor. The cells retain their ability to respond to contractile or relaxant agents that bypass receptors, for example, calcium ionophores and derivatives of cyclic nucleotides.

The technique of selective protection is particularly useful when two or more subtypes of the same receptor coexist on smooth muscle cells. Three neurokinin receptor types have been identified in this fashion in muscle cells from circular and longitudinal muscle layers of rat intestine.[52] Cells in which the NK-1 receptors were preserved following protection with selective NK-1 agonists or antagonists responded only to selective NK-1 agonists (i.e., substance P methyl ester) with contraction and an increase in [Ca^{2+}]$_i$. Muscle cells in which the NK-2 receptors were preserved following protection with selective NK-2 agonists or antagonists responded only to the selective NK-2 agonist, [β-Ala^8]NKA$_{4-10}$. Finally, muscle cells where only NK-3 receptors were preserved following protection with an NK-3 agonist responded only to the selective NK-3 agonist, senktide. The endogenous agonists, substance P (SP) and neurokinin A (NKA) interacted preferentially with NK-1 and NK-2 receptors, respectively. NK-2 receptors exhibited species differences with one subtype, NK-2b, present in rat and hamster and a different subtype, NK-2a, present in guinea pig, rabbit and human. The analysis of the various receptor types by selective protection clearly indicated the coexistence of three distinct neurokinin receptors, each separately coupled to Ca^{2+} mobilization and contraction. The same approach has been used to identify receptor subtypes for the following peptide and non-peptide transmitters and hormones: CCK and gastrin,[22] the bombesin-like peptides, gastrin releasing peptide (GRP) and neuromedin B,[23] neuropeptide Y (NPY),[94] motilin,[68] opioid peptides,[51,92] vasoactive intestinal peptide (VIP) and its homologue, pituitary adenylate cyclase-activating peptide (PACAP),[72,80,95] adenosine,[102,103] histamine,[89] acetylcholine[88] and serotonin.[55]

The technique of receptor protection is also applicable to radioligand binding. Opioid δ, κ, and μ receptors on intestinal circular muscle cells have been identified in this fashion pharmacologically and by radioligand binding.[51] As shown in Figure 3, when μ receptors were preserved using the μ-selective agonist, D-Ala[2], N-Me-Phe[4], Gly[5]-ol (DAMGO), only DAMGO elicited contraction in or bound with high affinity to muscle cells; when δ receptors were preserved using the δ-selective agonist, [D-Pen[2,5]]-enkephalin (DPDPE), only DPDPE elicited contraction in or bound with high affinity to muscle cells; finally, when κ receptors were preserved with the κ-selective agonist, U-69,593, only U-69,593 elicited contraction in or bound with high affinity to muscle cells. Here also, the technique clearly demonstrated the coexistence of three opioid receptor types separately coupled to contraction. Among the endogenous opioid peptides, dynorphin interacted preferentially with κ receptors, [Methionine]enkephalin with δ receptors and [Leucine]enkephalin with μ and to a lesser extent with δ receptors.

It is worth noting that the signalling pathway reflected, for example, in IP$_3$ formation and Ca^{2+} mobilization, for contractile agonists was not affected by procedures involved in receptor protection. The use of NEM at low concentration (1 μM) and for a short period (20 min) insured that only unprotected receptors were inactivated leaving intact the signal transduction apparatus of the cell.

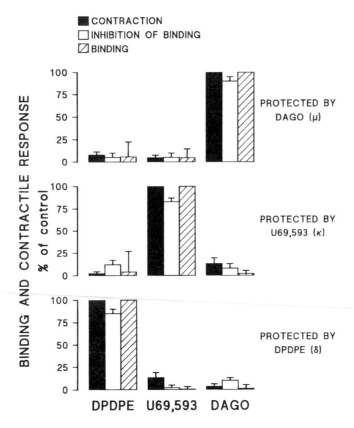

FIGURE 3 Contraction, specific binding of [^{3}H]ligand, and inhibition of binding of [^{3}H]ligand by unlabeled ligand in muscle cells from the rabbit intestine. Cells were enriched with only one opioid receptor type by the technique of receptor protection. Cells in which μ-receptors were protected with DAGO (upper panel), contracted only in response to DAGO, demonstrated specific binding of [^{3}H]DAGO only, and only unlabeled DAGO was able to inhibit binding. Cells in which κ-receptors were protected with U69,593 (middle panel), contracted only in response to U69,593, demonstrated specific binding of [^{3}H]U69,593 only, and only unlabeled U69,593 was able to inhibit binding. Cells in which δ-receptors were protected with DPDPE (lower panel), contracted only in response to DPDPE, demonstrated specific binding of [^{3}H]DPDPE only, and only unlabeled DPDPE was able to inhibit binding. (From *Am. J. Physiol.*, 263, G269, 1992, Figure 7. With permission.)

SIGNAL TRANSDUCTION PATHWAYS IN MUSCLE CELLS

The transduction of an external signal involves sequential activation of three membrane proteins: a membrane-spanning receptor, a GTP-binding protein (G protein) which couples the receptor to effector enzymes which act on membrane-bound, or cytoplasmic precursors to generate one or more messenger molecules. Isolated cell preparations have proven invaluable in identifying various steps in the signal transduction pathway in smooth muscle. The cellular homogeneity of cell suspensions enables measurements of biochemical changes in muscle cells. The cells can be permeabilized enabling the use of impermeant agents, such as GTPγS, GDPβS, IP_3 and even G protein and effector enzyme antibodies, to probe various steps in the signalling pathway. The cells retain enough receptors to enable them to maintain normal function. GTPγS has been used activate G protein directly and GDPβS to block G protein-dependent activation in muscle cells. The effect of some permeabilizing agents is reversible making it possible to insert an agent during a transient period of permeabilization after which the cell is re-sealed.

SECOND MESSENGERS MEDIATING CONTRACTION

Each step in the signalling cascade from receptor activation to the rise in intracellular calcium ($[Ca^{2+}]_i$) has been examined in isolated muscle cells. In cells isolated from the circular muscle layer of the intestine and stomach, Ca^{2+} mobilization is mediated by IP_3-dependent Ca^{2+} release from sarcoplasmic stores.[111,112,113] In these cells, contractile agonists, such as acetylcholine, substance P and cholecystokinin, stimulate preferentially hydrolysis of phosphatidylinositol 4,5-bisphosphate resulting in formation of IP_3 and diacylglycerol (Figure 4). Suppression of phosphoinositide hydrolysis by neomycin or U73,122 inhibits IP_3 formation, increase in $[Ca^{2+}]_i$ and contraction. Circular muscle cells possess high-affinity IP_3, heparin-sensitive receptors (Figure 5) that mediate Ca^{2+} release: addition of contractile agonists, GTPγS or IP_3

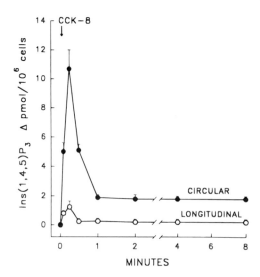

FIGURE 4 Kinetics of IP_3 production elicited by cholecystokinin (CCK-8) in suspensions of smooth muscle cells isolated from the circular and longitudinal muscle layers of guinea pig intestine. A similar pattern of rapid and preferential stimulation of IP_3 in circular muscle cells by contractile agents occurs in other mammalian species and other regions of the gut. (From *Am. J. Physiol.*, 261, G945, 1991, Figure 1. With permission.)

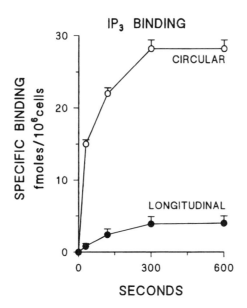

FIGURE 5   Kinetics of binding of [³H]IP₃ to permeabilized muscle cells isolated separately from the circular (open circles) and longitudinal (closed circles) muscle layers of rabbit intestine. (From *Am. J. Physiol.*, 266, C1421, 1994, Figure 4, lower. With permission.)

to permeabilized circular muscle cells causes Ca^{2+} release (measured in cells preloaded with $^{45}Ca^{2+}$; Figure 6), increase in $[Ca^{2+}]_i$ and contraction;[50,114] all these events are inhibited by the IP₃ antagonist, heparin.[114] The effects of GTPγS and agonists are inhibited additionally by the G protein inhibitor, GDPβS.[114] Depletion of Ca^{2+} stores by incubation of the cells with the sarcoplasmic Ca^{2+}/ATPase inhibitor, thapsigargin, in Ca^{2+}-free medium followed by restoration of Ca^{2+} abolishes agonist-induced Ca^{2+} mobilization in circular muscle cells thus confirming that the initial Ca^{2+} transient in these cells depends on Ca^{2+} release from intracellular stores and that this step is a prerequisite for subsequent Ca^{2+} mobilization.

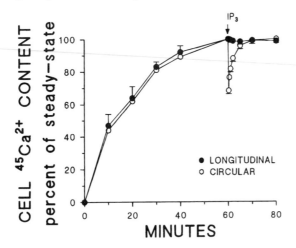

FIGURE 6   Net $^{45}Ca^{2+}$ efflux in response to IP₃ (10 μM) in permeabilized muscle cells isolated separately from the circular (open circles) and longitudinal (closed symbols) muscle layers of rabbit intestine. Intracellular Ca^{2+} stores were loaded by incubation in cytosolic medium containing $^{45}Ca^{2+}$; steady state was attained at 60 min. IP₃ caused release of Ca^{2+} from intracellular stores in circular but not longitudinal muscle. (From *Am. J. Physiol.*, 266, C1421, 1994, Figure 4, right. With permission.)

The G proteins and phospholipase C (PLC) isoforms to which they are coupled have been identified using a panel of G protein and phospholipase C antibodies and found to vary with agonist used.[103,115,116] Receptors for CCK are coupled mainly to activation of PLC-β1 and to a lesser extent, PLC-β3 via the α subunit of G_q. Receptors for adenosine (A_1 subtype), however, are coupled to activation of PLC-β3 via both the α and $\beta\gamma$ subunits of G_{i3}. The interactions with CCK and adenosine (or other receptors) results in IP_3 formation and IP_3-dependent Ca^{2+} mobilization.

In muscle cells isolated from the longitudinal muscle layer of rabbit, guinea pig and human intestine, Ca^{2+} mobilization is mediated by an IP_3-independent process.[50,111,114] Although phosphoinositide hydrolysis occurs in longitudinal muscle, the preferred substrate is phosphatidylinositol 4-monophosphate which generates diacylglycerol but not IP_3.[111] Suppression of phosphoinositide hydrolysis in this cell type has no effect on agonist-induced Ca^{2+} mobilization. The increase in cytosolic Ca^{2+} with agonists depends on an initial obligatory step involving influx of Ca^{2+} into the cell. Contraction and the increase in $[Ca^{2+}]_i$ in longitudinal but not circular muscle cells are abolished in Ca^{2+}-free medium or in the presence of Ca^{2+} channel blockers.[50,54,114] The initial influx of Ca^{2+} triggers release of Ca^{2+} from intracellular stores. These stores possess Ca^{2+} channels that are highly sensitive to Ca^{2+} and that bind both ryanodine (Figure 7) and cyclic ADP ribose with an affinity similar to that found in cardiac Ca^{2+} release channels.[50,117] In permeabilized longitudinal but not circular muscle, ryanodine and cADP ribose cause concentration-dependent release of Ca^{2+} (Figure 8). Small changes in ambient Ca^{2+} in the range of concentrations encountered within the cytosol (100–500 nM) cause Ca^{2+} release (i.e., Ca^{2+}-induced Ca^{2+} release) in longitudinal muscle cells.[50] Ca^{2+}-induced Ca^{2+} release occurs also in circular muscle cells but requires the presence of IP_3. After depletion of Ca^{2+} from intracellular stores in longitudinal muscle cells with thapsigargin, agonists elicit only transient, attenuated increases in $[Ca^{2+}]_i$ and contraction reflecting the component of Ca^{2+} influx only in the absence of subsequent Ca^{2+} release from intracellular stores.[50]

The mechanism responsible for the initial Ca^{2+} influx in longitudinal muscle involves G protein dependent activation of phospholipase A_2 (PLA_2) and generation of arachidonic acid.[118]

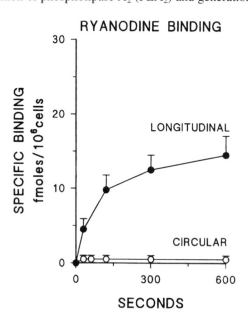

FIGURE 7   Kinetics of binding of [^{3}H]ryanodine to permeabilized muscle cells isolated separately from the circular (open circles) and longitudinal (closed circles) muscle layers of rabbit intestine. (From *Am. J. Physiol.*, 266, C1421, 1994, Figure 1, left. With permission.)

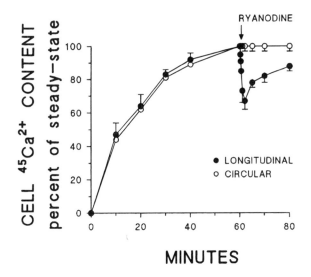

FIGURE 8 Net $^{45}Ca^{2+}$ efflux in response to ryanodine (10 μM) in permeabilized muscle cells isolated separately from the circular (open circles) and longitudinal (closed symbols) muscle layers of rabbit intestine. Intracellular Ca^{2+} stores were loaded by incubation in cytosolic medium containing $^{45}Ca^{2+}$; steady state was attained at 60 min. Ryanodine caused release of Ca^{2+} from intracellular stores in longitudinal but not circular muscle. (From *Am. J. Physiol.*, 266, C1421, 1994, Figure 4, upper. With permission.)

Contractile agonists cause an initial increase in arachidonic acid only in longitudinal muscle cells. Suppression of arachidonic acid release by selective PLA_2 inhibitors abolishes contraction and the increase in $[Ca^{2+}]_i$. Exogenous arachidonic acid causes contraction and an increase in $[Ca^{2+}]_i$ which can be abolished by Ca^{2+} channel blockers reflecting entry of Ca^{2+}. After depletion of Ca^{2+} from intracellular stores with thapsigargin, agonists, as noted above, and arachidonic acid elicit only transient, attenuated increases in $[Ca^{2+}]_i$ and contraction reflecting the component of Ca^{2+} influx only in the absence of subsequent Ca^{2+} release from intracellular stores.

Similar studies in isolated cells prepared from esophagus and lower esophageal sphincter (LES) suggest that Ca^{2+} mobilization in muscle from the sphincter, like those from the circular muscle layer of stomach and intestine, is mediated by IP_3-dependent Ca^{2+} release, whereas Ca^{2+} mobilization from muscle cells of the esophageal body depends on IP_3-insensitive Ca^{2+} influx.[3,5]

SECOND MESSENGERS MEDIATING RELAXATION

Relaxation of smooth muscle involves cAMP- and cGMP-dependent activation of protein kinases.[16,79,119,120] The kinases act by (i) inhibiting phosphoinositide metabolism and Ca^{2+} release from intracellular stores; (ii) stimulating Ca^{2+} uptake into the stores; (iii) decreasing the sensitivity of contractile proteins to Ca^{2+}, and (iv) by increasing (i.e., hyperpolarizing) membrane potential; the latter reflects the stimulation of plasmalemmal K^+ channels and inhibition of Ca^{2+} channels.[120,121,122]

Relaxant agents act variously to stimulate cAMP, cGMP or both cAMP and cGMP. β-adrenergic agonists and peptide histidine isoleucine (PHI) stimulate only cAMP, causing activation of cAMP-dependent protein kinase (cA-kinase), and at higher concentration, cross-activation of cGMP-dependent protein kinase (cG-kinase).[16,79,119] VIP and PACAP, on the other hand, cause an increase in both cAMP and cGMP, and stimulate both cA-kinase and cG-kinase at all concentrations (Figure 9).[16,79] Stimulation of cAMP results from activation of adenylate cyclase. Stimulation of cGMP and cG-kinase results from activation of a Ca^{2+}/calmodulin-sensitive constitutive nitric oxide synthase (NOS) located in smooth muscle plasma membranes.[15] The

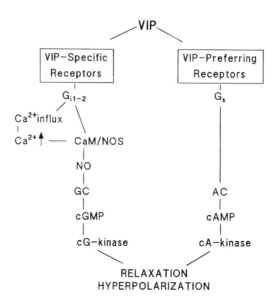

FIGURE 9 Signaling pathways activated by VIP. VIP interacts with VIP-preferring receptors to activate adenylate cyclase (AC) and generate cAMP, which, in turn activates cAMP-dependent protein kinase (cA-kinase). VIP interacts with VIP-specific receptors to induce G-protein coupled activation of a membrane-bound constitutive Ca^{2+}/calmodulin-dependent NO synthase (NOS) and generations of nitric oxide (NO). NO activates soluble guanylate cyclase (GC), leading to generation of cGMP and activation of cGMP-dependent protein kinase (cG-kinase). Both cA- and cG-kinase, separately and additively, induce relaxation and hyperpolarization of muscle cells. (*News in Physiol. Sci.*, 8, 195, 1993, Figure 2. With permission.)

process of activation of NOS is initiated by VIP/PACAP-mediated influx of Ca^{2+} and leads to a cascade involving generation of NO, activation of soluble guanylate cyclase, generation of cGMP and activation of cG-kinase. The steps in this cascade have been identified in isolated muscle cells from the stomach and intestine of several species, including human, dog, rat, guinea pig and rabbit.[8,16,78,79,123] As expected, NO generation is abolished by NOS inhibitors and Ca^{2+} channel blockers resulting in suppression of cGMP but not cAMP generation and resulting in partial inhibition of relaxation. Selective inhibitors of cA-kinase and cG-kinase cause partial inhibition of relaxation, and in combination, abolish relaxation.

The activity and location of smooth muscle NOS in the plasma membrane has been determined in membranes isolated from dispersed muscle cells.[15] NO generation in these membranes is induced by Ca^{2+} and is blocked by calmodulin and NOS inhibitors. GTPγS, VIP and PACAP selectively increase NO generation in a concentration-dependent fashion over and above Ca^{2+}-induced generation. The effect of VIP and PACAP is pertussis toxin sensitive and is selectively inhibited by antibodies to the α subunit of G_{i1-2}, clearly implying that smooth muscle NOS is a G protein-dependent regulatory enzyme.

Some peptide and non-peptide agonists are coupled to Ca^{2+} mobilization and/or inhibition of adenylate cyclase. In some instances, this occurs via distinct receptor subtypes (e.g., M_3 and M_2 muscarinic receptors; NPY Y_1 and Y_2 receptors)[88,94]; in other instances, the process occurs through the same receptors (e.g., adenosine A_1) coupled to different G protein subunits.[102]

ION CHANNELS IN SMOOTH MUSCLE CELLS

The plasma membrane of smooth muscle cells contains a variety of ion channels including passive ion-selective channels that regulate resting membrane potential and ion channels that are regulated (i.e. gated) by membrane potential (voltage-gated) and by various hormonal or neural agents (ligand-gated). The channels are usually selective for one ion such as Ca^{2+} or K^+, although some allow the passage of more than one ion (i.e. non-selective channels).

Ion channels in isolated smooth muscle cells of various regions of the gut have been studied by the patch clamp technique in which patches of plasmalemma can be electrically isolated by suction into the tip of a microelectrode where they form a tight seal.[4,6,12,13,39,40,44,74,91,124,125] This technique makes it possible to record current flow in one or a few channels in the patch. Patches can remain attached to the cell so that effects of ligands can be examined or the patch can be detached so that the inner (inside-out) or outer (outside-out) surface faces the medium. Detached patches are used to study the effects of intracellular messengers or changes in ion composition of the medium.

Application of these techniques have demonstrated the presence of voltage-gated Ca^{2+} channels in muscle cells from stomach and intestine which carry the inward Ca^{2+} current responsible for the upstroke of the fast action potential and the steady inward current observed during the plateau phase of the slow wave.[4,39,40,62,74,126,127] Several types of K^+ channels have also been identified in isolated smooth muscle cells. The most widely distributed is a high conductance Ca^{2+}-activated, voltage-sensitive K^+ channel.[6,40,74,127,128] These channels open when the membrane is depolarized and the levels of cytosolic Ca^{2+} are increased. The channels carry an outward current that drives membrane potential back towards the K^+ equilibrium potential. Thus, a stimulus that acts by inducing Ca^{2+} influx and membrane depolarization is terminated. Two additional K^+ channels have been identified in smooth muscle: a low conductance K^+ channel that opens during the prolonged depolarization such as occurs during the plateau phase of the slow wave,[74,125] and a channel with characteristics similar to that of K^+ channels in sympathetic neurons.[91,129,130] The latter is responsible for the outward current known as the M-current. High conductance non-selective voltage sensitive channels which carry K^+ and Na^+ currents have been also identified. These carry an inward depolarizing current that may be responsible for the pacemaker potential or prepotential that triggers the slow waves in some regions of the gut.

Ligand-gated channels have not been characterized to the same extent as voltage-gated channels. In smooth muscle undergoing rhythmic depolarization, agonists act to increase the influx of Ca^{2+} into the cell by way of ligand-gated and voltage-gated ion channels. In mammalian intestinal cells, depolarization is accompanied by an increase in membrane conductance which appears to reflect an increase in Ca^{2+} and other cationic inward currents and suppression of an outward K^+ current carried by Ca^{2+}-activated K^+ channels.[125]

The role of ion channels in contraction and relaxation is best examined in intact syncytia which undergo cyclical changes in membrane potential (i.e. slow waves). Slow waves that attain a critical level of depolarization can lead to opening of Ca^{2+} channels. This leads to Ca^{2+}-induced Ca^{2+} release, increase in $[Ca^{2+}]_i$ and a wave of contraction. Upon release, excitatory transmitters that activate Ca^{2+} or inhibit K^+ channels can cause a transient depolarization of membrane potential. Except in some regions where membrane potential is close to mechanical threshold, the depolarization is not sufficient to cause opening of Ca^{2+} channels and increase resting muscle tone. The main increase in $[Ca^{2+}]_i$ results from agonist-induced Ca^{2+} mobilization from intracellular stores as noted above. If the transient depolarization is superimposed over the depolarization induced by a slow wave, a larger wave of contraction ensues. Conversely, release of "inhibitory" transmitters, such as PHI, VIP and NO, acting via cA-and/or cG-kinase leads to inhibition of Ca^{2+} channel activity or stimulation of K^+ channel activity resulting in hyperpolarization of membrane potential. Hyperpolarization superimposed on resting membrane potential is unlikely to influence Ca^{2+} flux across the plasma membrane. However, when superimposed on a slow wave, it reduces the amplitude of the slow wave and prevents the opening of Ca^{2+} channels and thus, inhibits the wave of contraction.

SUMMARY AND CONCLUSIONS

Single cells and suspensions of muscle cells have been used effectively to characterize receptors pharmacologically as well as immunochemically by radioligand binding. Identification of receptor subtypes and their coexistence on the same cells have been facilitated by the development of selective receptor protection techniques that enable only one receptor subtype to be preserved. Suspensions of cells have also been used to define the signal transduction pathways involved in contraction and relaxation. Ca^{2+} mobilization in circular muscle was shown to depend on IP_3-dependent Ca^{2+} release whereas Ca^{2+} mobilization in longitudinal muscle was shown to depend on an initial Ca^{2+} influx that results in Ca^{2+}-induced Ca^{2+} release. The sarcoplasmic channels in circular and longitudinal muscle cells were shown to be different: those in circular muscle were sensitive to IP_3 whereas those in longitudinal muscle, akin to those in cardiac muscle, were sensitive to ryanodine and cADP ribose. Depending on the agonist, relaxation was shown to depend on activation of cAMP- and cGMP-dependent protein kinases. The cGMP pathway is selectively stimulated by VIP and PACAP and involves activation of a G protein-dependent constitutive NO synthase present in smooth muscle membranes.

ACKNOWLEDGMENT

Supported by grants DK15564 and DK28300 from the National Institutes of Diabetes, Digestive and Kidney Diseases.

REFERENCES

1. **Grider, J. R. and Makhlouf, G. M.,** Suppression of inhibitory neural input to colonic circular muscle by opioid peptides, *J. Pharmacol. Exp. Ther.,* 243, 205, 1987.
2. **Bauer, A. J. and Szurszewski, J. H.,** Effect of opioid peptides on circular muscle of canine duodenum, *J. Physiol. (Lond.), 434, 409, 1991.*
3. **Biancani, P. Hillemeier, C., Bitar, K. N., and Makhlouf, G. M.,** Contraction mediated by Ca^{2+} influx in esophageal muscle and by Ca^{2+} release in the LES, *Am. J. Physiol.* 253, G760, 1987.
4. **Sims, S. M., Vivaudou, M. B., Hillemeier, C., Biancani, P., Walsh, J. V., and Singer, J. J.,** Membrane currents and cholinergic regulation of K^+ current in esophageal smooth muscle cells, *Am. J. Physiol.* 258, G794, 1990.
5. **Biancani, P., Harnett, K. M., Sohn, U. D., Rhim, B. Y., Behar, J., Hillemeier, C., and Bitar, K. N.,** Differential signal transduction pathway in cat lower esophageal sphincter tone and response to ACh, *Am. J. Physiol.* 266, G767, 1994.
6. **Akbarali, H. I.,** K^+ currents in rabbit esophageal muscularis mucosae, *Am. J. Physiol.* 264, G1001, 1993.
7. **McHenry, L., Murthy, K..S., Grider, J. R., and Makhlouf, G. M.,** Inhibition of muscle cell relaxation by somatostatin: Tissue-specific, cAMP-dependent, pertussis toxin-sensitive. *Am. J. Physiol.,* 262, G45, 1991.
8. **Grider, J. R. and Jin, J-G.,** VIP-induced nitric oxide (NO) production and relaxation in isolated muscle cells of the gut in human and other mammalian species, *Gastroenterology,* 104, A515, 1993.
9. **Bitar, K. N., Burgess, G. M., Putney, J. W., and Makhlouf, G. M.,** Source of activator calcium in isolated guinea pig and human gastric muscle cells, *Am. J. Physiol.,* 250, G280, 1986.
10. **Bitar, K. N., Saffouri, B., and Makhlouf, G. M.,** Cholinergic and peptidergic receptors on isolated human antral smooth muscle cells, *Gastroenterology,* 82, 832, 1982.
11. **Ozaki, H., Zhang, L., Buxton, I. L. O., Sanders, K. M., and Publicover, N. G.,** Negative-feedback regulation of excitation-contraction coupling in gastric smooth muscle, *Am. J. Physiol.,* 263, C1160, 1992.

12. **Vogalis, F., Publicover, N. G., and Sanders, K. M.,** Regulation of calcium current by voltage and cytoplasmic calcium in canine gastric smooth muscle, *Am. J. Physiol.,* 262, C691, 1992.

13. **Sims, S. M.,** Cholinergic activation of a non-selective cation current in canine gastric smooth muscle is associated with contraction, *J. Physiol. (Lond.),* 449, 377, 1991.

14. **Collins, S. M.,** Calcium utilization by dispersed canine gastric smooth muscle cells, *Am. J. Physiol.,* 251, G181, 1986.

15. **Murthy, K. S. and Makhlouf, G. M.,** Vasoactive intestinal peptide/pituitary adenylate cyclase-activating peptide-dependent activation of membrane-bound NO synthase in smooth muscle mediated by pertussis toxin-sensitive G_{i1-2}, *J. Biol. Chem.,* 269, 15977, 1994.

16. **Murthy, K. S., Zhang, K-M., Jin, J-G., Grider, J. R., and Makhlouf, G. M.,** VIP-mediated, G-protein coupied Ca^{2+} influx activates a constitutive nitric oxide synthase and induces relaxation in dispersed gastric smooth muscle cells, *Am. J. Physiol.,* 265, G660, 1993

17. **Murthy, K. S., Jin, J-G., and Makhlouf, G. M.,** Inhibition of nitric oxide synthase activity in dispersed gastric muscle cells by protein kinase C, *Am. J. Physiol.,* 266, G161, 1994.

18. **Tomomasa, T., Hyman, P. E., Hsu, C. T., Jing, J., and Snape, W. J.,** Development of the muscarinic receptor in rabbit gastric smooth muscle, *Am. J. Physiol.,* 254, G680, 1988.

19. **Bitar, K. N. and Makhlouf, G. M.,** Relaxation of isolated gastric muscle cells by vasoactive intestinal peptide, *Science,* 216, 531, 1982.

20. **Bitar, K. N. and Makhlouf, G. M.,** Receptors on smooth muscle cells: characterization by contraction and specific antagonists, *Am. J. Physiol.,* 242, G400, 1982.

21. **Bitar, K. N. and Makhlouf, G. M.,** Measurement of function in isolated single smooth muscle cells, *Am. J. Physiol.,* 250, G357, 1986.

22. **Grider, J. R. and Makhlouf, G. M.,** Distinct receptors for cholecystokinin and gastrin on isolated cells of stomach and gallbladder, *Am. J. Physiol.,* 259, G184, 1990.

23. **Severi, C., Jensen, R. T., Erspamer, V., D'Arpino, L., Coy, D. H., Torsoli, A., and Delle Fave, G.,** Different receptors mediate the action of bombesin-related peptides on gastric smooth muscle cells, *Am. J. Physiol.,* 260, G683, 1991.

24. **Kurosawa, S., Hasler, W. L., Torres, G., Wiley, J. W., and Owyang, C.,** Characterization of receptors mediating the effects of dopamine on gastric smooth muscle, *Gastroenterology,* 100, 1224, 1991.

25. **Chijiiwa, Y., Kabemura, T., Misawa, T., Kawakami, O., and Nawata, H.,** Direct inhibitory effect of calcitonin gene-related peptide and atrial natriuretic peptide on gastric smooth muscle cells via different mechanisms, *Life Sci.,* 50, 1615, 1992.

26. **Chijiiwa, Y., Harada, N., Misawa, T., Yoshinaga, M., Kabemura, T., and Nawata, H.,** The direct contractile effect of gastrin releasing peptide on isolated gastric smooth muscle cells of the guinea pig, *Life Sci.,* 49, PL-173, 1991.

27. **Seidel, E. R. and Johnson, L. R.,** Contraction and [^{3}H]QNB binding in collagenase isolated fundic smooth muscle cells, *Am. J. Physiol.,* 245, G270, 1983.

28. **Maton, P. N., Sutliff, V. E., Zhou, Z-C., Collins, S. M., Gardner, J. D., and Jensen, R. T.,** Characterization of receptors for calcitonin gene-related peptide on gastric smooth muscle cells, *Am. J. Physiol.,* 254, G789, 1988.

29. **Menozzi, D., Gu, Z. F., Maton, P. N., and Bunnett, N. W.,** Inhibition of peptidases potentiates enkephalin-stimulated contraction of gastric muscle cells, *Am. J. Physiol.,* 261, G476, 1991.

30. **Zhang, L., Gu, Z. F., and Maton, P. N.,** Characterization of β-adrenoreceptors on smooth muscle cells from guinea pig stomach, *Am. J. Physiol.* 259, G436, 1990.

31. **Honda, T., Zhou, Z-C., Gu, Z-F., Kitsukawa, Y., Mrozinski, J. E., and Jensen, R. T.,** Structural analysis of CGRP receptors on gastric smooth muscle and pancreatic acinar cells, *Am. J. Physiol.,* 264, G1142, 1993.

32. **Behar, J., Rhim, B. Y., Thompson, W., and Biancani, P.,** Inositol trisphosphate restores impaired human gallbladder motility associated with cholesterol stones, *Gastroenterology,* 104, 563, 1993.

33. **Yu, P., DePetris, G., Biancani, P., Amaral, J., and Behar, J.,** Cholecystokinin-coupled intracellular signaling in human gallbladder muscle, *Gastroenterology,* 106, 763, 1994.

34. **Chijiiwa, K., Yamasaki, T., and Chijiiwa, Y.,** Direct contractile response of isolated gallbladder smooth muscle cells to cholecystokinin in patients with gallstones, *J. Surg. Res.,* 56, 434, 1994.

35. **Yamasaki, T., Chijiiwa, K., and Chijiiwa, Y.,** Direct contractile effect of motilin on isolated smooth muscle cells from human gallbladder, *J. Surg. Res.,* 56, 89, 1994.

36. **Severi, C., Grider, J. R., and Makhlouf, G. M.,** Identification of separate bombesin and tachykinin receptors on isolated muscle cells from canine gallbladder, *J. Pharmacol. Exp. Ther.,* 245, 195, 1988.

37. **Severi, C., Grider, J. R., and Makhlouf, G. M.,** Functional gradients in muscle cells isolated from the gallbladder cystic duct and common bile duct of the dog, *Am. J. Physiol.,* 255, G647, 1988.

38. **Severi, C., Grider, J. R., and Makhlouf, G. M.,** Characterization of opioid receptors on isolated canine gallbladder smooth muscle cells, *Life Sci.,* 42, 2373, 1988.

39. **Shimada, T.,** Voltage-dependent calcium channel current in isolated gallbladder smooth muscle cells of guinea pig, *Am. J. Physiol.,* 264, G1066, 1993.

40. **Zhang, L., Bonev, A. D., Nelson, M. T., and Mawe, G. M.,** Ionic basis of the action potential of guinea pig gallbladder smooth muscle cells, *Am. J. Physiol.,* 265, C1552, 1993.

41. **Bitar, K. N. and Makhlouf, G. M.,** Selective presence of opiate receptors on intestinal circular muscle cells, *Life Sci.,* 37, 1545, 1985.

42. **Micheletti, R., Grider, J. R., and Makhlouf, G. M.,** Identification of bombesin receptors on isolated muscle cells from human intestine, *Reg. Pept.,* 21, 219, 1988.

43. **Grider, J. R., Bitar, K. N., and Makhlouf, G. M.,** Identification of muscarinic M_2 receptors on single muscle cells of the human and guinea pig intestine, *Gastroenterology,* 93, 951, 1987.

44. **Farrugia, G., Irons, W. A., Rae, J. L., Sarr, M. G., and Szurszewski, J. H.,** Activation of whole cell currents in isolated human jejunal circular smooth muscle cells by carbon monoxide, *Am. J. Physiol.,* 264, G1184, 1993.

45. **Farrugia, G., Rae, J. L., Sarr, M. G., and Szurszewski, J. H.,** Potassium current in circular smooth muscle of human jejunum activated by fenamates, *Am. J. Physiol.,* 265, G873, 1993.

46. **Torihashi, S., Kobayashi, S., Gerthoffer, W. T., and Sanders, K. M.,** Interstitial cells in deep muscular plexus of canine small intestine may be specialized smooth muscle cells. *Am. J. Physiol.,* 265, G638, 1993.

47. **Botella, A., Delvaux, M., Frexinos, J., and Bueno, L.,** Comparative effects of galanin on isolated smooth muscle cells from ileum in five mammalian species, *Life Sci.,* 50, 1253, 1992.

48. **Botella, A., Delvaux, M., Bueno, L., and Frexinos, J.,** Intracellular pathways triggered by galanin to induce contraction of pig ileum smooth muscle cells, *J. Physiol. (Lond.)* 458, 475, 1992.

49. **Botella, A., Delvaux, M., Berry, P., Frexinos, J., and Bueno, L.,** Cholecystokinin and gastrin induce cell contraction in pig ileum by interacting with different receptor subtypes, *Gastroenterology,* 102, 779, 1992.

50. **Kuemmerle, J. F., Murthy, K. S., and Makhlouf, G. M.,** Agonist-activated, ryanodine-sensitive, IP_3-insensitive Ca^{2+} release channels in longitudinal muscle of intestine, *Am. J. Physiol.,* 266, C1421, 1994.

51. **Kuemmerle, J. F. and Makhlouf, G. M.,** Characterization of k, δ and μ opioid receptors in intestinal muscle cells by selective radioligands and receptor protection. *Am. J. Physiol.,* 263, G269, 1992.

52. **Hellstrom, P. M., Murthy, K. S., Grider, J. R., and Makhlouf, G. M.,** Coexistence of three tachykinin receptors coupled to one signalling pathway in intestinal muscle cells, *J. Pharmacol. Exp. Ther.,* 270, 236, 1994.

53. **Souquet, J. C., Bitar, K. N., Grider, J. R., and Makhlouf, G. M.,** Receptors for substance P on isolated intestinal smooth muscle cells of the guinea pig, *Am. J. Physiol.,* 253, G666, 1987.

54. **Grider, J. R. and Makhlouf, G. M.,** Contraction mediated by Ca^{2+} release in circular and Ca^{2+} influx in longitudinal intestinal muscle cells, *J. Pharmacol. Exp. Ther.,* 244, 432, 1988.

55. **Kuemmerle, J. F., Martin, D. C., Murthy, K. S., Kellum, J. M., Grider, J. R., and Makhlouf, G. M.,** Coexistence of contractile and relaxant 5HT receptors coupled to distinct signalling pathways in intestinal muscle cells: Convergence of the pathways on Ca^{2+} mobilization, *Molec. Pharmacol.,* 42, 1090, 1993.

56. **Harada, N., Chijiiwa, Y., Misawa, T., Yoshinaga, M., and Nawata, H.,** Direct contractile effect of motilin on isolated smooth muscle cells of guinea pig small intestine, *Life Sci.,* 51, 1381, 1992.

57. **Yoshinaga, M., Chijiiwa, Y., Misawa, T., Harada, N., and Nawata, H.,** Endothelin$_B$ receptor on guinea pig small intestinal smooth muscle cells, *Am. J. Physiol.,* 262, G308, 1992.

58. **Barocelli, E., Chiavarini, M., Ballabeni, V., Bordi, F., and Impicciatore, M.,** Interaction of selective compounds with muscarinic receptors at dispersed intestinal smooth muscle cells, *Br. J. Pharmacol.,* 108, 393, 1993.

59. **Thomas, E. A., Baker, S. A., and Ehlert, F. J.,** Functional role for the M_2 muscarinic receptor in smooth muscle of guinea pig ileum, *Molec. Pharm.,* 44, 102, 1993.

60. **Bitar, K. N. and Zhu, X-X.,** Expression of bombesin-receptor subtypes and their differential regulation of colonic smooth muscle contraction, *Gastroenterology,* 105, 1672, 1993.

61. **Post, J. M. and Hume, J. R.,** Ionic basis for spontaneous depolarization in isolated smooth muscle cells of canine colon, *Am. J. Physiol.,* 263, C691, 1992.

62. **Langton, P. D., Burke, E. P., and Sanders, K. M.,** Participation of Ca currents in colonic electrical activity, *Am. J. Physiol.,* 257, C451, 1989.

63. **Zhang, L., Horowitz, B., and Buxton, I. L. O.,** Muscarinic receptors in canine colonic circular smooth muscle, *Molec. Pharmacol.,* 40, 943, 1991.

64. **Zhang, L., Keef, K. D., Bradley, M. E., and Buxton, I. L. O.,** Action of alpha$_{2A}$-adrenergic receptors in circular smooth muscle of canine proximal colon, *Am. J. Physiol.,* 262, G517, 1992.

65. **Taniyama, K., Kuno, T., and Tanaka, C.,** Distribution of β-adrenoceptors associated with cAMP-generating system in cat colon, *Am. J. Physiol.,* 253, G378, 1987.

66. **Ringer, M. J., Hyman, P. E., Kao, H. W., Hsu, C. T., Tomomasa, T., and Snape, W. J.,** [^{3}H]QNB binding and contraction of rabbit colonic smooth muscle cells, *Am. J. Physiol.,* 253, G656, 1987.

67. **Ennes, H. S., McRoberts, J. A., Hyman, P. E., and Snape, W. J.,** Characterization of colonic circular smooth muscle cells in culture, *Am. J. Physiol.,* 263, G365, 1992.

68. **Hasler, W. L., Heldsinger, A., and Owyang, C.,** Erythromycin contracts rabbit colon myocytes via occupation of motilin receptors, *Am. J. Physiol.,* 262, G50, 1992.

69. **Bologna, S. D., Hasler, W. L., and Owyang, C.,** Down-regulation of motilin receptors on rabbit colon myocytes by chronic oral erythromycin, *J. Pharmacol. Exp. Ther.,* 266, 852, 1993.

70. **Bitar, K. N., Stein, S., and Omann, G. M.,** Specific G proteins mediate endothelin induced contraction, *Life Sci.,* 50, 2119, 1992.

71. **Xiong, Z., Sperelakis, N., Noffsinger, A., and Preiser, C. F.,** Changes in calcium channel current densities in rat colonic smooth muscle cells during development and aging, *Am. J. Physiol.,* 265, C617, 1993.

72. **Grider, J. R., Katsoulis, S., Schmidt, W. E., and Jin, J-G.,** Regulation of the descending relaxation phase of intestinal peristalsis by PACAP, *J. Autonom. Nerv. Syst.,* 50, 151, 1994.

73. **Grider, J. R. and Makhlouf, G. M.,** Enteric GABA: mode of action and role in the regulation of the peristaltic reflex, *Am. J. Physiol.,* 262, G690, 1992.

74. **Vogalis, F., Lang, R. J., Bywater, R. A. B., and Taylor, G. S.,** Voltage-gated ionic currents in smooth muscle cells of guinea pig proximal colon, *Am. J. Physiol.,* 264, C527, 1993.

75. **Obara, K.,** Isolation and contractile properties of single smooth muscle cells of the guinea pig tenia caeci, *Jpn. J. Physiol.,* 34, 41, 1984.

76. **Obara, K. and Yabu, H.,** Dual effect of phosphatase inhibitors on calcium channels in intestinal smooth muscle cells, *Am. J. Physiol.,* 264, C296, 1993.

77. **Mita, M. and Uchida, M. K.,** Muscarinic receptor binding and Ca^{2+} influx in the all-or-none response to acetylcholine of isolated smooth muscle cells, *Eur. J. Pharmacol.,* 151, 9, 1988.

78. **Grider, J. R., Murthy, K. N., Jin, J-G., and Makhlouf, G. M.,** Stimulation of nitric oxide from muscle cells by VIP: prejunctional enhancement of VIP release, *Am. J. Physiol.,* 262, G774, 1992.

79. **Jin, J-G, Murthy, K. S., Grider, J. R., and Makhlouf, G. M.,** Activation of distinct cAMP- and cGMP-dependent pathways by relaxant agents in isolated gastric muscle cells, *Am. J. Physiol.,* 264, G470, 1993.

80. **Jin, J-G, Katsoulis, S., Schmidt, W. E., and Grider, J. R.,** Inhibitory transmission in tenia coli mediated by distinct VIP and apamin-sensitive PACAP receptors, *J. Pharmacol. Exp. Ther.,* 270, 433, 1994.

81. **Bitar, K. N., Hillemeier, C., and Biancani, P.,** Differential regulation of smooth muscle contraction in rabbit internal anal sphincter by substance P and bombesin, *Life Sci.,* 47, 2429, 1990.

82. **Bagby, R. M., Young, A. M., Dodson, R. S., Fisher, B. A., and McKinnon, K.,** Contraction of single smooth muscle cells from Bufo marinus stomach, *Nature,* 234, 351, 1971.

83. **Ahmad, S., Allescher, H-D., Manaka, H., and Daniel, E. E.,** [³H]saxitoxin as a marker for canine deep muscular plexus neurons, *Am. J. Physiol.,* 255, G462, 1988.
84. **Collins, S. and Gardner, J. D.,** Cholecystokinin-induced contraction of dispersed smooth muscle cells, *Am. J. Physiol.,* 243, G497, 1982.
85. **Fay, F. S., Cooke, P. H., and Canaday, P. G.,** Contractile properties of isolated smooth muscle cells. In: *Physiology of Smooth Muscle,* eds. E. Bulbring and M. F. Shuba, 249, Raven Press, N. Y., 1976.
86. **Sims, S. and Janssen, L. J.,** Cholinergic excitation of smooth muscle, *NIPS* 8, 207, 1993.
87. **Singer, J. J. and Fay, F. S.,** Detection of contraction of isolated smooth muscle cells in suspension, *Am. J. Physiol.,* 232, C138, 1977.
88. **Murthy, K. S. and Makhlouf, G. M.,** Differential coupling of M_3 and M_2 muscarinic receptors to adenylate cyclase via distinct G protein subunits in dispersed muscle cells, *Gastroenterology,* 106, A828, 1994.
89. **Morini, G., Kuemmerle, J. F., Impicciatore, M., Grider, J. R., and Makhlouf, G. M.,** Coexistence of histamine H_1 and H_2 receptors coupled to distinct signal transduction pathways in isolated intestinal muscle cells, *J. Pharmacol. Exp. Ther.,* 264, 598, 1993.
90. **Morini, G., Barocelli, E., Impicciatore, M., Grider, J. R., and Makhlouf, G. M.,** Characterization of receptors for cholecystokinin on isolated intestinal muscle cells of the guinea pig, *Regl. Pept.,* 28, 313, 1990.
91. **Menozzi, D., Gardner, J. D., Jensen, R. T., and Maton, P. N.,** Properties of receptors for gastrin and CCK on gastric muscle cells, *Am. J. Physiol.,* 257, G73, 1989.
92. **Grider, J. R. and Makhlouf, G. M.,** Identification of opioid receptors on gastric muscle cells by selective receptor protection, *Am. J. Physiol.,* 260, G103, 1991,
93. **Zhang, L., Gu, Z. F., Pradhan, T., Jensen, R. T., and Maton, P. N.,** Characterization of opioid receptors on smooth muscle cells from guinea pig stomach, *Am. J. Physiol.,* 262, G461, 1992.
94. **Misra, S., Murthy, K. S., and Grider J. R.,** Characterization of distinct receptors and signaling pathways for neuropeptide Y (NPY) and related peptides on isolated gastric muscle cells, *Gastroenterology,* 104, A1053, 1993.
95. **Jin, J-G., Murthy, K. S., Grider, J. R., and Makhlouf, G. M.,** Characterization of PACAP receptors on dispersed gastric muscle cells of the rabbit, *Gastroenterology,* 106, A817, 1994.
96. **Chijiiwa, Y., Murthy, K. S., Grider, J. R., and Makhlouf, G. M.,** Expression of functional receptors for vasoactive intestinal peptide in freshly isolated and cultured gastric muscle cells, *Regl. Pept.,* 47, 223, 1993.
97. **Gu, Z. F., Pradhan, T., Coy, D. H., Mantey, S., Bunnett, N. W., Jensen, R. T., and Maton, P. N.,** Actions of somatostatins on gastric smooth muscle cells, *Am. J. Physiol.,* 262, G432, 1992.
98. **Gu, Z. F., Pradhan, T. K., Coy, D. H., and Jensen, R. T.,** Smooth muscle cells from guinea pig stomach possess high-affinity galanin receptors that mediate relaxation, *Am. J. Physiol.,* 266, G839, 1994.
99. **Kitsukawa, Y., Gu, Z. F., Hildebrand, P., and Jensen, R. T.,** Gastric smooth muscle cells possess two classes of endothelin receptors but only one alters contraction, *Am. J. Physiol.,* 266, G713, 1994.
100. **Eglen, R. M., Reddy, H., Watson, N., and Challiss, R. A. J.,** Muscarinic acetylcholine receptor subtypes in smooth muscle, *TIPS,* 15, 114, 1994.
101. **Kuemmerle, J. F., Murthy, K. S., and Makhlouf, G. M.** Co-expression of $5-HT_2$ and $5-HT_4$ receptors on human intestinal muscle cells coupled to distinct signaling pathways, *Gastroenterology,* 104, A537, 1993.
102. **Murthy, K. S., McHenry, L., and Makhlouf, G. M.,** Identification of a pertussis toxin (PTx)-sensitive adenosine A1 receptor coupled to Ca^{2+} mobilization and contraction in isolated intestinal muscle cells, *Gastroenterology,* 104, A842, 1993.
103. **Murthy, K. S. and Makhlouf, G. M.,** Adenosine A_1 receptor-induced PI hydrolysis, Ca^{2+} mobilization and contraction are mediated by $G_{i\alpha3}/G_{\beta\gamma}$ coupled to a distinct PLC-β isoform (PLC-β_3), *Gastroenterology,* 106, A828, 1994.
104. **DeLegge, M., Murthy, K. S., Grider, J. R., and Makhlouf, G. M.,** Characterization of distinct receptors for peptidyl leukotrienes LTC_4 and LTD_4/LTE_4 coupled to the same signalling pathway in isolated gastric muscle cells, *J. Pharmacol. Exp. Ther.,* 266, 857, 1993.

105. **Maggi, C. A., Patacchini, R., Giachetti, P. R., and Giachetti, A.,** Tachykinin receptors and tachykinin antagonists, *J. Autonomic. Pharmacol.* 13, 23, 1993.

106. **Von Schrenck, T., Wang, L. H., Coy, D. H., Villanueva, M. L., Mantey, S., and Jensen, R. T.,** Potent bombesin receptor antagonists distinguish receptor types, *Am. J. Physiol.,* 259, G468, 1990.

107. **Chen, C. K., McDonald, T. J., and Daniel, E. E.,** Galanin receptor in plasma membrane of canine small intestine circular muscle, *Am. J. Physiol.* 266, G113, 1994.

108. **Mao, Y. K., Wang, Y. F., and Daniel, E. E.,** Distribution and characterization of vasoactive intestinal polypeptide binding in canine lower esophageal sphincter, *Gastroenterology* 105, 1370, 1993.

109. **Kostka, P., Ahmad, S., Berezin, I., Kwan, C. Y., Allescher, H. D., and Daniel, E. E.,** Subcellular fractionation of the longitudinal smooth muscle/myenteric plexus of dog ileum: Dissociation of the distribution of two plasma membrane marker enzymes, *J. Neurochem.,* 49, 1124, 1987.

110. **Collins, S. W. and Crankshaw, D. S.,** Identification of putative muscarinic receptors in isolated smooth muscle cells from canine gastric corpus by contraction studies and [^{3}H] quinuclidinyl benzilate binding, *Gastroenterology,* 84, 1128, 1983.

111. **Murthy, K. S. and Makhlouf, G. M.,** Phosphoinositide metabolism in intestinal smooth muscle: preferential production of Ins (1,4,5)P$_3$ in circular muscle cells, *Am. J. Physiol.,* 261, G945, 1991.

112. **Murthy, K. S., Grider, J. R., and Makhlouf, G. M.,** InsP$_3$-dependent Ca^{2+} mobilization in circular but not longitudinal muscle cells of intestine, *Am. J. Physiol.,* 261, G937, 1991.

113. **Bitar, K. N., Bradford, P., Putney, J. W., and Makhlouf, G. M.,** Stoichiometry of contraction and Ca^{2+} mobilization by inositol 1,4,5-trisphosphate in isolated gastric smooth muscle cells, *J. Biol. Chem.,* 261, 16591, 1986.

114. **Murthy, K. S., Grider, J. R., and Makhlouf, G. M.,** Receptor-coupled G-proteins mediate contraction and Ca^{2+} mobilization in isolated intestinal muscle cells, *J. Pharmacol. Exp. Ther.,* 260, 90, 1992.

115. **Murthy, K. S. and Makhlouf, G. M.,** Functional characterization of phosphoinositide-specific phospholipase C-β1 and β3 in intestinal smooth muscle, *Am. J. Physiol.,* In press, 1994.

116. **Murthy, K. S. and Makhlouf, G. M.,** Identification of phospholipase-β as the main isoenzyme responsible for G protein-coupled hydrolysis of phosphoinositides in intestinal muscle cells, *Gastroenterology,* 102, A747, 1992.

117. **Kuemmerle, J. F. and Makhlouf, G. M.,** Activation of ryanodine receptor/Ca^{2+} channels in longitudinal muscle cells by cyclic ADP ribose: Endogenous modulator of Ca^{2+} release, *Gastroenterology,* 106, A821, 1994.

118. **Murthy, K. S. and Makhlouf, G. M.,** Agonist-mediated G protein-coupled activation of PLA$_2$ generates arachidonic acid (AA) and triggers Ca^{2+} influx in longitudinal muscle cells, *Gastroenterology,* 106, A828, 1994.

119. **Gu, Z. F., Jensen, R. T., and Maton, P. N.,** A primary role for protein kinase A in smooth muscle relaxation induced by adrenergic agonists and neuropeptides, *Am. J. Physiol.,* 263, G360, 1992.

120. **Murthy, K. S., Severi, C., Grider, J. R., and Makhlouf G. M.,** Inhibition of inositol 1,4,5-trisphosphate (IP$_3$) production and IP$_3$-dependent Ca^{2+} mobilization by cyclic nucleotides in isolated gastric muscle cells, *Am. J. Physiol.,* 264, G967, 1993.

121. **Kume, H., Takai, A., Tokuno, H., and Tomita, T.,** Regulation of Ca^{2+}-dependent K$^+$ channel activity in tracheal myocytes by phosphorylation, *Nature,* 341, 152, 1989.

122. **Furukawa, K., Oshima, N., Tawada-Iwata, Y., and Shigekawa, M.,** Cyclic GMP stimulates Na$^+$/Ca^{2+} exchange in vascular smooth muscle cells in primary culture, *J. Biol. Chem.,* 266, 12337, 1991.

123. **Murthy, K. S., Jin, J-G., and Makhlouf, G. M.,** VIP-induced activation of NO synthase in circular muscle cells of dog colon, *Gastroenterology,* 106, A545, 1994.

124. **Benham, C. D. and Bolton, T. B.,** Patch-clamp studies of slow potential-sensitive potassium channels in longitudinal smooth muscle cells of rabbit jejunum, *J. Physiol. (Lond.),* 340, 469, 1983.

125. **Bolton, T. B., Lang, R. J., Takewaki, T., and Benham, C. D.,** Patch and whole-cell voltage clamp of single mammalian visceral and vascular smooth muscle cells, *Experimentia,* 41, 887, 1985.

126. **Ganitkevich, V. Y., Shuba, M. F., and Smirnov, S. V.,** Potential-dependent calcium inward current in a single smooth muscle cell of the guinea pig tenia caeci, *J. Physiol. (Lond.)* 381, 1, 1986.

127. **Mitra, R. and Morad, M.,** Ca^{2+} and Ca^{2+}-activated K^+ currents in mammalian gastric smooth muscle cells, *Science,* 229, 269, 1985.

128. **Benham, C. D., Bolton, T. B., Lang, R. J., and Takewaki, T.,** Calcium-activated potassium channels in single smooth muscle cells of rabbit jejunum and guinea pig mesenteric artery, *J. Physiol. (Lond.)* 371, 45, 1986.

129. **Sims, S. M., Singer, J. J., and Walsh, J. V.,** Cholinergic agonists suppress a potassium current in freshly dissociated smooth muscle cells of the toad, *J. Physiol. (Lond.)* 367, 503, 1985.

130. **Sims, S. M., Clapp, L. H., Walsh, J. V., and Singer, J. J.,** Dual regulation of M current in gastric smooth muscle cells: β-adrenergic-muscarinic antagonism, *Pflugers Arch.,* 417, 291, 1990.

11 In Vitro Electrophysiological Methods in Gastrointestinal Pharmacology

James J. Galligan

INTRODUCTION

This chapter will focus on techniques used to study electrophysiological properties of gastrointestinal smooth muscle and enteric neurons *in vitro*. The information provided is a basic introduction and overview of each method. As part of this introduction, the technical and theoretical problems associated with electrophysiological studies of smooth muscle and neurons will be discussed.

ELECTROPHYSIOLOGY OF GASTROINTESTINAL (GI) SMOOTH MUSCLE

Studies of GI smooth muscle are accomplished in two types of preparations: 1) intact tissues obtained from experimental animals or humans and 2) dispersed smooth muscle cells. Electrophysiological studies of GI smooth muscle in intact tissues are complicated by several functional and structural properties of these preparations.

MULTIFUNCTIONAL COMPONENTS OF INTACT GI PREPARATIONS

GI tissues contain multiple cell types. In addition to smooth muscle cells, there are nerves and non-neuronal cells which can affect smooth muscle electrical activity. Nervous elements include cell bodies and terminals of myenteric and submucosal neurons and the terminals of extrinsic, sympathetic, parasympathetic and sensory nerves which are capable of releasing neurotransmitter during the course of most *in vitro* experiments. Spontaneous or evoked release of neurotransmitter can alter electrical properties of GI smooth muscle and the investigator needs to account for neurotransmitter-induced effects. However, for many experiments, nerves in the preparation are to the investigator's advantage as studies of neuromuscular transmission are the focus of the study. Using appropriate stimulus parameters and drugs, the investigator can study the electrophysiological basis for neuromuscular transmission in the GI tract.[1,2]

GI smooth muscle exhibits rhythmic electrical activity called slow waves or electrical control activity.[3,4,5] The apparently spontaneous rhythmic activity may arise from the cyclic activity of specialized cells called interstitial cells of Cajal.[6] The interstitial cells may induce cyclic electrical activity in GI smooth muscle cells via direct electrical coupling.[7] In intact preparations of GI smooth muscle, nerve stimulation or drugs which mimic or block the action of nerves could affect the activity of interstitial cells and thereby indirectly alter smooth muscle electrical activity.

It is assumed that electrical activity of smooth muscle in a given layer is homogenous but a number of studies have shown that this assumption is not valid. For example, in dog colon, circular muscle cells close to the myenteric plexus have a resting membrane potential near -45 mV and exhibit spontaneous potential oscillations which cycle at a frequency of 20/min. Circular muscle cells near the submucosal border have a resting membrane potential of -70 mV and exhibit slow waves which cycle at a frequency of 5/min.[8,9] Methods which record electrical activity of bulk circular muscle would not detect heterogeneity in resting membrane potential or cyclic activity and would record only the sum of these electrical activities.

ELECTRICAL COUPLING BETWEEN GI SMOOTH MUSCLE CELLS

GI smooth muscle cells are connected by low resistance gap junctions.[1,10] Gap junctions permit passive current spread through the muscle layer which behaves as a functional syncytium and synchronizes the activity of large groups of cells.[1,3–5,11] Coupling complicates measurement of electrophysiological properties of smooth muscle cells in intact preparations. The response to a current pulse injected into single smooth muscle cells, either by a microelectrode or via the action of a neurotransmitter, is dissipated 3 dimensionally throughout the group of coupled cells so that the passive or active properties of single cells can not be measured.[1,12] Methods have been developed that take advantage of electrical coupling to measure smooth muscle membrane potential and resistance in intact preparations.

EXTRACELLULAR SPACE AND SURFACE TO VOLUME RATIO

GI smooth muscle has a large surface to volume ratio.[13,14] Small changes in ion permeability can lead to local extracellular or intracellular accumulation of ions (particularly K^+) near the membrane of individual cells. The extracellular fluid between individual muscle cells also has limited exchange with the bulk extracellular solution used during *in vitro* experiments. Limited exchange and local increases or depletion of ions near the membrane of smooth muscle cells result in ionic gradients that are different from those calculated based on concentrations in the bulk extracellular fluid.[13,14]

SUCROSE GAP

SINGLE SUCROSE Gap

The single sucrose gap method was introduced by Stampfli[15] who used it to study frog myelinated nerves and this method was adapted for studies of electrical activity in GI smooth muscle.[16,17] Szurszewski has provided a detailed discussion of the practical and theoretical issues associated with use of the sucrose gap method for measurements of membrane potential.[18]

The sucrose gap technique takes advantage of electrical coupling between smooth muscle cells and records *relative* changes in potential between two groups of smooth muscle cells separated by a flowing stream of a nonionic sucrose solution (Figure 1A). A 10% w/v sucrose solution with a high specific resistance (>2 megohms/cm) flows around a segment of the smooth muscle preparation. The flowing sucrose solution forms a zone of high extracellular resistance and all current must flow across the tissue membrane or along the longitudinal axis of muscle fibers. One end of the tissue is depolarized by a high K^+ solution and the potential difference between the depolarized tissue and the test tissue is measured. Drugs can be added to the flowing Krebs solution bathing the test tissue or this tissue can be stimulated electrically to study nerve-mediated changes in membrane potential. As originally designed, the single sucrose gap measured only relative changes in membrane potential. Recently, the single sucrose gap has been modified to measure membrane potential and resistance.[19]

DOUBLE SUCROSE GAP

The double sucrose gap measures membrane potential and resistance simultaneously.[18] Two flowing sucrose solutions are used to isolate a node of smooth muscle (Figure 1B). The node width should be less than 1 length constant (~1 mm) so that smooth muscle cells within the node are isopotential. The two ends of the smooth muscle strip are polarized using a high K^+ solution. The potential difference between the node and one end of the tissue is measured while the potential in the node can be changed by current pulses passed between the second polarized end and the node. Using Ohm's Law ($V = IR$), the amplitude of electrotonic potentials produced by constant current pulses will yield a measurement of membrane resistance of smooth muscle cells within the node during nerve- mediated or drug-induced responses. As the electrical activity of an intact strip of GI smooth muscle is studied, the contractile activity of the strip can be measured during sucrose gap recordings (Figure 1B). This capability has functional utility when trying to relate changes in electrical activity to smooth muscle motor activity.[18]

When configured with the appropriate electronics, the double sucrose gap can be used to voltage clamp the potential of smooth muscle cells in the node (Figure 1C).[18,20] An excellent review of the practical and theoretical advantages and limitations of voltage clamping using the double sucrose gap has been provided previously by Bolton et al. and the reader is referred to this review for a detailed discussion of voltage clamp using the double sucrose gap.[21] As with potential measurements, the node width when voltage clamping should be less than 1 length constant to increase the probability that the node remains isopotential. However, as the procedures used to prepare a strip of smooth muscle for double sucrose gap recordings damage some cells in the preparation, small nodal widths (< 0.2 mm) contain a greater fraction of damaged smooth muscle cells and are associated with large increases in series resistance. For voltage clamp, the optimal node width is 0.5 mm.[18,20,21] When microelectrodes are inserted into cells within the node it has been shown that there is reasonable agreement between potential measurements made with intracellular electrodes and those made between the polarized tissue and the node. Furthermore, it has also been demonstrated that cells within the node under optimal conditions are all at similar membrane potentials.[20,22] Therefore, measurements of conductance associated with changes in membrane potential or with the action of neurotransmitters or drugs can be made under voltage clamp conditions when slowly developing currents are studied (>100 ms).[20] In addition, the properties of agonist- or neurotransmitter-regulated channels can be studied under conditions when contributions of voltage-operated channels are minimized.[20]

The single and double sucrose gap can provide reasonably accurate measurements of membrane potential and resistance of GI smooth muscle. These measurements provide important information when the investigator is attempting to determine mechanisms of drug, hormone or

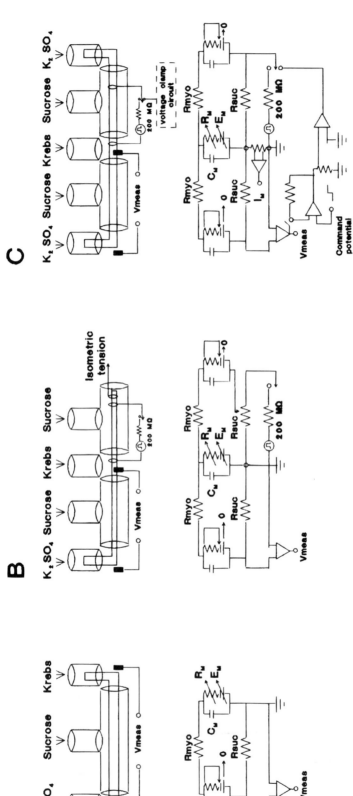

FIGURE 1 Schematic representation of single and double sucrose gap methods. A. Single sucrose gap. Upper, a muscle strip extends from the Krebs solution through the sucrose solution into an isotonic K_2SO_4 solution. All solutions flow continuously. The length of the sucrose gap is 7-10mm. Lower, equivalent circuit of the experimental arrangement. V_{meas}, measured potential difference between the test gap and the K_2SO_4 solution, R_m, C_m and V_m are membrane resistance, capacitance and potential respectively. R_{suc}, resistance of the sucrose solution; R_{myo}, longitudinal resistance of the smooth muscle. B. Double sucrose gap. Upper, a second sucrose gap containing a stimulating electrode has been added. The distance between stimulating electrodes is 10mm, width of tissue exposed to Krebs solution is 0.5 - 0.9 mm. Lower, equivalent circuit for the double sucrose gap. C. Double sucrose gap for voltage clamp. Upper, a second pool of depolarizing K_2SO_4 solution has been added to the double sucrose gap and a current supplying electrode is positioned in this gap. The width of the tissue exposed to Krebs solution is 0.1 - 0.15 mm. Lower, equivalent circuit of the experimental arrangement. (Modified from reference 18. With permission.)

neurotransmitter action on GI smooth muscle. Although, recordings can be maintained for several hours, exposure of muscle strips to sucrose solutions of low ionic strength depletes intracellular ions in the exposed tissue and ion depletion limits the duration of tissue viability.[18]

MICROELECTRODE RECORDINGS FROM INTACT TISSUES

Types of Microelectrodes

Two types of microelectrodes have been used to record electrical activity from smooth muscle *in vitro;* extracellular glass "pressure electrodes" and intracellular microelectrodes. Extracellular electrodes were first used by Bortoff and co-workers[23] to record slow waves from gastric smooth muscle. Capillary tubing or fire-polished microelectrodes filled with physiological saline solutions record electrical activity of smooth muscle cells when the electrodes are pressed firmly against the muscle layer. Extracellular recordings measure the potential difference between the tissue under the electrode and the bath ground. Extracellular electrodes are appropriate for recording slow waves and action potentials. When multiple electrodes are used, propagation of myoelectric events throughout the tissue can be studied in detail.[23,24] In addition, extracellular electrodes can record electrical activity from actively contracting tissues. However, extracellular electrodes do not directly measure membrane potential, resistance or the ionic basis for changes in electrical activity. Studies using intracellular microelectrodes provide this information.

Bulbring first applied intracellular microelectrode recording methods to the study of GI smooth muscle in her studies of guinea pig taenia coli.[25] Intracellular microelectrodes are glass electrodes filled with a 1–3 M KCl solution. Smooth muscle cells are impaled by advancing the microelectrode into the muscle layer using a micromanipulator until there is a sudden drop in electrode tip potential. Certain criteria must be met before an impalement of a cell is considered successful. These criteria include a membrane potential more negative than -50 mV that is stable for more than 5 minutes.

One of the main difficulties encountered with intracellular recordings is that muscle movement frequently dislodges the microelectrode. Many investigators take no special precautions to minimize movements of the muscle but it is possible to inhibit contractions in order to increase the duration of intracellular impalements. Lowering the temperature of the superfusing solution (<34 C),[22,26] using a hypertonic extracellular solution[27] or adding dihydropyridine calcium channel antagonists to the extracellular solutions[28–30] are treatments that minimize muscle movements during intracellular recordings.

TISSUE PREPARATION FOR INTRACELLULAR RECORDINGS

Esophageal Smooth Muscle

Smooth muscle cells in opossum esophagus and lower esophageal sphincter have been studied using intracellular microelectrodes.[26,31] The esophagus and a portion of the stomach are removed from the donor animal and the tissue is placed in physiological salt solution. The esophagus is cut open along its long axis and pinned flat in dissecting dish with the mucosal surface up. The dissecting dish is lined with a transparent silastic elastomer (Sylgard[R], Dow Corning, Midland, MI) and fine dissecting pins are used to fix the tissue in place. The mucosa and submucosa are removed using fine forceps and a scalpel and small strips of tissue are transferred serosal surface up to a recording chamber.

Gastric Smooth Muscle

Extracellular and intracellular electrical activity have been recorded from circular and longitudinal muscle cells in the stomach of cat,[23] dog,[24,32,33] guinea pig[34] and human[33] and from the muscularis mucosae of the dog stomach.[35] A portion of the stomach is cut open along the greater or lesser curvature and the tissue is pinned flat in a dissecting dish. The mucosal layer is removed by gentle scraping with forceps or a scalpel. The remaining tissue is transferred to a small recording chamber lined with Sylgard® and the tissue is pinned flat. In guinea pig stomach, the tissue is pinned serosal side up and microelectrodes are inserted directly into the longitudinal muscle or passed through the longitudinal muscle layer to impale circular muscle cells.[34] In canine stomach, transverse or longitudinal sections of tissue can be cut so that muscle cells at specific depths along the circular muscle layer can be impaled (Figure 2).[32]

Small Intestinal Smooth Muscle

Microelectrode recordings of electrical activity have been obtained from smooth muscle cells in small intestine of several species, including humans.[3,36-38] In most experiments, full thickness preparations of intestine are pinned flat in a recording chamber with the serosal surface up. Intracellular microelectrodes are inserted directly into longitudinal smooth muscle cells or the electrode is passed through the longitudinal muscle layer into the underlying circular muscle. Extracellular recordings from the longitudinal muscle can be obtained by pressing the electrode directly against the longitudinal muscle while a portion of the longitudinal muscle must be dissected away to expose a small area of circular muscle for circular muscle recordings.

In addition to basic studies of electrical behavior of smooth muscle cells and their innervation, preparations of guinea pig ileum have been used in conjunction with microsurgical techniques to study the length and polarity of projections of excitatory and inhibitory motorneurons along the small intestine.[28,39] In these studies, ascending and descending pathways in the myenteric plexus were surgically interrupted by severing the longitudinal-muscle myenteric plexus around

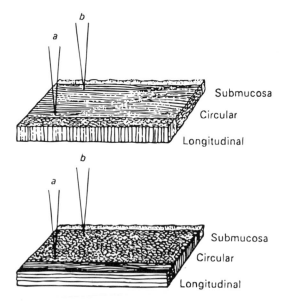

FIGURE 2   Cross-sectional preparations of gastric antral muscle. Top, preparation cut parallel to the circular muscle fibers; Bottom, preparation cut perpendicular to the circular muscle fibers. Cells can be impaled close to the myenteric plexus (a) or submucosa (b) with separate electrodes. (From Bauer, A. J., et al., *J. Physiol.*, 366, 221, 1985. With permission.)

the circumference of the ileum. Several days after surgery, which is sufficient time to allow severed axons to degenerate, the operated segment and surrounding tissue were removed from the animal and prepared for intracellular recording from smooth muscle cells. By recording the amplitude of excitatory or inhibitory junction potentials evoked by electrical stimulation (see below) at various distance oral and aboral to the lesion it is possible to estimate the length of projections of motorneurons. Guinea pig ileum has also been used to study reflex activation of excitatory or inhibitory motorneurons.[29,40] Reflexes were activated in two ways. In one set of experiments the mucosa was exposed by opening the intestine at either end of an intact segment.[29] The mucosa in the exposed end was stroked by a fine brush and intracellular recordings were obtained from smooth muscle cells in the intact segment. In another kind of experiment, a segment of ileum was pinned flat with the mucosal surface up. The preparation was positioned over two inflatable balloons which could distend the segment wall without deforming the mucosa while the mucosa could be compressed with a sponge without balloon distention.[40] Recordings were obtained from smooth muscle at the oral or aboral ends of the preparation.

Colonic Smooth Muscle

Microelectrode studies of electrical activity colonic smooth muscle have been done in tissues obtained from guinea pig,[27,41] cat,[42] dog,[8,9,11] mouse[43] and humans[44–46]. A segment of colon is cut open along the mesenteric attachment and pinned flat in a dissecting dish as described above. The mucosa is stripped away using forceps. A small piece of dissected colon with the longitudinal muscle layer up is transferred to a recording dish. In guinea pig and mouse colon microelectrodes are inserted directly into longitudinal muscle cells or passed through the longitudinal muscle into the circular muscle layer. Extracellular electrodes can be pressed directly against the longitudinal muscle or onto the circular muscle after a small section of longitudinal muscle is removed. In dog colon, the tissue can be cut and pinned flat in such a way as to make recordings from smooth muscle cells at different points along the thickness of the circular muscle layer.[8,9] This latter method is similar to that described above for dog stomach (Figure 2).

MEASUREMENTS OF MEMBRANE RESISTANCE

Electrical coupling between GI smooth muscle cells complicates measurements of input resistance when using intracellular microelectrodes. Most amplifiers used for intracellular electrophysiological recordings have circuitry that permits simultaneous measurement of membrane potential and current injection into the cell through the microelectrode. However, current passed through the recording microelectrode into the impaled cell spreads through the syncytium in 3 dimensions and measurements of resistance in a single cell are inaccurate.[12] Abe and Tomita[27] developed an apparatus that can polarize a length of tissue in the longitudinal axis and the potential response to polarizing currents is recorded at various distances from the polarizing electrode (Figure 3). The validity of this method is based on the assumption that the passive electrical properties of a strip of smooth muscle behave according to the predictions of cable equations developed for current spread in axons.[47] Studies by Abe and Tomita[27] and others have shown that this assumption is generally valid for strips smooth muscle.[11,12,48] Using the Abe and Tomita chamber, measurements of length and time constants of smooth muscle can be obtained using cable equations and the amplitude of electrotonic potentials evoked by polarizing current pulses is used to measure input resistance of smooth muscle.[11,12,48] Accurate measurements of length and time constants are obtained only when the length of polarized tissue is longer than 3-length constants.[48] In addition, the amplitude of the current pulses should be relatively small (< 0.25 V/cm) to avoid activation of nerves or voltage-dependent conductances and the duration of the pulses should be sufficiently long (several seconds) to

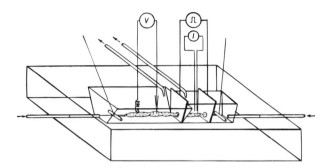

FIGURE 3 Recording and stimulating arrangement for partition method for polarizing smooth muscle cells in intact muscle strips. The muscle chamber is divided into two parts using stimulating electrodes. The stimulating electrodes are silver or platinum foil plates separated by a distance of 10 mm. The chamber are perfused separately with Krebs solution. (From Abe, Y. and Tomita, T., *J. Physiol.*, 196, 87, 1968. With permission.)

allow the membrane potential change to reach steady state. Finally, the polarity of the pulses should be alternated to avoid polarization of the stimulating electrodes.[48] When appropriate precautions are taken, extracellular polarization of the smooth muscle preparation provides accurate measurements of membrane resistance, length constant and time constant when intracellular microelectrodes are used to record membrane potential responses.

NERVE STIMULATION

Nerves can be stimulated electrically in a number of ways. First, when using the Abe-Tomita chamber,[27] the polarizing electrodes can stimulate nerve pathways that project in the long axis of the tissue. High stimulus strengths (> 25 V/cm) and short pulse durations (≤ 0.5 ms) selectively stimulate the nerves without directly depolarizing muscle cells.[48] Secondly, transmural stimulation using electrodes made of Ag/AgCl wire or platinum wire or foil is accomplished by positioning electrodes on either side of the long axis of the tissue; this arrangement stimulates all nerve fibers in the tissue.[34,45] Nerves can also be stimulated transmurally by positioning one electrode in the bath several centimeters from the recording electrode while the second stimulating electrode is positioned on the tissue near the recording electrode.[49,50] Finally, nerve fibers with longitudinal or circumferential orientations can be selectively stimulated by appropriate placement of transmural electrodes.[28,39] Stimulating electrodes positioned above and below the tissue at one end will stimulate all axons that project from the site of stimulation in the long axis of the tissue. By positioning the transmural electrodes in transverse arrangement, nerve fibers projecting from the site of stimulation in the circumferential axis of the tissue can be stimulated selectively.[28,39] The portions of the electrodes that extend beyond the width or length of the tissue should be insulated with a nonconducting material to minimize current spread into the bath.

DRUG APPLICATION

Drugs can be applied in two ways. Drugs can be added in known concentrations to the superfusing physiological salt solution. Under these conditions the drug reaches a known concentration in the bath and is in equilibrium with the site of action. Equilibrium conditions are essential for quantitative studies of drug-receptor interactions. In addition, as most drugs are selective for a site of action in a limited range of concentrations, drug concentration in the tissue must be known when attempting to study receptors or mechanisms of drug action.

Some drugs can be applied locally. For example, nitric oxide solutions can be applied locally to the smooth muscle using a syringe or local perfusion system.[37] As nitric oxide is unstable, addition to the oxygenated superfusing solution decreases the activity of applied nitric oxide. Local application preserves activity but the drug concentration at the site of action is unknown and not at equilibrium.

RECORDINGS FROM DISPERSED SMOOTH MUSCLE CELLS

GENERAL CONSIDERATIONS

Many of the problems associated with electrophysiological recordings from smooth muscle cells in intact tissues have been resolved using isolated, dispersed cells. Preparations of isolated smooth muscle cells contain few neurons or other cell types which can alter myoelectric activity. As the cells are dispersed, electrotonic coupling is eliminated and ion accumulation or depletion at the membrane surface is also limited due to free exchange with the extracellular medium. However, dispersion of smooth muscle cells can be associated with its own set of problems. Dispersion requires enzyme treatment to dissolve the connective tissue binding smooth muscle cells into bundles. Enzymatic dispersion may affect cell surface receptors, the extracellular portions of ion channels or the structural integrity of the sarcolemma. Despite these concerns, the membrane properties and pharmacological responses of the smooth muscle are preserved after enzymatic dispersion and most measurements of smooth muscle properties (time constant, length constant, etc.) obtained from studies in intact tissues are similar to those obtained from isolated cells.[3,12]

DISPERSION OF SMOOTH MUSCLE CELLS

Most currently used enzymatic methods are based on procedures developed by Bagby et al.[51] for dispersion of smooth muscle cells from the stomach of *Bufo marinus* and Sanders[52] has reviewed the development and evaluation these methods.

Electrophysiological recordings have been a variety of GI smooth muscle cells from different species, including opossum esophagus,[53] toad stomach,[54] guinea pig stomach,[55,56] dog stomach,[57] guinea pig ileum,[58,59] guinea pig taenia coli,[60] rabbit jejunum,[61,62] dog small intestine,[63] dog colon[64,65] and cat colon.[66] Tissues are removed from donor animals and the mucosa and submucosal layers are removed as described above. Longitudinal and circular muscle layers are separated and muscle strips are cut using a scalpel. Muscle cells are dispersed after incubation of tissues in collagenase-containing solutions for varying periods of time. The collagenase-containing medium is usually Ca^{2+}-free to limit collagenase activity and to keep smooth muscle cells in a relaxed state.[52] Trypsin inhibitors in the incubation medium are included to block the activity of any trypsin contamination of collagenase preparations. Healthy smooth muscle cells are phase bright, when viewed with phase contrast microscopy, and relaxed. Electrical stimulation, exposure to high K^+ solutions or agonists induce contractions of healthy smooth muscle cells.[52]

CONVENTIONAL INTRACELLULAR RECORDINGS

Initial studies of dispersed gastric smooth muscle cells of *Bufo* were accomplished using conventional, high resistance (> 100 megohms), KCl-filled microelectrodes.[54] Input resistance was determined by measuring the amplitude of voltage responses evoked by current pulses passed through the recording microelectrode. Input resistance was often as high as 3 gigaohms. With high resistance cells, leakage currents produced by the intracellular electrometer must be monitored as even small currents cause marked changes in the apparent membrane potential of the cell. These experiments were done using extracellular solutions that contained elevated Ca^{2+} concentrations (20 mM) which improved stability of impalements and increased membrane input resistance.[54]

Conventional microelectrodes have been used to voltage clamp freshly isolated smooth muscle cells from toad stomach.[67-69] Single and two electrode voltage clamp methods were used to study the properties of voltage-activated currents and drug- and neurotransmitter-induced changes in these currents.

WHOLE CELL PATCH CLAMP RECORDINGS

One advantage of using dispersed smooth muscle cells is that high resistance (gigaohm) seal patch clamp methods can be applied to these cells.[52] Gigaohm seals require a cell surface free of connective tissue or other debris and enzymatic dispersion permits direct contact between the cell membrane and the patch electrode.[70] As whole cell recording pipettes are low resistance (<10 megohms), the frequency response characteristics and large current passing capabilities optimize voltage clamping conditions.[70] Large currents with a fast time course can be studied with more accuracy using the whole cell configuration vs. voltage clamping with a single conventional intracellular microelectrode.

The whole cell patch pipette dialyzes the intracellular content of the cell with the pipette content. Intracellular solutions generally contain K^+ (140–160 mM) as the primary permeant ion. EGTA is added to the intracellular solution to buffer resting intracellular Ca^{2+} to approximately 100 nM. Drugs, enzymes, or membrane-impermeable substances can be applied directly to the cytoplasm and the intracellular processes controlling smooth muscle electrical activity can be manipulated by the investigator.[70] While dialysis of the intracellular space is an important tool for some studies, the pipette solution can dilute important intracellular contents and disrupt cell function. A modified whole cell technique using a perforated patch can minimize intracellular dialysis when this is not an important component of the experiment. In addition to the normal components of the intracellular solution, nystatin or amphotericin B can be added to the pipette solution as perforating agents.[62,71] The perforated patch technique maintains the high resistance seal, low access resistance of the whole cell method while minimizing intracellular dialysis.

SINGLE CHANNEL RECORDINGS

There are three configurations of the patch clamp method for recording the activity of single ion channels.[52,70] The *cell-attached* configuration measures the activity of channels in a patch of membrane on an intact cell. When using the cell-attached configuration, the intracellular mechanisms which control channel activity are intact and treatments which alter channel activity must be applied *via* the patch pipette or must use a diffusible intracellular transduction pathway when applied outside the patch pipette. The *inside-out* configuration uses an excised patch of membrane from the cell with the intracellular face of the membrane patch exposed to the extracellular solution. Intracellular constituents which regulate ion channel activity are lost but the investigator has control of the content of the solution exposed to the intracellular surface of the membrane. The *outside-out* configuration uses an excised membrane patch with the intracellular surface of the membrane exposed to the pipette solution. Drugs or other substances are applied to the extracellular surface *via* the extracellular solution. All three configurations have been used to study the activity of single K^+ channels from longitudinal smooth muscle cells of rabbit jejunum,[62] gastric smooth muscle cells from toad stomach,[72] and circular smooth muscle cells from dog colon.[73]

METHODS USED TO STUDY ENTERIC NEURONS

A brief history of the development and application of electrophysiological methods for studies of enteric neurons has been provided by Wood.[74] In general, three methods have been used to study enteric neurons: 1) intracellular electrophysiological recordings in intact preparations; 2) extracellular recordings in intact preparations and 3) conventional and patch clamp methods in acutely dissociated and primary cultures of enteric neurons.

INTACT TISSUE PREPARATIONS

Myenteric Plexus

Electrophysiological recordings have been obtained from myenteric neurons in guinea pig,[75–80] cat,[81–83] rabbit[84] and rat[85] small intestine, guinea pig stomach[86,87] and from guinea pig,[88,89] mouse[90] and human[91] colon. In experiments on myenteric neurons from rat, rabbit and guinea pig GI tissues, the longitudinal muscle-myenteric plexus is prepared by opening the intestinal or gastric tissue along the mesenteric attachment and pinning the tissue flat with the mucosal surface up in a Sylgard®-lined petri dish. The mucosa, submucosa and circular muscle layers are stripped away using forceps and fine scissors under a dissecting microscope. The best intracellular recordings are obtained from ganglia which are free of overlying circular muscle. A 5 mm² piece of longitudinal muscle-myenteric plexus is transferred to a recording chamber made of a small square of plexiglass in which a rectangular window ($\sim$20 $\times$ 40 mm) has been cut in the middle. A glass coverslip (#1 thickness) is attached to the plexiglass window using silicone rubber and the well formed by the plexiglass-silicone-coverslip is filled with Sylgard® to a depth of 0.5 mm. The preparation is pinned flat in the recording chamber with the longitudinal muscle layer down using small stainless steel pins (0.05 mm diameter) cut from stainless steel wire (Goodfellow Industries, Malvern, PA). An upright or inverted microscope can be used to view individual ganglia and the preparation is sufficiently transparent to allow observation of ganglia at magnifications of 200–400 $\times$ without the use of vital stains. Contrast enhancing optics such as phase contrast or modulation contrast optics are useful in identifying ganglia and in positioning microelectrodes on the ganglion surface (Figure 4).

Preparations of myenteric plexus from mouse colon and cat small intestine are obtained by first opening a segment of intestine along the mesenteric attachment pinning the tissue flat with the mucosa down. The longitudinal muscle layer is carefully stripped away leaving the myenteric plexus attached to the circular muscle layer. This preparation of cat intestine is sufficiently thick that individual ganglia can not be visualized with out the use of a vital stain such as a 0.1% solution of methylene blue.[81–83]

Immobilization of Myenteric Ganglia

As myenteric ganglia adhere to a muscle layer, spontaneous, nerve-mediated or drug-induced contractions will dislodge microelectrodes during intracellular recordings from individual neurons. However, ganglia can be immobilized either mechanically or pharmacologically. Individual ganglia can be mechanically immobilized in two ways. Firstly, fine, L–shaped wires are clamped down onto the muscle on either side of a myenteric ganglion. The inter-wire separation is adjusted to a width that is just wider than a myenteric ganglion. The "pressure feet" are positioned using a micromanipulator.[76,92] Secondly, small diameter (10 μm) stainless steel pins are pushed

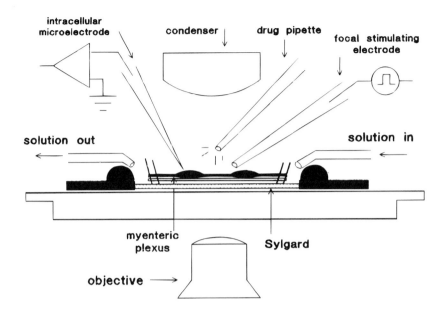

FIGURE 4   Schematic representation of arrangement used to record from myenteric neurons using conventional intracellular microelectrodes. The recording chamber containing the preparation is positioned on the stage of an inverted microscope. The preparation is attached to the Sylgard®-lined base of the chamber using stainless steel pins. The preparation is superfused continuously with a physiological salt solution and drugs can be added to this solution or can be applied directly onto the neuron using a small pressure pipette. Nerve fibers are stimulated using an electrode positioned on an interganglionic nerve strand.

through the muscle layer into the underlying Sylgard at close intervals along the length of the ganglia.[75] Both methods minimize movement of individual ganglia but interconnecting nerve strands can be damaged and studies of synaptic inputs to neurons in the isolated ganglion can be compromised. A non-mechanical approach is to add 1 μM of the dihydropyridine calcium channel antagonists, nifedipine or nicardipine, to the physiological salt solution superfusing the preparation.[87,90,93,94] The dihydropyridine antagonists block voltage-operated calcium channels in the muscle and block contractions. Dihydropyridine antagonists do not change the resting membrane properties of myenteric neurons, action potentials or alter synaptic transmission.[90,94] However, the possibility remains that dihydropyridine antagonists have as yet unidentified actions on enteric neurons.

Submucous Plexus

Most studies of submucosal neurons have been done using preparations of guinea pig small intestine, cecum and colon.[95–99] A small piece of intestine is cut open along the mesenteric border and pinned flat in a Sylgard®-lined petri dish with the mucosal surface up. The mucosa is scraped off using forceps and a 5 mm² piece of submucosa is cut away using fine scissors. The submucosal preparation is transferred to the recording chamber described above and any adhering circular muscle should be stripped away using fine forceps. Visualization of submucosal ganglia is difficult due to their small size and irregular arrangement in the submucosal layer and a microscope equipped with phase contrast or differential interference optics is helpful in visualizing submucosal ganglia. As there is little muscle associated with the submucosa, there are no movements of this layer which can dislodge microelectrodes.

Gall Bladder Neurons

Intracellular electrophysiological recordings have been obtained from ganglia in the gall bladder of guinea pigs[100] and opossum.[101] In order to expose the ganglia, the gall bladder is cut open and pinned flat in a Sylgard®-lined Petri dish and the mucosa, submucosa and muscle layers are stripped away using fine forceps and a dissecting microscope. The ganglia which reside below the serosal layer are pinned flat in a small recording chamber.

Pancreatic Neurons

Intracellular recordings have been obtained from individual neurons in cat pancreas.[102] The pancreas and attached nerve bundles can be dissecting from the animal and pinned flat in a Sylgard®-lined recording chamber and individual ganglia can be observed using a dissecting microscope.

CONVENTIONAL INTRACELLULAR ELECTROPHYSIOLOGICAL METHODS

The first intracellular recordings from enteric neurons were obtained from guinea pig myenteric neurons. Most subsequent work has used modifications of methods developed by Hirst and co-workers,[77] Nishi and North[75] and Wood and colleagues.[76]

MICROELECTRODES

Intracellular recordings are obtained using microelectrodes filled with 1–3 M KCl with an optimum tip resistance of 80–120 megohms. Relatively high resistance electrodes provide the highest rate of success as enteric neurons do not tolerate impalements with low resistance electrodes.

Membrane Potential Recordings

Current clamp methods control current flow across the neuronal membrane and measure voltage responses to currents provided by the intracellular electrometer or by the action of neurotransmitters or drugs. Intracellular electrometers are equipped with circuitry that allows simultaneous current passing and membrane potential measurement with a single microelectrode. The amplifiers use a bridge circuit or operational amplifier that allows neutralization of microelectrode tip resistance and capacitance. Details of these procedures and circuits are provided in the operations manual of the recording device. Constant current pulses are used to measure membrane input resistance and the membrane time constant during intracellular recordings. Input resistance is measured as the voltage drop across the membrane during an intracellular current pulse. The contribution of electrode resistance to the voltage drop during an applied current pulse must be nullified using the bridge balance circuit of the intracellular amplifier. In addition, the electrotonic potential must reach a steady state value and it must be of sufficiently long duration that it will reach steady state after treatments that increase input resistance. Electrotonic potentials should be relatively small (<10 mV) to ensure that only passive membrane properties are measured.

Single Electrode Voltage Clamp (SEVC)

Voltage clamp is a powerful tool for studying voltage- and agonist-activated ion channels in enteric nerves. Conventional voltage clamping requires two intracellular microelectrodes to measure potential and to supply the clamp current. As enteric neurons are relatively small ($\leq$ 30 μm) and in intact preparations single neurons are not visible, impalement of enteric neurons with two microelectrodes is not practical. However, SEVC methods have been used to study currents in enteric nerves. SEVC uses a feedback amplifier that permits alternating membrane potential measurement and current passing. The head stage amplifier is close to the impaled neuron to increase the frequency response performance of the circuit. It is critical that the voltage drop at the headstage is monitored on an oscilloscope to ensure that the feedback circuit is operating properly.[103]

Microelectrodes are most often the limiting factor when using SEVC. A low resistance electrode ($<$ 60 megohms) is optimal as fast switching frequencies can be used and large currents can be passed through the microelectrode. However, low resistance electrodes decrease the rate of successful impalements in enteric nerves. The investigator needs to compromise between the advantages of low resistance electrodes for optimal SEVC and the need for a higher resistance electrode for long term impalements. Microelectrode performance can be improved by reducing electrode capacitance by coating the electrode shank with hydrophobic material such as Sylgard®. Alternatively, the level of the superfusing solution in the recording chamber bath can be reduced to the minimum needed to maintain the preparation.

Even when conditions are optimum for SEVC, the investigator is limited in the types of currents that can be studied reliably. As the circuitry alternates between current passing and potential measurement, currents with fast kinetics such as voltage-gated sodium currents can not be adequately controlled using SEVC with high resistance microelectrodes.[103] However, currents with slower kinetics such as Ca^{2+} [104] and K^+ currents[105–107] and a hyperpolarization-activated cation current[108] have been studied in enteric neurons using SEVC methods.

Electrical Stimulation of Nerve Fibers

Electrical stimulation of interganglionic nerve fibers is accomplished using transmural or focal electrodes. Nerves can be stimulated transmurally using platinum or Ag/AgCl wire bipolar electrodes positioned above and below one end of the tissue.[77,90,95,97] The portions of the wire not in contact with the tissue are insulated with a nonconducting material to prevent current spread into the bath.[77] Transmural stimulation excites long pathways projecting from the site of stimulation to the impaled neuron. Focal electrodes are made of a Krebs solution-filled pipette (tip diameter 20–60 μm) in which a Ag/AgCl wire is inserted (Figure 4).[75,94,98] Focal stimulation can also be accomplished using bipolar tungsten, Ag or platinum wires positioned over an interganglionic nerve strand.[76] Focal stimulation excites short and long pathways entering a ganglion. However, as the electrode is positioned over only one nerve bundle all inputs to a given neuron may not be stimulated. In addition, as a focal electrode is usually positioned within 200 μm of the impaled neuron, current spread can directly excite impaled neurons or antidromically activate their processes.[75] Focal stimulating electrodes have also been used to stimulate interganglionic connectives in gall bladder[100,101] and pancreatic[102] ganglia.

In guinea pig stomach, vagal nerve fibers providing input to myenteric neurons can be selectively stimulated by dissecting the vagal trunks away from the esophagus and placing the vagus nerve over bipolar platinum wire electrodes. With this arrangement it is possible to identify specific gastric myenteric neurons which receive direct vagal input.[109]

Regardless of the type of electrodes, pulse durations of 1 ms or less are used to stimulate presynaptic nerves. The current intensity need to evoke a synaptic response can vary from 100 μA up to 10 mA. Single shocks will evoke fast synaptic potentials in most enteric neurons. Fast synaptic potentials often have a duration of less than 50 ms and most fast synaptic potentials in the enteric nervous system are mediated by acetylcholine acting at nicotinic cholinergic receptors.[74] Trains of high frequency ($\geq$ 10 Hz) stimuli will elicit slow synaptic potentials that can last several seconds to several minutes in many enteric neurons. The slow synaptic potentials may be mediated by a number of peptide and non-peptide neurotransmitters.[74]

Distention-Evoked Synaptic Potentials

In addition to using electrical stimuli to evoke synaptic responses, mucosal stroking has been used to evoke fast and slow synaptic responses in segments of guinea pig small intestine.[93] The method used in these studies is similar to that described above for mechanical mucosal stimulation evoked junction potentials in circular and longitudinal smooth muscle. A segment of ileum is cut open an pinned flat in a recording chamber. The mucosa, submucosa and circular muscle are removed from a small segment of the preparation in order to expose a few myenteric ganglia (Figure 5). Single neurons were impaled with microelectrodes and synaptic responses were evoked in many neurons when the mucosa was stroked with a fine brush.[93]

Drug Application

In order to study drug action on electrical and synaptic behavior of enteric neurons, suitable methods of drug application are needed. Drugs can be added to the superfusing Krebs solution by using reservoirs of control and drug-containing solutions connected in series through a system of 3-way stopcocks. Superfusion applies a known concentration of drug to the tissue and equilibrium can be achieved; both conditions are important when using quantitative pharmacological methods to characterize specific receptors mediating a response. However, superfusion requires prolonged drug-application, washout times and long-term impalements. In addition, desensitization of responses can occur during superfusion before peak responses have been reached.

Some of the problems with drug application by superfusion can be overcome with local drug application. Drugs can be applied locally to neurons in several ways. Iontophoresis is used to eject charged drugs from a small tipped electrode positioned near the neuron.[75] The latency and duration of iontophoretic responses are short (ms) and iontophoresis can be used to mimic the amplitude and time course of fast synaptic potentials. Using iontophoresis, it is difficult to control the amount of drug ejected and the drug concentration at the receptor can only be estimated. In addition, the agonist is not in equilibrium with the receptor and iontophoresis is not appropriate for quantitative analysis of drug/receptor interactions. Finally, some drugs are not ionized at physiological pH and the solution must be acidified or alkalinized to get the drug in an ionized form appropriate for iontophoresis. A set of control experiments is then required

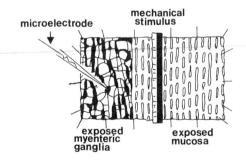

FIGURE 5   Schematic drawing of experimental preparation for recording synaptic potentials evoked by mechanical stimulation of the mucosa. A segment of guinea-pig small intestine was opened along its mesenteric border and pinned serosal surface down in an organ bath. The mucosa, submucosa and circular muscle were dissected from the myenteric plexus at either the oral or the anal end of the segment. Neurons were impaled in the cleared myenteric plexus. The preparation was stimulated by stroking the exposed mucosa with a mechanically driven brush. Note that the drawing is not to scale; the recording site was usually 4–12 mm from the point at which the brush first touched the mucosa, and the brush moved away from the recording site during a stimulus. (From Bornstein, et al., *J. Neuroscience*, 11: 505, 1991. With permission.)

to ensure that the buffer solution itself does not produce any effects. A second method for local drug application uses pressure ejection from a pipette positioned near the impaled neuron (Figure 4). The pipette tip diameter is 10–20 μm and a controlled pulse of nitrogen is used to eject small quantities of drug from the pipette. The pressure ejection pipette can not be positioned as close to the neuron as an iontophoresis electrode as the pressure pulse can dislodge the microelectrode. Response latencies and durations are longer than those obtained with iontophoresis. The concentration of drug at the receptor site is also unknown and is not in equilibrium with the receptor. Therefore as with iontophoresis, pressure ejection of drugs is not appropriate for quantitative pharmacological studies. Pressure ejection is useful for studies of synaptic transmission as the pressure response can mimic the latency, amplitude and time course of many slow synaptic events.

A fourth method of drug application combines the advantages of local application and superfusion techniques. Several pieces of small diameter capillary tubing (200 μm) are glued together side by side. The proximal end of each tube is connected to small reservoirs of drug containing solution. The tubes are mounted on a micromanipulator and the multi-barrel apparatus is positioned within 200 μm of impaled neurons.[110] Flow is controlled by a stopcock and the solutions are gravity fed. By adjusting the flow rate and position of the tubes, equilibrium conditions can be established quickly (< 1 s) and different concentrations of drug or agonist/antagonist combinations can be applied by moving the apparatus so that different drug-containing tubes are positioned over the neuron. This arrangement permits quantitative analysis of drug/receptor interactions in a short period of time. In intact preparations of myenteric or submucosal plexus most experiments are done at 36°C. This requires that the drug-containing solutions in the capillary tubes also be warmed to 36°C.

INTRACELLULAR RECORDING FROM SUBMUCOSAL ARTERIOLES

The small diameter (< 100 μm) arterioles residing in the submucosa are the resistance vessels whose diameter is an important determinant of GI blood flow. Submucosal arterioles are innervated by extrinsic vasoconstrictor and vasodilator nerves and by intrinsic enteric vasodilator nerves. The electrophysiological basis for vasoconstriction has been studied in detail using arterioles in guinea pig ileum submucosa.[111,112] The submucosal preparation is made as described above. Smooth muscle cells of an arteriole are impaled with high resistance 1–3 M KCl-filled microelectrodes. The resting membrane potential of submucosal arterioles is between –55 and –70 mV and stable recordings are possible even in the presence of some contractile activity in the arteriole. Junction potentials are evoked by focal stimulation of perivascular nerves.

Hirst and Neild[112] and Finkel et al.[113] have described a method that is suitable for voltage clamp analysis of electrophysiological events in arteriolar smooth muscle. As with other types of smooth muscle, arteriolar smooth muscle cells are electrotonically coupled. It is necessary then to shorten the length of arteriole so that the segment under study is isopotential. This was accomplished by cutting a segment of arteriole to less than 200 μm in length; i.e. less than 1 length constant. Under these conditions Hirst and Neild demonstrated that the isolated segment of arteriole was isopotential. SEVC clamp methods can then be applied to electrophysiological analysis of events occurring in the isolated segment of arteriole.[113]

EXTRACELLULAR ELECTROPHYSIOLOGICAL METHODS

Wood has provided an excellent review and discussion of extracellular recording methods and the type of information derived from these recordings. Extracellular recordings are used only rarely at present the reader is referred to the chapter by Wood for detailed information regarding this method.[74]

ENTERIC NEURONS IN CULTURE

GENERAL CONSIDERATIONS

Conventional electrophysiological methods have provided a great deal of information concerning the physiology of enteric neurons but there are limitations to these methods. Detailed studies of fast currents using SEVC are limited by the slow frequency response SEVC and the small clamp currents that can be passed by the high resistance microelectrodes needed to record from enteric neurons. In addition, application of drugs directly into the intracellular compartment is limited by low diffusion from the tip of high resistance electrodes. As with other kinds of neurons, these difficulties have been circumvented using patch clamp methods for studying enteric neurons.[70] Low resistance patch pipettes facilitate accurate recordings of large, fast currents and permit dialysis of the intracellular space with drugs added in known concentrations to the pipette solution. Patch clamp methods have also been used to study single ion channels in enteric neurons.

Enteric ganglia are surrounded by a basement membrane. This membrane prevents formation of the high resistance seal between the neuron and the patch pipette required for patch clamp recordings. Therefore it is necessary to disrupt this membrane in order to expose neurons. Two methods have been used to achieve this goal. First, patch clamp recordings have been obtained from acutely dispersed neurons from guinea pig ileum and cecum. Secondly, primary neuronal cultures have been used.

Acutely dispersed or cultured neurons are useful for certain kinds of studies of enteric neurophysiology. However, the investigator needs to be aware that dispersed or cultured neurons may have different properties from neurons in intact preparations. The neurochemistry of enteric nerves is very labile and removing these cells from their normal environment can induce marked changes in the electrophysiological or neurochemical properties of enteric neurons. Intracellular electrophysiological studies have established that cultured neurons retain many of the electrophysiological and pharmacological properties of neurons in intact preparations but the possibility remains that cultured neurons have been altered in ways that have not yet been identified.

ACUTE DISPERSION OF ENTERIC NEURONS

A number of studies have used acutely dispersed myenteric ganglia from guinea pig ileum[114] or submucous neurons from guinea pig ileum and cecum.[110,115–117] The myenteric or submucosal plexus is prepared from ileum or cecum as described above for conventional intracellular recordings. Tissues are then incubated in a collagenase-containing, Ca^{2+}/Mg^{2+} free Krebs solution, triturated through a fire-polished pasteur pipette and plated onto poly-l-lysine coated coverslips in tissue culture medium. The cells are allowed to settle and attach to the coverslips for 5–24 hours. Neurons are present in small clumps with the surface few neurons exposed to the extracellular medium. Although synaptic contacts are disrupted under these conditions, this preparation in conjunction with the whole cell patch clamp configuration has been used to study voltage-gated currents,[114] mechanisms of α_2 adrenergic, somatostatin and opioid-mediated hyperpolarizations[117] and inhibition of calcium currents in submucous neurons.[110] In addition, single 5-HT_3 receptor/channels have been studied using the cell-attached configuration of the patch clamp method.[115]

CULTURES OF ENTERIC NEURONS

Willard has provided a review of the history of the development and application of cultured enteric neurons particularly for electrophysiological studies.[118] The methods used for primary and explant cultures of enteric neurons from the small intestine, cecum and large intestine have been developed by several groups and have used tissues from newborn and adult rats,[119–121] guinea pigs,[121,122] rabbits[121] and humans.[123]

Explant Cultures

Small pieces of intestine or taenia coli from guinea pigs are placed in a physiological salt solution containing collagenase and incubated 3–5 h at 37 C. After incubation the myenteric plexus or submucous plexus can be dissected from the remaining layers using fine forceps and a dissecting microscope. After isolating the nerve plexus, this tissue is transferred onto glass coverslips which are placed in tissue culture chambers. The coverslips are either uncoated or coated with poly-l-lysine or collagen. The explants are maintained at 37°C in 5% CO_2 atmosphere and are grown in tissue culture medium containing 10% fetal calf serum.[121]

Primary Cultures of Dissociated Neurons

Methods for primary cultures of myenteric neurons are based on those developed by Nishi and Willard[119,124,125] for new born rats and modified by others.[126] Segments of longitudinal muscle-myenteric plexus are cut into small pieces and placed in small volumes of Ca^{2+}/Mg^{2+}-free Krebs solution containing collagenase, trypsin or dispase. The tissues are incubated with enzyme-containing solution (30 minutes at 36°C) and then triturated through successively smaller-tipped, fire-polished pasteur pipettes. The suspension is centrifuged and the supernatant is discarded. The cells are resuspended in tissue culture medium and plated out on collagen or poly-l-lysine glass coverslips. The cultures are grown in serum-supplemented tissue culture medium that contains a mitotic inhibitor to limit fibroblast proliferation. The medium also contains streptomycin/penicillin to inhibit bacterial growth. The cultures are grown in an incubator in a 5% CO_2 atmosphere. After 5–7 days, myenteric neurons can be observed as single neurons or in small groups of 4–8 cells. When viewed using phase contrast microscopy, neurons are recognized as round phase-bright cells that have extended processes (Figure 6). Many of these processes contact other neurons and form functional synaptic contacts (see below).

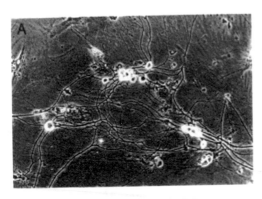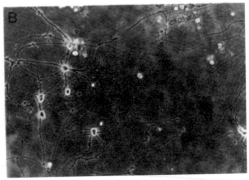

FIGURE 6 Photomicrographs of myenteric neurons in primary culture. A. Myenteric neurons are phase bright and extend numerous processes which contact other neurons (magnification 200×). B. Neurons similar to those in A but at 100× magnification.

Conventional Intracellular Recordings

Intracellular microelectrodes have been used to record from myenteric neurons in explant and dissociated cultures of guinea pig cecum,[127] rat[124,125] and human small intestine.[123] The basic methods for intracellular recordings are similar to those used for neurons in intact preparations. The neuron-containing culture dish is mounted on the stage of an inverted microscope and superfused with warmed Krebs solution. Neurons are impaled with KCl (1–3 M) containing electrodes.

Whole Cell Patch Clamp Recordings

Low resistance (<10 megohms) micropipettes are filled with an intracellular solution of appropriate composition for the particular studies. Some enteric neurons express a Ca^{2+}-activated K^+ channel which mediates a long-lasting spike afterhyperpolarization and contributes to the resting membrane potential.[106] When the intracellular Ca^{2+} concentration increases this channel is activated. Intracellular resting Ca^{2+} should be buffered to 100 nM using appropriate concentrations of added calcium and EGTA in order to limit resting activation of the Ca^{2+}-activated K^+ channel and the accompanying membrane hyperpolarization. A concentration of 2.9 mM added calcium with 5 mM EGTA will yield a free Ca^{2+} concentration of 100 nM.[128]

Drug Application and Synaptic Transmission

Myenteric neurons in primary culture extend processes and establish synaptic contacts with other neurons. While it is uncertain if the contacts made in culture are identical to those formed *in vivo*, transmission between connected pairs of neurons is a powerful system for studying synaptic transmission. Willard has used this system to establish that a single neuron can release more than one neurotransmitter and that the transmitter released is dependent on the stimulus parameters used to evoke synaptic responses.[129,130] Synaptically-connected neurons were identified by random sampling of pairs of neurons. Alternatively, the fluorescent dye, Lucifer Yellow (0.12%), was added to the intracellular pipette solution to fill a neuron with the dye. After several minutes the processes of the filled cell can be traced using fluorescence microscopy and neurons contacted by fluorescent fibers were impaled with a microelectrode. The whole cell patch electrode was used to apply depolarizing current pulses to evoke action potentials in the presynaptic neuron and subsequent synaptic responses in the post-synaptic cell. In addition to direct depolarization of a single presynaptic neuron, axons can be stimulated extracellularly using a focal stimulating electrode as described above for stimulation of nerves in intact tissues.

Drugs can be applied by superfusion, by pressure ejection from a fine-tipped pipette positioned near the impaled neuron or by iontophoresis directly onto the impaled neuron (see above for discussion of these methods).

Single Channel Recordings

The activity of single agonist-activated K^+ channels[116] and 5-HT_3 receptors[115] has been studied in acutely dissociated submucous neurons of guinea pig ileum and cecum using outside-out patches. In the case of 5-HT_3 receptors, single channel studies demonstrated that the 5-HT_3 receptor is a ligand-gated ion channel similar to the nicotinic acetylcholine receptor as there could be no intracellular transduction mechanism between receptor and ion channel in the cell-free patch. Channel activation by 5-HT also did not require the presence of ATP or GTP in the pipette solution bathing the intracellular face of the membrane patch supporting the conclusion of a direct coupling between the agonist binding site and the channel.[115]

In studies of norepinephrine-, somatostatin- and enkephalin- activated K^+ channels it was found that each agonist increased channel activity in cell-free patches but there was an absolute requirement for GTP in the pipette solution. Therefore although there was close coupling between receptor and channel, there was an intermediate GTP-dependent step.[116]

SUMMARY AND CONCLUSIONS

There are several methods to study the electrophysiological properties of GI smooth muscle and enteric nerves *in vitro*. These methods use intact tissues or dispersed cells. GI smooth muscle cells are electrotonically coupled and electrical changes spread passively throughout the muscle layers. The single sucrose gap method takes advantage of electrotonic coupling and allows the investigator to measure relative changes in membrane potential following nerve stimulation or drug-treatment. The double sucrose gap method allows the investigator to voltage clamp a small node of muscle cells to make detailed studies of conductance changes induced by nerve stimulation or drugs. The sucrose gap measures the average potential or current in a group of smooth muscle cells. Intracellular microelectrodes directly measure membrane potential of smooth muscle and can discriminate differences in electrical activity of groups cells within a layer of smooth muscle. In order to measure changes in membrane conductance using intracellular microelectrodes, large extracellular electrodes are required to provide the polarizing currents needed to elicit electrotonic potentials for measurement of membrane resistance. This arrangemnt permits the investigator to study the electrophysiological basis for neuromuscular transmission in GI tissues. In order to eliminate the problems associated with electrotonic coupling, isolated dispersed smooth muscle cells have been used to study the membrane properties of individual cells. Conventional intracellular microelectrodes and patch clamp methods can be applied to dispersed smooth muscle cells. Patch clamp methods include the whole cell configuration for recording macroscopic currents and for intracellular dialysis of individual muscle cells. Intracellular dialysis in the whole cell configuration is an important tool for studying signal transduction. Cell-free patches of smooth muscle membrane are used to study the behavior of single ion channels in smooth muscle.

The electrophysiological properties of enteric neurons can be studied in intact preparations of GI tissues or in acutely dispersed or cultured neurons. In intact preparations, intracellular microelectrodes are commonly used to study single neurons. Intracellular microelectrodes can be used to measure membrane potential using current clamp methods or membrane currents using single electrode voltage clamp methods. Synaptic transmission can be studied in intact tissues using focal or transmural electrodes to electrically excite nerve fibers in the enteric plexuses. Extracellular electrophysiological methods are rarely used at present. Enzymatically-dispersed or cultured enteric neurons also provide a useful system for studying enteric neurophysiology. Intracellular microelectrodes and patch clamp methods are used to record from dispersed or cultured neurons. Acutely dispersed cells allow the investigator to use patch clamp methods to study signal transduction or the activity of single channels in enteric nerves. Cultured enteric neurons are also useful for these studies; however enteric neurons in culture establish synaptic contacts with other cells. This phenomenon allows the investigator to make detailed studies of the electrophysiological pre- and post-synaptic processes responsible for synaptic transmission in the gut.

REFERENCES

1. **Bennett, M. R.,** *Autonomic neuromuscular transmission.* Cambridge University Press, Cambridge, 1972.

2. **Hoyle, C. H. V. and Burnstock, G.,** Neuromuscular transmission in the gastrointestinal tract, in *Handbook of Physiology—Section 6 The Gastrointestinal System Part 1.* Schultz S. G., Wood, J. D. and Rauner, B. B., Eds., Oxford University Press, New York, 1989 chap. 13.

3. **Bolton, T. B.,** Electrophysiology of the intestinal musculature, in *Handbook of Physiology—Section 6 The Gastrointestinal System Part 1.* Schultz S. G., Wood, J. D. and Rauner, B. B., Eds., Oxford University Press, New York, 1989 chap. 6.

4. **Sanders, K. M. and Publicover, N. G.,** Electrophysiology of the gastric musculature, in *Handbook of Physiology—Section 6 The Gastrointestinal System Part 2.* Schultz S. G., Wood, J. D. and Rauner, B. B., Eds., Oxford University Press, New York, 1989 chap. 5.

5. **Sanders, K. M. and Smith, T. K.,** Electrophysiology of colonic smooth muscle, in *Handbook of Physiology—Section 6 The Gastrointestinal System Part 2.* Schultz S. G., Wood, J. D. and Rauner, B. B., Eds., Oxford University Press, New York, 1989 chap. 7.

6. **Thuneberg, L.,** Interstitial cells of Cajal, in *Handbook of Physiology—Section 6 The Gastrointestinal System Part 1.* Schultz S. G., Wood, J. D. and Rauner, B. B., Eds., Oxford University Press, New York, 1989 chap. 10.

7. **Langton, P., Ward, S. M., Carl, A., Norell, M. A. and Sanders, K. M.,** Spontaneous electrical activity of interstitial cells of Cajal isolated from canine proximal colon. *Proc. Natl. Acad. Sci. (USA)* 86, 7280, 1989.

8. **Smith, T. K., Reed, J. B. and Sanders, K. M.,** Origin and propagation of electrical slow waves in circular muscle of canine proximal colon. *Am. J. Physiol.* 252, C215, 1987.

9. **Smith, T. K., Reed, J. B. and Sanders, K. M.,** Interaction of two electrical pacemakers in muscularis of canine proximal colon. *Am. J. Physiol.* 252, C290, 1987.

10. **Gabella, G.,** Structure of intestinal musculature, in *Handbook of Physiology—Section 6 The Gastrointestinal System Part 1.* Schultz S. G., Wood, J. D. and Rauner, B. B., Eds., Oxford University Press, New York, 1989 chap. 2.

11. **Huizinga, J. D., Shin, A. and Chow, E.,** Electrical coupling and pacemaker activity in colonic smooth muscle. *Am. J. Physiol.* 255, C653, 1988.

12. **Tomita, T., Katayama, N., Tokuno, H. and Somiya, H.,** Electrotonic potential in smooth muscle in: *Cell Interactions and Gap Junctions.* CRC Press, Boca Raton, FL pp. 267,

13. **Casteels, R., Droogmans, G. and Raeymaekers, L.,** Distribution and exchange of electrolytes in gastrointestinal muscle cells, in *Handbook of Physiology—Section 6 The Gastrointestinal System Part 1.* Schultz S. G., Wood, J. D. and Rauner, B. B., Eds., Oxford University Press, New York, 1989 chap. 3.

14. **Brading, A. F.,** Ionic distribution and mechanisms of transmembrane ion movements in smooth muscle, in *Smooth muscle: an assessment of current knowledge.* Bulbring, E., Brading, A. F., Jones, A. W. and Tomita, T., Eds., University of Texas Press, Austin, 1981 chap. 3.

15. **Stampfli, J.,** A new method for measuring membrane potentials with external electrodes. *Experientia* 12, 508, 1954.

16. **Burnstock, G. and Straub, R. W.,** A method for studying the effects of ions and drugs on the resting and action potentials in smooth muscle with external electrodes. *J. Physiol.* 140: 156, 1958.

17. **Burnstock, G.,** The effects of acetylcholine on membrane potential, spike frequency conduction velocity and excitability in the taenia coli of guinea-pig. *J. Physiol.* 143: 165, 1958.

18. **Szurszewski, J. H.,** Recording of electrical activity of smooth muscle by means of the sucrose gap, in *Proceedings of the Fourth International Symposium on Gastrointestinal Motility.* Daniel, E. E., Ed., Mitchell Press, Vancouver, 1974, p 409.

19. **Hoyle C. H. V.,** A modified single sucrose-gap: junction potentials and electrotonic potentials in gastrointestinal smooth muscle. *J. Pharmacol. Methods* 18, 219, 1987.

20. **Bolton, T. B.,** Effects of stimulating the acetylcholine receptor on the current voltage relationships of the smooth muscle membrane studied by voltage clamp of potential recorded by microelectrode. *J. Physiol.* 250, 175, 1975.

21. **Bolton, T. B., Tomita, T. and Vassort, G.,** Voltage clamp and the measurement of ionic conductances in smooth muscle, in *Smooth muscle: an assessment of current knowledge.* Bulbring, E., Brading, A. F., Jones, A. W. and Tomita, T., Eds., University of Texas Press, Austin, 1981 chap. 2.

22. **Kuriyama, H. and Tomita, T.,** The action potential in the smooth muscle of the guinea pig taenia coli and ureter studied by the double sucrose-gap method. *J. Gen. Physiol.* 55, 147, 1970.

23. **Bortoff, A. and Sachs, F.,** Electrotonic spread of slow waves in circular muscle of small intestine. *Am. J. Physiol.* 218, 576, 1970.

24. **Publicover, N. G. and Sanders, K. M.,** Myogenic regulation of propagation in gastric smooth muscle. *Am. J. Physiol.* 248, G512, 1985.

25. **Bulbring, E.,** Membrane potentials of smooth muscle fibres of the taenia coli of the guinea pig. *J. Physiol.* 125, 302, 1954.

26. **Crist, J., Surprenant, A. and Goyal, R. K.,** Intracellular studies of electrical membrane properties of opossum esophageal circular smooth muscle. *Gastroenterology* 92, 978, 1987.

27. **Abe, Y. and Tomita, T.,** Cable properties of smooth muscle. *J. Physiol.* 196, 87, 1968.

28. **Smith, T. K., Furness, J. B., Costa, M. and Bornstein, J. C.,** An electrophysiological study of the projections of motor neurones that mediate non-cholinergic excitation in the circular muscle of the guinea pig small intestine. *J. Auton. Nerv. Syst.* 22, 115, 1988.

29. **Smith, T. K. and Furness, J. B.,** Reflex changes in circular muscle activity elicited by stroking the mucosa: an electrophysiological analysis in the isolated guinea-pig ileum. *J. Auton. Nerv. Syst.* 25, 205, 1988.

30. **Smith, T. K., Bornstein, J. C. and Furness, J. B.,** Distention evoked ascending and descending reflexes in the circular muscle of guinea pig ileum. *J. Auton. Nerv. Syst.* 29, 203, 1990.

31. **Conklin, J. L., Du, C., Murray, J. H. and Bates, J. N.,** Characterization and mediation of inhibitory junction potentials from opossum lower esophageal sphincter. *Gastroenterology* 104, 1439, 1993.

32. **Bauer, A. J., Reed, J. B. and Sanders, K. M.,** Slow wave heterogeneity within the circular muscle of the canine gastric antrum. *J. Physiol.* 366, 221, 1985.

33. **El-Sharkawy, T. Y., Morgan, K. G. and Szurszewski, J. H.,** Intracellular electrical activity of canine and human gastric smooth muscle. *J. Physiol.* 279, 291, 1978.

34. **Komori, K. and Suzuki, H.,** Distribution and properties of excitatory and inhibitory junction potentials in circular muscle of the guinea pig stomach. *J. Physiol.* 370, 339, 1986.

35. **Morgan, K. G., Angel, F., Schmalz, P. F. and Szurszewski, J. H.,** Intracellular electrical activity of muscularis mucosae of the dog stomach. *Am. J. Physiol.* 249, G256, 1985.

36. **Bolton, T. B.,** On the nature of the oscillations of the membrane potential (slow waves) produced by acetylcholine or carbachol in intestinal smooth muscle. *J. Physiol.* 216 403, 1971.

37. **Stark, M. E., Bauer, A. J., Sarr, M. G. and Szurszewski J. H.,** Nitric oxide mediates inhibitory nerve input in human and canine jejunum. *Gastroenterology* 104, 388, 1993.

38. **Bauer, A. J., Sarr, M. G. and Szurszewski, J. H.,** Opioids inhibit neuromuscular transmission in circular muscle of human and baboon jejunum. *Gastroenterology* 101, 870, 1991.

39. **Bornstein, J. C., Costa, M., Furness, J. B. and Lang, R. J.,** Electrophysiological analysis of projections of enteric inhibitory motorneurones in the guinea pig small intestine. *J. Physiol.* 370, 61, 1986.

40. **Yaun, S. Y., Furness, J. B., Bornstein, J. C. and Smith, T. K.,** Mucosal distortion by compression elicits polarized reflexes and enhances responses of the circular muscle to distention in the small intestine. *J. Auton. Nerv. Syst.* 35, 219, 1991.

41. **Furness, J. B.,** An electrophysiological study of the innervation of the smooth muscle of the colon. *J. Physiol.* 205, 549, 1969.

42. **Christensen, J., Caprilli, R. and Lund, G. F.,** Electrical slow waves in circular muscle of the cat colon. *Am. J. Physiol.* 217, 771, 1969.

43. **Bywater, R. A. R., Small, R. C. and Taylor, G. S.,** Neurogenic slow depolarizations and rapid oscillations in the membrane potential of circular muscle of mouse colon. *J. Physiol.* 413, 505, 1989.

44. **Koch, T. R., Carney, J. A., Go, V. L. W. and Szurszewski, J. H.,** Spontaneous contractions and some electrophysiologic properties of circular muscle from normal and sigmoid colon of ulcerative colitis. *Gastroenterology* 95, 77, 1988.

45. **Koch, T. R., Carney, J. A., Go, V. L. W. and Szurszewski, J. H.,** Inhibitory neuropeptides and intrinsic inhibitory innervation of descending human colon. *Dig. Dis. Sci.* 36, 712, 1991.

46. **Keef, K. D., Du, C., Ward, S. M., McGregor, B. and Sanders, K. M.,** Enteric inhibitory neural regulation of human colonic circular muscle: role of nitric oxide. *Gastroenterology* 105, 1009, 1993.

47. **Hodgkin, A. L. and Rushton, W. A. H.,** The electrical constants of a crustacean nerve fibre. *Proc. Roy. Soc.* B 133, 444, 1946.

48. **Bywater, R. A. R. and Taylor, G. S.,** The passive membrane properties and excitatory junction potentials of the guinea pig vas deferens. *J. Physiol.* 300, 303–316, 1980.

49. **Bauer, V. and Kuriyama, H.,** Evidence for non-cholinergic non-adrenergic transmission in the guinea-pig ileum. *J. Physiol.* 330, 95, 1982.

50. **Hidaka, T. and Kuriyama, H.,** Responses of the smooth muscle membrane of guinea pig jejunum elicited by field stimulation. *J. Gen. Physiol.* 53, 471, 1969.

51. **Bagby, R. M., Young, A. M., Dotson, R. S., Fisher, B. A. and McKinnon, K.,** Contraction of single smooth muscle cells from Bufo marinus stomach. *Nature* 234, 351, 1971.

52. **Sanders, K. M.,** Electrophysiology of dissociated gastrointestinal muscle cells, in *Handbook of Physiology—Section 6 The Gastrointestinal System Part 1.* Schultz S. G., Wood, J. D. and Rauner, B. B., Eds., Oxford University Press, New York, 1989 chap. 4.

53. **Sims, S. M., Vivadou, M. B., Hillemeier, C., Biancani, P., Walsh, J. V. and Singer, J. J.,** Membrane currents and cholinergic regulation of K^+ current in esophageal smooth muscle cells. *Am. J. Physiol.* 258, G794, 1990.

54. **Singer, J. J. and Walsh, J. V.,** Passive properties of single freshly isolated smooth muscle cells. *Am. J. Physiol.* 239, C153–C161, 1980.

55. **Mitra, R. and Morad, M.,** A uniform enzymatic method for dissociation of myocytes from hearts and stomachs of vertebrates. *Am. J. Physiol.* 249, H1056, 1985.

56. **Katzka, D. A. and Morad, M.,** Properties of calcium channels in guinea-pig gastric myocytes. *J. Physiol.* 413, 175, 1989.

57. **Vongalis, F. and Sanders, K. M.,** Cholinergic stimulation activates a non-selective cation current in canine pyloric circular smooth muscle cells. *J. Physiol.* 429, 223, 1990.

58. **Droogmans, G. and Callewaert, G.,** Ca^{2+}-channel current and its modification by the dihydropyridine agonist Bay k 8644 in isolated smooth muscle cells. *Pflugers Arch.* 406, 259, 1986.

59. **Zholos, A. V., Baidan, L. V. and Shuba, M. F.,** Properties of the late transient outward current in isolated intestinal smooth muscle cells of the guinea-pig. *J. Physiol.* 443, 555, 1991.

60. **Ganitkevich, V. Ya., Shuba, M. F. and Smirnov, S. V.,** Potential dependent calcium inward current in a single isolated smooth muscle cell of the guinea pig taenia caeci. *J. Physiol.* 380, 1, 1986.

61. **Ohya, Y., Terada, K., Kitamura, K. and Kuriyama, H.,** Membrane currents recorded from a fragment of rabbit intestinal smooth muscle cell. *Am. J. Physiol.* 251, C335, 1986.

62. **Benham, C. D., and Bolton, T. B.,** Patch-clamp studies of slow potential-sensitive potassium channels in longitudinal smooth muscle cells of rabbit jejunum. *J. Physiol.* 340, 469, 1983.

63. **Farrugia, G., Rae, J. L. and Szurszewski, J. H.,** Characterization of an outward potassium current in canine jejunal circular smooth muscle and its activation by fenamates. *J. Physiol.* 468, 297, 1993.

64. **Langton, P. D., Burke, E. P. and Sanders, K. M.,** Participation of Ca currents in colonic electrical activity. *Am. J. Physiol.* 257, C451, 1989.

65. **Cole, W. C. and Sanders, K. M.,** Characterization of macroscopic outward currents of canine colonic myocytes. *Am. J. Physiol.* 257, C461, 1989.

66. **Bielefeld, D., Hume, J. R. and Krier, J.,** Action potentials and membrane currents of isolated smooth muscle cells of cat and rabbit colon. *Pflugers Arch.* 415, 678, 1990.

67. **Walsh, J. V. and Singer, J. J.,** Voltage clamp of single freshly isolated dissociated smooth muscle cells: current-voltage relationships for three currents. *Pflugers Arch.* 390, 207, 1981.

68. **Sims, S. M., Singer, Joshua, J. J. and Walsh, J. V.,** Antagonistic adrenergic-muscarinic regulation of M current in smooth muscle cells. *Science* 239, 190, 1988.

69. **Sims, S. M., Singer, J. J. and Walsh, J. V.,** Cholinergic agonist suppress a potassium current in freshly dissociated smooth muscle cells of the toad. *J. Physiol.* 367, 503, 1985.

70. **Hamill, O. P., Marty, A., Neher, E., Sakmann, Sigworth, F. J.,** Improved patch clamp techniques for high resolution current recording from cells and cell-free membrane patches. *Pflugers Arch.* 391, 85, 1981.

71. **Horn, R. and Marty, A.,** Muscarinic activation of ionic currents measured by a new whole cell recording method. *J. Gen. Physiol.* 92, 145, 1988.

72. **Singer, J. J. and Walsh, J. V.,** Characterization of calcium- activated potassium channels in single smooth muscle cells using the patch clamp technique. *Pflugers Arch.* 408, 98, 1987.

73. **Carl, A. and Sanders, K. M.,** Ca^{2+}-activated K channels of canine colonic myocytes. *Am. J. Physiol.* 257, C470, 1989.

74. **Wood J. D.,** Electrical and synaptic behavior of enteric neurons, in *Handbook of Physiology— Section 6 The Gastrointestinal System Part 1.* Schultz S. G., Wood, J. D. and Rauner, B. B., Eds., Oxford University Press, New York, 1989 chap. 14.

75. **Nishi, S. and North, R. A.,** Intracellular recording from the myenteric plexus of the guinea-pig ileum. *J. Physiol.* 231, 471–491, 1973.

76. **Wood, J. D. and Mayer, C. J.,** Intracellular study of electrical activity of Auerbach's plexus in guinea pig-small intestine. *Pflugers Arch.* 374, 265–275, 1978.

77. **Hirst, G. D. S., Holman, M. E. and Spence, I.,** Two types of neurones in the myenteric plexus of duodenum in guinea pig. *J. Physiol.* 236, 303–326, 1974.

78. **Williams, J. T. and North, R. A.,** Extracellular recording from the guinea pig myenteric plexus and the action of morphine. *Eur. J. Pharmacol.* 45, 23–33, 1977.

79. **Dingeldine, R. and Goldstein, A.,** Effect of synaptic transmission blockade on morphine action in the guinea pig myenteric plexus. *J. Pharmacol. Exp. Ther.* 196, 97, 1976.

80. **Sato, T., Takayanagi, I., and Takagi, K.,** Pharmacological properties of electrical activities obtained from neurons in Auerbach's plexus. *Jap. J. Pharmacol.* 23, 665, 1973.

81. **Wood, J. D.,** Electrical activity from single neurons in Auerbach's plexus. *Am. J. Physiol.* 219, 159, 1970.

82. **Ohkawa, H. and Prosser, C. L.,** Electrical activity in myenteric and submucous plexuses of cat intestine. *Am. J. Physiol.* 222, 1412, 1972.

83. **Wood, J. D.,** Intracellular study of effects of morphine on electrical activity of myenteric neurons in cat small intestine. *Gastroenterology* 79, 1222, 1980.

84. **Yokoyama, S., Ozaki, T. and Kajitsuka, T.,** Excitation conduction in Auerbach's plexus of rabbit small intestine. *Am. J. Physiol.* 232, E100, 1977.

85. **Brookes, S. J. H., Ewart, W. R. and Wingate, D. L.,** Intracellular recordings from cells in the myenteric plexus of the rat duodenum. *Neuroscience* 24, 297, 1988.

86. **Schemann, M. and Wood, J. D.,** Electrical behaviour of myenteric neurones in the gastric corpus of the guinea-pig. *J. Physiol.* 417, 501, 1989.

87. **Tack, J. F. and Wood, J. D.,** Electrical behaviour of myenteric neurones in the gastric antrum of the guinea-pig. *J. Physiol.* 447, 48, 1992.

88. **Wade, P. R. and Wood, J. D.,** Electrical behavior of myenteric neurons in guinea pig distal colon. *Am. J. Physiol.* 254, G522, 1988.

89. **Tamura, K. and Wood, J. D.,** Electrical and synaptic properties of myenteric plexus neurones in the terminal large intestine of the guinea pig. *J. Physiol.* 415, 275, 1989.

90. **Furukawa, K., Taylor, G. S. and Bywater, R. A. R.,** An intracellular study of myenteric neurons in the mouse colon. *J. Neurophysiol.* 55, 1395, 1986.

91. **Brookes, S. J. H., Ewart, W. R. and Wingate, D. L.,** Intracellular recordings from myenteric neurones in the human colon. *J. Physiol.* 390, 305, 1987.

92. **Erde, S. M., Sherman, D. and Gershon, M. D.,** Morphology and serotonergic innervation of physiologically identified cells of the guinea pig's myenteric plexus. *J. Neuroscience* 5, 617, 1985.

93. **Bornstein, J. C., Furness, J. B., Smith, T. K. and Trussell, D. C.,** Synaptic responses evoked by mechanical stimulation of the mucosa in morphologically characterized myenteric neurons of the guinea pig ileum. *J. Neuroscience* 11, 505, 1991.

94. **Galligan, J. J., Surprenant, A., Tonini, M. and North, R. A.,** Differential localization of 5-HT_1 receptors on myenteric and submucosal neurons. *Am. J. Physiol.* 255, G603, 1988.

95. **Hirst, G. D. S. and Silinsky, E. M.,** Some effects of 5-hydroxytryptamine, dopamine and noradrenaline on neurones in the submucous plexus of guinea-pig small intestine. *J. Physiol.* 251, 817–832, 1975.

96. **Hirst, G. D. S. and McKirdy, H. C.,** Synaptic potentials recorded from neurones of the submucous plexus of guinea pig small intestine. *J. Physiol.* 249, 369–384, 1975.

97. **Surprenant, A.,** Slow excitatory synaptic potentials recorded from neurones of guinea-pig submucous plexus. *J. Physiol.* 351, 343–361, 1984.

98. **Mihara, S., Katayama, Y. and Nishi. S.,** Slow synaptic potentials in neurones of submucous plexus of guinea pig caecum and their mimicry by noradrenaline and various peptides. *Neuroscience* 4, 1057, 1985.

99. **Frieling, T., Cooke, H. J. and Wood, J. D.,** Synaptic transmission in submucosal ganglia of guinea pig distal colon. *Am. J. Physiol.* 260, G842, 1991.

100. **Mawe, G. M.,** Intracellular recording from neurones of the guinea-pig gall-bladder. *J. Physiol.* 429, 323, 1990.

101. **Bauer, A. J., Hanani, M., Muir, T. C. and Szurszewski, J. H.,** Intracellular recordings from gallbladder ganglia of opossums. *Am. J. Physiol.* 260, G299, 1991.

102. **King, B. F., Love, J. A. and Szurszewski, J. H.,** Intracellular recordings from pancreatic ganglia of the cat. *J. Physiol.* 419, 379, 1989.

103. **Finkel, A. and Redman, S. J.,** Theory and operation of a single electrode voltage clamp. *J. Neurosci. Meth.* 11, 101, 1984.

104. **Hirst, G. D. S., Johnson, S. M. and van Helden, D. F.,** The calcium current in a myenteric neurone of the guinea pig-ileum. *J. Physiol.* 361, 297, 1985.

105. **Galligan, J. J., North, R. A. and Tokimasa, T.,** Muscarinic agonists and potassium currents in guinea pig myenteric neurons. *Br. J. Pharmacol.* 96, 193, 1989.

106. **North, R. A. and Tokimasa, T.,** Persistent calcium-activated potassium current and the resting properties of guinea-pig myenteric neurones. *J. Physiol.* 386, 333, 1987.

107. **Mihara, S., North, R. A. and Surprenant, A.,** Somatostatin increases an inwardly rectifying potassium conductance in guinea-pig submucous plexus neurones. *J. Physiol.* 390, 335, 1987.

108. **Galligan, J. J., Tatsumi, H., Shen, K.-Z., Surprenant, A. and North, R. A.,** Cation current activated by hyperpolarization (I_H) in guinea pig enteric neurons. *Am. J. Physiol.* 259, G966, 1990.

109. **Schemann, M. and Grundy, D.,** Electrophysiological identification of vagally innervated enteric neurons in guinea pig stomach. *Am. J. Physiol.* 263, G709, 1992.

110. **Surprenant, A., Shen, K.-Z., North, R. A. and Tatsumi, H.,** Inhibition of calcium currents by noradrenaline, somatostatin and opioids in guinea pig submucosal neurones. *J. Physiol.* 481, 585, 1990.

111. **Hirst, G. D. S.,** Neuromuscular transmission in arterioles of guinea pig submucosa. *J. Physiol.* 273, 263–275, 1977.

112. **Hirst, G. D. S. and Neild, T. O.,** An analysis of excitatory junctional potentials recorded from arterioles. *J. Physiol.* 280, 87–104, 1978.

113. **Finkel, A. S., Hirst, G. D. S. and van Helden, D. F.,** Some properties of excitatory junction currents recorded from submucosal arterioles of guinea pig ileum. *J. Physiol.* 351, 87, 1984.

114. **Baidan, L. V., Zholos, A. V., Shuba, M. F. and Wood, J. D.,** Patch-clamp recording in myenteric neurons of guinea pig small intestine. *Am. J. Physiol.* 262, G1074, 1992.

115. **Derkach, V., Surprenant, A. and North, R. A.,** 5-HT$_3$ receptors are membrane ion channels. *Nature* 339, 706–709, 1989.

116. **Shen, K.-Z., North, R. A. and Surprenant, A.,** Potassium channels opened by noradrenaline and other transmitters in excised membranes patches of guinea pig submucosal neurones. *J. Physiol.* 445, 581–599, 1992.

117. **Tatsumi, H., Costa, M., Schimerlik, M. and North, R. A.,** Potassium conductance increased by noradrenaline, opioids, somatostatin and G-proteins: whole cell recording from guinea pig submucous neurons. *J. Neuroscience* 10, 1675, 1990.

118. **Willard, A. L. and Nishi, R.,** Enteric neurons in culture, in *Handbook of Physiology—Section 6 The Gastrointestinal System Part 1.* Schultz, S. G., Wood, J. D. and Rauner, B. B., Eds., Oxford University Press, New York, 1989 chap. 9.

119. **Nishi, R. and Willard, A. L.,** Neurons dissociated from rat myenteric plexus retain differentiated properties when grown in cell culture. I. Morphological properties and immunocytochemical localization of transmitter candidates. *Neuroscience* 16, 187–199, 1985.

120. **Jessen, K. R., McConnell, J. D., Purves, R. D., Burnstock, G. and Chamley-Campbell, G.,** Tissue culture of mammalian enteric neurons. *Brain Res.* 152, 573, 1978.

121. **Jessen, K. R., Saffrey, M. J. and Burnstock, G.,** The enteric nervous system in tissue culture. I. Cell types and their interactions in explants of the myenteric and submucous plexus from guinea pig, rabbit and rat. *Brain Res.* 262, 17–35, 1983.

122. **Saffrey, M. J., Bailey, D. J. and Burnstock, G.,** Growth of enteric neurones from isolated myenteric ganglia in dissociated cell culture. *Cell Tiss. Res.* 265, 527, 1991.

123. **Maruyama, T.,** Two types of spike generation of human Auerbach's plexus cells in culture. *Neuroscience Letters* 25, 143, 1981.

124. **Willard, A. L. and Nishi, R.,** Neurons dissociated from rat myenteric plexus retain differentiated properties when grown in cell culture. II. Synaptic interactions and modulatory effects of neurotransmitter candidates. *Neuroscience* 16, 213–221, 1985.

125. **Willard, A. L. and Nishi, R.,** Neurons dissociated from rat myenteric plexus retain differentiated properties when grown in cell culture. III. Synaptic interactions and modulatory effects of neurotransmitter candidates. *Neuroscience* 16, 213, 1985.

126. **Hirning, L. D., Fox, A. P. and Miller, R. J.,** Inhibition of calcium currents in cultured myenteric neurons by neuropeptide Y: evidence for direct receptor/channel coupling. *Brain Res.* 532, 120, 1990.

127. **Hanani, M., Baluk, P. and Burnstock, G.,** Myenteric neurons express electrophysiological and morphological diversity in tissue culture. *J. Auton. Nerv. Syst.* 5, 155, 1982.

128. **Bartfi, T.,** Preparation of metal-chelate complexes and the design of steady state kinetic experiments involving metal nucleotide complexes. in *Advances in Cyclic Nucleotide Research*, G. Brooker, P. Greengard, G.A. Robison Eds, Raven Press, NY, 10, 219, 1979.

129. **Willard, A. L.,** A vasoactive intestinal peptide-like cotransmitter at cholinergic synapses between rat myenteric neurons in cell culture. *J. Neuroscience* 10, 1025, 1990.

130. **Willard, A. L.,** Substance P mediates synaptic transmission between rat myenteric neurones in cell culture. *J. Physiol.* 426, 453, 1990.

12 Gastrointestinal Sphincter Function

Kenneth R. DeVault and Satish Rattan

INTRODUCTION

The gastrointestinal tract while functioning as whole in the transport and digestion of ingested material is physiologically partitioned into subdivisions by a series of sphincters. The esophagus begins at the striated muscle upper esophageal sphincter (UES) and extends to the smooth muscle lower esophageal sphincter (LES) while the stomach is the defined proximally by the LES and distally by the pylorus. The biliary tree is separated from the small intestine by the sphincter of Oddi (SO) and the small intestine itself is bordered by the pylorus and the ileocecal sphincter (ICS). The most distal portion, the colon, begins at the ICS and continues to the exit of the gastrointestinal tract at the anal sphincters [the smooth muscle internal anal sphincter (IAS) and the striated external anal sphincter (EAS)].

These sphincters have two major functions: To remain in a tonic contractile state in the resting condition to serve as barriers to the free flow of gastrointestinal contents from one area to another, and to undergo relaxation in response to an appropriate reflex in coordination with the normal progression of gastrointestinal contents in the distal direction.

Although of vital importance, the exact control mechanisms for the normal function of these sphincters are not known, nor is the pathophysiology of various disorders affecting the sphincters. The broad approaches used to study and facilitate understanding of sphincteric function include: 1) Intraluminal pressure measurement, 2) Strain gauge recording, 3) Electrophysiologic changes in smooth muscle, 4) Isometric tension in smooth muscle strips, 5) Morphometric analysis of isolated smooth muscle cells.

The purpose of this chapter is to provide an overview of the general techniques of sphincter evaluations. Specific examples of the use of these techniques in the study of gastrointestinal sphincters will be discussed. We will concentrate on two sphincters from which the majority of data is available, the LES and IAS. Most of the following observations can be applied to other sphincter systems as well.

INTRALUMINAL PRESSURE MEASUREMENTS

Intraluminal pressure measurement or manometry is a mainstay in the study of gastrointestinal motility in general and *in vivo* sphincter function in particular. These methods are valuable, especially because of the simplicity, reliability and reproducibility of manometric measurements. Manometric studies have been attempted for nearly 100 years, yet it was not until the development of low-compliance perfusion systems that accurate measurements could be obtained.[1,2] The two

0-8493-8304-8/96/$0.00+$.50

normal functions of a sphincter, tone and relaxation, can be studied using manometry both in human and animal subjects.

BASAL SPHINCTER PRESSURE

The tone and length of a sphincter contribute to its competency. This can be measured using any one of several manometry systems. In order to determine the length and amplitude of the high pressure zone within a sphincter the most common technique is that of pulling a manometry device across the sphincter. This can be a steady pull or step wise (station pull-through) technique. An example of a station pull-through of the human lower esophageal sphincter is presented in Figure 1. In this technique the recording port of the catheter is pulled across the sphincter in steps of a given size (0.5–1 cm in the human LES). The pressure slowly increases from baseline indicating entrance into the sphincter, a high pressure zone is reached, then the catheter passes from the sphincter. The length of the sphincter is the distance from the beginning of the increase in pressure to the return to baseline while the resting pressure is usually defined as the pressure of the high pressure zone.

In the LES, respiratory changes may influence both tonic and phasic pressure components. The tonic component is the steady state increase in pressure from baseline independent of rhythmic fluctuations. The phasic activity on the other hand represents rhythmic fluctuations over and above the tonic pressures and may be partly related to respiration due to the contribution of the crural diaphragm to the LES. A major portion of sphincteric tone is myogenic in nature.

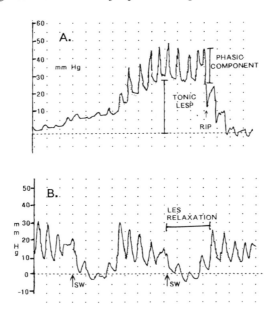

FIGURE 1 Examples of the manometric evaluation of the human lower esophageal sphincter. A. A station pull-thought of the lower esophageal sphincter demonstrates the recording port to be pulled into the high pressure zone of the LES and then into the esophageal body. The point of transition from positive or intraabdominal pressure fluctuations to negative or intrathroacic fluctuations is the respiratory inversion point (RIP). There is both a phasic and a tonic component to the sphincter pressure. Sphincter pressure can be measured at the lowest portion of the phasic component (end expiratory) which would be 25 mm Hg in this case. It also can be measured at the highest portion (end inspiratory), 45 mm Hg or at mid expiratory (about 35 mm Hg). B. In this demonstration of LES relaxation the catheter is placed into the LES (mid expiratory pressure approximately 20 mm Hg) and a series of wet swallows (SW) are given. The LES relaxes to a level of less than 0 mm Hg which is a normal response.

The sphincteric pressure in the resting state, its changes in response to swallowing or other physiological and pharmacological stimuli can be expressed either from tonic pressure (end expiratory), mid respiratory pressure or from the top of the respiratory excursions (end inspiratory) as illustrated in Figure 1A. The method used is the choice of the investigator but should remain consistent within given studies.

SPHINCTER RELAXATION

The evaluation of sphincter relaxation as measured manometrically is much more difficult. When single, unidirectional recording ports are placed within a sphincter, a fall in pressure consistent with relaxation may sometimes be manometrically indistinguishable from migration of the catheter out of the sphincter (movement artifact). Techniques have been developed to control for catheter movement artifact. The Dent Sleeve is a specially constructed manometry catheter with a 3–6 cm segment at the distal end covered with a thin flexible membrane.[3] When the sleeve is placed across a sphincter, an average of the maximum pressure changes in the sphincter at a given time and its relaxation can be obtained.

A solid-state sphincter transducer has been developed. This transducer has the advantage of measuring pressures in a 360 degree area and has enough length to hopefully remain within the sphincter during relaxation.[4] The advantages and disadvantages of each system will be discussed in the following section. The changes in sphincter pressure can be quantified by examining the effects of different agonists and antagonists on the tone of the sphincter under identical experimental conditions and by using each animal or subject as its own control. A typical tracing of human LES relaxation is presented in Figure 1B.

In order to investigate the nature of inhibitory neurotransmitters responsible for the relaxation of a sphincter, it is essential to devise an alternative physiological stimulus which will mimic the relaxation of the sphincteric smooth muscle in a fashion similar to the physiological reflex (e.g. swallowing in the case of LES and defecation reflex in the case of IAS). The quantification of the sphincteric relaxation is particularly valuable in the evaluation of potency of agonists and antagonists in the quantitative alteration of sphincter relaxation.

The best examples of alternative stimuli to mimic the swallowing induced relaxation of the LES are esophageal balloon distension and electrical stimulation of vagus nerve.[5] Swallowing can also be elicited by pharyngeal stimulation or superior laryngeal nerve stimulation in lightly anesthetized animals. By using these alternative stimuli, a graded LES response to either varying volumes of distention or vagal stimulation parameters can be evaluated before, during, and after the administration of a test agent. The IAS relaxation can be induced by the rectoanal reflex (which mimics defecation reflex) using different volumes of rectal balloon distention and by varying parameters of sacral nerve stimulation.[6,7]

Study of the other sphincters in intact subjects may suffer due to lack of a well defined stimulus to reproducibly mimic the relaxation comparable to that with the physiologic reflex. Other methodological factors influencing measurements of gastrointestinal sphincter pressure which should be kept in mind include catheter diameter, perfusion fluid, accommodation, body position, bolus type, and frequency of stimulation. These can be minimized by carefully controlling the experimental conditions.

PERFUSED MANOMETRY CATHETERS VERSUS SOLID STATE SYSTEMS

Intraluminal pressures can be monitored using either low-compliance perfused catheter systems or by the use of solid state intraluminal transducers. A water perfused system consists of a multilumen catheter assembly with small openings at different levels on the individual catheter. Each catheter is perfused with bubble-free water by a pneumohydraulic low-compliance pump. Each recording catheter in turn is connected to a pressure transducer with its output to a chart recorder or computer for analysis.

When using a water perfusion system the pressures recorded will be from a small discrete zone depending upon the size of the open tip (approximately 1 mm). This may be useful for the recording of intraluminal pressures from small sphincters such as the sphincter of Oddi. The other advantage of the small tip is that it can distinguish the physiological behavior of very small segments of the larger sphincters and may help characterize different areas of a given sphincter. Since these catheters have no internal electronics they are economical, often disposable and can be custom designed for the specific experiment on a short notice.

While modern low-compliance pneumohydraulic systems for the perfused catheters provide reliable pressure measurement using a relatively low flow of bubble-free water one should keep in mind certain technical problems associated with water perfused systems. These problems include the possibility of tube leaks with water spillage and the presence of air bubbles anywhere in the system. In addition with longer studies the source of fluid must be refilled which may introduce air-bubbles and artifact. Also since the column of fluid in the catheter may influence the pressures recorded, the subject's position must be controlled carefully. These difficulties can usually be overcome with adequate planning and preparation. Another theoretical issue is the effect of the infused water on the sphincter itself. This could exert a local effect at the perfusion port or a local reflex especially after accumulation of large amounts of fluid in an adjacent organ. For example, in a study of a sphincter using 4 perfusion ports with a flow rate of 0.3 ml/min the hourly perfusion rate would be 72 ml. In human studies, this may not cause a problem except in the case of the sphincter of Oddi where the flow rate of perfusion has been associated with an increased incidence of post-manometry pancreatitis compared to standard dye studies of the bile ducts.[8] In small animals, this can be a problem especially in longer studies. Attempts to minimize this include limiting the number of ports to monitor sphincter pressures and length of the study, and including extra idle nonperfused ports to aspirate the excess fluid from the parts proximal or distal to the recording site.

Another disadvantage of the water perfusion relates to one of the above mentioned advantages. The precise location of the port of the catheter in the sphincter may create problems related to catheter movement. This is of particular importance with the quantitative evaluation of sphincter relaxation. For example, in recording intraluminal pressures from the LES in response to swallowing or vagal stimulation, the contraction of longitudinal muscle may cause proximal movement of the LES and esophagus resulting in "false" relaxation.

The influence of movement has been addressed with perfused sleeves such as the Dent Sleeve which measures pressure over 3–6 cm. Since the wide span of the sleeve may assure the relationship of the recording device with the sphincter, the impact of movement artifact may be less. With the sleeve catheter however, other artifacts may be induced including falsely elevated pressures secondary to adjacent nonsphincteric changes in pressure. The sleeve records the averages of maximal pressures at a given time. If one is monitoring LES relaxation during swallowing, the swallowing associated contraction in the esophageal body may complicate the results.

The other limitation of the sleeve catheter is that it may not allow recording from the discrete zone of the sphincter and the pressures recorded represent averages of the highest pressures recorded in the area. Furthermore, since flexible material is used for the construction of the sleeve, the sharp and brisk contraction of high amplitude may lead to the spread of pressures in the sleeve thus minimizing the recording of the true high pressures at a given point.

An alternative approach to record the intraluminal pressures keeping in view the strengths of the perfused catheters and to overcome the concern of the possible displacement of the relationship of recording tip from the sphincter has been developed.[9] This experimental setup

(Figure 2) allows the anchoring of the catheter assembly inside the LES. If there is any movement of the sphincter, the setup helps to maintain the relationship between the recording device and the sphincter.

Using the above described setup, Figure 3A gives examples of typical recording of basal LES pressures and its changes in responses to vagal stimulation, local intramural stimulation (LES stimulation) and esophageal distension. The LES stimulation is meant to stimulate the intramural myenteric inhibitory neurons. Figures 3B and 3C exemplify the responses to isoproterenol and bethanechol respectively, before and after the neurotoxin tetrodotoxin (TTX). It is well known that TTX blocks the neural conduction without significantly affecting smooth muscle activity. In these sets of experiments TTX was used to establish that the neural blockade abolished the LES relaxation in response to vagal stimulation, LES stimulation and esophageal distension (Figure 3A). Conversely, TTX failed to affect the resting tone in the LES and its changes to both the inhibitory agonist isoproterenol (Figure 3B) and excitatory agonist bethanechol (Figure 3C). These experiments for the first time suggested that resting tone in the LES is primarily due to myogenic properties of the sphincteric smooth muscle. Since then the experimental design described above has been used for a variety of physiological and pharmacological studies. The approach however is applicable only in the acute *in vivo* experiments in the animals.

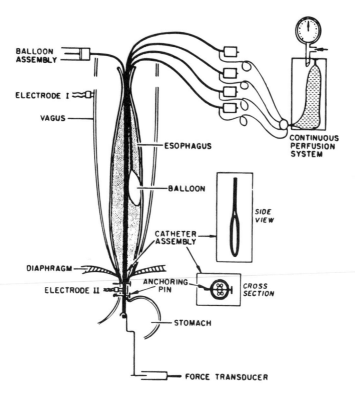

FIGURE 2   Experimental setup showing the catheter assembly of four polyvinyl catheters with a specially designed terminal part. The insert (side view) shows the central core of soft polyvinyl tubing. Anchoring pins are used to anchor the assembly to the lower esophagus after laparotomy. The tip of the catheter is attached to the force transducer by a stainless steel support through a small opening in the stomach. Electrode I, placed on the distal end of the vagus after cervical vagotomy, was used to produce vagal stimulation. Electrode II, inserted in the region of the LES, was used to produce local stimulation of neurons in the LES. The balloon assembly was used to produce reflex LES response to esophageal distention. The arrangement for continuous perfusion of catheters is also shown. (From Goyal and Rattan, *Gastroenterology,* 71, 62, 1976. With permission.)

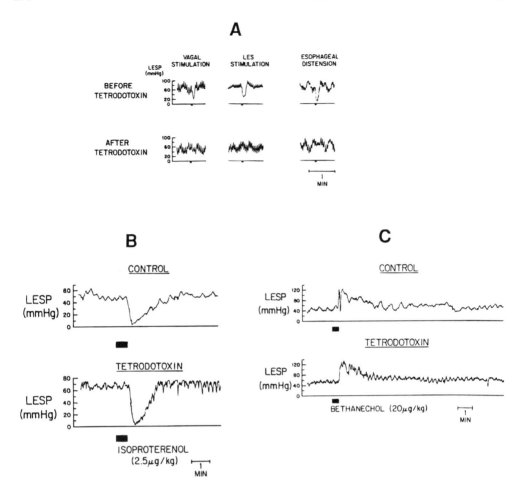

FIGURE 3 A. Examples of LES responses to various stimuli before and after tetrodotoxin. Note that vagal stimulation, LES stimulation, and esophageal distension all caused a fall in sphincter pressure before tetrodotoxin, and that all of these responses were blocked after tetrodotoxin. B. Effect of isoproterenol on LESP before and after tetrodotoxin. Note that tetrodotoxin treatment did not modify the fall in sphincter pressure caused by isoproterenol. C. Effect of bethanechol on LESP before and after tetrodotoxin. Note that tetrodotoxin treatment did not modify the sphincter contraction due to bethanechol. (From Goyal and Rattan, *Gastroenterology,* 71, 62, 1976. With permission.)

The primary alternative to perfused catheter systems is an intraluminal solid state pressure monitoring device. These intraluminal transducers have been used for several years,[10] but have received recent attention secondary to the development of improved microtransducers contained on a soft flexible catheter. Advantages of this system include the direct, position independent measurement of pressures making subject position less important. The lack of water perfusion may allow better long-term studies, and the faster response time of these transducers is especially important in the evaluation of faster striated muscle sphincters such as the upper esophageal (cricopharyngeal) sphincter.[4,11]

Recording from sphincters has been improved further with the recent development of a specialized solid state transducer that senses pressure circumferentially over 360 degrees. This consists of a silastic circumferential annulus filled with a viscous fluid that surrounds a single miniature titanium strain gauge. The pressure exerted by the sphincter is then transmitted through the fluid to the transducer. This provides an advantage when measuring asymmetrical sphincters such as the UES, EAS, and possibly the diaphragmatic component of the LES. A perfusion port measures pressures over a 1 mm area, while a unidirectional solid state transducers measures over 3 mm, a circumferential measures over 6 mm and a Dent sleeve over 30–60 mm. These differences can be used to better characterize entire sphincters (using circumferential or Dent sleeve) or specific quadrants or areas of a sphincter (using unidirectional or perfusion port). While the initial high cost of solid state catheters is a major disadvantage, they may be quite durable if cared for properly.

The output from either of these systems can be recorded on a physiograph and/or downloaded to a computer for analysis. The solid state systems are particularly well suited to computer analysis.

USE OF MANOMETRY IN SPECIFIC STUDIES OF SPHINCTER CONTROL

Intrinsic tonic myogenic activity contributes primarily to the basal pressure of the LES. A series of experiments using classic agents that effect autonomic nerves have provided important information and a prototypical method of study of sphincter function. Alpha-adrenergic agents and beta antagonists increase LES pressure while alpha-blockers and beta agonists decrease it. TTX has no effect on basal pressure[9] (Figure 3). LES relaxation on the other hand is neurally mediated since it is abolished by TTX. This neural mediation appears to not involve the classical adrenergic and cholinergic transmitters since blockade of these two systems has no effect on relaxation.[12] Because of this, the term nonadrenergic, noncholinergic (NANC) is used.[13]

These methods have been applied to examine the specific nature of NANC inhibitory neurotransmitters or mediators for the LES relaxation, and actions of many neuropeptides and other neurohumoral substances considered to effect LES function. Similar studies have been performed in the IAS demonstrating that the resting pressures in the anal canal are primarily due to myogenic properties of the IAS.[6] This conclusion was based on the following observations described in Figure 4.

These experiments were performed in the opossums where the intraluminal pressures from the high pressure zone of the anal canal were recorded using a water perfused catheter assembly. In addition, the electromyographic (EMG) activity of the EAS was recorded using bipolar metallic hook electrodes. In order to mimic the defecation reflex-induced fall in the anal canal pressures, rectal balloon distension (RBD) to simulate anorectal inhibitory reflex was used. As shown in Figure 4I, RBD in the awake animals caused the expected fall in high pressures in the anal canal accompanied with the increased EMG activity in the EAS. The changes in these parameters were not modified by α-chloralose which is a long duration, safe and stable anesthetic (eliminating the frequent redosing of short acting anesthetic). However, the use of the α-chloralose plus neuromuscular blocking agent pancuronium caused a complete obliteration of EMG activity of the EAS without any effect on either the basal pressures in the anal canal or its relaxation in response to RBD. These data suggested that the EAS and other surrounding skeletal muscles may not play a significant role in the basal pressures in the anal canal. Therefore, the anal canal pressures recorded in the presence of pancuronium are termed as the IAS pressures.

As shown further in Figure 4II, the pretreatment of the animal with the α-adrenoceptor antagonist also had no significant effect on the resting pressures. The data negate an important contribution of sympathetic drive towards the basal IAS pressures. The observations have been supported by the subsequent studies where specific α-adrenoceptor antagonist prazosin[14] in selective doses and catecholamine depletor guanethidine[15] had no significant effect on the resting IAS pressures. There is significant data to show that the parasympathetic innervation may also not play a significant role in the maintenance of resting sphincteric tone. The data shown in Figure 4III further showed that TTX had no notable effect on the resting IAS pressures in

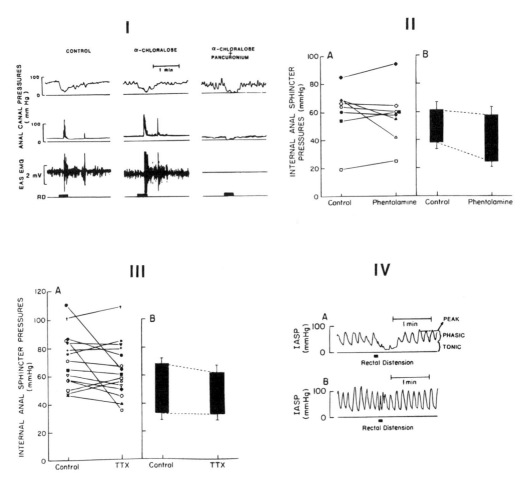

FIGURE 4   I. Representative tracings to show influence of α-chloralose and combination of α-chloralose and pancuronium on anal canal pressures and electromyograph (EMG) of external anal sphincter (EAS). Control represents recordings from awake animals. *Top:* pressures recorded from anal canal at level of highest pressures. *Middle:* pressures from lower end of anal canal. *Bottom:* recording of EMG from the EAS. *Horizontal bars* at bottom represent duration of rectal distention (RD). Note that none of treatments had any significant effect on resting pressures or relaxation to RD of anal canal at upper level (*top*). α-Chloralose had no effect on resting contractile and electrical activity. Increase in contractile and electrical activity in response to RD was also not affected. Combination of α-chloralose and pancuronium had no apparent effect on resting pressures in anal canal at lower level but did cause obliteration of ongoing EMG activity of EAS and intermittent increase in pressures at lower level of the anal canal.

II. Influence of phentolamine on anal canal pressures. A: peak pressures in anal canal zone where highest pressures before and after phentolamine were recorded in different animals. B: means ± SE of peak (top of *dark bars*) and tonic (bottom of *dark bars*) pressures before and after phentolamine. Mean values on dark bars are joined by *dotted lines* for direct comparison. Peak pressures were not modified by phentolamine, however, tonic pressures after phentolamine were slightly but significantly lower than those of controls.

III. Influence of tetrodotoxin (TTX) on resting anal canal pressures. A: influence of TTX on peak pressures in zone of anal canal showing highest pressures in 15 animals. Some animals showed trend toward a fall, others, toward a rise in pressure. B: means ± SE of peak (top of *dark bars*) and of tonic pressures (bottom of *dark bars*). The data show that TTX failed to modify peak and tonic pressures in anal canal ($P > 0.05$).

IV. Influence of TTX on anal canal relaxation in response to rectal distension (RD). *A:* in controls RD caused an immediate fall in resting anal canal pressures, which returned to predistension levels following deflation of balloon, *B:* TTX administration, on the other hand, caused obliteration of the anal canal response to rectal distention. (From Culver and Rattan, *Am. J. Physiol.,* 251, G765, 1986. With permission.)

different animals investigated. The dose of TTX used in these experiments was appropriate since it abolished the IAS relaxation in response to RBD (Figure 4IV).

The use of intraluminal perfused catheters to record the sphincter pressures has been valuable to characterize the nature of the inhibitory neurotransmitters (in response to an appropriate intact reflex) in the gut. Using this approach in the LES and IAS *in vivo* in opossums, a number of studies have identified the role of VIP[12,16] and NO[17,18,19] as inhibitory neurotransmitters in the gastrointestinal tract. The details of the experiments leading to those conclusions have been given later in the chapter.

The approach has also served well to determine the actions, sites of action, the receptor type involved and role of a number of neuropeptides and other neurohumoral substances in the function as outlined later in the chapter. A number of concepts evolved in the sphincters in turn are important in the understanding of the pathophysiology and in therapeutic approaches of the rest of the gastrointestinal motility disorders.

Intraluminal pressure measurement has the advantage of studying an intact organism and allows for the simultaneous evaluation of muscle and nerve function. It may however be difficult to discriminate between myogenic and neurogenic factors. An additional factor in the evaluation of potential neurotransmitters is the difficulty in the correlation between pharmacologic dosages, serum concentrations and the actual concentration of peptide at the cellular site of action. For example, intraarterial substance P results in an immediate, but short lived contraction of the LES.[20] Whether this is of physiologic significance or if it is an epiphenomena of a supraphysiologic dose is not known since determination of the actual concentration of substance P at the neuromuscular junction is unknown. Manometry is of course the only method for study of intact humans and allows for chronic experiments both in animals and humans.

EXTRALUMINAL STRAIN GAUGE RECORDING

A limitation of intraluminal pressure recording is the artifact potentially caused by the introduction of an intraluminal device. This is of particular importance in the study of sphincters with small internal diameters such as the sphincter of Oddi, various pediatric sphincters in humans and in smaller animal models. Serosal strain gauges may offer an alternative to intraluminal manometry bypassing intraluminal manipulation of the sphincter.[21,22] This also is an important technique in chronic animal studies and allows study without the potential confounding factor of anesthesia. Use of a chronic preparation is particularly valuable when day to day follow-up of the animal is needed especially in the case of chronic drug studies. Anesthetics are a problem when studying gastrointestinal reflexes and should be avoided when possible.

Despite these potential advantages there are significant limitations of extraluminal strain gauge recording. A relatively major surgical procedure is required for the placement of the strain gauge. Major surgery may alter sphincter function for an unknown period of time and could potentially produce long-term dysfunction by disruption of both intrinsic and extrinsic innervation. Considerable surgical skill is needed to efficiently place the gauges avoiding an unacceptably high failure rate. The gauges also must be durable enough to complete chronic experiments. A more serious consideration is the possibility that external gauges may not accurately reflect intraluminal pressure changes experienced by the traveling food or liquid bolus.

MEASUREMENT OF ISOMETRIC TENSION OF ISOLATED SMOOTH MUSCLE STRIPS

While manometric evaluation of the sphincter in an intact organism is ideal in many experiments, other studies are not possible using that approach. These include studies where manipulation would not allow the organism to survive the study, application of certain rare and expensive biologically active substances, and when determination of actual function of individual muscle layers is desired. Measurement of *in vitro* isometric tension of isolated smooth muscle strips is a method of overcoming some of these limitations of manometry. Dose response curves are less difficult to construct using this method and are the corner stone of pharmacologic research.

The isolated smooth muscle strip preparation of the sphincter is crucial to investigate: 1) the nature of inhibitory neurotransmitter; 2) the myogenic factors characteristically important for the maintenance of the resting tone of the smooth muscle; 3) the neural and humoral factors responsible for the modulation of the sphincteric smooth muscle function; 4) the biochemical pathways responsible for smooth muscle relaxation.

The specific details of the methods for the preparation of the smooth muscle strips, recording of the isometric tension, the appropriate parameters for the electrical field stimulation (EFS) to elicit nerve stimulation, the method to construct dose response curve before and after the appropriate antagonists have been described in a number of publications from our laboratory.

The sphincteric smooth muscle strips are easily recognizable based on their functions. They develop spontaneous tone and undergo relaxation in response to the appropriate parameters of EFS (3 mA; 0.5 to 1 ms pulse duration; varying frequency from 0.5 to 20 Hz for 1 to 4 sec train duration). The field stimulation is delivered in the muscle bath via two platinum electrodes placed on the either side of the smooth muscle. Quantification of sphincteric smooth muscle relaxation to different frequencies is important in the investigation of the nature of NANC neurotransmitter and to determine the potency of different agents and modulators of the resting tone and the neurally-mediated smooth muscle relaxation. The IAS smooth muscle strips responses to different stimulus frequencies are shown in Figure 5I. Interestingly, TTX caused almost complete obliteration of the EFS-induced relaxation of IAS smooth muscle strips (Figure 5II) without causing any change in the resting tone. Data like this and the lack of modification of the resting tone in the LES and IAS smooth muscle strips in the presence of different neurohumoral antagonists led to the hypothesis that the resting tone in the sphincter is largely due to myogenic properties. The EFS-induced relaxation of the sphincteric smooth muscle strips has been characterized to be NANC in nature since the adrenergic and cholinergic antagonists had no significant effect on the relaxation.

Sphincteric smooth muscle strips studies also have been very helpful in the characterization of the nature of the NANC inhibitory neurotransmitters. Using this approach, the experiments suggested the involvement of VIP[16,18,23,24] and NO[17,18,19,25] as inhibitory neurotransmitters in the sphincters. The details of the experiments leading to those conclusions have been described later in the chapter.

Studies in isolated sphincteric smooth muscle strips are important to determine the actions, sites of action, receptor type involved and role of a number of neuropeptides and other neurohumoral substances in the sphincter function and in structure activity relationship studies. The studies are also valuable in investigating the nature of secondary messengers in the relaxation of the sphincteric smooth muscle in response to NANC nerve stimulation and the inhibitory neurotransmitters.[26,27] Some of the specific studies are described in the later part of the chapter.

The preparations of the isolated smooth muscle strips can also be exploited to examine the role of free intracellular Ca^{2+} $[Ca^{2+}]_i$ in the resting tone of the sphincter and in the smooth muscle contraction and relaxation.[28] Two common methods to determine the resting levels of $[Ca^{2+}]_i$ using the isolated smooth muscle strips preparations are, aequorin[29] and Fura-2.[30]

The aequorin method involves the loading of the isolated smooth muscle strips with the photoprotein aequorin by transiently increasing the permeability of the smooth muscle cells. The aequorin bioluminiscence and the tension signals are recorded simultaneously by using a light-tight apparatus. Using this approach, it was found that the tonic smooth muscle of the LES is characterized by higher levels of $[Ca^{2+}]_i$ as compared to the nontonic smooth muscle

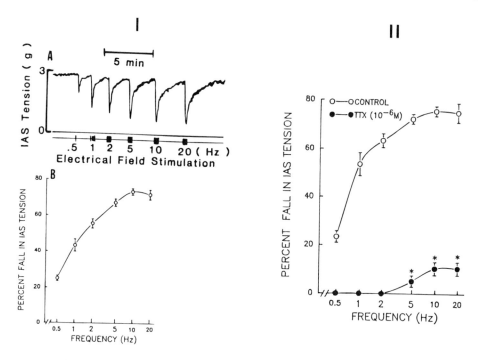

FIGURE 5 I. Frequency-dependent fall in resting tension of internal anal sphincter (IAS) by electrical field stimulation (EFS) (40 V; 2 ms for 4-s train). *A:* actual recording from a typical experiment showing graded fall in resting tension of IAS smooth muscle in response to stepwise increase in frequency from 0.5 to 20 Hz. Note that maximal fall in IAS tension was observed with 10 Hz. *B:* frequency-response curve showing incremental fall in IAS tension in response to varying frequencies of EFS. Each point represents mean ± SE of 8 observations.

II. Influence of TTX on percent fall in resting IAS tension in response to varying frequencies of EFS at 40 V; 2 ms for 4-s train. Each point represents a mean ± SE of 6 observations. Note that inhibitory responses of EFS at lower frequencies were abolished by TTX and antagonism of responses at other frequencies was significant ($P < 0.05$). (From Moummi and Rattan, *Am. J. Physiol.,* 255, G571, 1988. With permission.)

of the esophageal body. Furthermore, the changes in the levels of $[Ca^{2+}]_i$ coincided with the characteristics of the smooth muscle contraction. For example, the transient smooth muscle contraction of the esophageal body was accompanied by the transient increases in $[Ca^{2+}]_i$. Conversely, the LES contraction in response to bethanechol was of protracted nature with the similar changes in $[Ca^{2+}]_i$.[28] The changes in relation to the relaxation of the sphincteric versus the nonsphincteric smooth muscle in response to the candidate NANC inhibitory neurotransmitter and NANC nerve stimulation remain to be investigated.

The Fura-2 method also allows the simultaneous recording of isometric tension of isolated smooth muscle strips and $[Ca^{2+}]_i$ using a specific Ca^{2+} analyzer or by adapting an appropriate spectrofluorometer for the purpose. Measurement of $[Ca^{2+}]_i$ in isolated smooth muscle strips and isolated smooth muscle cells is done by the method of Asaki and Karaki.[30] Since the circular smooth muscle strips of the sphincter may represent a mixture of diverse types of cells, the light signal may not be a true representation of smooth muscle cells alone. This could be resolved by recording of Fura-2 signals from isolated smooth muscle cells. Dispersed smooth muscle cells may be obtained by the method established by Bitar and Makhlouf.[31] This technique of recording Ca^{2+} signals from the smooth muscle cells involves: a) loading of cells with fura-2; b) recording of fluorescence signals; and, c) quantification of $[Ca^{2+}]_i$.

The sphincteric smooth muscle strips are tied at both ends with silk sutures. One end is attached to the quvette type tissue analysis attachment and the other to an isometric muscle transducer which is connected to a Dynograph recorder for recording the isometric tension of the smooth muscle strips and the fluorescence signals. The quvette containing the tissue is filled with oxygenated physiological Krebs' solution (pH 7.4). The smooth muscle strip is then subjected to optimal tension (L_0) and allowed to equilibrate for one hour. The smooth muscle is loaded with Fura-2AM (10 uM) for 2 hours. After this, the muscle strip is washed for 20 to 30 minutes with oxygenated Krebs' solution until the fluorescence values at 340 and 380 nm are stabilized.

The fluorescence of Fura-2-Ca^{2+} is measured with a fluorometer specially designed to measure the fluorescence of living tissues. In this method, the muscle strip is illuminated alternately (48 Hz) with two excitation wavelengths (340 and 380 nm) and the fluorescence emitted at 500 nm is collected on the face of a photomultiplier tube. The amount of fluorescence emitted, and the ratio (R340/380) are calculated by a computer. This ratio (R340/380) is an indication of the relative $[Ca^{2+}]_i$.[32,33]

$[Ca^{2+}]_i$ is calculated from the following equation.

$$[Ca^{2+}]_i = K_d \frac{R-R_{min}}{R_{max}-R} \times B$$

For Fura-2 and Ca^{2+} in physiological solution at 37°C, K_d is taken to be 224 nM as suggested by Grynskiewicz et al.[32]. R_{max} and R_{min} are determined by the addition of ionomycin (1 uM) and EGTA (4 mM) to the tissue respectively[33]. The amount of background fluorescence is measured at the end of the experiment by adding 5 mM $MnCl_2$. In sphincteric smooth muscle strips, the resting tone is defined by determining the "zero baseline" at the end of the experiment by the treatment of the tissues with 5 mM EDTA, the Ca^{2+} chelator.

There are major advantages of isolated smooth muscle strips studies. The actions of different neural stimuli, neurohumoral substances and other pharmacological agents can be investigated directly on the smooth muscle without the influence of the central nervous system, extrinsic nerves, the adrenal medullary release of catecholamines, other extrinsic influences and hormones. The preparations allow incubation with antisera and antagonists. An additional advantage of muscle strip studies is that the similar experiments can be performed simultaneously on different sphincteric tissues from the same animal. The obvious disadvantage is that the changes are recorded from the isolated segments and may not provide complete information of the full spectrum of neural pathways involved in the *in vivo* physiological reflexes.

MORPHOMETRIC ANALYSIS OF ISOLATED SMOOTH MUSCLE CELLS

Both of the techniques discussed to this point, intraluminal manometry and measurement of isometric using smooth muscle strips, study muscle function with a variable amounts of associated nerve tissue and other nonneuronal nonmuscle tissue cells. Smooth muscle function can be inferred from the use of TTX. Recently, dispersed smooth muscle cells have been studied to overcome this limitation.[31] Advantages of isolated smooth muscle cells include the decreased diffusion barriers allowing direct interaction of the test substance with pure smooth muscle cells specimens without innervation and cell-to-cell coupling.[34] The technique allows the evaluation of the effects of both the contractile and relaxant agents on the resting state of the cells. The methods involve the isolation of the smooth muscle cells and measurement of cell length.

ISOLATION OF THE SMOOTH MUSCLE CELLS

The methods for isolation of sphincteric muscle cells are similar to those for other gastrointestinal smooth muscle (See Chapter 10). The respective sphincteric tissues from the appropriate animal are dissected out and the mucosa and the longitudinal muscle layer are removed by sharp dissection, while the tissue are kept in oxygenated Krebs' physiological solution. The circular smooth muscle is cut into small strips (~ 2 cm long and 2 mm wide). The individual smooth muscle cells are isolated by two successive incubations under oxygen (at 31°C) in Krebs' buffer (pH 7.4) containing 0.1% collagenase (CLS type II, Worthington Biochemicals), 0.01% soybean trypsin inhibitor, Basal Medium Eagle amino acids solution with L-glutamine (Gibco, 1X final conc.) and vitamin mixture (Gibco, 1X final conc.). After the first 30 minutes incubation, the incubation medium is replaced with fresh medium and the incubation continued for another 30 minutes. At the end of second incubation, the medium is filtered through a Nitex (500 um) and the tissues are washed with 50 mL of enzyme-free Krebs' buffer. The tissues are then incubated in the fresh Krebs' buffer at 31°C for 30 minutes during which time the smooth muscle cells are spontaneously dispersed into the medium. The cells are isolated by filtering the medium through a Nitex (500 um). The same procedure is followed for the isolation of smooth muscle cells from the longitudinal muscle layer after the removal of circular smooth muscle layer.

MEASUREMENT OF CELL LENGTHS

Individual cell lengths are measured by micrometry using phase contrast microscopy. The cells are treated with the known concentration of the contractile agonist for 30 seconds after which the cells were fixed by adding acrolein (final conc. 1%). The mean cell length of cells is measured randomly and the percent decrease in the cell length by the agonist is calculated. In order to examine the effect of the relaxant agent on the cell length, the muscle cells are first treated with the relaxant agent for 60 seconds followed by bethanechol for 30 seconds after which the cells are fixed with acrolein. The mean length of cells is measured and the percent inhibition of bethanechol-induced contraction by the relaxant agent is calculated. Isolated smooth muscle cells can be used to determine the role of $[Ca^{2+}]_i$ and other second messengers in excitation-contraction coupling and in the differential behavior of cells obtained from tonic versus nontonic smooth muscle cells. Using this method, combined with isolated smooth muscle strips studies, important conclusions addressing intracellular basis for the resting tone in the LES and IAS were made.[35,36,37] The major determinant of the resting tone in the LES and IAS may be higher levels of $[Ca^{2+}]_i$ in the smooth muscle cells. Furthermore, the higher levels of $[Ca^{2+}]_i$ may be under the influence of higher basal levels of inositol 1,4,5-trisphosphate (IP_3) in sphincteric smooth muscle cells. The reduced levels of IP_3 and lower levels of $[Ca^{2+}]_i$ may correlate with the decrease in the level of basal tone in the cats affected with reflux esophagitis by the esophageal perfusion of 0.1 N HCL. Whether these basic findings can explain the pathophysiology of human hypotensive or hypotonic LES and the reflux esophagitis remains to be investigated.

Although very important for the determination of actions of agents directly at the smooth muscle cells, isolated cells can not be used for the examination of the effects of the endogenously released neurotransmitter substances in response to neural stimulation.

ELECTROPHYSIOLOGIC CHANGES IN SMOOTH MUSCLE

Characteristic changes in electrical potentials have been demonstrated in the stomach, small and large intestines. These so called migrating motor complexes have characteristic smooth muscle electrophysiological changes. These changes can be recorded extracellularly with simple extraluminal electrodes but greater accuracy can be found with intracellular recording. The intracellular electrical activity of sphincteric smooth muscle is less well characterized, but can and has been studied. This technique allows even minor changes in resting membrane activity to be recorded as well as any spike potentials, but requires considerable expertise and equipment limiting its applications to address specific questions. Although even more cumbersome, the more modern and precise method of single ion channel recording with the patch clamp technique provides an excellent potential to understand the intracellular basis of changes in gastrointesinal motility. The advantages and disadvantages of each technique (extracellular, intracellular and patch clamp) will be discussed in the following sections.

EXTRACELLULAR RECORDING

Extracellular recording has the advantage of being noninvasive and simple in comparison to the other techniques. This recording has been attempted extracorporally in the case of the electrogastrogram, but recording from specific sphincters requires either a surgically placed extraserosal electrode or intraluminal electrodes.[38] These techniques have rarely been applied to sphincteric regions of humans. The electrical myographic (EMG) activity of different sphincters has been successfully employed.[39,40,41,42,43,44]

The recording of the EMG activity requires a surgical approach for the implantation of appropriate electrodes. The experiments may be done either under an acute or chronic setting. Chronic studies require at least two weeks to allow for the complete recovery from the surgical procedure. The advantage of the chronic experiments is that one can carry out the studies in an awake animal without the use of an anesthetic letting the animal move about freely.[40]

Overall, the EMG activity may not offer a significant practical advantage over intraluminal pressure recording to quantify the sum total changes in the sphincteric activity. This is because unlike nonsphincteric tissues, the sphincteric smooth muscles exhibit spontaneous tone which allow the monitoring of both contractile and relaxant effects on the basal intraluminal pressures. Furthermore, there is considerable correlation between changes in the EMG activity and changes in the basal sphincter pressures.

The EMG activity of the LES has been distinctly characterized by the presence of continuous spike activity.[39] In response to the contractile agent, there was an increase in the spike activity corresponding to the rise in the LES pressures. Conversely, there was a cessation of the spike activity in response to the relaxant agonist like isoproterenol or the neural stimulation that causes the relaxation of the sphincter.

The major advantage of the recording of the EMG activity is that it may help in pinpointing the structures responsible for certain components of sphincteric activity. This is possible only by examining the electrical behavior of individual structures or smooth muscle layer of the sphincteric zone in relation to the mechanical activity. The recording of mechanical activity of the sphincters on the other hand provides the sum total of activity and may not be able to identify the exact structures responsible for the actual activity.

INTRACELLULAR AND PATCH CLAMP RECORDING

Intracellular recording may serve an important purpose to provide specific information on sphincter function. This is especially important in the investigations of the nonsphincteric function. For example, the descending inhibition of esophageal smooth muscle preceding a peristaltic sequence is not apparent by manometry or extracellular electrical recording of the esophageal body since it has no resting tone and is already fully relaxed. The relaxation of the sphincter segment on the other hand is easy to document because of the presence of the resting tone. The inhibition of the nonsphincteric segment e.g., the esophageal body can however be demonstrated by the recording of intracellular electrical events (hyperpolarization).[45,46]

Because of the presence of the resting tone in the sphincteric smooth muscles, the changes recorded by either of the methods may lead to the same conclusion in *in vivo* and *in vitro* experiments. Considering the simplicity of the methods to record the mechanical changes *in vivo* and *in vitro,* and because of the lack of significant disparity in the outcome from that of the intracellular electrical recording, the latter has not gained much popularity in the sphincteric studies. Furthermore, because of the presence of significantly higher levels of connective tissue in the tissues, the penetration of the micro-tip glass electrode is rather difficult in the sphincteric smooth muscles.[45]

An alternative useful approach is to record the relative changes in the membrane potentials *in vivo* both in the sphincteric and nonsphincteric smooth muscles of the esophagus.[47] Such technique may not provide the specific information on the resting membrane potentials and absolute changes in membrane potentials in individual smooth muscle cell. However, it provides a useful tool to determine the relative changes in the membrane potentials in response to a specific stimulus or a physiological reflex. Whether the same approach can be employed in different sphincters of the gastrointestinal tract to record relative changes in membrane events in response to different neurohumoral agonists and the neural stimulation is not known.

Intracellular recording of the electrical events of the LES,[45] canine fundus[48] and guinea-pig IAS[49] suggest clear differences in the resting membrane potentials (RMP) of the sphincteric as compared to their adjoining smooth muscles. The RMP of the sphincteric zones is usually less negative, that means closer to the threshold action potential for the spike activity and the contraction. This suggests fundamental differences in the behavior of the sphincteric and nonsphincteric smooth muscles' ionic control mechanisms, ionic channels and other events taking place inside or across the smooth muscle cells. The recording of the intracellular electrical activity provides additional information on the electropharcomechanical coupling in the smooth muscle cells of the sphincter and insights into the pathophysiology of sphincteric dysfunction.

The most recent electrophysiological technique of patch clamp may help in the revelation of the basic mechanisms underlying differences in the control mechanisms of these two types of smooth muscles. The method for recording ion current flow through single channels has provided important information in the study of gastrointestinal smooth muscle cells. In this approach, a micropipette with a diameter of 1–2 m is placed against the isolated smooth muscle cell membrane. The membrane is then pulled into the pipette and the activity is recorded from a single channel in the "patch". Unfortunately, this method to examine sphincteric function has not been exploited.

EXAMPLES OF PHARMACODYNAMIC INFORMATION OBTAINABLE FROM THE STUDY OF GASTROINTESTINAL SPHINCTERS

The underlying tonic state of the gastrointestinal sphincters provide a unique opportunity for the study of drugs on gastrointestinal motility. Both inhibitory and excitatory agents can be easily evaluated without additional pharmacological or mechanical intervention of the organ system. In the nonsphincteric regions of the gut, which are not tonic, there is no consistent reproducible activity. This makes the quantitative study of these regions (especially of relaxation) more difficult. Therefore, the smooth muscle sphincters are ideal to investigate the nature of nonadrenergic, noncholinergic (NANC) inhibitory neurotransmitters, the structure/activity relationship of receptor subtypes, the modulatory action of neurohumoral substances and the biochemical mechanisms responsible for smooth muscle tone and relaxation.

For a substance to be considered as a NANC inhibitory neurotransmitter for a sphincter several conditions must be met:

1. The candidate substance should produce a relaxation in the sphincteric smooth muscle similar to that produced by NANC nerve stimulation.
2. The sphincteric muscle should relax in response to the candidate substance by its direct action at the sphincteric smooth muscle.
3. Specific antagonists which block the effect of the candidate substance should also block sphincteric relaxation caused by NANC nerve stimulation.
4. The candidate substance should be present in the myenteric neurons and should be released in response to NANC nerve stimulation.
5. Biochemical pathways and electrophysiological events leading to sphincter smooth muscle relaxation in response to NANC nerve stimulation and the candidate substance should correlate.

In order to prove or disprove these points, pharmacologic tools (agonists and/or antagonists) have been developed. The specificity of these tools is only relative and must be understood when evaluating results of pharmacologic studies. The specificity of the antagonist must be confirmed by its ability to selectively block the effect of the respective agonist, but not modify significantly the actions of another unrelated agonist which has a similar effect to the test agonist.

Using these criteria, studies on the IAS and LES ruled out the significant contribution of a number of classical and putative neurotransmitters as the sphincteric inhibitory neurotransmitter, including norepinephrine, acetylcholine, dopamine and ATP.[13,50] After several other possible transmitters were discarded, VIP was investigated.[12] VIP caused dose-dependent fall in the IAS pressure. Furthermore, the fall in IAS pressure in response to VIP was resistant to the actions of TTX suggesting a direct inhibitory action of the neuropeptide on the IAS smooth muscle. The direct action of VIP on different gastrointestinal smooth muscles has been confirmed on isolated smooth muscle cells.

In vitro studies showed that NO causes a fall in the resting tension of the IAS similar to NANC nerve stimulation.[51] The fall in the resting tension of the IAS by NO was concentration-dependent and was resistant to TTX. The effect of a nitric oxide synthase (NOS) (enzyme for the biosynthesis of NO) inhibitor on the NANC nerve-mediated relaxation of the IAS was tested next. The selective NOS inhibitor N^G-nitro-L-arginine (L-NNA) caused concentration-dependent suppression of the neurally-mediated IAS relaxation. The L-NNA suppressed relaxation of the IAS in response to neural stimulation was reversible by the NO precursor L-arginine in a concentration-dependent manner.

Furthermore, the IAS responses to L-NNA and L-arginine were stereoselective since D-NNA and D-arginine failed to have any effects.

The data of the experiments *in vivo* studies is similar to that of *in vitro* studies. The NO generator sodium nitroprusside caused fall in the IAS pressure which was resistant to TTX. The NOS inhibitor L-NNA caused concentration-dependent suppression of IAS relaxation in response to rectal balloon distension.

The IAS relaxation in response to different NANC neural stimuli (sacral nerve stimulation, local intramural stimulation and the ganglionic stimulant DMPP) were equally attenuated by L-NNA. All of the suppressant responses of L-NNA were reversible by L-arginine. The data showing the involvement of NO in the relaxation of IAS are similar to those from other laboratories in the IAS and LES.[18,19,25,52]

A number of neuropeptides including VIP have been localized to fibers innervating the gastrointestinal sphincters' smooth muscle. VIP has been demonstrated to be present in increased concentrations in sphincters as compared to the adjacent nonsphincteric smooth muscle regions.[53] Interestingly, VIP-immunoreactive neurons have been shown to be present in the normally functioning sphincteric neurons. Furthermore, such VIP-immunoreactive neurons are either absent or drastically reduced in the smooth muscle sphincters which fail to undergo appropriate relaxation in response to the appropriate reflex in patients affected with achalasia[54] and Hirschsprungs' disease.[55] It is of further interest that these patients experienced a fall in the LESP and an improvement in the sphincteric relaxation with VIP infusion.[56] These data provide further support for VIP as an inhibitory neurotransmitter in the LES. Evidence for VIP release in response to NANC nerve stimulation in the LES was provided by studies of Biancani and colleagues.[23]

Supportive evidence for the role of NO as an inhibitory neurotransmitter in the sphincters include the presence of NADPH diaphorase activity in the IAS of the opossum.[57] The release of NO in response to NANC nerve stimulation was recently shown by Chakder and Rattan.[58]

Similar to the absence of VIP-immunoreactive neurons in certain disease entities affecting the sphincters, data exists for the NOS containing myenteric neurons in different parts of the gut. For example, NOS containing neurons shown to be present in the normal pylorus were found to be absent in specimens obtained from pyloric stenosis patients.[59] Furthermore, subsequent studies by the same group[60] demonstrated the presence of NOS positive neurons in colonic specimens from controls. However, NOS positive neurons were missing in the aganglionic segments of the colon obtained from Hirschsprungs' disease patients. There is no data from the IAS specimens of either normals or the diseased individuals. Although a selective absence or dysfunction related to any neuropeptide in a disease state does not prove its role in the disease, the observations may point in the direction of dependence of a specific sphincter function on the neuropeptide and NOS.

Studies involving measurements of second messengers for the relaxation of the IAS smooth muscle in response to NANC nerve stimulation, using VIP and NO have suggested a common biochemical pathways for the smooth relaxation i.e. cAMP and cGMP.[27] Both cAMP and cGMP are involved as secondary messengers for smooth muscle relaxation by the activation of adenylyl and guanylyl cyclases respectively. Based on pharmacological studies, previous studies in our laboratory in the LES and IAS had suggested the presence of both adenylyl and guanylyl cyclases.[26,61,62] Furthermore, the data suggested the involvement of adenylyl and guanylyl cyclases in sphincteric smooth muscle relaxation in response to NANC nerve stimulation and different agents. The concept of VIP and NO as inhibitory neurotransmitters/mediators and the involvement of both cAMP and cGMP has been supported in a number of other sphincteric as well as nonsphincteric gastrointestinal tissues.

The similar nature of second messengers in smooth muscle relaxation in response to NANC nerve stimulation, VIP and NO may also suggest an interaction between VIP and NO. The interaction between VIP and NO was further tested by investigating the influence of the NOS inhibitor on the IAS relaxation by VIP. Interestingly, the fall in the resting tone of the IAS caused by VIP was significantly suppressed by the NOS inhibitor L-NNA.[17] On the other hand, the inhibitory effects of isoproterenol (which works primarily via adenylyl cyclase stimulation) and atrial natriuretic factor (ANF) (which works primarily via guanylyl cyclase stimulation) were not modified by the NOS inhibitor. The experiments with isoproterenol and ANF suggest specificity of action of the NOS inhibitor. Furthermore, the fall in IAS tone with VIP was partially accompanied by the release of NO.[58] The source of the NO release in response to VIP however is not exactly known. There are a large number of studies supporting the concept of an interaction of VIP with NO and of the involvement of both VIP and NO in the NANC nerve-mediated relaxation of the gastrointestinal smooth muscle.

Whether VIP and NO can explain all of the NANC nerve-mediated sphincteric relaxation is not exactly known. Interestingly, In the IAS, recent studies suggest the possibility of carbon monoxide (CO) as another inhibitory mediator.[63] The relative contribution of VIP, NO and CO in the relaxation of the gastrointestinal smooth muscle sphincters remains to be determined. Whether NO and CO serve as the actual inhibitory neurotransmitters or mediators in the gastrointestinal smooth muscle sphincters remains to be resolved. There are a number of examples to show the hyperpolarization response to both NANC nerve stimulation and VIP in the sphincteric as well as the nonsphincteric smooth muscle cells.[48] It is also of interest that recent studies examining VIP gene expression scanning the entire gastrointestinal tract revealed the characteristic higher expression of VIP mRNA in all the smooth muscle sphincters.[64] Such data support the concept of VIP-rich innervation of the gastrointestinal sphincters.[53]

An additional use of gastrointestinal sphincters studies is the investigation of receptors and receptor subtypes and to investigate the structure-activity-relationship of different agents. The heterogeneity of muscarinic receptors was found first in the LES based on the following observations. Vagal stimulation-induced LES relaxation was only partially antagonized by lower doses of the classical muscarinic antagonist atropine. This antagonism was however clearly evident when vagal stimulation-induced LES relaxation was examined in the presence of the nicotinic antagonist hexamethonium. Moreover, the predominant effect of the muscarinic ganglionic agonist (McN-A-343) when given close-intraarterially in the region of the LES, was to cause the relaxation of the LES. Interestingly, the relaxant action of McN-A-343 was antagonized by TTX and lower doses of atropine. Conversely, the commonly used muscarinic agonist, bethanechol caused contraction of the LES. The contractile effect of bethanechol on LES was resistant to antagonism by TTX but was blocked by atropine. These data led to the hypothesis of heterogeneity of muscarinic receptor types.[65] One type present on the myenteric ganglia in the vagal inhibitory pathway and the other directly on the smooth muscle cells of the LES. Furthermore, these studies in the LES led to the concept of not only nicotinic but also the specific type of muscarinic receptor in the synaptic transmission in the vagal inhibitory pathway of the LES. Since then, the heterogeneity of muscarinic receptors has been reported in different sphincteric and nonsphincteric areas of the gastrointestinal tract and other organs. These heterogeneity of muscarinic receptors was later recognized to play a significant physiological role in a variety of tissues in the gastrointestinal tract and other organs systems. To date, five different types of muscarinic receptors have been characterized and cloned and the data is summarized in a recent review article.[66]

Likewise, the LES and IAS preparations have been used to identify receptor types and subtypes for a number of neurohumoral agents; 5-hydroxytryptamine,[67] histamine,[68] opioids,[69,70] cholecystokinin,[71] neuropeptide Y,[15] galanin[72] and CGRP,[73] and VIP and PHI[74].

The studies examining the detailed structure-activity-relationship in the IAS reveal the diverse actions of neuropeptides and help to clarify divergent actions in various portions of the gut.[72] The characteristic differences in the actions of closely related neuropeptides VIP and PHI in the IAS suggested for the first time distinct differences in the types of receptors activated by each of these neuropeptides in gut smooth muscle.[74] These conclusions have been confirmed by recent studies in other regions of the gastrointestinal tract.[75]

Regarding structure-activity-relationships, two studies in the IAS dealing with the effects of VIP[76] and galanin[72] are worth mentioning. Even a slight change in the structure of VIP (VIP 1–28) caused the loss of biological activity of the neuropeptide. Interestingly, the C-terminal portions of the molecule (VIP 2–28 and VIP 10–28) although devoid of biological activity had the ability to bind to the IAS smooth muscle receptor. The binding of VIP and analogs was determined by receptor binding experiments. Furthermore, these C-terminal fragments were found to be competitive antagonists of VIP. In addition, the specific function of galanin depends upon specific portions of the neuropeptide. The C-terminal portion (galanin 15–29) caused an increase in IAS tension while the N-terminal portion (galanin 1–10) exhibited an inhibitory effect on the IAS. Further analysis revealed that the inhibitory actions of galanin 1–10 were partly neurally-mediated, and the excitatory actions of galanin 15–29 were direct on the IAS smooth muscle. Interestingly, the predominant effects of full molecule of galanin on the IAS were inhibitory.

Sphincteric preparations have also been used to investigate the modulatory actions of neuropeptides and other endogenous substances in the gastrointestinal tract. This important aspect of sphincteric studies may be typified by an *in vivo* study that examines the role of neuropeptide Y (NPY) in the IAS.[15] Our studies in the IAS showed two sites of actions of NPY, one on the IAS smooth muscle and the other at the myenteric NANC inhibitory neurons in the IAS. NPY receptors on the IAS smooth muscle were apparent by the inability of different neurohumoral antagonists and tetrodotoxin to attenuate the excitatory actions of NPY. NPY receptors at the myenteric NANC inhibitory neurons were examined by eliciting the rectoanal inhibitory reflex by rectal balloon distension. These NPY receptors may be comparable to NPY_1 and NPY_2 and similar in location to those of α_1- and α_2-adrenoceptors in the IAS.[77]

OTHER CONSIDERATIONS IN STUDY OF SPHINCTERS

The sphincter of Oddi (SO) is a sphincter with a very narrow lumen. This presents a challenge in the recording of intraluminal pressures. Solid state transducers have thus far not been made in small enough sizes to record, limiting the techniques to perfused catheters which may produce an artifact in these small sphincters. In humans and large animals a catheter may be placed in the SO using the technique of endoscopic retrograde cholangiography (ERCP). This approach is not practical in some animal models including the opossum which is the most commonly used animal model. In addition, if too rapid an infusion rate is used then post procedural pancreatitis is more likely.[78] In animal studies the catheter can be placed via an incision in the common bile duct or duodenal lumen and then advanced into the sphincter.

The pylorus while not as easily studied as the esophageal or anal sphincters, has an important function and can be studied in many of the ways above mentioned. In intact humans and lab animals, a catheter can be placed across the pylorus, although with some difficulty, and manometric tracings can be obtained.[79] Contraction of the pylorus alone, isolated pyloric pressure waves (IPPW's), has been reported to occur during both active mixing of the gastric contents and during the solid phase of gastric emptying.[80] There is good correlation between manometric abnormalities in the pylorus and antropyloric segment compared to radioisotope gastric emptying studies.[81] As in the LES and other sphincters, sleeve devices have been fashioned to better define the pyloric pressure profile, although the experience is limited.[82] Like other sphincters, myoelectrical and contraction studies can be performed on isolated strips of pyloric muscle.[83]

Evaluation of the ileocecal sphincter (ICS) in intact animals using intraluminal manometry is difficult. A method of evaluation using an open preparation with a manometry catheter placed into the ICS from a colonic incision has been reported.[84] Using this technique the various opioid receptors at the ICS (μ, κ, δ, σ) have been studied.[85] Muscle strips obtained from the ileocecal valve demonstrate tonic activity like the other sphincters and can be studied using the previously described techniques.[86]

Using *in vivo* and *in vitro* studies, different concepts developed in the LES and IAS have been reproduced in the sphincter of Oddi, pylorus and the ICS. In these sphincters, both VIP and NO have been shown to be involved as inhibitory neurotransmitters or mediators. Different receptors and subtypes to a number of neurohumoral substances have been shown. Furthermore, the modulatory role of a number of neuropeptides and other neurohumoral substances resembling those in the LES and IAS have been demonstrated.

THE CHOICE OF AN ANIMAL MODEL

While no animal model may replace humans, with small compromises one can come fairly close to an appropriate model. The choice of the animal should be one that can most accurately reflects the human condition. For example, in the study of the LES, if human and primate subjects are excluded, the opossum may be an excellent choice. Interestingly enough the opossum is also an excellent model of the IAS.[87] Sometimes the choice of an animal model may depend on the strategic location of the sphincteric apparatus. The SO in the opossum may not be the most similar to the human, but its extraduodenal location both makes it accessible to study and allows the muscle to be studied without the interference of pressure changes caused by the duodenal musculature. Expense also is a consideration. Common lab rats would be ideal, but differences in muscle composition (striated LES in rats) and size issues make their study less than optimal. Primates would be a good choice, but there are ethical concerns in their use as well as cost issues. The opossum and cat appear to be the best models for the study of most gastrointestinal sphincters.

ISSUES OF VARIABILITY

Intra- and intersubject, intra- and interspecies, and individual smooth muscle strip variation must be a constant consideration in physiologic and pharmacologic studies. Intraspecies variability can only be controlled for by keeping in mind the issues outlined in the preceding section. Much of the other variability can be minimized by using each preparation, be it animal or even individual smooth muscle strip as its own control. In order to assure normal function in an *in vivo* preparation the response to the intact reflex (e.g. swallowing in the LES and rectoanal reflexes in the IAS) should be recorded and serve as the baseline for pharmacologic manipulation.

SUMMARY AND CONCLUSIONS

The main methods for the pharmacological studies of the sphincter are: intraluminal pressures recording (using perfused catheters manometry and solid state) *in vivo,* recording of isometric tension *in vitro,* extracellular EMG activity *in vivo* and intracellular electrical activity *in vitro.*

The choice of the methodology depends on the type of the question to be addressed and the information sought for the action of the drugs in relation to the sphincter function. For example, if the pharmacological study calls for the investigation of the drug at the neural pathways controlling a particular sphincter function, the initial studies have to be carried *in vivo* and intraluminal pressures recording would be choice of methodology. For the pharmacological analysis of the motor (contractile and relaxant) actions of the drug at the neuromuscular level of the sphincter, the isometric tension recording of the sphincteric smooth muscle strips *in vitro* alone or combined with *in vivo* studies would be the choice. Carefully planned studies with the judicious use of pharmacological tools applied on these *in vivo* and *in vitro* studies help in sorting out a wide variety of issues. These issues may pertain anywhere from the role and actions of an agent in question on the reflex pathway, the nature of the inhibitory neurotransmitter, to the receptor site of action of a particular agent. The combination of these approaches may allow one to narrow down the site of action of the drug. These methods have also served an excellent purpose to characterize the nature of the receptor types and subtypes, and the nature of the putative inhibitory neurotransmitters.

Once the site of action in response to a certain agent has been narrowed down, it may be confirmed by the use of other approaches e.g. the isolated smooth muscle cells and the recording of the extracellular and intracellular activities from the structure under scrutiny. To further resolve the issues, one may examine the release of the neurotransmitter substance in question and perform histological examination of the sphincteric specimens for the substance of interest. In order to understand the role of the appropriate ionic channels in the regulation of the function of the sphincter and its changes in response to the specific agent, one may take the advantage of the patch clamp approach.

Manometry, however, (whether done by the use of perfused catheters or the solid state intraluminal device) remains the mainstay of the study in human sphincters and is a bridge between the animal and human studies. Such studies are invaluable for pathophysiological investigations of the sphincter function.

The use of any of the approaches to examine sphincteric function and drug action requires an understanding of different disciplines including Anatomy, Neurophysiology and Pharmacology. It is very important to understand the specific use and the limitation of different methods, and established pharmacological tools to unravel the actions of unknown agents on the sphincter function. Continued progress in the understanding of the sphincteric function will provide important clues to the pathophysiology and therapeutic regimen of not only the sphincteric but also of other gastrointestinal motility disorders.

REFERENCES

1. **Meltzer, S. J.,** Recent experimental contributions to the physiology of deglutition, *NY State J Med* 59, 389, 1894.
2. **Pope, C. E.,** A dynamic test of sphincter strength: its application to the lower esophageal sphincter, *Gastroenterology* 52, 770, 1967.
3. **Dent, J., Chir, B.,** A new technique for continuous sphincter pressure measurement, *Gastroenterology* 71, 263, 1976.
4. **Castell, J. A., Dalton, C. B., Castell, D. O.,** Effects of body position and bolus consistency on the manometric parameters and coordination of the upper esophageal sphincter and pharynx, *Dysphagia* 5, 179, 1990.
5. **Sugarbaker, D. J., Rattan, S., Goyal, R. K.,** Swallowing induces sequential activation of esophageal longitudinal smooth muscle. *Am J Physiol* 247, G515, 1984.
6. **Culver, P. J., Rattan, S.,** Genesis of anal canal pressures in the opossum, *Am J Physiol* 251, G765, 1986.
7. **Rattan, S., DeVault, K.,** Role of peptides in the function and dysfunction of the internal anal sphincter, *Regulatory Peptides* 3, 29, 1991.
8. **Cannon, D. A., Geenan, J. E., Hogan, W. J., Venu, R. P., Johnson, G. K., Schmalz, M. J.,** Pancreatitis following sphincter-of-Oddi manometry: A prospective evaluation of possible risk factors. *Gastroenterology* 104, A351, 1993.
9. **Goyal, R. K., Rattan, S.,** Genesis of basal sphincter pressure: Effect of tetrodotoxin on lower esophageal sphincter pressure in opossum in vivo. *Gastroenterology* 71, 62, 1976.
10. **Humphries, T. J., Castell, D. O.,** Pressure profile of esophageal peristalsis in normal humans as measured by direct intraesophageal transducers, *Am J Dig Dis* 22, 641, 1977.
11. **Castell, J. A., Dalton, C. B.,** Esophageal manometry, in *The Esophagus*, Castell, D. O., Ed., Little, Brown and Co. Boston 143, 1992.
12. **Goyal, R. K., Rattan, S., Said, S. I.,** VIP as a possible neurotransmitter of non-cholinergic, non-adrenergic inhibitory neurons, *Nature* 288, 378, 1980.
13. **Rattan, S.,** The non-adrenergic non-cholinergic innervation of the esophagus and the lower esophageal sphincter, *Arch Int Pharmacodyn* 280, 62, 1986.
14. **Yamato S, Rattan S.** Role of alpha adenoreceptors in opossum internal anal sphincter. *J Clin Invest* 86, 424, 1990.
15. **Nurko, S., Rattan, S.,** Role of neuropeptide Y in opossum internal anal sphincter. *Am J Physiol* 258, G59, 1990.
16. **Nurko, S., Rattan, S.,** Role of vasoactive intestinal polypeptide in the internal anal sphincter of the opossum, *J Clin Invest* 81, 1146, 1988.
17. **Rattan, S., Chakder, S.,** Role of nitric oxide as a mediator of internal anal sphincter relaxation, *Am J Physiol* 262, G107, 1992.
18. **Yamato, S., Saha, J. K., Goyal, R. K.,** Role of nitric oxide in lower esophageal sphincter relaxation to swallowing. *Life Sciences* 50, 1263, 1992.

19. **O'Kelly, T., Brading, A., Mortensen, N.** Nerve mediated relaxation of the human internal anal sphincter: the role of nitric oxide. *Gut* 34, 689, 1993.

20. **Sandler, A. D., Maher, J. W., Weinstock, J. V., Schmidt, C. D., Schlegel, J. F., Jew, J. Y., Williams, T. H.,** Tachykinins in the canine gastroesophageal junction, *Am J Surg* 161, 165, 1991.

21. **Rostad H.** Colonic motility in the cat. I. Extraluminal strain gage technique. Influence of anesthesia and temperature. *Acta Physiol Scand* 89, 79, 1973.

22. **Pascaud, X. B., Genton, M. J. H., Bass, P.,** A miniture transducer for recording of intestinal motility in unrestrained chronic rats. *Am J Physiol* 235, E532, 1978.

23. **Biancani, P., Walsh, J. H., Behar, J.** Vasoactive intestinal polypeptide. A neurotransmitter for lower esophageal sphincter relaxation. *J Clin Invest* 73, 963, 1984.

24. **Biancani, P., Walsh, J. H., Behar, J.,** Vasoactive intestinal peptide: A neurotransmitter for relaxation of the rabbit internal anal sphincter, *Gastroenterology* 89, 867, 1985.

25. **Tottrup, A., Knudsen, M. A., Gregersen H.,** The role of the L-arginine-nitric oxide pathway in relaxation of the opossum lower oesophageal sphincter. *Br J Pharmacol* 104, 113, 1991.

26. **Rattan, S., Moummi, C., Chakder, S.,** CGRP and ANF cause relaxation of opossum internal anal sphincter via different mechanisms, *Am J Physiol* 269, G764, 1991.

27. **Chakder, S., Rattan, S.,** Involvement of both cAMP and cGMP in relaxation of internal anal sphincter by neural stimulation, VIP and NO, *Am J Physiol* 264, G702, 1993.

28. **Rattan, S., Goyal, R. K.,** Free intracellular calcium ($[Ca^{2+}]_i$) in unstimulated and stimulated lower esophageal sphincter (tonic) and esophageal body (phasic) smooth muscle. *Gastroenterology* 91, 1064, 1986.

29. **Neering, I. R., Morgan, K. G.,** Use of aequorin to study excitation-contraction coupling in mammalian smooth muscle. *Nature (Lond)* 288, 585, 1980.

30. **Abe, A., Karaki, H.,** Effect of forskolin on cytosolic Ca^{++} level and contraction in vascular smooth muscle. *J Pharmacol Exp Ther* 249, 895, 1989.

31. **Bitar, K. N., Makhlouf, G. M.,** Receptors on smooth muscle cells: characterization by contraction and specific antagonists. *Am J Physiol* 242, G400, 1982.

32. **Grynkiewicz, G., Poenie, M., Tsien, R. Y.,** A new generation of Ca++ indicators with greatly improved fluorescence properties. *J Biol Chem* 260, 3440, 1985.

33. **Sato, K., Ozaki, H., Karaki, H.,** Changes in cytosolic calcium level in vascular smooth muscle strip measured simultaneously with contraction using fluorescent calcium indicator fura 2. *J Pharmacol Exp Ther* 246, 294, 1988.

34. **Makhlouf, G. M.,** Isolated smooth muscle cells of the gut, in *Physiology of the gastrointestinal tract,* Johnson, L. R., Ed., Raven Press, NY, NY. 555, 1987.

35. **Biancani, P., Hillemeier, C., Bitar, K. N., Makhlouf, G. M.,** Contraction mediated by Ca^{2+} influx in esophageal muscle and by Ca^{2+} release in the LES. *Am J Physiol* 253, G760, 1987.

36. **Hillemeier, C., Bitar, K. N. Marshall, J. M., Biancani, P.,** Intracellular pathways for contraction in gastroesophageal smooth muscle cells. *Am J Physiol* 260, G770, 1991.

37. **Bitar, K. N., Hillemeier, C., Biancani, P., Balazovich, K. J.,** Regulation of muscle contraction in rabbit internal anal sphincter by protein kinase C and Ins (1,4,5)P3. *Am J Physiol* 260, G537, 1991.

38. **Abell, T. L., Malagelada, J. R.,** Electrogastrography. Current assessment and future perspectives, *Dig Dis Sci* 33, 982, 1988.

39. **Asoh, R., Goyal, R. K.,** Electrical activity of the opossum lower esophageal sphincter in vivo. Its role in the basal sphincter pressure. *Gastroenterology* 74, 835, 1978.

40. **Sarna, S. K.,** In vivo myoelectric activity: methods, analysis, and interpretation. In *Handbook of Physiology, The gastrointestinal system,* Wood, J. D., Ed. American Physiological Society, Bethesda 817, 1989.

41. **Monges, H., Salducci, J., Naudy, B., Ranier, F., Gonella, J., Bouvier, M.,** The electrical activity of the internal anal sphincter: a comparative study in man and cats. In: *Gastrointestinal Motility,* Christensen, J., Ed., Raven, New York 495, 1980.

42. **Toouli, J., Dodds, W. J., Honda, R., Sarna, S., Hogan, W. J., Komarowski, R. A., Linehan, J. H., Arndorfer, R. C.,** Motor function of the opossum sphincter of Oddi. *J Clin Invest* 71, 208, 1983.

43. **Ouyang, A., Snape, W. J., Cohen, S.,** Myoelectric properties of the cat ileocecal sphincter. *Am J Physiol* 240, G450, 1981.

44. **Bouvier, M., Gonella, J.,** Nervous countrol of the internal anal sphincter of the cat. *J Physiol Lond* 310, 457, 1981.

45. **Decktor, D. L., Ryan, J. P.,** Transmembrane voltage of opossum esophageal smooth muscle and its response to electrical stimulation of intrinsic nerves. *Gastroenterology* 82, 301, 1981.

46. **Conklin, J. L., Du, C.,** Guanylate cyclase inhibitors: effect on inhibitory junction potentials in esophageal smooth muscle. *Am J Physiol* 263, G87, 1992.

47. **Rattan, S., Gidda, J. S., Goyal, R. K.,** Membrane potential and mechanical responses of the opossum esophagus to vagal stimulation and swallowing. *Gastroenterology* 85, 922, 1983.

48. **Szurszewski, J. H.,** Electrical basis for gastrointestinal motility. In: *Physiology of the Gastrointestinal Tract.* Johnson, L. R., Ed., Raven, New York 1435, 1981.

49. **Lim, S. P., Muir, T. C.,** Neuroeffector transmission in the guinea-pig internal anal sphincter: an electrical and mechanical study. *Euro J Pharmacol* 126, 17, 1986.

50. **Rattan, S., Shah, R.,** Influence of purinoceptors' agonists and antagonists on opossum internal anal sphincter, *Am J Physiol* 255, G389, 1988.

51. **Rattan, S., Sarkar, A., Chakder, S.,** Nitric oxide pathway in rectoanal inhibitory reflex of opossum internal anal sphincter. *Gastroenterology* 103, 43, 1992.

52. **Murray, J., Du, C., Ledlow, A., Bates, J. N., Conklin, J. L.,** Nitric oxide: mediator of nonadrenergic noncholinergic responses of opossum esophageal muscle. *Am J Physiol* 261, G401, 1991.

53. **Alumets, J., Schaffalitzky de Mckadell, O., Fahrenkrug, J., Sundler, F., Hakanson, R., Uddman, R.,** A rich VIP nerve supply is characteristic of sphincters. *Nature* 280, 155, 1979.

54. **Aggestrup, S., Uddman, R., Sundler, F., Fahrenkrug, J., Hakanson, R., Rahbek, H. J., Sorensen, Hambraeus, G.,** Lack of vasoactive intestinal polypeptide nerves in esophageal achalasia, *Gastroenterology* 84, 924, 1983.

55. **Tsuto, T., Okamura, H., Fukui, K., Obata, H. L., Terubayashi, H., Iway, N., Majima, S., Yanaihara, N., Ibata, Y.,** An immunohistochemical investigation of vasoactive intestinal polypeptide in the colon of patients with Hirschsprung's disease, *Neurosci Lett* 34, 57, 1982.

56. **Guelrud, M., Rossiter, A., Souney, P. F., Rossiter, G., Fanikos, J., Mujica, V.,** The effect of vasoactive intestinal polypeptide in the lower esophageal sphincter in achalasia, *Gastroenterology* 103, 377, 1992.

57. **Lynn, R. B., Sankey, S. L., Chakder, S., Rattan, S.,** Colocalization of NADPH—diaphorase staining and VIP immunoreactivity in neurons in opossum internal anal sphincter. *Dig Dis Sci* 40, 78, 1995.

58. **Chakder, S., Rattan, S.,** Release of nitric oxide by activation of nonadrenergic noncholinergic neurons of internal anal sphincter. *Am J Physiol* 264, G7, 1993.

59. **Vanderwinden, J. M., Mailleux, P., Schiffmann, S. N., Vanderhaeghen, J. J., De Laet, M. H.,** Nitric oxide synthase activity in infantile hypertrophic pyloric stenosis. *New Eng J Med* 327, 511, 1992.

60. **Vanderwinden, J. M., De Laet, M. H., Schiffmann, S. N., Mailleux, P., Lowenstein, C. J., Snyder, S. H., Vanderhaeghen, J. J.,** Nitric oxide synthase distribution in the enteric nervous system of Hirschsprung's disease. *Gastroenterology* 105, 969, 1993.

61. **Rattan, S., Moummi, C.,** Influence of stimulators and inhibitors of cyclic nucleotides on lower esophageal sphincter. *J Pharmacol Exp Ther* 248, 703, 1989.

62. **Moummi, C., Rattan, S.,** Effect of Methylene blue and N-Ethlmaleimide on internal anal sphincter relaxation. *Am J Physiol* 255, G571, 1988.

63. **Rattan, S., Chakder, S.,** Inhibitory effect of CO on internal anal sphincter: heme oxygenase inhibitor inhibits NANC relaxation. *Am J Physiol* 265, G799, 1993.

64. **Bandyopadhyay, A., Chakder, S., Lynn, R. B., Rattan, S.,** Vasoactive intestinal polypeptide gene expression is characteristically higher in opossum gastrointestinal sphincters. *Gastroenterology* 107, 1911, 1994.

65. **Rattan, S., Goyal, R. K.,** Neural control of the lower esophageal sphincter: Influence of the vagus nerves. *J Clin Invest* 54, 899, 1974.

66. **Wess, J.,** Molecular basis of muscarinic acetylcholine receptor function. *Tr Pharmacol Sci.* 14, 308, 1993.

67. **Rattan, S., Goyal, R. K.,** Effects of 5-Hydroxytryptamine on the lower esophageal sphincter in vivo. Evidence for multiple sites of action. *J Clin Invest* 59, 125, 1977.

68. **Rattan, S., Goyal, R. K.,** Effects of histamine on the lower esophageal sphincter in vivo: evidence for action at three different sites. *J Pharm Exp Ther* 204, 334, 1978.

69. **Rattan, S., Goyal, R. K.,** Identification and localization of opioid receptors in the opossum lower esophageal sphincter, *J Pharmacol Exp Ther* 224, 391, 1983.

70. **Barnette, M. S., Grovs, M., Manning, S. D., Callahan, J. F., Barone, F. C.,** Inhibition of neuronally induced relaxation of canine lower esophageal sphincter by opioid peptides, *Euro J Pharmacol* 182, 363, 1990.

71. **Rattan, S., Goyal, R. K.,** Structure-activity relationship of subtypes of cholecystokinin receptors in the cat lower esophageal sphincter. *Gastroenterology* 90, 94, 1986.

72. **Chakder, S., Rattan, S.,** Effects of galanin on the opossum internal anal sphincter: structure-activity relationship. *Gastroenterology* 100, 711, 1991.

73. **Chakder, S., Rattan, S.,** Antagonism of calcitonin gene-related peptide (CGRP) by human CGRP-(8-37): role of CGRP in internal anal sphincter relaxation. *J Pharmacol Exp Ther* 256, 1019, 1991.

74. **Nurko, S., Dunn, B. M., Rattan, S.,** Peptide histidine isoleucine and vasoactive intestinal polypeptide cause relaxation of opossum internal anal sphincter via two distinct receptors. *Gastroenterology* 96, 403, 1989.

75. **Murthy, K. S., Zang, K. M., Jin, J. G., Makhlouf, G. M.,** Characterization of distinct VIP- and PHI-preferring receptors and VIP- and PHI-specific receptors on dispersed gastric muscle cells. *Gastroenterology* 104, A843, 1993.

76. **Chakder, S., Rattan, S.,** The entire VIP molecule is required for the activation of the VIP receptor: Functional and binding studies on opossum internal anal sphincter smooth muscle. *J Pharmacol Exp Ther* 266, 392, 1993.

77. **Yamato, S., Rattan, S.,** Role of alpha adrenoceptors in opossum internal anal sphincter. *J Clin Invest* 86, 424, 1990.

78. **Toluli, J., Roberts-Tompson, I. C., Dent, J., Lee, J.,** Manometric disorders in patients with suspected spincter of Oddi dysfunction. *Gastroenterology* 88, 1243, 1985.

79. **Malagelada, J. R., Stanghellini, V.,** Manometric evaluation of functional upper gut symptoms, *Gastroenterology* 88, 1223, 1985.

80. **Houghton, L. A., Read, N. W., Heddle, R., Horowitz, M., Collins, P. J., Chatterton, B., Dent, J.,** Relationship of the motor activity of the antrum, pylorus and duodenum to gastric emptying of a solid-liquid mixed meal, *Gastroenterology* 94, 1285, 1988.

81. **Camilleri, M., Brown, M. L., Malagelada, J. R.,** Relationship between impaired gastric emptying and abnormal gastrointestinal motility, *Gastroenterology* 91, 94, 1986.

82. **Horowitz, M., Dent, J.,** Disordered gastric emptying: mechanical basis, assessment and treatment, in *Buillere's Clinical Gastroenterology: Practical Issues in Gastrointestinal Motor Disorders,* Vol 5. Dent, J. Ed. Billere Tindall, London, 371, 1991.

83. **Sanders, K. M., Vogalis, F.,** Organization of electrical activity in the canine pyloric canal, *J Physiol* 416, 49, 1989.

84. **Ouyang, A., Clain, C. J., Snape, W. J., Cohen, S.,** Characterization of opiate mediated responses of the feline ileum and ileocecal sphincter, *J Clin Invest* 69, 507, 1982.

85. **Ouyang, A., Vos, P., Cohen, S.,** Sites of activity of u-, k- and o- opiate receptor agonists at the feline ileocecal sphincter. *Am J Physiol* 254, G224, 1988.

86. **Boeckxstaens, G. E., Pelckmans, P. A., Rampart, M., Verbeuren, T. J., Herman, A. G., Van Maercke, Y. M.,** Nonadrenergic noncholinergic mechanisms in the ileocolonic junction, *Arch Int Pharmacodyn* 303, 270, 1990.

87. **Christensen, J., Stiles, M. J., Rich, G. A., Sutherland, J.,** Comparative anatomy of the myenteric plexus of the distal colon in eight mammals. *Gastroenterology* 86, 706, 1984.

13 Assessment of CNS Control of Gastrointestinal Motility

Lionel Bueno

INTRODUCTION

The existence of an egemonial control of gut motility was suspected from evidence of colics resulting from anxiety or fear. However, the first evidence that the brain may be a target site of actions of drugs to alter gastrointestinal motility or transit concerns the influence of intracerebroventricular (ICV) administration of morphine in rats. In parallel, numerous studies have shown that electrical stimulation of the hypothalamic area affects gastric and intestinal contractions in anaesthezed animals. For example, stimulation of the paraventricular nucleus (PVN) decreases intragastric pressure[1] while phasic antral contractions are induced by the electrical stimulation of the lateral hypothalamus (LH).[2]

The characterization in brain structures of a large number of peptides known to influence gastrointestinal motility has provided new impetus for the evaluation of their role at cerebral and spinal levels in the control of gut motility. The first evidence that a hypothalamic factor may affect gastrointestinal motility by acting primarily on the central nervous system (CNS) was given in 1977 by Smith et al.[3] who showed that thyrotropin releasing hormone (TRH) administered by ICV route stimulates colonic motility in the anaesthezed rabbit. The use of intracerebroventricular cannula to inject directly peptides into the cerebrospinal fluid has permitted to largely improve our knowledge concerning drugs and neuropeptides acting centrally on gastrointestinal transit and motility in awake animals. Furthermore, the use of microcannulas directed into nuclei and microiontophoretic deposit of substances have largely contributed to this improvement of our knowledge. We review herein the role of brain structures and neurotransmitters in the course of gut motility not only in physiological conditions but also in experimentally induced pathological states.

PATTERNS OF GI MOTILITY AND DIGESTIVE STATUS

STOMACH

In many species manometric recordings of antral motility during fasting or interdigestive period exihibit a cyclic pattern of high-amplitude contractions grouped in phases lasting 20–90 minutes separated by periods of quiescence and appearing at 90–120 minutes intervals (Figure 1). The fundamental characteristic of fundic motility is the presence of a steady resting potential of the smooth muscle cells with no regular fluctuations (slow waves) at least in dog and man.[4–5] The other important property of the proximal stomach is the receptive relaxation, mediated by inhibitory neurons in vagal nerves,[6] which enables it to receive readily boluses of food from the oesophagus. The patterns of contractile activity of the canine gastric corpus and antrum

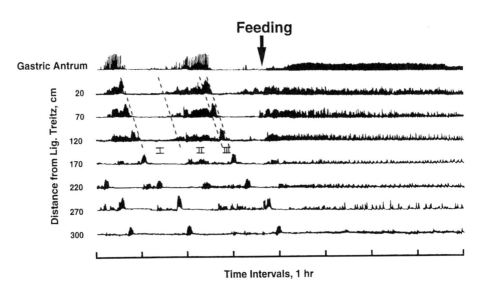

FIGURE 1 Organization of gastrointestinal motility in awake dogs recorded by chronically implanted strain-gauge. In fasted state, the motility is organized in migrating myoelectric complex (MMC) propagated from the duodenum to the ileum and comprising 3 phases: 1: quiescience, 2: irregular, 3: regular activity. This cyclic pattern is disrupted by feeding for a duration depending from the nature of food.

consist of a series of high-amplitude contractions for 15–25 minutes followed by a long lasting (70–110 min) motor quiescence. By analogy with the nomenclature used for the small intestine (see below) this pattern has been divided in three successive periods: phase 1: quiescence, phase 2: moderate activity, and phase 3: maximal activity. The contractions of the corpus and the antrum are coordinated; a slow concentration of the corpus lasting about 30 seconds is associated with three to five more rapid contractions of the antrum.[7] After a meal, the digestive pattern is characterized by steady low-amplitude contractions (4–5 per min) in the gastric antrum with no significant motor activity in the gastric body. An intermediate pattern characterized by contractions of the body and higher amplitude contractions of the antrum, together with the steady postprandial contractions, is present for a variable period before the gastric motility returns to a typical fasted state.

Such a pattern of gastric motility has been found in the dog[8] and in man.[9] In the rat[10] and the rabbit[11] there is no cyclic organization of the gastric motility, and feeding induces an increase of both amplitude and frequency of contractions.

SMALL INTESTINE

The basic motor pattern of many animal species investigated consists of migrating motor (or myoelectric) complexes (MMC), first identified as "a caudad band of large-amplitude action potentials starting in the duodenum and traversing the small bowel".[12] Each MMC corresponds to three consecutive phases: phase 1 has little or no contractile activity (quiescent phase), phase 2 has intermittent and irregular contractions, while the contractions of phase 3 occur at their maximal rate, which is determined by the frequency of the slow waves. The duration of phase 3 activity is relatively constant, but that of other phases varies from cycle to cycle, depending on the flow of digesta.[13] According to the animal species, the duration of intestinal MMC cycle varies between 60–120 minutes intervals except in rats in which MMC occurs at 15–20 minutes intervals.[14]

Feeding is accompanied by a disruption of this intestinal MMC to give a "postprandial" pattern characterized by the irregular occurence of small-amplitude contractions similar to those observed during phase 2 of the MMC[15] (Figure 1).

This disruption of the MMC pattern and its replacement by a "fed" pattern is related to multiple factors, including the energy content of the meal, the nature of nutrients and the frequency of meals and is mediated through mixed neural and humoral factors. In dogs, it has been established that there is a linear relationship between the duration of the postprandial state of gut motility and the energy content of a meal.[16]

However, non-nutrient factors are also involved in the postprandial disruption of the MMC pattern, since sham-feeding significantly delays the next phase 3 in man.[17] On the other hand, meal frequency modulates the effects of feeding on small intestinal motility. For example, in pigs[18] or in rats,[19] ingestion of a daily large meal disrupts the MMC for several hours, while under *ad libitum* conditions the MMC frequency is similar to that observed in the fasted state in pigs and is only reduced in rats during the night, which corresponds to a period of intense ingestion. However, in adult as well as in neonatal pigs, feeding a standard meal only induces a 1 hour delay in the onset of the next phase 3.[20]

LARGE INTESTINE

A universal pattern analogous to that observed for the small intestine has not been found for the large bowel. A common feature of the colon in all mammalian species investigated is a duality of the contractile activity: tonic contractions corresponding to myoelectrical events characterized by short spike bursts. However, the spatial and temporal organization of these two kinds of contractions which form the colonic motor pattern is peculiar in each mammalian species investigated. This pattern is independent of colonic anatomy and of the traditional regimen of the animal species, but gross similarities exist within species producing moulded faeces in pellets such as the rabbit or the sheep.[21]

In dogs high-amplitude colonic contractions are grouped in phases lasting 4–6 minutes and appearing at a rate of 2–3 per hour in the fasted state with an increase in frequency (4 or 5 per hour) during the 10 hours after a daily meal.[22] In man the most typical characteristic of colonic motility, not seen in animals, consists of a very low activity during the night time.[23] After a 3000–4000 kJ meal the frequency of colonic contractions is increased for 2–3 hours. Such an increase in colonic motility after a meal seems to be a common feature.

ACCESS TO BRAIN STRUCTURES

LOCALIZATION OF BRAIN CENTERS

It has been known for many years that the nucleus tractus solitarius is the major projecting site of vagal afferent fibers which in turn projects to the dorsal motor nucleus of the vagus (DMNV) a major site of efferent vagal fibers.[24–26] However, other brain structures may influence such vago-vagal reflexes either through a direct effect of motorneurons of the DMNV or by modulating the neuronal activity at NTS level.[27] (Figure 2) Electrophysiological technics reveal the presence of neuronal connections between the hypothalamus and the NTS[28] and microstimulations of the NTS induce both ortho-and antidromic activation of median and lateral hypothalamus[29] while electrical stimulation of the PVN activates neurons of the NTS[30] (Figure 2).

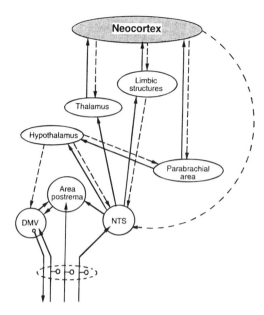

FIGURE 2   Representation of the main connections of brain structures involved in vagal afferent and efferent control of gut motility. Note that it corresponds to a general schema related to observations performed in various animal species but numerous interspecific differences exist in the distribution of projecting neurons.

HYPOTHALAMUS AND CONNECTIONS TO THE BRAINSTEM

The hypothalamus receive afferent messages from both parasympathetic and sympathetic afferent fibers as well as from circulating or locally released neuropeptides and hormones. Retrograde labelling have shown that there are many connections between the VMH, PVN, LHA and DMH (Figure 3) and that the DMH is a major interconnecting site between the VMH and LHA.

Periaqueducal gray matter (PAG) is the major projecting site from VMH[31-32] and PAG nucleus appears to be a major relay from the VMH to the DVC[33] but also to the reticular formation[34] (Figure 3).

In contrast LHA projects directly to the DVM but also through several nucleus such as PAG, nucleus ambigus or other hypothalamic sites including parvocellular reticular nucleus (RPC).[35]

CENTRAL AFFERENT NEURONS TO THE NTS

In addition to peripheral afferents from cranial nerves, the NTS receives projecting neurons from many brain structures (Figure 2).

Among them bilateral projections from nucleus ambigus[36] and from parabrachial nucleus,[37] two nuclei playing a major regulatory role in the control of the autonomic nervous system and receiving spinal afferents. The NTS also receives several projections from several nuclei of the raphe pallidus, dorsalis and obscurus with predominant inputs from raphe magnus[38] most of them containing serotonin and constitute one of the major ways of nociceptive messages.[39]

However, the most proeminant projections to the NTS coming from the hypothalamus particularly are from the dorsomedial part and the paraventricular nuclei (PVN) as well as from the ventral regions.[40] Electrophysiological evidence indicates an interaction between descending

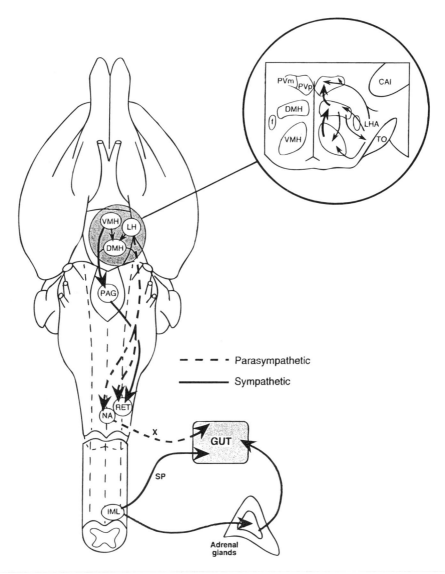

FIGURE 3 Main intrahypothalamic connections and sympathetic and parasympathetic efferent pathways to the gut. VMH: ventromedian hypothalamus; LH: lateral hypothalamic, DMH: dorsomedian hypothalamus, PAG: periaqueductal gray matter; NA: nucleus ambigus, ret: reticular formation, IMG: inferior mesenteric ganglion; SE: splanchnic nerves.

PVN[41] neurons and vagal motor of the DMN as well as NTS. Microstimulation of the PVN enhances neuronal response of NTS neurons to gastric distension while its destruction sharply reduces the sensitivity of vago-vagal reflexes.[41]

Other structures, such as the central part of the amygdala involved in the control of emotional states often associated with abnormalities of gut motility, also project to the NTS.[42–43]

In addition to these pleiotropic connections, the NTS contains most of the classical neurotransmitters found active on gastrointestinal motility when injected centrally such as Ach, 5-HT and catecholamines but also neuropeptides like CCK_8, NPY, Substance P, somatostatin and opioids. Moreover, immunohistochemistry has revealed that the pathways connecting the PVN to the DVC contain peptides including also vasopressin, oxytocin and TRH.[44]

Functional Evidence of Hypothalamic Control of Gut Motility

Stomach

In 1965, Folkow and Rubinstein,[45] following several pioneering experiments performed 60 years ago, confirmed that electrical stimulation of the LHA induces a vagally mediated gastric relaxation. This inhibition was demonstrated to persist under atropine and spinal cord section and not selective from the stimulation of the LHA.[46] In contrast, the electrical stimulation of the VMH induces a gastric hyperkinesia while those of the PVN is followed by an inhibition of phasic contractions.[1] More generally, the stimulation of the anterior nuclei of the hypothalamus stimulates gastric motility through both a decrease of vagal cholinergic tone[46] and an increase in sympathetic discharges.[47–48]

However, it has also been recently reported that electrical stimulation of the nucleus ambigus with low-current, high-frequency electrical stimulation increases the force of antral contractions. It was also found that stimulation of the LHA in cats with 1mA, 10Hz and 8 ms increases the force of antral contractions without increasing acid output suggesting that the two phenomenon are not correlated and that the gastric motor effects are not secondary to cardiovascular effects.[49]

Small Intestine and Colon

The literature concerning the effects of hypothalamic stimulation on small intestine motility still remains controversial. In general, electrical stimulation of many hypothalamic areas activates intestinal or colonic motility but these effects are preceded by a transient or prolonged inhibition in cats.[50–51] This primary inhibition is not detected in anaesthetized dogs and only the activation of few areas of the anterior hypothalamus is able to stimulate colonic motility[52] while a marked stimulation of small intestine motility is obtained only after stimulation of the LHA.[45] In contrast, in awake cats, it was found that the stimulation of the dorsal nuclei of the hypothalamus is always associated with a stimulation of colonic motility; however, the technic used to stimulate these nuclei and the parameters chosen were far to be as selective than that used in more recent studies.[53]

Methods of Investigations

With the discovery of brain neuropeptides, numerous studies have been focused on the determination of their role in the regulation of gut motility. In this issue several methods have been introduced from intracerebroventricular to iontophoretic administration for determination of the active sites, as well as, the identification of activated brain structures by expression of proonctogene-like C-Fos, C. Jun and Krox 24.

In addition, the retrograde or anterograde labelling of afferent and efferent fibres, several techniques of selective surgical deafferentation at nodose ganglion or at bulbar level[54] as well as nerve cooling or chemical deafferentation with capsaicin destroying selectively C. fibers, recently have been introduced.[55]

Intraventricular Injections or Perfusion

Most of the published works were performed using cannula chronically inserted into the lateral ventricle of the brain, allowing injected substances to penetrate brain from the inner surface.

The major risk of drug leakage back into the subarachnoid space through the needle track is limited by the placement of the end of the cannula 1–2 mm above the upper wall of the ventricle; the injection being performed through a tube introduced into the cannula penetrating the ventricle. The passage of substances, injected from lateral ventricle to the third and fourth ventricles, is related to the volume injected (Figure 4). For example, the apomorphine injection into lateral ventricle of the brain in cats produces vomiting by action on the area postrema, which is situated at the end of the fourth ventricle for the same amount, only when it is diluted into 0.25 ml but not 0.1 ml of saline.[56] Consequently, the volumes used for injection into lateral ventricle of the brain have to be adjusted between a minimal and maximal values according to the species investigated (Table 1).

Perfusions may be performed in anaesthetized animals either by infusion into the lateral ventricle and outflow collection from cisterna magna or directly with better and selective supraspinal drainage from the rostral end of the aqueduct limiting the contact of drugs to the inner surface of lateral and third ventricles.[57]

In such conditions, a 1 to 10 ratio active doses, injected ICV and IV respectively, strongly suggests a CNS target site, but a possible spinal site of action may be determined by comparing the active dose injected intrathecally and ICV. Independently of the short half-life of many peptides injected centrally and their rapid appearance in the peripheral circulation after ICV administration,[58] ICV infusion is more adequate than bolus injection for testing the effects of centrally administered neuropeptides. For example, CCK_{8s} infused ICV at a rate of 0.3 nmole/min is enough to produce a disruption for the MMC pattern in fasted rats while 1 μmole is the minimal active bolus injection in the same ventricle.[59]

MICROINJECTIONS INTO THE NUCLEI

Microinjection may be performed in chronically prepared animals while microintophoretic deposits are made in anesthetized animals.

Stainless-steel guide cannulas 200–300 μm in diameter (gauge 23) with obturators are generally used in awake animals. They are lowered just above the nuclei investigated according to brain atlas. Injections are performed through 30 gauge stainless-steel injector cannulas inserted into the guide cannulas. The injectors are constructed so that their tip extend 1 mm beyond the end of the guide cannulas (Figure 5). The injectors are connected by a polyethylene tube (PE-10) to a 10 μl syringe mounted on an infusion pump. In rats, volumes of 50 nl are commonly used. Polyvinyl tubes are not recommended due to adhesion of some peptides. Distilled apyrogenic water containing or not bovine serum albumin (4%) is commonly used. The possible thermogenic effects of saline (NaCl 9%) injected ICV limits its use.

The microintophoretic technique allows substances to be applied in the vicinity of a small group of neurons. Most commonly the multibarreled micropipettes has an overall size of 4–5 μm [i.e. 1 μm (barrel)]. The barrels used for drug or peptide delivers are filled either with NaCl solution, and their resistance should not exceed 120 MΩ, they can contain different drugs or concentrations of the same drugs in order to perform administrations according to the phoretic current applied.[60]

INVESTIGATIONS ON PATHWAYS INVOLVED

The role of the vagus in either afferent or efferent transmission from the CNS may be investigated by temporal cooling of the vagus, a technique originally described in dogs.[61] Results obtained after chronic bilateral section of the vagus at cervical or thoracic levels may be considered with caution as well as those obtained just after section associated with a temporary hypervagotonia.

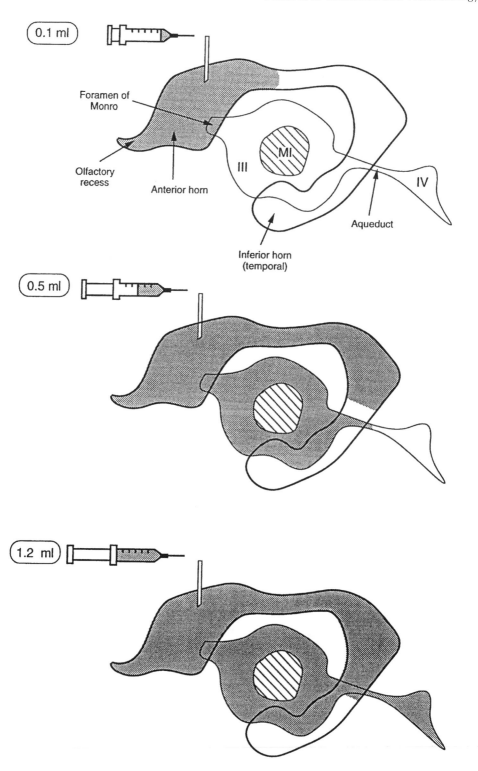

FIGURE 4 Diagrams illustrating the distribution of a drug injected into the lateral ventricle of the canine brain according to the volume injected. The tip of out flowing cannula is indicated by two vertical bars: The grey area corresponds to the distribution of injected substances. III and IV: 3^{d} and 4th ventricles, MI: massa intermedia.

TABLE 1
Minimal and Maximal Volumes Admitted for Intracerebroventricular Administrations (Lateral Ventricle) to Reach the Third Ventricle (Minimum) Without Detectable Consequences on Intraventricular Pressure (Maximum)

	Volumes (μl)	
	Min	Max
Mouse	0.5	2
Rat	2	10
Cat	200	400
Dog	400	800
Sheep	500	1000

In the cooling *technic*, the vagus nerves are exteriorized at cervical level in a skin loop and vagal blockade is performed by circulation of absolute ethanol at $-2°C$ through copper cooling jackets placed around the skin loop. This technique has been largely used to evaluate the role of the CNS in the control of intestinal MMC pattern[62] and has also being applied to cool the vagus at intrathoracic level.[63] However this technique does not permit identification of the type of vagal fibers involved: afferent *vs* efferent. The use of capsaicin which exerts a long-term sensory receptor blocking action acting mainly of C fibers has been successfully used in

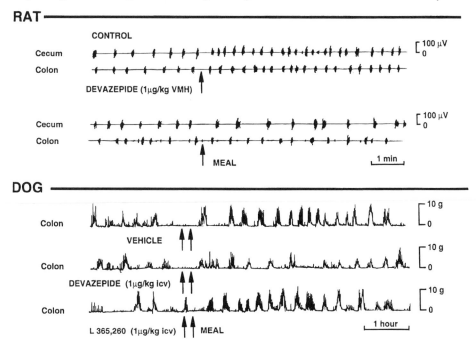

FIGURE 5   Central modulation of the colonic motor response to feeding by CCK antagonists in rats and dogs. Upper part: direct record of myoelectrical activity of the proximal colon in rats. Note that the increase in the frequency of spike-bursts associated to eating is suppressed after bilateral administration of 50 ng of devazepide (a CCK_A antagonist) into the VMH. Lower part: record of colonic contractions in awake dog using strain-gauges placed on the transverse colon showing the delayed food-induced colonic hyperkinesia which is suppressed after ICV administered devazepide but not L 265360, a selective CCK_B antagonist.

functional investigations of sensory pathways.[64] In the digestive tract, capsaicin sensitive afferent innervation is evident.[55] In rats capsaicin is administered either systemically, daily during 4 days to reach a total dose of 125 mg/kg[65] or perivagally, after *in vivo* isolation of the vagus at cervical level under anaesthesia and atropinization.[66] The comparison of the responses between systemic and perivagal treatments permits identification of the sensory pathways involved.

ROLE OF THE CNS IN THE CONTROL OF GUT MOTOR PATTERNS

The brain contains highly specific binding sites for many peptides located in areas involved in the control of gut motility. A large number of these peptides have been found to influence gastric emptying and intestinal transit when injected centrally (Table 2).

PUTATIVE BRAIN ACTIVE PEPTIDES

Hypothalamic Releasing Hormones

Thyrotropin-releasing hormone (TRH) and corticotropin-releasing hormone (CRH) are largely distributed in hypothalamic areas that control gut motility. Furthermore, localization of TRH and its receptors are well correlated with the sites of origin of vagal preganglionic neurons that innervate the stomach, as well as with the termination of gastric vagal afferent pathways, particularly in the tractus solitarius. Central administration of TRH enhances gastric emptying of a methylcellulose meal in rats,[67] and nutritive meal in mice.[68] Accelerated intestinal transit is observed after administration of TRH in the medial and lateral nuclei of the hypothalamus.[69] Accordingly, intracisternal injection of TRH markedly stimulates gastrointestinal motility in anesthetized rats, and in conscious animals, increases the amplitude and duration of phasic contractions of the corpus. Stimulation of the amplitude of antral contractions was also observed

---

TABLE 2
Comparative CNS Influence of Several Peptides on Gastrointestinal and Colonic Transit

Peptides		Gastric emptying	Intestinal transit	Colonic transit	Site of action	Species
Opioid peptides	μ	−	−	−	Cerebral (Hyp), spinal	Mice, rats, dogs
	δ	−	−	−	Spinal	Rats, mice
	κ	0/−	0	−	Spinal	Rats, mice
TRH		+	+	+	Cerebral (Hyp)	Rats, cats, rabbits
CRF		−	−	+	Cerebral (Hyp)	Rats, dogs
Bombesin		−	−	−	Cerebral (DVC) NTS/spinal	Mice
Calcitonin		−	−	ND	Cerebral (DVC)	Rats
CGRP		−	−	ND	Cerebral (DVC), spinal	Rats
Neurotensin		−	−	ND	Cerebral (PAG)	Rats
CCK8		−	−	ND	Cerebral (Hyp, DVC)	Mice

ND, Not Determined; Hyp, Hypothalamic nucleus; DVC, Dorsal Vagal Complex; PGM, Periaqueducal Grey Matter.
Adapted from Buens and Fioramonti (1991)[96].

after ICV administration of TRH in sheep.[70] Duodenal spike activity is also stimulated after central injection of TRH in rats,[71] sheep,[70] and rabbits.[72]

Microinjection techniques have allowed localizing TRH sites of action in the dorsal motor nucleus of the vagus, the nucleus tractus solitarius, nucleus ambiguus and in the raphe, but not in the postrema area and other medullary nuclei.[73–74] Stimulation of gastric contractile activity elicited by central administration of TRH is abolished after vagotomy and in atropinized rats;[75] moreover, ICV injection of TRH stimulates gastric vagal efferent discharges in the rat, suggesting that TRH acts in the dorsal vagal complex to stimulate preganglionic vagal efferent neurons which in turn synapse with myenteric cholinergic excitatory neurons. Using microdialysis, it was recently shown that CNS administration of TRH increases the release of serotonin and dopamine in the gastric interstitial fluid and serotonin appears to play a major role in the genesis of centrally administered TRH-induced gastric ulceration.[76]

TRH appears to be one of the central mediators of gastric injuries associated with cold restraint stress,[77] but its role in other experimental stressful situations, often associated with slowing of gastric emptying, is not supported by experimental data.

The motor effects of TRH are not limited to the upper gut and it also stimulates colonic transit with occurence of diarrhea associated with peripheral serotonin release in rabbits.[69] Similarly, ICV administration of TRH enhances defecation in conscious rats.[78]

CRH was first described as a hypothalamic factor regulating pituitary ACTH secretion. Its location, in both the hypothalamus and in the area of the brain controlling gut motility suggested a physiological role in the regulation of gastrointestinal motor events. CRH also plays an important role in the supraspinal regulation of gastrointestinal motility and transit. Both gastric emptying and intestinal transit are altered by central administration of CRH in rats, mice and dogs.[67]

The first evidence that CRH injected centrally affects gastrointestinal motility was obtained in dogs. Intracerebroventricular administration of ovine CRF suppresses the gastric activity fronts corresponding to MMC for several hours without affecting jejunal motility.[79] However, when injected postprandially, CRF does not affect greatly gastric motility,[80] but delays the occurence of the fasted pattern i.e., MMC at intestinal level. Administration of CRH in rats inhibits the fundic motor response to intracisternal administration of the TRH analog RX77368.[77] In rats intracisternal or ICV injection of CRH reduces gastric emptying of a non-nutritive liquid meal associated with a decrease of small bowel transit and an enhancement of colonic transit and fecal output.[81–83] Similarly in dogs, CRH injected into the third ventricle also delays gastric emptying of a liquid protein meal, while in mice, ICV injection of CRF increases gastric emptying of a milk meal.[84] Such opposite effects of centrally administered CRH on gastric emptying in rats and mice has been attributed to the differences in species; however, in most of the studies, including those performed in rats, a non-caloric meal was used for the measurement of gastric emptying while a nutritive meal was used in mice (Table 2). According to the different effects of CRF on gastrointestinal motility in relation to the digestive status, a crucial role of the meal composition in the effects of CRH on gastric emptying has to be considered.

Pretreatment with a ganglionic or noradrenergic blocker as well as vagotomy suppress the CRH-induced delay in gastric emptying and intestinal transit while vagotomy alone is able to prevent the effects of CRF on colonic transit.[81,82]

All these results suggest that the centrally mediated effects of CRH on gastrointestinal motility are not uniform; they depend at least on the species, the digestive segment considered, and the basal motor profile. They also differ from proposed pathways for mediating CRH-induced inhibition of gastric acid secretion which involve efferent fibres of the sympathetic nervous system, and in part, a vasopressin-dependent pathway, but not the parasympathetic nervous system, adrenal epinephrine release or opiate-sensitive pathways.[82]

Blockade of the effects of CRH on gastric motility after vagotomy in dogs[83] as well as the inability of central CRH to alter gastric emptying in vagotomized rats strongly suggests that the vagus is involved. Central administration of CRH modulates the parasympathetic outflow from the brain regulating gastric functions[85] to produce vagal excitation. However, the failure of CNS administration of atropine, or pirenzepine, to block CRH induced gastric motor inhibition (unpublished observations) is not in agreement with this hypothesis.

OPIOID PEPTIDES

A number of studies have suggested that μ and δ opioid receptor subtypes are involved in both the cerebral and spinal cord structures controlling gut motility (Table 2). However, it is also clear that the ratio of central to peripheral sites of action depends upon the species and the digestive state considered. The central antipropulsive effects of selective μ opiate agonists like DAGO (D-Ala^2, N-methylphe, gly^5-ol enkephalin) are reversed by naloxone and vagotomy; in contrast, the highly selective cyclic enkephalin analogue DPDPE (D-pen^2, pen^5 enkephalin), acting selectively on δ receptors, is inactive on intestinal transit when administered by ICV injection; although DPDPE does inhibit colonic transit in mice. Taken together these data indicate that the centrally mediated inhibitory action of opiates on gastric and intestinal transit appears to be selectively mediated through the μ receptor subtype whereas both μ and δ subtypes may be involved in the inhibition of colonic transit in rodents.[86]

In dogs ICV administration of DALAMIDE (D-Ala$_2$, Met$_5$-enkephalinamide), but not DADLE (D-Ala$_2$, D-Leu$_5$-enkephalinamide), alters gastrointestinal motility inhibiting cyclic contractions of the antrum with concomitant stimulation of intestinal motility. It has been demonstrated that the periaqueductal gray matter is a site of action of the enkephalin analog, FK 33824 with selective μ receptor affinity and β-endorphin to inhibit intestinal transit, but the δ agonist DALAMIDE microinjected into the same area of the brain does not affect intestinal transit in rats. Slowing of gastric emptying induced by CNS administration of Metenkephalin acting through μ receptors is probably related to an inhibition of gastric motility; a decrease in gastric, but not intestinal, motility index is observed after ICV administration of Damamide in fasted rats.[87]

Dynorphin 1–13 as well as selective kappa agonists injected ICV or microinjected into the opiate-sensitive area of the brain have no effect on intestinal transit. This suggests that this opioid peptide is not important in the CNS regulation of gut motility in basal conditions. However, kappa opioid agonists are able to act centrally to suppress stress-induced gastric hypomotility (see § Va).

Porreca et al.[88] have shown that the spinal cord is an independent site of action for the influence of opiates on gastrointestinal transit. Indeed, morphine injected intrathecally after spinal cord transection still inhibits gastrointestinal transit in mice and rats. However, in mice, intrathecal injection of the δ agonist DPDPE is as active as DAGO, a selective μ agonist, in influencing intestinal transit, suggesting that opiate-induced inhibition of intestinal transit by spinal action may result from activation of both μ and δ receptor subtypes. Concerning the location of supraspinal sites of action for the opiates, it has been suggested that μ receptor agonists act in the periaqueducal grey matter to inhibit intestinal transit.[89] Moreover, the midline thalamus and the lateral and dorsal hypothalamus are responsive to morphine-induced inhibition of intestinal transit whereas the amygdala, caudate nucleus and frontal cortex are not active sites. Moreover, the antitransit effect of morphine applied into the periaqueducal area requires the integrity of the serotonergic pathways and is not vagally mediated.[89]

OTHER NEUROPEPTIDES

Several peptides including bombesin, calcitonin, calcitonin gene-related peptide (CGRP), cholecystokinin (CCK), neuropeptide Y (NPY), neurotensin, oxytocin, somatostatin and substance P influence gastrointestinal transit and/or the fed and fasted patterns of gastrointestinal motor activity when injected centrally (Table 2) but little information concerning the mechanisms and the sites of action is at present available.

The neurohumoral mechanisms involved in the effects of these peptides are different. While the inhibition of gastric emptying elicited by ICV administration of bombesin is reversed by vagotomy,[90] that of calcitonin is abolished by ganglionic blockade but not by vagotomy, hypophysectomy, adrenalectomy or by sympathetic blockade.[91] In contrast the effects of CGRP are abolished after adrenalectomy, while bombesin requires an intact pituitary adrenal axis.[92] Slowing of intestinal transit induced by central administration of neurotensin or CGRP is suppressed after vagotomy[90] and the centrally-mediated intestinal motor effects of neurotensin are blocked by antidopaminergic substances acting on D2 receptor subtype.[93]

Finally, the lateral and medial hypothalamus and limbic system are proposed to be the sites of action of TRH for the acceleration of intestinal transit while the periaqueducal grey matter may be responsible for the antitransit effects of neurotensin as for enkephalins. Most of these effects have been shown to be vagally mediated, but the nature of the vagal fibres involved remain to be determined.

INITIATION OF THE FED PATTERN

Among the peptides released after feeding, CCK8, insulin and neurotensin induced a "fed-like" pattern when injected centrally (Table 3). Cholecystokinin is present in cell bodies and fibres within the hypothalamus with the highest levels being found in the para- and periventricular nuclei and high affinity binding sites in the ventromedial hypothalamic nucleus. Exogenous CCK8 introduced into the cerebrospinal fluid could reach CCK8 terminals in the hypothalamic area and act at these sites to affect intestinal motility as suggested by MMC disruption following ICV administration.[59] However, CCK8 applied iontophoretically stimulates neurons of the dorsal vagal nucleus which influence gastrointestinal motility. Recently, it was shown that the ventrome-dial hypothalamus (VMH) is also one of the major sites of action of CCK8 to initiate the fed pattern. Microinfused into the VMH in rats, CCK8 (50 ng) disrupts the MMC pattern while the same amount injected into the LHA is not active.[94] Furthermore, the CCK_A receptor antagonist L364,718 injected bilaterally prior to feeding into the VMH, consistently reduced the duration of the "fed pattern" confirming that CCK8 is involved at hypothalamic (VMH) level in main-

TABLE 3
Non-Peptidergic Drugs Acting at CNS Level to Modulate the Pattern of Migrating Myoelectric Complex in the Duodenum-Jejunum

MM initiation	MMC disruption	Frequency	Duration
M_1 agonists			
α_2 agonists	α_2 agonists	Benzodiazepines	Opioids
D_1, D_2 agonists	H_2 agonists	M_3 agonists	NK_1 agonists
$5HT_{1A}$ agonists	$5TH_2$, $5HT_3$ agonists	α_2 agonists	$5HT_3$ agonists
$GABA_A$ agonists	$GABA_B$ agonists	$5HT_4$ agonists	
H_1, H_3 agonists	Benzodiazepines	Indomethacin	
Prostaglandins E_2	$IL1\beta$	CCK_A agonists	
Platelet-activating factor	H_2 agonist		
A_1, A_2 adenosine Analogues	L-NAME		
Opioids (μ)			

taining the postprandial duodenal motor pattern.[95] The origin of active CCK8 is not clear, since CCK8 released into the blood stream after feeding is not supposed to cross the blood-brain barrier. It is also known that CCK8 from nerve terminals is released at hypothalamic level after a meal. It is possible, however, that feeding may induce a late CCK8 release in the CNS. More recently, it was also shown that CCK8 injected into the VMH mimicked the stimulatory effects of feeding on colonic motility.[95] The fact that a CCK$_A$ antagonist injected bilaterally into the VMH prior to feeding abolishes the colonic motor response to feeding strongly supports the hypothesis that CCK8 is involved not only in the adaptation of intestinal motility to fed state, but also to the related changes in colonic motility (Figure 6).

RECOVERY OF THE FASTED MMC PATTERN

Administered by ICV injection at fentomolar doses, calcitonin restores the MMC pattern after feeding in rats and dogs. Radiolabeled calcitonin administered parentally binds specifically to sites in the hypothalamus and immunoreactive calcitonin is present in the hypothalamus and cerebrospinal fluid. This leads to the possibility of some physiological involvement for calcitonin in the postprandial recovery of the MMC pattern and agrees with its centrally mediated effects on gastric emptying and intestinal transit. Such premature recovery of the fasting pattern may be responsible for slowing of gastric emptying.

Other brain peptides like CGRP, neurotensin and enkephalins, but also non-peptidic substances (Table 3) are able to restore the fasted pattern in "fed" rats and to shorten the duration of postprandial pattern in rats and dogs.[96] These peptides are known for their inhibitory effect

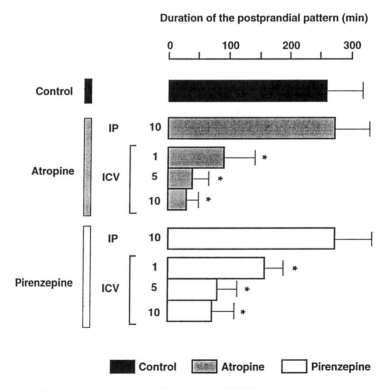

FIGURE 6 Brain cholinergic modulation of the duration of the postprandial motor pattern after a chow pellet meal (6g) in 15 h fasted rats previously treated ICV or IP with atropine and pirenzepine (adapted from ref. 100). Note that the reduction is observed for ICV administration and is equivalent for the two antimuscarinic agents.

on gastric emptying of liquid test meals, all of them being detected in brain regions supposed to be involved in the control of gut motility. Many non-peptidic substances probably act by modulating their release at the corresponding activated pathways to the brainstem.

NON-PEPTIDERGIC NEUROTRANSMITTERS

For many years classical neurotransmitters such as acethylcholine (Ach) or adrenaline deposits in hypothalamic nuclei are known to induce changes in gastric motility in anesthetized rats. Recent investigations have confirmed that these neurotransmitters and others (dopamine, serotonin, histamine etc.) play a role in the supraspinal regulation of gut motility.

Acethylcholine

Numerous studies have revealed that Ach and its receptors are present in NTS and hypothalamic neurons.[97–99] Cholinergic stimulation of certain areas of the brain affect colonic motility suggesting the involvement of cholinergic transmission in the activation of both excitatory and inhibitory hypothalamic neurons regulating digestive motility.[52]

M_1 and M_2 receptors have been evidenced in the rat brain with a differential anatomical localization, adding evidence for a distinct functional role of these two receptor populations in brain function.[99]

Using selective M_1 or M_2 agonists and antagonists it was shown that muscarinic receptors are probably involved in the disruption of the jejunal MMC pattern induced by a meal in rats (Figure 6), and that these effects are linked to activation of M_2 receptor subtype.[100] In contrast, postprandial stimulation of colonic motility related to central release of CCK mainly involved M_3 receptor subtype.[95]

Catecholamines

Catecholaminergic binding sites are present in the vagal dorsal motor nucleus and the tractus solitarius which contains gastrointestinal afferents and efferents;[101] moreover, most of the binding sites correspond to α_2 presynaptic receptors[102] and dopaminergic type D_2 receptors.[103] Several subgroups of neurons have been identified[104] and centrally administered clonidine is known to inhibit intestinal[105] as well as colonic[106] transit in rats. Concerning intestinal motility, it was shown that central administration of clonidine or naphazoline, which poorly crosses the blood-brain barrier, induces a fed-like pattern in fasted rats while α_2 antagonists like yohimbine, which increases central adrenergic outflow, restore a MMC pattern typical of the fasted state in fed rats[107] (Figure 7). Furthermore, the disruption of the cyclic activity induced by feeding is altered after ICV treatment with DSP_4, a selective noradrenergic neurotoxic agent.[107]

The *locus caeruleus* (L. C.) is one possible important noradrenergic nucleus participating in the modulation of intestinal pattern, since lesions induced by local injections of 6-hydroxydopamine alter the periodicity of MMC;[108] a major role of this nucleus is confirmed by the absence of any alteration of motor pattern induced by bilateral lesions of the central segmental tract which carries ascending noradrenergic axons from the medullary and pontine cell groups outside the L. C. (Figure 8).

All these results suggests the involvement of supraspinal adrenergic compound in the regulation of intestinal motility under physiological circumstances. Finally, we hypothetize from these results that a balance between central noradrenergic and cholinergic activity may be responsible for the adaptation of the intestinal motor pattern to the digestive state. Colonic motility also appears to be under a central noradrenergic control. Yohimbine, an α_2-adrenoceptor antagonist, as well as SKF 86466 which poorly crosses the blood brain barrier, strongly stimulate

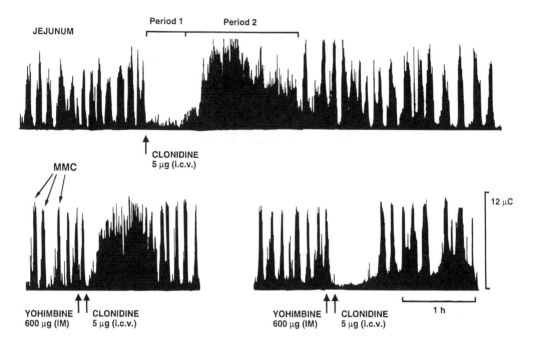

FIGURE 7 Central noradrenergic influences on the pattern of myoelectric activity (integrated record) of the jejunum in fasted rats. Clonidine, an α_2 adrenergic agonist disrupts the MMC pattern with a primary inhibitory phase and a delayed induction of a "fed-like" pattern. Injected systemically (IM) yohimbine abolishes the primary inhibitory phase while administered ICV it restores the MMC pattern without affecting the primary inhibition.

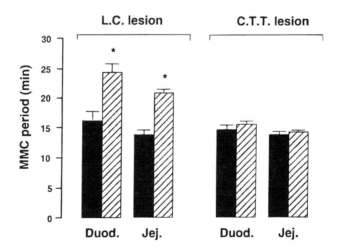

FIGURE 8 Comparative influence of lesions of the locus caeruleus (LC) and central tegmental tract (CTT) induced by 6-OHDA on the duration of duodenal (duod) and jejunal (jej) migrating myoelectric complex in rats. Treatment is associated with a drastic noradrenergic depletion in the two nuclei but influencing intestinal motor pattern only for the LC.

colonic motility when injected centrally in dogs and these effects are mediated through the vagus since they are suppressed after bilateral vagotomy.[109]

Dopamine

CCK8 and dopamine[110] or neurotensin (NT) and dopamine[111] are colocalized in several brain areas particularly mesencephalic neurons and hypothalamus involved in the control of gastrointestinal and colonic motility. Moreover DA neurons of the DVC have dendritic branches distributed in the NTS.[112]

Dopamine injected ICV mimics the effects of both calcitonin and neurotensin on the small intestine, i.e. a delay or a blockade in the occurence of postprandial disruption of duodenal and jejunal fed pattern.[93]

The central effects of NT and [D-Trp$_{11}$] NT, a potent agonist at NT receptors, involved dopaminergic neurons since they are blocked by haloperidol and (+) SCH 23390, a selective D$_1$ receptor antagonist, suggesting the participation of D$_1$ receptors.[93] Dopamine also participates in the supraspinal control of colonic motility since DA, as well as selective D$_1$ (SKF 38383) or D$_2$ (quinpirole) receptor agonist injected ICV, increases the frequency of colonic contractions. Furthermore, such dopaminergic activation may be involved in stress-induced colonic motor hyperkinesia.[113]

Histamine

Neurochemical, neurophysiological and pharmacological evidence[114-115] has given great support to the theory that histamine is a neurotransmitter in the CNS.

Several studies[116-118] have shown that the highest concentrations of histamine are found in the ventral posterior hypothalamus where there are histaminergic neurons from which arise widespread projections distributed to various regions of the brain.[119]

Histamine injected centrally exhibits opposite effects from those observed after systemic administration increasing the frequency of MMC in the fasted state and restoring MMC pattern in the fed state.[120] While the peripheral effects are antagonized by H$_1$ (chlorpheniramine), and to a lesser extent, H$_2$ (cimetidine) receptor antagonists, the centrally mediated effects of histamine are easily blocked by a selective H$_3$ receptor antagonist (thioperamide) and reproduced by R-α methylhistamine and H$_3$ agonist.[120]

Serotonin

The role of 5-HT in the regulation of gut motility is pleitropic due to a wide array of 5HT receptor types[121] which are distributed on both nerves and muscles[122,123] as well as in the CNS.[124]

Presence of 5HT$_{1A}$ and 5HT$_2$ receptor subtypes[125] in the area postrema as well as 5HT$_3$ in several animal species[126,127] is well documented, but binding sites of 5HT are also present in other brain nuclei such as the hypothalamus and the NTS.[126,128]

Several studies performed in sheep have shown evidence that 5HT$_2$ and 5HT$_3$ receptor subtypes are both involved in the inhibition of forestomach induced by centrally administered 5-HT.[129-130] However, central 5HT$_{1A}$ receptors appear to mediate inhibition of gastric motility associated with duodenal distension.[131]

Evidence that hypothalamic 5HT$_3$ receptors are involved in the physiological regulation of gastric motility is supposed by the increase in gastric emptying of radio-opaque spheres in fasted guinea-pig after injection of ICS 205930 into the perifornical area of the hypothalamus and its antagonism of the slowing effects of 2-methyl 5HT injected in the same area.[132]

The effects seem to be mediated through the vagus,[133] however, 5HT$_3$ receptors were described to be present along the entire length of noradrenergic fibers within spinal ganglia as well as spinal cord itself.[134]

Other Mediators

γ-aminobutyric acid (GABA) is a major inhibitory transmitter of the brain[135] and its centrally mediated effects are mediated by two subtypes of GABA receptors, namely $GABA_A$ and $GABA_B$ receptors which can be distinguished by appropriate agonists and antagonists. Many studies have evaluated the role of GABA receptors at peripheral level in the control of gut motor events. Indeed, injected systemically, $GABA_B$ agonist like baclofen induces relaxation in the guinea-pig ileum and colon[136] and stimulates gastric motility in rats.[137]

Recent results suggest that, in rats, only $GABA_B$ receptor subtype is involved in the centrally mediated effects of GABA on gastrointestinal motility consisting of an increase in duodenal and jejunal motor activity (Figure 9). These effects are probably mediated through the stimulation of brain muscarinic receptors at a site yet to be precised, but do not involve adrenergic and opiate receptors.[138]

In contrast, in other species like sheep, both $GABA^A$ and $GABA_B$ receptor subtypes were supposed to be involved also at CNS level in the inhibition of forestomach motility associated with colonic motor stimulation.[139]

In other species like dogs, $GABA_A$ agonist like muscimol are efficient when injected ICV to suppress the gastric motor inhibition induced by an acoustic stress and this effect is related to the blockade of the release of CRH in response to a stressful stimulus.[80]

The purine nucleoside adenosine is also an important endogenous regulator of the antonomic nervous system and adenosine receptors are involved in a variety of gastrointestinal functions including gastric secretion[140] and intestinal motility.[141,142]

However, adenosine and its analogues bind on two receptor subtypes, A_1 and A_2 inhibiting or activating adenylate cyclase respectively.[143] In rats, adenosine or three potent analogues NECA, CHA and RPIA alters intestinal motility and transit when injected ICV. NECA, the

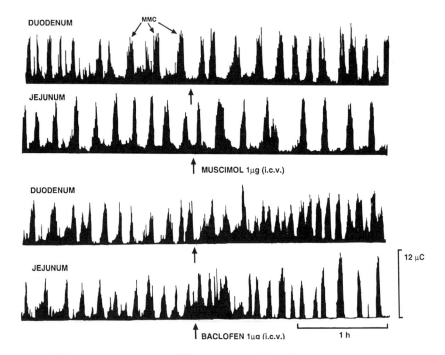

FIGURE 9 Supraspinal GABAergic modulation of duodeno-jejunal myoelectrical activity in fasted rats. The $GABA_A$ agonist muscimol injected ICV does not affect the cyclic pattern of MMC while baclofen, a $GABA_B$ agonist as well as GABA itself transiently disrupts this pattern and secondarily affects its cyclic occurrence, this effect being selectively blocked by phaclofen, a selective $GABA_B$ antagonist (not shown).

most potent adenosine analogue acting at A_2 subtype receptor, has more potent slowing effects on intestinal transit, but these effects are also obtained with CHA and RPIA which both bind to A_1 receptor. The central origin of these effects is confirmed by their blockade by IP injection of 8 PT an adenosine receptor antagonist crossing the blood brain barrier but not by 8 SPT which does not penetrate the brain.[144] As for histamine, the centrally-mediated effects of adenosine on intestinal motility are opposite to those observed after peripheral administration.

Most of these neurotransmitters are also found active on colonic motility in rats and dogs particularly those influencing the release of CCK8 or modulating central adrenergic or dopaminergic pathways (Table 4).

INFLAMMATORY MEDIATORS

Prostaglandins mediate the responses at neuroendocrine junctions in the preoptic area at the anterior hypothalamus that are involved in thermoregulation and fever. There is now evidence that prostaglandins are involved in other neuroendocrine responses and ICV administration of prostaglandin E_2 (PGE_2) causes tachycardia and a rise in blood pressure confirming that the pressure response to parental PGE_1 and PGE_2 is partially mediated by the central nervous system. This pressure response has been attributed to a prostaglandin-induced activation of adrenergic or cholinergic neurons rather than being considered a reflex reaction to the prostaglandin-induced hyperthermia.[145] Prostaglandins also participate in the regulation of hypothalamic and adenohypophyseal hormone secretions and centrally administered prostaglandins affect gastrointestinal function; injected ICV prostaglandins inhibit forestomach motility in goat,[146] insulin-stimulated gastric secretion in rats[147] and cause anorexia in rats.[148]

In rats, ICV administration of prostaglandin E_2 restores a normal MMC pattern in fasted rats[149] and dogs.[150] These effects are centrally mediated and involves a calcium dependant mechanism. In dogs, oral administration of synthetic prostaglandin E_1 (misoprostol) or prostaglandin E_2 (enprostil) analogues before a meal induces postprandial MMC on the jejunum through a mechanism involving central prostaglandin receptors.[151] Moreover, the effects of some peptides injected centrally such as calcitonin, seem related to the central release of PGE_2. Accordingly, the effects of calcitonin injected centrally on both feeding behavior (anorexia) and

---

TABLE 4
Non-Peptides Substances Acting on the Brain to Influence Colonic Motility or Transit in Rats and Dogs

Stimulation	Inhibition
RAT	
σ ligands	CCK_A receptor antagonists
$5HT_{1A}$ agonists	D_2 antagonists
α_2 antagonists	opioids (mu)
PGs (EP_1, EP_3) analogues	
D_1 and D_2 agonists	
DOG	
α_2 antagonists	CCK_A receptor antagonists
$5HT_2$ and $5HT_3$ agonists	D_2 antagonists
PGs analogues	
Opioids (mu)	

gut motility, i.e. MMC recovery, are suppressed after previous ICV administration of indomethacin or piroxicam, two cyclooxygenase inhibitors.[149]

Interleukin 1 (IL_1), one of the major cytokines found in brain structures and particularly at
hypothalamus level[152] when administered centrally at much lower doses than when administered
peripherally, can elicit a number of physiological and behavioral changes similar to that seen
following infection, such as fever.[153] It also induces effects characteristic of stress, such as
activation of the hypothalamo-pituitary-adrenal axis,[154] brain catecholaminergic system, and
peripheral sympathetic nervous system.[155]

IL_1 can also influence gut functions and recently it was found that the effects of $IL_1\beta$ can
be mainly ascribed to a central action. While the caeco-colonic motor stimulation is related to
the CNS release of CRH, the effects of $IL_1\beta$ on small intestinal motility, i.e. the recovery of
the MMC pattern in fed rats, is linked to the central release of PGE_2, since they are blocked
by previous treatment with indomethacin, as well as with a PGE_2 antagonist, SC 19220, acting
at EP_2 receptor subtype.[156] (Table 5).

DRUGS ACTING IN PHYSIOPATHOLOGICAL MODELS

STRESS-INDUCED ALTERATIONS OF GI MOTILITY

The role of the brain in the genesis of stress-induced gastrointestinal and colonic motor
alterations has been extensively reviewed.[157] The evidence that the CNS release of CRF is
directly involved in the initiation of digestive motor disturbances induced by different stressors
was first obtained in rats[83,158] and in mice,[84] (Table 6).

In this last species, pretreatment with ICV administration of antiserum against rat CRF, as
well as α-helical CRF_{9-41} considered to be a CRF antagonist, is able to prevent the increase in
gastric emptying of a milk meal induced by acoustic and cold stress at doses that block the
effects produced by ICV administration of CRF.[84]

This result was confirmed in rats on which cerebroventricular administration of α-helical
CRF_{9-41}, but not of the CRF fragment CRF_{1-20}, prevented the gastrointestinal secretory and
motor (transit) responses elicited by partial body restraint, (Table 6). Moreover, α-helical CRF_{9-41}
prevented the abdominal surgery-induced inhibition of gastric emptying.[159]

TABLE 5

**Comparative Influence of Interleukin Receptor Antagonist Protein (IRAP),
Indomethacin (a Cox-Inhibitor), SC 19220 (EP_1 Antagonist) and α-Helical CRF
(CRF antagonist) on Centrally Administered Interleukin 1β-induced Small Intestinal
and Colonic Motor Alterations**

	IL-1β/ICV (15 ng) +			
	IRAP (10 μg)	Indomethacin (200 μg)	SC 19220 (50 μg)	α helical CRF (10 μg)
Duodenum	+	+	+	−
Colon	+	−	N.D.	+

+: Suppression; − No effect; N.D.: Not Determined.

TABLE 6
Evidence for CRF Involvement in Stress-Induced Alterations of Transit

Species	Stressful stimulus	Method	Route	Gastric emptying	Intestinal transit	Colonic transit	Ref.
Rat	W.R.S.	α-helical	IV/ICV	—	unblocked	blocked	83
Mice	A.S. + A.S.	Antiserum	ICV/IV	blocked	blocked	—	84
	A.S. + C.S.	α-helical	ICV	blocked	blocked	—	80
Rat	P.R.S.	α-helical	ICV	blocked	blocked	blocked	158
Rat	S.S.	α-helical	ICV	blocked	—	—	159

A.S.: acoustic stress; C.S.: cold stress; W.R.S.: wrapping restraint stress; P.R.S.: partial restraint stress; S.S.: surgical stress; ICV: intracerebroventricular; IV: intravenous.

UPPER GUT

A cascade of hormonal releases and the subsequent activation of the ANS are associated with the CNS release of CRF such as peripheral adrenergic activation, and release of β endorphin, release of vasopressin or activation of central cholinergic pathways.

In dogs, acoustic stress selectively inhibits the gastric MMC without affecting intestinal motility with a concomitant increase in plasma cortisol, and these effects are mimicked by central injection of CRF. Anxiolytic substances such as diazepam as well as a GABAergic agonist, muscimol, block the acoustic stress-induced gastric hypomotility.[80] They act at the CNS level to block the effects of acoustic stress on gastric motility and plasma cortisol levels by inhibiting the release of CRF.

In rats, opioid peptides, more particularly κ agonists such as dynorphin, act through specific receptors to inhibit CRF release from the hypothalamus. In dogs, intracerebroventricular administration of the selective non peptide κ opioid agonists, U50488 and ethylketocyclazocine (EKC) block acoustic stress-induced gastric hypomotility and hypercortisolemia.[160] These effects, as those of benzodiazepines, are linked to an inhibition of central CRF release rather than a direct action on the pituitary or adrenal glands.

It is important to note that benzodiazepines, GABAergic substances, or κ opiate agonists that inhibit the gastric response to stress by inhibiting the central release of CRF, also block the autonomic, endocrine and behavioral responses to CRF that are considered to be an adaptive bodily reaction to stressful situations.

LOWER GUT

Several substances block both emotional stress-induced increase in colonic motility and CRF-induced colonic hyperkinesia, indicating that they act on the CRF-mediating pathway rather than on the central release of CRF in response to stress.

In rats, emotional stress (E. S.) produced by conditioned fear to receive electric footshocks, increases dopamine turnover in mesoprefrontal neurons that arising from the ventral tegmental area (A10).[161] Emotional stress also increases colonic motility; the central injection of a dopamine D1 antagonist (SCH 23 390) blocks the emotional stress-induced colonic motor change, but dopamine D2 antagonist (sulpiride) is inactive at the same dosage;[113] when given intraperitoneally, a 10 times higher dose of SCH 23 390 is required to produce the same blocking effect, which suggests that dopamine is involved at the level of the central nervous system level in the colonic response to stress.

Vasopressin potentiates the CRF-induced ACTH release[162] and in our model of emotional stress-induced colonic hyperkinesia a vasopressin (AVP) antagonist injected intracerebroventricularly blocks the emotional stress- and CRF-induced increase in colonic motility in rats. Since vasopressin injected centrally also stimulates colonic motility, it is suggested that release of vasopressin in the central nervous system in response to stressful stimuli is responsible for the colonic motor disturbances.[163] These results point to the following pathway; stress activates the central release of CRF, which activates the central dopaminergic pathway that then activates the vasopressinergic system which stimulates the colonic motility (Figure 10).

Neuropeptide Y and sigma ligands, such as d-NANM or (+)-N-cyclopropylmethyl-N-methyl-1,4-diphenyl-1-1-ethyl-but-3-en-1-ylamine, hydrochloride (JO 1784),[164] when centrally administered block both stress-and CRF-induced colonic hyperkinesia in rats.[165,166] The inhibitory effect of NPY and JO 1784 on emotional stress-induced colonic hyperactivity is blocked by BMY 14082, a putative sigma antagonist. It was also found that buspirone[167] and 8-OH-DPAT[168] act at CNS level to block the stress-induced colonic motor excitation (Figure 10).

Some effects of sigma agonists and $5HT_{1A}$ agonists are linked to the CNS release of CCK, and we found that the "visceral" anxiolytic effects of these compounds are blocked by CCK antagonists selective for CCK_A receptor subtype.[169] Moreover, CCK_A agonists are also able to block the effects of emotional stress on colonic motility by reducing the activation of central dopaminergic pathways in limbic structures where they are interfering.[170]

Finally, these results lead to the conclusion that two kinds of substances can modulate the CRF-induced changes in gastrointestinal motility: The first type acts directly at the receptor level; these are substances such as α-helical CRF_{9-41}, dopamine D1 antagonists, and vasopressin antagonists that interfere with CRF, dopaminergic and vasopressin receptors, to block the stress- and CRF-induced gastrointestinal motor disturbances. The second type of substances act on

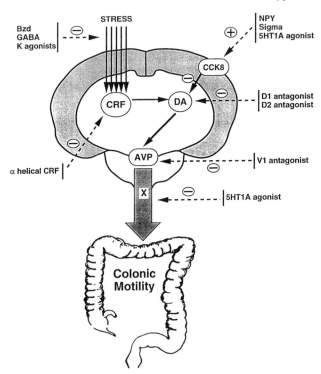

FIGURE 10   Schematic representation of the centrally activated pathways responsible of emotional stress-induced alteration of colonic motility and central target sites of drugs to modulate this colonic motor response.

pathways that modulate the release of CRF and the mediating pathways through which it stimulates colonic motility. For instance, benzodiazepines, GABA and κ agonists prevent the central release of CRF in response to stress and inhibit not only stress-induced gastrointestinal motor disturbances, but also cortisol release and the concomitent body reactions to stress. Some other substances such as sigma ligands or NPY act centrally to activate CCK nervous and/or to release CCK that in turn modulates the dopaminergic system. The $5HT_{1A}$ agonists act peripherally probably through afferent pathways to stimulate the central activation of CCK neurons or its release (Figure 10).

In this issue, the amygdala projects both to the hypothalamus mainly the VMH[171] and to the NTS and appears to be one major modulatory site of hypothalamo-mediated CRF activation of DVC consistently. CCK agonists, such as A 71378, acting mainly on CCK_A receptor subtype microinfused into the central amygdala are able to suppress stress-induced activation of colonic motility while CCK_B agonists, such as A 63387, are unable to reproduce such effects. Furthermore destruction of the amygdala by Ibotenic acid suppresses the "visceral" anti-stress effects of CCK_{8s} injected into the central amygdala (Figure 11).

INTESTINO-INTESTINAL INHIBITORY REFLEX

Numerous studies have shown that afferent fibers from abdominal vagus and splanchnic nerves participate to enterogastric inhibitory reflex induced by local distension. In dogs, the afferent pathway involved a nonadrenergic noncholinergic mechanism, and in the ferret, this inhibitory reflex is mediated by adrenergic pathways[172] and also the vagus.[173] Recently, it has been shown that this long reflex, which involves brain structures, as evidenced by C-Fos, C-Jun and Krox-24 expressions,[174] may be modulated by both peripheral and central neuropeptides or mediators. Serotonin appears to be a major candidate to modulate this enterogastric inhibitory reflex through different receptors subtypes. In sheep, activation of both $5HT_{1A}$ and $5HT_2$ receptor subtypes are involved at the brain level in this enterogastric reflex, since the ICV administration of $5HT_{1A}$ (spiroxatrine) and $5HT_2$ (ritanserin) receptor antagonists are able to block the inhibitory reflex, while $5HT_3$ receptors are involved only at peripheral level located on afferent sensitive fibers (Figure 12).

High densities of 5HT binding sites are present in the area postrema, including $5HT_{1A}$ and $5HT_2$ as well as $5HT_3$ receptor subtypes. In rats, ritanserin has been shown to have antinociceptive properties in the writhing test when injected subcutaneously, and these effects are inhibited by intrathecal application of ritanserin or methysergide,[175] activating descending monoaminergic pathways in the spinal cord. These results are in agreement with an action of ritanserin at the supraspinal level to activate pain-modulating descending serotonergic pathways and in agreement with the observation that ritanserin has analgesic effects in experimental tests of pain in humans.[176] The fact that spiroxatrine, a selective $5HT_{1A}$ antagonist, blocks the forestomach and antrum motor inhibition when injected centrally may result from activation of 5HT transmission modulated by presynaptic $5HT_{1A}$ receptors, which inhibit the spinomedullary pathways mediating the intestinointestinal inhibitory reflex, as in the mediation of analgesia and descending spinal inhibition by 5HT.[177] In agreement with this hypothesis, histochemical analyses have identified numerous serotonergic neurons projecting to the nucleus tractus solitarius, particularly from the nucleus raphe magnus and nucleus raphe dorsalis.[38]

EXPERIMENTAL ILEUS

In experimental ileus produced by surgical procedure or peritonitis, the inhibition of gastric activity is also under the control of supraspinal structures and neuromediators.

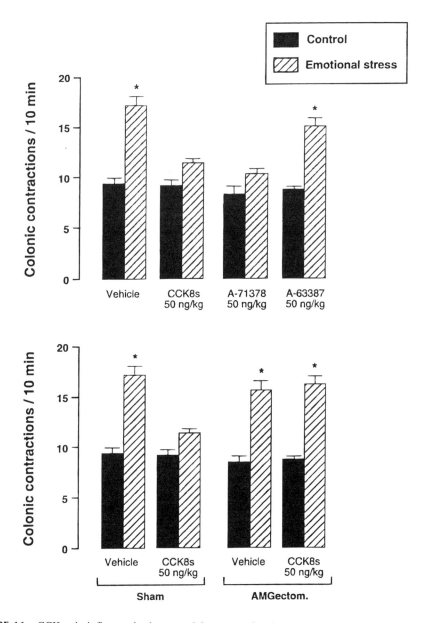

FIGURE 11 CCKergic influence in the amygdala on emotional stress-induced colonic hyperkinesia. Upper panel: emotional stress (fear to receive electric footshocks) is associated with an increase in the frequency of colonic contractions which is blocked by CCK_{8s} as well as A 71378, a CCK_A agonist, but not by A 63387, a CCK_B agonist, injected into the central nucleus of the amygdala. Lower panel: compared with sham operated animals, amygdalectomy using ibotenic acid does not affect stress-induced colonic hyperkinesia but suppresses the antagonistic influence of CCK_{8s}.

In rats, the inhibition of intestinal MMC following laparotomy is suppressed by yohimbine, an α_2 adrenergic blocker; the ratio of the active doses by ICV and IP route is in agreement with a central site of action while the α_1 antagonist, prazosin acts peripherally to suppress such inhibitory reflex.[178]

More recently it was shown that gastric and intestinal motor inhibition induced by abdominal surgery or peritonitis involved brain structures and are mediated through the CNS release of

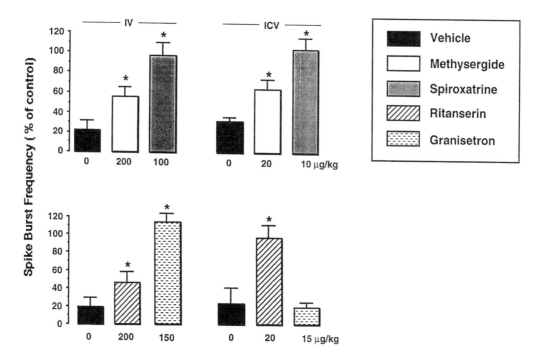

FIGURE 12   Comparative influence of central (ICV) vs peripheral (IV) administrations of 5HT receptor antagonists on gastric (abomasal) motor inhibition induced by duodenal distension in sheep (ref. 174). Note that spiroxatrine (5HT$_{1A}$ antagonist), methysergide (5HT$_1$/5HT$_2$ antagonist) and ritanserin (5HT$_2$ antagonist) are active at a 10 times lower dose by ICV then IV route to block such inhibitory reflex while granisetron (5HT$_3$ antagonist) is active only when injected systemically.

CRF, since ICV administration of α-helical CRF$_{9-41}$, a CRF antagonist suppress their effects on gastrointestinal motility.[159,179]

SUMMARY AND CONCLUSIONS

The brain appears to be the major structure controlling gut motility. The brain can adapt gut motility to physiological digestive state and to situations associated with stress or inflammation.

Nearly all classical brain neurotransmitters and many neuropeptides found in the CNS participate in such supraspinal regulation of gut motor function. The hypothalamus and the brainstem are the main target, modulatory sites, but the mechanisms of transduction to the periphery are multiple.

A change in the balance between central noradrenergic and cholinergic tones is one of the major features associated with the switching between the fed/fasted intestinal motor patterns, while CCK$_8$ and dopamine are the major candidates for long-term CNS modulation of colonic motility. Serotonin is highly involved in the brain modulation of intestinal motor adaptative reflex from the lower to the upper gut; CRH, vasopressin and IL$_1$ are directly involved in the changes associated with external stimuli. But, many structures and mechanisms involved in the brain-gut dialogue remain to be discovered.

There are increasing evidences that the brain plays a major role in the control of gut motility and particularly to adjusting propulsive function to the digestive state, but also to adapting the gut to situations associated with stress, inflammation or alterations in absorption processes.

Many peptides or neurotransmitters found in both brain and gut are localized in supraspinal structures associated with the control of gut motility. Microinjections into different brain areas have permitted localization of the brain targets of different hypothalamic peptides, opioid peptides (enkephalin, dynorphin), CCK_8 and bombesin involved in the changes from fasted (MMC) to fed pattern of small intestine motility. A balance between cholinergic and noradrenergic activity in the brainstem appears to be the key to the abrupt switching from one to an other.

Stress is associated with changes in gastric and colonic motility; both TRH and CRH released in different brain nuclei are responsible of these motor alterations. The colonic hyperkinesia being associated with supraspinal activation of dopaminergic pathways associated with vasopressin release in the brainsterm and amygdala appears to be a target site to drugs for modulating such activated pathways.

Brain serotonin, cytokines and prostaglandins are also involved in a number of motor adaptative reflexes from the lower to the upper gut. Their modulation may also be considered in motor dysfunction associated with hypersensitivity of the gut. Improvement of our knowledge of the brain-gut dialogue may offer new targets for future drugs in the treatment of functional bowel disorders.

REFERENCES

1. **Sakaguchi, T., and Ohtake, M.,** Inhibition of gastric motility induced by activation of the hypothalamic paraventricular nucleus, *Brain Res,* 335, 365, 1985.
2. **Fengs, H. S., Brobeck, J. R., and Brooks, F. P.,** Lateral hypothalamic sites in cats for stimulation of gastric antral contractions, *Clin Invest Med,* 10, 140, 1987.
3. **Smith, J. R., Lahann, T. R., Chesnut, R. M., Carino, M. A., and Horita, A.,** Thyrotropin-releasing hormone: stimulation of colonic activity following intracerebroventricular administration, *Science,* 196, 660, 1977.
4. **Kelly, K. A., Code, C. F., and Elveback, L. R.,** Patterns of canine gastric electrical activity, *Am J Physiol,* 217, 461, 1969.
5. **Hinder, R. A., and Kelly, K. A.,** Human gastric pacesetter potential. Site of origin, spread, and response to gastric transection and proximal gastric vagotomy, *Am J Surg,* 133, 29, 1977.
6. **Abrahamsson, H.,** Studies on the inhibitory nervous control of gastric motility, *Acta Physiol Scand,* 390, S 1, 1973.
7. **Gill, R. C., Pilot, M. A., Thomas, P. A., and Wingate, D. L.,** Organization of fasting and postprandial myoelectric activity in stomach and duodenum of conscious dogs, *Amer J Physiol,* 249, G655, 1985.
8. **Itoh, Z., Aizawa, I., Takeuchi, S., and Takayanagi, R.,** Diurnal changes in gastric motor activity in conscious dogs, *Dig Dis Sci,* 22, 117, 1977.
9. **Rees, W. D., W., Malagelada, J. R., Miller, L. J., and Go, V. L. W.,** Human interdigestive and postprandial gastrointestinal motor and gastrointestinal hormone patterns, *Dig Dis Sci,* 527, 321, 1982.
10. **Buéno, L., Ferre, J. P., Fioramonti, J., and Ruckebusch, M.,** Control of the antral motor response to feeding by gastric acid secretion in rats, *J Physiol (London),* 325, 43, 1982.
11. **Deloof, S., and Rousseau, J. P.,** Specific effects of thoracic vagotomy on the electrical activity of the gastric antrum and pylorus in rabbits, *Quart J Exp Physiol,* 70, 491, 1985.
12. **Szurszewski, J. H.,** A migrating electric complex of the canine small intestine, *Am J Physiol,* 217, 1757, 1969.
13. **Ruckebusch, Y., and Buéno, L.,** Migrating myoelectrical complex of the small intestine. An intrinsic activity mediated by the vagus, *Gastroenterology,* 73, 1309, 1977.
14. **Ruckebusch, M., and Fioramonti, J.,** Electrical spiking activity and propulsion in small intestine in fed and fasted rats, *Gastroenterology,* 68, 1500, 1975.
15. **Code, C. F., and Marlett, J. A.,** The interdigestive myoelectric complex of the stomach and the small bowel of dogs, *J Physiol (London),* 246, 298, 1975.

16. **De Wever, I., Eeckhout, C., Vanrappen, G., and Hellemans, J.,** Disruptive effect of test meals on interdigestive motor complex in dogs, *Am J Physiol,* 235, E661, 1978.

17. **Defilippi, C., and Valenzuela, J. E.,** Sham feeding disrupts the interdigestive motility complex in man, *Scand J Gastroenterol,* 16, 977, 1981.

18. **Ruckebusch, Y., and Buéno, L.,** The effect of feeding on the motility of the stomach and small intestine in the pig, *Br J Nut,* 35, 397, 1976.

19. **Ruckebusch, M., and Ferre, J. P.,** Origine alimentaire des variations nycthémérales de l'activité électrique de l'intestin grêle chez le rat, *C R Soc Biol,* 167, 2005, 1973.

20. **Burrows, C. F., Merritt, A. M., and Tash, J.,** Jejunal myoelectrical activity in the conscious neonatal pig, *J Physiol (London),* 374, 349, 1986.

21. **Fioramonti, J.,** Etude comparée des fonctions motrices du gros intestin, (A comparative study of large intestine motor functions) Doctoral Thesis, University of Toulouse, 1981.

22. **Fioramonti, J., and Buéno, L.,** Diurnal changes in colonic motor profile in conscious dogs, *Dig Dis Sci,* 28, 257, 1983.

23. **Frexinos, J., Buéno, L., and Fioramonti, J.,** Diurnal changes in myoelectric spiking activity of the human colon, *Gastroenterology,* 88, 1104, 1985.

24. **Paintal, A. S.,** A study of gastric strech receptors, *J Physiol (London)* 126, 255, 1954.

25. **Iggo, A. F.,** Gastric mucosal chemoreceptors with vagal afferent fibers in the cat, *Q J Exp Physiol,* 42, 398, 1957.

26. **Contreras, R. J., Beckstead, R. M., and Norgren, R.,** Central projections of trigeminal, facial glossopharyngeal, and the vagus nerves: an autoradiographic study in the rat, *J Auton Nerv Syst,* 6, 303, 1982.

27. **McCann, M. J., and Rogers, R. C.,** Central modulation of the vago-vagal reflex: Influence on gastric function, in *Brain-Gut Interaction,* Taché, Y., and Wingate, D., Eds., CRC Press, Boca Raton, 1991, pp. 57.

28. **Rogers, R. C., and Hermann, G. E.,** Vagal afferent stimulation-evoked gastric secretion suppressed by paraventricular nucleus lesion, *J Auton Nerv Syst,* 13, 191, 1985.

29. **Barber, W. D., Yuan, C. S., and Burks, T. F.,** What does the proximal stomach tell the brain?, in *Nerves and the Gastrointestinal Tract,* Singer, M. V., and Goebell, H., Eds., MTP Press, London, 1988, pp. 721.

30. **Rogers, R. C., and Nelson, D. O.,** Neurons of the vagal division of the solitary nucleus activated by the paraventricular nucleus of the hypothalamus, *J Auton Nerv Syst,* 10, 193, 1984.

31. **Grofova, J., Ottersen, O. P., and Rinvik, E.,** Mesencephalic and diencephalic afferents to the superior colliculus and periacqueducal gray substance demonstrated by retrograde axonal transport of horseradish peroxidase in the cat, *Brain Res,* 146, 205, 1978.

32. **Morrell, J. I., Greenberger, L. M., and Pfaff, D. W.,** Hypothalamic, other diencephalic,and telencephalic neurons that project the dorsal midbrain, *J Comp Neurol,* 201, 589, 1981.

33. **Weaver, F. C.,** Localization of parasympathetic preganglionic cell bodies innervating the pancreas within the vagal nucleus and nucleus ambiguus of the rat brainstem: evidence of dual innervation based on retrograde axonal transport of horseradish peroxidase, *J Auton Nerv Syst,* 2, 61, 1980.

34. **Kalia, M., and Fuxe, K.,** Rat medulla oblongata. I Cytoarchitectonic considerations, *J Comp Neurol,* 233, 285, 1985.

35. **Ter Horst, G. J., Luiten, P. G. M., and Kuipers, F.,** Descending pathways from hypothalamus to dorsal motor vagus and ambiguus nuclei in the rat, *J Auton Nerv Syst,* 11, 59, 1984.

36. **Portillo, F., and Pasaro, R.,** Axonal projections to the ventrolateral nucleus of the solitary tract revealed by double labelling of retrograde fluorescent markers in the cat, *Neurosci Lett,* 76, 280, 1987.

37. **Bystrzycka, E. K.,** Afferent projections to the dorsal and ventral respiratory nuclei in the medulla oblongata of the cat studied by the horseradish peroxidase technique, *Brain Res,* 185, 59, 1980.

38. **Schaffar, N., Kessler, J. P., Bosier, O., and Jean, A.,** Central serotoninergic projections to the nucleus tractus solitarii: evidence from a double labeling study in the rat, *Neuroscience,* 26, 951, 1988.

39. **Besson, J. M., Guilbaud, G., Abdelmoumene, M., and Chaouch, A.,** Physiologie de la nociception, *J Physiol (Paris),* 78, 7, 1982.

40. **Willett, C. J., Rutherford, J. G., Gwyn, D. G., and Leslie, R. A.,** Projections between the hypothalamus and the dorsal vagal complex in the cat: an HRP and autoradiographic study, *Brain Res Bull,* 18, 63, 1987.

41. **Rogers, R. C., and Hermann, G. E.,** Gastric-vagal solitary neurons excites by paraventricular nucleus microstimulation, *J Auton Nerv Syst,* 14, 351, 1985.

42. **Gray, T. S., and Magnuson, D. J.,** Neuropeptide neuronal efferents from the bed nucleus of the stria terminalis and central amygdaloid nucleus to the dorsal vagal complex in the rat, *J Comp Neurol,* 262, 365, 1987.

43. **Rogers, R. C., and Fryman, D. L.,** Direct connections between the central nucleus of the amygdala and the nucleus of the solitary tract: an electrophysiological study in the rat, *J Auton Nerv Sys,* 22, 83, 1988.

44. **Sofroniew, M. V., and Schrell, U.,** Evidence for a direct projection from oxytocin and vasopressin neurons in hypothalamic paraventricular nucleus to the medulla oblongata: immunohistochemical visualization of both horseradisch peroxidase transported and the peptide produced by the same neurons, *Neurosci Lett,* 22, 211, 1981.

45. **Folkow, B., and Rubinstein, E. H.,** Behavioural and autonomic patterns evoked by stimulation of the lateral hypothalamic area in the cat, *Acta Physiol Scand,* 65, 292, 1965.

46. **Lisander, B.,** The hypothalamus and vagally mediated gastric relaxation, *Acta Physiol Scand,* 93, 1, 1975.

47. **Jansson, G., and Lisander, B.,** On adrenergic influence on gastric motility in chronically vagotomized cats, *Acta Physiol Scand,* 76, 463, 1969.

48. **Delbro, D., and Lisander, B.,** The interrelations between hypothalamically induced changes in sympathetic discharge to gastrointestinal and cardiovascular systems, *Acta Physiol Scand,* 101, 165, 1977.

49. **Fengs, H. S., Lynn, R. B., and Brooks, F. B.,** How does the brain modify gastric contractions independently of gastric acid secretion, in *Nerves and the Gut,* Singer, M. V. and Goebell H., Eds., MTP Press LTD, Lancaster, 1989, 183.

50. **Strom, G., and Uvnäs, B.,** Motor responses of gastrointestinal tract and bladder to topical stimulation of the frontal lobe, basal ganglia and hypothalamus in the cat, *Acta Physiol Scand,* 21, 90, 1950.

51. **Rostad, H.,** Colonic motility in the cat. IV. Peripheral pathways mediating the effects induced by hypothalamic and mesencephalic stimulation, *Acta Physiol Scand,* 89, 154, 1973.

52. **Boom, R., Chavez-Ibarra, G., Del Villar, J. J., and Hernandez-Pron, R.,** Changes in colonic motility indiced by electrical and chemical stimulation of the forebrain and hypothalamus in cats, *Int J Neuropharmacol,* 4, 169, 1965.

53. **Thomas, J. E., and Baldwin, M. V.,** Pathways and mechanisms of regulation of gastric motility, in *Handbook of Physiology, Section 6: Alimentary Canal, Vol. 4,* Code, C. F., Ed., American Society, Washington, DC, 1968.

54. **Smith, G. P., Jerome, C., and Norgren, R.,** Afferent axons in abdominal vagus mediate satiety effect of cholecystokinin in rats, *Am J Physiol,* 249, R638, 1985.

55. **Holzer, P., Schluet, W., Lippe, I. T., and Sametz, W.,** Involvement of capsaicin-sensitive sensory neurons in gastrointestinal function, *Acta Physiol Hung,* 69, 403, 1987.

56. **Borison, H. L.,** Effect of ablation of medullary emetic chemoreceptor trigger zone on vomiting responses to cerebral intraventricular injection of adrenaline, apomorphine and pilocarpine in the cat, *J Physiol,* 147, 172, 1959.

57. **Bhattacharya, B. K., and Feldberg, W.,** Perfusion of cerebral ventricles: effects of drugs on outflow from the cisterna and aqueduct, *Brit J Pharmacol,* 13, 156, 1958.

58. **Passaro, E., Debas, H., Oldendorf, W., and Yamada, T.,** Rapid appearence of intraventricularly administered neuropeptides in the peripheral circulation, *Brain Res,* 241, 335, 1982.

59. **Buéno, L., and Ferré, J. P.,** Central regulation of intestinal motility by somatostatin and cholecystokinin octapeptide, *Science,* 216, 1427, 1982.

60. **Stone, T. W.,** Microiontophoresis and pressure ejection, in *Methods in Neuroscience, IBRO Handbook Series, Vol. 8,* Smith A. D., Ed., John Wiley & Sons, New York, 1985.

61. **Phillipson, E. A., Murphy, E., Kozar, L. F., and Schultze, R. K.,** Role of vagal stimuli in exercise ventilation in dogs with experimental pneumonitis, *J Appl Physiol,* 39, 76, 1975.

62. **Hall, K. E., El-Sharkawy, T. Y., and Diamant, N. E.,** Vagal control of migrating motor complex in the dog, *Am J Physiol,* 243, G276, 1982.
63. **Gleysteen, J. J., Sarna, S. K., and Myrvik, A. L.,** Canine cyclic motor activity of stomach and small bowel: The vagus is not the governor, *Gastroenterology,* 88, 1926, 1985.
64. **Jancso, N., Jancso-Gabor, A., and Szolcsanyi, J.,** Direct evidence for neurogenic inflammation and its prevention by denervation and by pretreatment with capsaicin, *Br J Pharmacol,* 31, 138, 1967.
65. **Holzer, P.,** Capsaicin: cellular targets, mechanism of action and selectively for thin sensory neurons, *Pharmacol Rev,* 43, 143, 1991.
66. **Raybould, H. E., and Taché, Y.,** Cholecystokin inhibits gastric motility and emptying via a capsaicin-sensitive vagal pathway in rats, *Am J Physiol,* 255, G242, 1988.
67. **Taché, Y., Stephens, R. L, and Ishikawa, T.,** Stress-induced alterations of gastrointestinal function: involvement of brain CRF and TRH, in *IV New Frontiers of Stress Research,* Weiner, H., Florin, L., Helhammer, D., and Murison, M., Eds., Hans Uber, 1988, chap. 1.
68. **Diop, L., Pascaud, X., Junien, J. L., and Buéno, L.,** CRF triggers the CNS release of TRH in stress-induced changes in gastric emptying, *Am J Physiol,* 260, G39, 1991.
69. **Carino, M. A., and Horita, A.,** Localization of TRH-sensitive sites in rat brain mediating intestinal transit, *Life Sci,* 41, 2663, 1987.
70. **Ruckebusch, Y., and Malbert, C. H.,** Stimulation and inhibition of food intake in sheep by centrally-administered hypothalamic releasing factors, *Life Sci,* 38, 929, 1986.
71. **Tonove, T., and Nomoto, T.,** Effect of intracerebroventricular administration of thyrotropin-releasing hormone upon the electroenteromyogram of rat duodenum, *Eur J Pharmacol,* 58, 369, 1979.
72. **Lahann, T. R., and Horita, A.,** Thyrotropin-releasing hormone: centrally mediated effects on gastrointestinal motor activity, *J Pharmacol Exp Ther,* 222, 66, 1982.
73. **Rogers, R. C., and Hermann, G. E.,** Oxytocin, oxytocin antagonist, TRH and hypothalamic paraventricular nucleus stimulation effects on gastric motility, *Peptides,* 8, 505, 1987.
74. **Garrick, T., Stephens, R., and Ishikawa, T.,** TRH-analogue, RX 77368, microinjected into the dorsal vagal complex and nucleus ambiguus stimulates gastric contractility in the rat, *Am J Physiol,* 256, G1010, 1989.
75. **Garrick, T., Buack, S., Veiseh, A., and Taché, Y.,** Thyrotropin-releasing hormone (TRH) acts centrally to stimulate gastric contractility in rats, *Life Sci,* 40, 649, 1987.
76. **Kolve, E., Stephens, R., Walsh, J. H., and Taché, Y.,** Intracisternal injection of the stable TRH analogue increases serotonin and dopamine levels in the gastric interstitial fluid in the rat, *Gastroenterology,* 96, 266, 1989.
77. **Taché, Y., Garrick, T., and Raybould, H.,** Central nervous system action of peptides to influence gastrointestinal motor function, *Gastroenterology,* 98, 517, 1990.
78. **Beleslin, D. B., Jovanovic Micic, D., Samardzic, R., and Terzic, B.,** Studies of thyrotropin-releasing hormone (TRH)-induced defecation in cats, *Pharmacol Biochem Behav,* 26, 639, 1987.
79. **Buéno, L., and Fioramonti, J.,** Effects of corticotropin-releasing factor, corticotropin and cortison on gastrointestinal motility in dogs, *Peptides,* 7, 73, 1986.
80. **Gué, M., and Buéno, L.,** Diazepam and muscimol blockade of the gastrointestinal motor disturbances induced by acoustic stress in dogs, *Eur J Pharmacol,* 131, 123, 1986.
81. **Lenz, H. J., Burlage, M., Raedler, A., and Greten, H.,** Central nervous system effects of corticotropin-releasing factor on gastrointestinal transit in the rat, *Gastroenterology,* 94, 598, 1988.
82. **Taché, Y., Maeda-Hagiwara, M., and Tirkelson, C. M.,** Central nervous system action of corticotropin-releasing factor to inhibit gastric emptying in rats, *Am J Physiol,* 253, G241, 1987.
83. **Williams, C. L., Villar, R. G., Peterson, J. M., and Burks, T. F.,** Stress-induced changes in intestinal transit in the rat: a model for the irritable bowel syndrome, *Gastroenterology,* 94, 611, 1988.
84. **Buéno, L., and Gué, M.,** Evidence for the involvement of corticotropin-releasing factor in the gastrointestinal disturbances induced by acoustic and cold stress in mice, *Brain Res,* 441, 1, 1988.
85. **Brown, M. R., Fischer, L. A., Rivier, J., Spiess, J., Rivier, C., and Vale, W.,** Corticotropin-releasing factor: effects on the sympathetic nervous system and oxygen consumption, *Life Sci,* 30, 207, 1982.

86. **Porreca, F., Mosberg, H. I., Hurst, R., Hruby, V. J., and Burks, T. F.,** Roles of mu, delta and kappa opiod receptors in spinal and supraspinal mediation of gastrointestinal transit effects on hot-plate analgesia in the mouse, *J Pharmacol Exp Ther,* 230, 341, 1984.

87. **Buéno, L., and Fioramonti, J.,** Action of opiates on gastrointestinal function, *Baillière's Clinical Gastroenterology,* 2, 123, 1988.

88. **Porreca, F., Filla, A., and Burks, T. F.,** Spinal cord-mediated opiate effects on gastrointestinal transit in mice, *Eur J Pharmacol,* 86, 135, 1982.

89. **Parolaro, D., Crema, G., Sala, M., Santagostino, A., Giognoni, G., and Gori, E.,** Intestinal effect and analgesia: evidence for different involvement of opioid receptor subtypes in periaqueductal grey matter, *Eur J Pharmacol,* 120, 95, 1986.

90. **Porreca, F., and Burks, T. F.,** Centrally administered bombesin affects gastric emptying and small and large bowel transit in the rat, *Gastroenterology,* 85, 313, 1983.

91. **Lenz, H. J.,** Calcitonin and CGRP inhibit gastrointestinal transit via distinct neuronal pathways, *Am J Physiol,* 254, G920, 1988.

92. **Gmereck, D. E., and Cowan, A.,** Pituitary-adrenal mediation of bombesin-induced inhibition of gastrointestinal transit in rats, *Reg Peptides,* 9, 299, 1984.

93. **Fargeas, M. J., Fioramonti, J., and Buéno, L.,** Involvement of dopamine in the central effect of neurotensin on intestinal motility in rats, *Peptides,* 11, 1169, 1990.

94. **Liberge, M., Arruebo, P., and Buéno, L.,** CCK$_8$ neurons of the ventromedial (VMH) hypothalamus mediate the upper gut motor changes associated with feeding in rats, *Brain Res,* 508, 118, 1990.

95. **Liberge, M., Arruebo, M. P., and Buéno, L.,** Role of hypothalamic CCK$_8$ in the colonic motor response to a meal in rats, *Gastroenterology,* 100, 441, 1991.

96. **Buéno, L., and Fioramonti, J.,** CNS peptidergic regulation of gut motility, in *Brain-gut interactions,* Taché, Y., and Wingate, D., Eds., CRC Press, Boca Raton, USA, 1991, pp. 231.

97. **Helke, C. J., Handelmann, G. E., and Jacobowitz, D. M.,** Choline acetyltransferase activity in the nucleus tractus solitarius: regulation by the afferent vagus nerve, *Brain Res Bull,* 10, 433, 1983.

98. **Simon, J. R., Oderfeld-Nowak, B., Felten, D. L., and Aprison, M. H.,** Distribution of choline acetyltransferase, acetylcholinesterase, muscarinic receptor binding, and choline uptake in discrete areas of the medulla oblongata, *Neurochem Res,* 6, 497, 1981.

99. **Wamsley, J. K., Lewis, M. S., Young, W. S. III., and Kuhar, M. J.,** Autoradiographic localization of muscarinic cholinergic receptors in rat brainstem, *J Neurosci,* 1, 176, 1981.

100. **Fargeas, M. J., Fioramonti, J., and Buéno, L.,** Central muscarinic control of the pattern of small intestinal motility in rats, *Life Sci,* 40, 1709, 1987.

101. **Robertson, H. A., and Leslie, R. A.,** Noradrenergic alpha 2 binding sites in vagal dorsal motor nucleus and nucleus tractus solitarius: autoradiographic localization, *Can J Physiol Pharmacol,* 63, 1190, 1985.

102. **Flügge, G., Jurdzinski, A., Brandt, S., and Fuchs, E.,** Alpha2-adrenergic bindings sites in the medulla oblongata of tree shrews demonstrated by in vitro autoradiography: Species related differences in comparison to the rat, *J Comp Neurol,* 297, 253, 1990.

103. **Yang, R. H., Oarashi, Y., Wyss, J. M., and Chen, Y. F.,** Dopamine D2 receptors in the posterior region of the nucleus tractus solitarius mediate the central pressor action of quipirole (LY171555), *Brain Res Bull,* 24, 97, 1990.

104. **Mittendorf, A., Denoroy, L., and Flügge, G.,** Anatomy of the adrenergic system in the medulla oblongata of the tree shrew: PNMT immunoreactive structures within the nucleus tractus solitarii, *J Comp Neurol,* 274, 178, 1988.

105. **Ruwart, M. J., Klepper, M. S., and Rush, B. D.,** Clonidine delays small intestinal transit in the rat, *J Pharmacol Exp Ther,* 212, 487, 1980.

106. **Theodorou, V., Fioramonti, J., and Buéno, L.,** Central α2-adrenergic control of colonic transit in rats, *J Gastrointestinal Mot,* 1, 85, 1989.

107. **Fargeas, M. J., Fioramonti, J., and Buéno, L.,** Involvement of central noradrenergic pathways in the control of intestinal motility in rats, *Neurosci Lett,* 90, 297, 1988.

108. **Bonaz, B., Martin, L., Beurriand, E., Manier, M., Hostein, J.,** and Feuerstein, Locus ceruleus modulates migrating myoelectric complex in rats, *Am J Physiol,* 262, G1121, 1992.

109. **Fioramonti, J., Berlan, M., Fargeas, M. J., and Buéno, L.,** Yohimbine stimulates colonic motility through a central action in conscious dogs, *J Gastroint Mot,* 4, 137, 1992.

110. **Hökfelt, T., Rehfeld, J. F., Skirbol, L., Ivemark, B., Golstein, M., and Markey, M.,** Evidence of coexistence of dopamine and CCK in mesolimbic neurons, *Nature (London),* 285, 476, 1980.

111. **Palacios, J. M., and Kuhar, M. J.,** Neurotensin receptors are located on dopamine containing neurons in rat midbrain, *Nature,* 294, 587, 1981.

112. **Armstrong, D. M., Ross, C. A., Pickel, V. M., Joh, T. H., and Reis, D. J.,** Distribution of dopamine-, noradrenaline-, and adrenaline- containing cell bodies in the rat medulla oblongata demonstrated by the immunocytochemical localization of catecholamines biosynthetic enzymes, *J Comp Neurol,* 212, 173, 1982.

113. **Buéno, L., Gué, M., Fabre, C., and Junien, J. L.,** Involvement of central dopamine and D1 receptors in stress-induced colonic motor alterations in rats, *Brain Res Bull,* 29, 135, 1992.

114. **Green, J. P., Johnson, C. L., and Weinstein, H.,** Histamine as a neurotransmitter, in *A generation of progress,* Lipton, M. A. et al., Eds., Raven Press, New York, 1978, pp. 319.

115. **Schwartz, J. C., Pollard, H., and Quach, T. T.,** Histamine as a neurotransmitter in mammalian brain: neurochemical evidence, *J Neurochem,* 35, 26, 1980.

116. **Taylor, K. M., and Snyder, S. H.,** Histamine in rat brain: sensitive assay of endogenous level, formation in vivo and lowering by inhibitions of histidine decarboxylase, *J Pharmacol Exp Ther,* 173, 619, 1971.

117. **Brownstein, M. J., Saavedra, J. M., Palkovits, M., and Axelrod J.,** Histamine content of hypothalamic nuclei of the rat, *Brain Res,* 77, 151, 1974.

118. **Palacios, J. M., Wamsley, J. K., and Kuhar, M. J.,** The distribution of histamine H1-receptors in the rat brain: an autoradiographic study, *Neuroscience,* 6, 15, 1980.

119. **Watanabé, T., Taguchi, Y., Shiosaka, S., Tanaka, J., Kubota, H., Terano, Y., Tohyama, M., and Wada, H.,** Distribution of the histaminergic neuron system in the central nervous system of rats: a fluorescent immunohistochemical analysis with histidine decarboxylase as a marker, *Brain Res,* 295, 13, 1984.

120. **Fargeas, M. J., Fioramonti, J., and Buéno, L.,** Involvement of different receptors in the central and peripheral effects of histamine on intestinal motility in the rat, *J Pharm Pharmacol,* 41, 534, 1989.

121. **Bradley, P. B., Engel, G., Fenuik, W., Fozard, J. R., Humphrey, P. P. A., Middlemiss, D. N., Mylecharane, E. J., Richardson, B. P., and Saxena, P. R.,** Proposals for the classification and nomenclature of functional receptors for 5-Hydroxytryptamine, *Neuropharmacol,* 25, 563, 1986.

122. **Costa, M., and Furness, J. B.,** The sites of action of 5-Hydroxytryptamine in nerve muscle preparations from the guinea-pig small intestine and colon, *Br J Pharmacol,* 65, 237, 1979.

123. **Johnson, S. M., Katayama, Y., and North, R. A.,** Multiple actions of 5-Hydroxytryptamine on myenteric neurones of the guinea-pig ileum, *J Physiol (London),* 304, 459, 1980.

124. **Jacobs, B. L., and Azmitia E. C.,** Structure and function of the brain serotonin system, *Physiol Rev,* 72, 165, 1992.

125. **Pazos, A., Probst, A., and Palacios, J. M.,** Serotonin receptors in the human brain III. Autoradiographic mapping of serotonin-1 receptors, *Neuroscience,* 21, 97, 1987.

126. **Waeber, C., Dixon, K., Hoyer, D., and Palacios, J. M.,** Localization by autoradiography of neuronal 5HT$_3$ receptors in mouse CNS, *Eur J Pharmacol,* 151, 351, 1988.

127. **Barnes, J. M., Barnes, N. M., Costall, B., Ironside, J. W., and Naylor, R. J.,** Identification and characterization of 5-Hydroxytryptamine recognition sites in human brain tissue, *J Neurochem,* 53, 1787, 1989.

128. **Pratt, G. D., and Bowery, N. G.,** The 5HT$_3$ receptor ligand {^{3}H}—BRL 43694 binds to presynaptic sites in the nucleus tractus solitarius of the rat, *Neuropharmacology,* 28, 421, 1989.

129. **Veenendaal, G. H., Woutersen-Van, N., and Van Miert, A. S. J.,** Responses of goat ruminal musculature to bradykinin and serotonin *in vitro* and *in vivo, Am J Vet Res,* 41, 479, 1980.

130. **Sorraing, J. M., Fioramonti, J., and Buéno, L.,** Central and peripheral serotonergic control of forestomach motility in sheep, *J Vet Pharmacol & Ther,* 8, 312, 1985.

131. **Brikas, P., Kania, B. F., Fioramonti, J., and Buéno, L.,** Central and peripheral serotonergic influences on viscerovisceral inhibitory reflex during duodenal distension in sheep, *Dig Dis Sci,* 38, 1079, 1993.

132. **Costall, B., Kelly, M. E., Naylor, R. J., Tan, C. C. W., and Tattersall, F. D.,** 5-Hydroxytryptamine M receptor antagonism in the hypothalamus facilitates gastric emptying in the guinea-pig, *Neuropharmacology,* 25, 1293, 1986.

133. **Costall, B., Gunning, S. J., Naylor, R. J., and Tyers, M. B.,** The effect of GR 38032F, a novel 5-HT$_3$ receptor antagonist, on gastric emptying in the guinea-pig, *Br J Pharmacol,* 91, 263, 1987.

134. **Roberts, M. H. T., Sizer, A. R., and Rees, H.,** 5-Hydroxytryptamine and neuronal activity in the dorsal horn of the spinal cord, in *Serotonin and Pain,* Besson, J. M., Ed., Elsevier, Amsterdam, 1990, chap. 85.

135. **Curtis, D. R., and Johnston, G. A. R.,** Amino acid transmitters in the mammalian central nervous system, *Rev Physiol Biochem Exp Pharmacol,* 69, 97, 1974.

136. **Giotti, A., Luzzi, S., Maggi, C. A., Spagnesi, S., and Silletti, L.,** Modulatory activity of GABA$_B$ receptors on cholinergic tone in guinea-pig distal colon, *Br J Pharmacol,* 84, 883, 1985.

137. **Andrews, P. L. R., and Lawes, I. N. C.,** Interactions between splanchnic and vagus nerves in the control of mean intragastric pressure in the ferret, *J Physiol (London),* 351, 473, 1984.

138. **Fargeas, M. J., Fioramonti, J., and Buéno, L.,** Central and peripheral action of GABA$_A$ and GABA$_B$ agonists on small intestine motility in rats, *Eur J Pharmacol,* 150, 163, 1988.

139. **Brikas, P., Buéno, L., and Fioramonti J.,** Central and peripheral β-adrenergic influences on reticulorumen and upper-gut myoelectrical activity in sheep, *J Vet Pharmacol Therap,* 12, 430, 1989.

140. **Scarpignato, C., Tramacere, R., Zappia, L., and Del Soldato, P.,** Inhibition of gastric acid secretion by adenosine receptor stimulation in the rat, *Pharmacology,* 34, 264, 1987.

141. **Gaion, R. M., Dorigo, P., Trolese, B., Borin, E., Adami, R., and Gambarotto, L.,** Involvement of P1-purinoreceptors in the relaxing effect of adenosine in rat duodenum, *J Auton Pharmacol,* 8, 135, 1988.

142. **Feit, C., and Roche, M.,** Action of adenosine on intestinal motility after experimental mesenteric ischaemia in the dog, *Gastroenterol Clin Biol,* 12, 803, 1988.

143. **Van Calker, D., Muller, M., and Hamprecht, B.,** Adenosine regulates via two different types of receptors the accumulation of cAMP in cultured brain cells, *J Neurochem,* 33, 999, 1979.

144. **Fargeas, M. J., Fioramonti, J., and Buéno L.,** Central and peripheral actions of adenosine and its analogues on intestinal myoeletric activity and propulsion in rats, *J Gastrointest Mot,* 2, 121, 1990.

145. **Chiu, K. Y., and Richardson, J. S.,** Effects of central and peripheral postraglandins on heart rate and blood pressure of rats, *Proc Can Fed Biol Soc,* 22, 48, 1979.

146. **Van Miert, A. S. J., Van Duick, C. T., and Woutersen-Van, N.,** Effects of intracerebroventricular injection of PGE$_2$ and 5HT on body temperature, heart rate and rumen motility of conscious goats, *Eur J Pharmacol,* 92, 143, 1983.

147. **Purunen, J.,** Central nervous system effects of arachidonic acid, PGE$_2$, PGF$_2$, PGD$_2$ and PGI$_2$ on gastric secretion in the rat, *Br J Pharmacol,* 80, 255, 1983.

148. **Baile, C. A., Simpson, C. W., Bean, S. M., and Jacobb, H. J.,** Prostaglandins and food intake of rats. A component of energy balance regulation? *Physiol Behav,* 10, 1077, 1973.

149. **Fargeas, M. J., Fioramonti, J., and Buéno, L.,** Prostaglandin E2: a neuromodulator in the central control of gastrointestinal motility and feeding behavior by calcitonin, *Science,* 225, 1050, 1984.

150. **Buéno, L., Fargeas, M. J., Fioramonti, J., and Primi, M. P.,** Central control of intestinal motility by prostaglandins: A mediator of the actions of several peptides in rats and dogs, *Gastroenterology,* 88, 1888, 1985.

151. **Staumont, G., Fioramonti, J., Frexinos, J., and Buéno, L.,** Oral prostaglandin analogues induce intestinal migrating motor complexes after a meal in dogs: evidence for a central mechanism, *Gastroenterology,* 98, 888, 1990.

152. **Lechan, R., Toni, R., Clark, B., Gannon, J., Shaw, A., Dinarello, C., and Reichkin, S.,** Immunoreactive interleukin-1β localization in rat forebrain, *Brain Res,* 514, 135, 1990.

153. **Dinarello, C. A.,** Interleukin 1, *Rev Infect Dis,* 6, 51, 1984.

154. **Berkenbosch, F., Van Oers, J., Del Rey, A., Tilders, F., and Besedovsky, H.,** Corticotropin releasing factor-producing neurons in the rat activated by interleukin-1, *Science,* 238, 524, 1987.

155. **Rivier, C., and Vale, W.,** In the rat, interleukin-1α and -β stimulate adrenocorticotropin and catecholamine release, *Endocrinology,* 125, 3096, 1989.

156. **Fargeas, M. J., Fioramonti, J., and Buéno, L.,** Central action of Interleukin 1 on intestinal motility in rats, *Gastroenterology,* 104, 377, 1993.

157. **Buéno, L.,** Stress and upper gut motility dosorders: mechanisms involved, in *Non-Ulcer Dyspepsia: Pathological and Therapeutic Approaches,* Galmiche, J. P., Jian, R., Mignon, M., Eds., John Libbey Eurotext, Paris, 1991, 59.

158. **Lenz, H. J., Raedler, A., Greten, H., Vale, W. W., and Rivier, J. E.,** Stress-induced gastrointestinal secretory and motor responses in rats are mediated by endogenous corticotropin-releasing factor, *Gastroenterology,* 95, 1510, 1988.

159. **Taché, Y., Kolve, E., Stephens, R., and Rivier, J.,** Role of brain CRF in mediating surgical stress induced inhibition of gastric function in the rat, 7th International symposium on gastrointestinal hormones, Shizuoka, 1988.

160. **Gué, M., Honde, C., Pascaud, S., Junien, J. L., Alvinerie, M., and Buéno, L.,** CNS blockade of acoustic stress-induced gastric motor inhibition by K-opiate agonists in dogs, *Am J Physiol,* 254, G802, 1988.

161. **Kaneyuki, H., Yokoo, H., Tsuda, A., Yoshisa, M., Mizuli,Y., Yamada, M., and Tanaka, M.,** Psychological stress increases dopamine turnover selectively in mesoprefrontal dopamine neurons of rats: Reversal by diazepam, *Brain Res,* 557, 154, 1991.

162. **Gillies, G. E., Linton, E. A., and Lowry, P. J.,** Corticotropin releasing activity of the new CRF is potentiated several times by vasopressin, *Nature Lond,* 299, 355, 1982.

163. **Buéno, L., Gué, M., and Delrio, C.,** CNS vasopressin mediates emotional stress and CRH-induced colonic motor alterations in rats, *Am J Physiol,* 262, G427, 1992.

164. **Roman, F. J., Pascaud, X., Martin, B., Vauche, D., and Junien, J. L.,** JO 1784, a potent and selective ligand for rat and mouse brain sigma sites, *J Pharm Pharmacol,* 42, 439, 1990.

165. **Jimenez, M., and Buéno, L.,** Inhibitory effects of neuropeptide Y (NPY) on CRF and stress-induced caecal motor response in rats, *Life Sci,* 47, 205, 1990.

166. **Junien, J. L., Gué, M., and Buéno, L.,** Neuropeptide Y and sigma ligand (JO 1784) act through a Gi protein to block the psychological stress and corticotropin-releasing factor-induced colonic motor activation in rats, *Neuropharmacology,* 30, 1119, 1991.

167. **Martinez, J. A., and Buéno, L.,** Buspirone inhibits corticotropin-releasing factor and stress-induced cecal motor response in rats by acting through 5-HT1A receptors, *Eur J Pharmacol,* 202, 379, 1991.

168. **Gué, M., Alary, C., Delrio, C., Junien, J. L., and Buéno, L.,** Comparative involvement of $5HT_1$, $5HT_2$ and $5HT_3$ receptors in stress-induced colonic motor alterations in rats, *Eur J Pharmacol,* 233, 193, 1993.

169. **Gué, M., Junien, J. L., Delrio, C., and Buéno, L.,** Neuropeptide Y and sigma ligand (JO1784) suppress stress-induced colonic motor disturbances in rats through Sigma and cholecystokinin receptors, *J Pharmacol Exp Ther,* 261, 850, 1992.

170. **Lane, R. F., Blaha, C. D., and Phillips, A. G.,** In vivo electrochemical analysis of cholecystokinin-induced inhibition of dopamine release in nucleus accumbens, *Brain Res,* 397, 204, 1986.

171. **Ricardo, J. A., and Koh, T. E.,** Anatomical evidence of direct projections from the nucleus of the solitary tract to the hypothalamus, amygdala, and other forebrain structures in the rat, *Brain Res,* 153, 1, 1978.

172. **Andrews, P. L. R., and Wood, K. L.,** Systemic baclofen stimulates gastric motility and secretion via a central action in the rat, *Br J Pharmacol,* 89, 461, 1986.

173. **Davison, J. S., Hodges, M., and Dickson, V.,** The enterogastric reflex in the ferret, *Dig Dis Sci,* 29, 558, 1984.

174. **Lantéri-Minet, M., Isnardon, P., de Pommery, J., and Menetrey, D.,** Spinal and hindbrain structures involved in visceroception and visceronociception as revealed by the expression of Fos, Jun and Krox-24 proteins, *Neuroscience,* 55, 737, 1993.

175. **Barber, A., Harting, J., and Wolf, H. P.,** Antinociceptive effects on the $5-HT_2$ antagonist ritanserin in rats: evidence for an activation of descending monoaminergic pathways in the spinal cord, *Neurosci Lett,* 99, 234, 1989.

176. **Sandrini, G., Alfonsi, E., De Rysky, C., Marini, S., Facchinen, F., and Nappi, G.,** Evidence of serotonin-S_2 receptor involvement in analgesia in humans, *Eur J Pharmacol,* 130, 311, 1986.

177. **Willis, W. D.,** Control of nociceptive transmission in the spinal cord, in *Progress in Sensory Physiology Monograph 3,* Ottoson, D., Ed., Berlin, Springer-Verlag, 1982, pp. 159.

178. **Sagrada, A., Fargeas, M. J., and Buéno, L.,** Involvement of alpha-1 and alpha-2 adrenoceptors in the postlaparotomy intestinal motor disturbances in the rat, *Gut,* 28, 955, 1987.
179. **Rivière, P. J. M., Pascaud, X., Chevalier, E., Le Gallou, B., and Junien, J. L.,** Fedotozine reverses ileus induced by surgery or peritonitis: action at peripheral κ-opiod receptors, *Gastroenterology,* 104, 724, 1993.

14 Evaluation of Antimotion Sickness Drugs

John J. Stewart and Charles D. Wood

INTRODUCTION

Brand and Perry reviewed testing methods for antimotion sickness drugs in 1966 and concluded "..that there is only one valid way of determining whether a compound is effective as a treatment for motion sickness, and that is to test it in a properly designed field study in man."[1] Today, the emphasis is on laboratory studies rather than field tests. Availability of laboratory motion devices and the development of motion sickness rating scales encouraged research in this area and brought some degree of standardization among different laboratories. In addition, animal tests no longer involve only dogs, cats and monkeys. The house musk shrew *(Suncus murinus),* which exhibits emetic behavior when exposed to motion, is a good animal model for motion sickness research. Even the rat, which cannot vomit and therefore is not normally considered for studies of motion sickness, exhibits certain motion-induced behaviors. At least two of these behaviors may be useful for testing antimotion sickness drugs. New animal models and standardized laboratory methods may advance this area, which has seen few major breakthroughs in the recent past.

Our treatment of this subject is not exhaustive. We describe only the most important methods and techniques available, and focus on those methods which are most practical for the average investigator. Excellent reviews on the topic of motion sickness are available and provide important background information on this interesting topic.[2-4]

HISTORY

Although the first account of motion sickness was not recorded, it was almost certainly associated with sea travel. In fact, the symptoms of motion sickness were so closely associated with the sea that the condition was originally called "seasickness." In 1881, Irwin suggested that what was called "seasickness" was a general response to motion and occurred in other situations besides sea travel.[5] Sir Frederick Banting is credited with popularizing the term "motion sickness" at the beginning of World War II.[16]

Our modern understanding of motion sickness began in 1882 when James demonstrated that a functional vestibular apparatus was essential for the development of motion sickness.[7] Previously, many theories sought to explain motion sickness and to identify the anatomical structures responsible for it. Reason and Brand describe a major class of theories popular at the end of the Nineteenth Century as "blood and guts" theories.[8] In brief, these theories attributed motion sickness either to reduced cerebral blood flow, or sensations arising from movement of the abdominal viscera. When the vestibular organs were proven to be an absolute necessity for motion sickness, it was popular to attribute motion sickness to excessive vestibular stimulation.

The Vestibular Overstimulation Theory persisted into the mid-Twentieth Century but failed to explain a number of observations, including the development adaptation and the development of motion sickness in stationary subjects presented with a disorienting visual scene.[9]

Today, the most popular theory of motion sickness is the Sensory Conflict or Sensory Rearrangement Theory. The Sensory Conflict Theory evolved over the past 30 years and involved the research and writings of many investigators. This theory suggests that motion sickness results from a conflict between present and anticipated sensory input. Reason,[10] borrowing from the work of von Holst[11] and Held,[12] suggested that each motion experience generates a neural trace of paired sensory input and motor commands. The degree to which this neural trace is incorporated in memory varies with the stimulus intensity and duration. Especially intense or long-duration stimuli consolidate more readily and become the dominate trace for future comparisons. When spatial receptors, the eyes, vestibular apparatus and the non-vestibular proprioceptors, receive a unique pattern of input, neural circuits compare the present sensory experience with the primary neural store. A conflict generates a signal proportional to the discrepancy. This signal activates the processes responsible for motion sickness symptoms. This theory explains protective adaptation and how discordant visual stimuli can induce motion sickness. A major weakness of the Sensory Conflict Theory, however, is its failure to identify the anatomic structures involved in motion sickness and its inability to explain the actions and mechanisms of antimotion sickness drugs.[13]

Three events in this century had a major impact on antimotion sickness drug research. The first was the Second World War, where the need to transport soldiers by boats and planes became a matter of national security. Many important studies were conducted at this time and the era was marked by a gradual development of standardized laboratory testing methods and a greater understanding of experimental variables in motion sickness research.[1] Research in Britain, the United States and Canada focused on the belladonna alkaloids, principally scopolamine, which is still one of the most effective drugs known. Another milestone was a chance observation by Gay and Carliner in 1947. While evaluating the antihistamine dimenhydrinate for use in hives and allergies, they prescribed the drug to a female patient who suffered from urticaria and chronic motion sickness. To their surprise, the drug not only alleviated the urticaria, but also allowed the patient to travel by car without the usual motion sickness.[14] The third important event was the development of the U.S. manned-space program. Only when spacecraft became larger and allowed greater crew mobility did space motion sickness (SMS) become a problem for U.S. astronauts.[15] Reduced crew performance and the possibility of equipment failure from vomitus, made SMS an important safety issue. As a result, the National Aeronautics and Space Administration (NASA) launched a major research effort to find effective countermeasures for SMS. NASA support allowed Dr. Ashton Graybiel and his colleagues at the U.S. Naval Aerospace Medical Institute in Pensacola, Florida, to add enormously to our knowledge of motion sickness. NASA's efforts recently culminated in what appears to be a major breakthrough in the treatment of SMS. The magic bullet long sought by NASA, turned out to be a magic needle. Intramuscularly administered promethazine appears to be the most effective remedy for SMS tested thus far.[16]

VESTIBULAR ANATOMY AND PHYSIOLOGY

The vestibular organs, eyes and non-vestibular proprioceptors all play a role in the development of motion sickness. Of these, the vestibular apparatus is the most important. Motion sickness does not occur in the absence of vestibular function.[17] Because of its crucial role, the vestibular apparatus is described below.

The vestibular apparatus lies in the inner ear and consists of the non-auditory membranous labyrinth. The membranous labyrinth is filled with a viscous fluid called endolymph. The movement of endolymph is sensed in five specialized areas *viz.* three semicircular canals and two otolith structures. The semicircular canals sense angular, while the otoliths sense linear acceleration. Vestibular output engages complex reflexes that maintain balance, posture and stationary vision in a motion environment.

THE SEMICIRCULAR CANALS

The superior, inferior and horizontal semicircular canals are approximately perpendicular to one another. The superior canals are tilted forward and approximately 45 degrees outward, while the inferior canals are tilted slightly backward and approximately 45 degrees outward. The canals are arranged so that the superior canal on one side is in the same plane as the inferior canal on the contralateral side. The horizontal canals on both sides are in the same plane (Figure 1).

Each canal ends in a specialized sensing area called an ampulla. The ampulla contains hair cells that synapse with fibers of the eight cranial nerve. Each hair cell contains a number of cilia which are emersed in a gelatinous capsule called the cupula. The movement of endolymph deforms the cupula and hence the cilia. When the cilia are bent in one direction, the firing rate of the vestibular fibers associated with those hair cells increase. When bent in the opposite direction, the basal firing rate of the fibers decrease. If a subject rotates around the vertical axis to a constant rotational velocity, the endolymph and cupula of the horizontal canals eventually reach a stable position and the initial change in nerve firing ceases. If the rotation is terminated abruptly, the endolymph and cupula move in the opposite direction. Signals of opposite "polarity" are sent during angular acceleration and deceleration.

OTOLITHS

The otolith organs, the utricle and saccule, sense linear acceleration. The sensing hair cells in each organ are contained in a small area called a macula. Each macula is covered by a

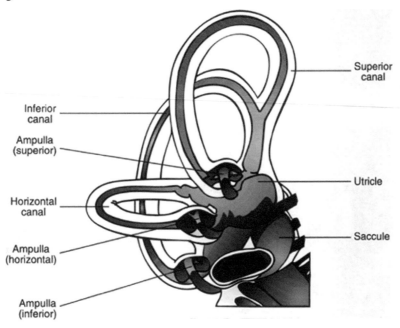

FIGURE 1 The vestibular apparatus consists of five sensing areas: 3 semicircular canals and 2 otoliths. The canals are responsive to angular and the otoliths to linear accelerations.

gelatinous layer which contains small particles of calcium carbonate, called otoliths. Forces act on the otoliths, which in turn deform the hair cells. The macula of the utricle is positioned horizontally, while the macula of the saccule is oriented vertically. The hair cells of the otolith organs are not oriented in one direction and as a result, they sense linear acceleration in various directions. The pattern of afferent fiber firing encodes the direction and force of linear translation.

CENTRAL NERVOUS SYSTEM CONNECTIONS

Fibers originating from the vestibular receptors innervate the vestibular nuclear complex (VNC). The VNC consists of superior, lateral, medial and inferior vestibular nuclei. Second-order neurons from the VNC extend to various reticular nuclei, the fastigial nuclei, the uvula and the flocculonodular lobes of the cerebellum. Some primary fibers in the vestibular nerve also pass to these areas. A major descending output from the VNC, the lateral vestibulospinal tract, arises from the lateral vestibular nuclei to influence the activity of motor neurons at all levels of the spinal cord. The ascending component of the medial longitudinal fasciculus derives mainly from the superior and medial vestibular nuclei and innervates the oculomotor nuclei. This fiber tract is mainly responsible for the vestibuloocular reflex described below. Readers interested in a further discussion of the physiology of the vestibular receptors are referred to textbooks by Guyton[18] and Berne and Levy.[19]

Another CNS area involved in motion sickness is the central emetic apparatus which consists of two anatomically close but functionally distinct areas, the chemoreceptor trigger zone (CTZ) and the vomiting center (VC). The CTZ lies on the floor of the fourth ventricle in the area postrema and senses chemical stimuli. The area bristles with pharmacological receptors and a large effort in antiemetic drug research has been devoted to finding drugs that act on these receptors. The VC is more lateral in the reticular formation, among centers responsible for the control respiration, cardiovascular and salivary gland function. The major pathway for the production of motion sickness is thought to includes the VCN, the cerebellum and the VC. Based on studies in dogs and monkeys,[20,21] the CTZ was once thought to be important in the development of motion sickness. The implication was that the CTZ could serve as a pharmacological target for antimotion sickness drugs. However, Borison[22] disproved the role of the CTZ in motion sickness which explains why typical antiemetic drugs, such as those used for toxic or chemotherapy induced vomiting, are not effective antimotion sickness drugs.

The above discussion of the neural pathways and sensory receptors is deceptively simple. We know for example that the vision and proprioceptor output interact in complex ways with vestibular input. Vision can either enhance or reduce the motion sickness potential of a motion experience (see below). Smell and taste[23,24] alter motion sickness susceptibility. Psychogenic factors, like anticipation of sickness or anxiety, also modify susceptibility. These factors become important sources of variability in drug testing protocols.

SYMPTOMS

Motion sickness is probably best known for the terminal symptoms of nausea and vomiting. However, a constellation of symptoms usually occurs before activation of the emetic reflex. Dizziness, nystagmus, pallor, sweating, salivation and headache also occur. Symptom recognition and development are important for many drug testing procedures.

Although subjects vary in the intensity and pattern of motion sickness symptoms, several characteristic symptoms almost always occur. Dizziness and nystagmus are two of the earliest signs. Both are said to be of vestibular, probably semicircular canal origin. The nystagmus results from the connections between the semicircular canals, VCN and oculomotor nuclei described previously. This pathway constitutes the vestibuloocular reflex which is designed to maintain visual fixation while the head moves. For example, the vestibuloocular reflex is activated when a subject rotates horizontally, around a vertical axis. Because of the inertia of the endolymph, the fluid moves slower than the walls of the canal structures. Eventually the endolymph shifts in the direction of head rotation and deforms the cupula in each canal in that direction. This results in the relatively slow movement of eyes in the direction opposite to the rotation. This movement compensates for the head movement and allows the eye to fixate on a distant point in the field of view. With continued head rotation, however, the eye eventually reaches the limit of rotation. At that point, the eye rotates rapidly back in the direction of rotation to pick another distant point for visual fixation and the process begins again. These alternating slow and rapid eye movements are called nystagmus. If rotation continued at an unchanging velocity, the endolymph in each horizontal canal would cease to move relative to the canal structures. At that point, the cupula would be maximally deformed, and would no longer signal acceleration. Nystagmus would cease until the rotation terminated abruptly. At that point, each cupula would move in the opposite direction. A postrotatory period of nystagmus would then occur, with the rapid and slow phases of eye movements opposite to their initial directions. A number of studies have tested drug effects on the intensity and duration of postrotatory nystagmus.

Another fairly consistent symptom is pallor or a color change, especially visible in the face. Pallor is caused by vasoconstriction and has the effect of turning the skin pale white or green. This is a relative color change and it is often necessary to have a good visual impression of the subject's appearance, or a means to compare the subject's coloration before and during testing. Darker skinned individuals acquire a yellowish appearance, especially around the mouth areas.

Sweating is another consistent motion sickness symptom. Initially, the sweating occurs in the so-called arousal areas, such as the palms of the hands. Sweating in these regions is usually associated with emotional arousal and anxiety provoking situations. Eventually, however, the sweating occurs in the thermal areas, such as the dorsal aspects of the hand and arms, where sweating is provoked by hot conditions.[25]

Salivation is highly variable from subject to subject during the development of motion sickness. Although usually associated with the psychic experience of nausea, increased saliva production can occur before nausea. Studies attempting to quantify the salivary gland flow, however, often record decreased production during motion sickness. Salivary protein concentration increases in subjects categorized as moderately or severely motion sick.[26]

Headache is another inconsistent symptom of motion sickness. When it occurs, however, it tends to be frontal and may persist for some time after the termination of motion sickness stimuli.

Graybiel and Knepton[27] identified a symptom complex associated with motion sickness that they called the sopite syndrome. As the name suggests, the symptoms center around drowsiness and yawning, and are associated with a disinclination to work and social interaction. The sopite syndrome can occur either before or after the appearance of other motion sickness symptoms, but more often occurs intertwined with other symptoms of motion sickness. The authors speculate that the sopite syndrome may be responsible for reports of depression and suicides that appear in the motion sickness literature.

The rate of symptom development varies with susceptibility. Reason and Graybiel[28] described the relationship between susceptibility and rate of symptom development. They found that the most susceptible individuals lose their sense of well-being rapidly and symptoms developed almost linearly with time. More resistant subjects remained well longer, and in general, their symptoms accumulate slowly. However, once symptoms developed in resistant subjects, they progress to severe sickness rapidly. The investigators called this phenomenon "avalanche". In general, the longer an individual remains unaffected by the motion stimuli, the more precipitous will be their deterioration once symptoms develop.

QUANTIFICATION OF MOTION SICKNESS

Assessment of antimotion sickness drugs requires some measure of motion sickness. Investigators have developed three general approaches to the problem. One approach is to rely exclusively upon measurable signs of motion sickness. Pallor,[29] peripheral blood flow,[30] heart rate, finger pulse volume, respiratory rate,[31] eye torsion,[32] skin conductance[33] and others can be measured with the appropriate instrumentation. Although these measurable quantities do change in motion sick subjects, it is not clear that they show a direct relationship to the degree of sickness present. These measures, however, do offer quantification and limit subject and investigator bias. For the most part, however, total reliance on objective measures of motion sickness symptoms is not adequate. Clearly, the subject has much to offer the investigator by describing the subjective feelings associated with motion sickness and drug therapy. Another approach therefore, is to allow the subject to rate the degree of sickness experienced or subjective sensations with minimal input from the investigative team. Several "sickness" or "well-being" scales have been developed where the subject ranks his or her relative sickness or discomfort. The subject may be presented with a standard stimulus to use for comparison.[34] Thus, the subject would be asked to compare their well-being on some scale with that experienced during the standard stimulus. Obviously, these methods work best with an intelligent, articulate and reliable subject population. Another approach, and one with considerable merit, is to combine both objective and subjective symptoms into one numerical score. In this way the subject provides a subjective assessment of his feelings, while one or more investigators independently evaluate the objective signs and symptoms present.

In laboratory studies of motion sickness, the stimulus and rating scale can be applied in two ways. One way is to assess the degree of motion sickness after the application of a fixed, standard motion stimulus. The standard motion stimulus should be in the mild to moderate range, so that most subjects reach an advanced level on the chosen rating scale during control conditions (see below). Because stimulus intensity and duration can often be controlled within narrow limits, the variability in such an experiment is mainly associated with the assessment of symptoms and the rating scale. The other approach is to fix the endpoint and vary the intensity and/or duration of the stimulus. When this is done, the stimulus parameters become a quantitative scale indicating the degree of stimulus tolerated or subject susceptibility. The major advantage of fixing the level of motion sickness and varying the stimulus intensity is that for most laboratory testing circumstances, the stimulus intensity and duration are much more accurately determined than the degree of motion sickness present. Variability in the standard motion sickness endpoint can be minimized by providing a training session before the actual tests. This training session allows the subject to experience the subjective feeling(s) associated with the endpoint. The investigators can then request that the subject remember the subjective feelings and continue subsequent tests until those same feelings occur. The training session also allows the laboratory personnel to assess the order, intensity and duration of symptom development for each subject. Experienced laboratory personnel look for similarities and differences between individuals and can become quite skilled at predicting a subject's endpoint after several tests. If every subject can reach approximately the same endpoint on all tests, then the variability between subjects can be removed by statistical methods.

The question of an appropriate endpoint is an important one. Emesis or actual vomiting is sometimes advocated as the only truly reproducible endpoint of motion sickness.[1,8] We believe that the inherent problems associated with a vomiting endpoint make it unacceptable for drug screening purposes. For example, the use of an vomiting endpoint might limit subject availability. Subjects who would ordinarily participate in a motion sickness test, might not do so if actual emesis was the endpoint achieved in each test. Institutional committees that oversee human research might be reluctant to approve a protocol that includes vomiting. Vomiting is not without risk, as choking and aspiration are possible. Vomiting can also become a conditioned response, making the data unreliable. In our view, emesis should not be used as an experimental endpoint, especially since endpoints short of vomiting are reproducible and avoid the pitfalls described above.

Wood and his colleagues[35] were the first to suggest that certain combinations of motion sickness symptoms have a certain quantitative value. In 1968, Graybiel and colleagues[36] proposed the most useful and well-known motion sickness symptom scale yet devised. After years of watching subjects develop motion sickness symptoms, Graybiel and his colleagues defined five levels of motion sickness based upon a numerical symptom scale as shown in Table I. Symptoms were graded, assigned a numerical value and summed to determine the level of motion sickness present.

There are several characteristics of the Graybiel Motion Sickness Symptom Scale that deserve comment. First, although most of the symptoms are readily observable by the investigators, some, like dizziness, headache, flushing and the subjective gastric complains must be obtained from the subject. What is unique and ingenious about the Graybiel scale is that it combines both objective and subjective signs of motion sickness into one numerical result. In other words, both the subject and the investigative personnel work together to score the level of motion sickness present. We should also comment on the gastric symptoms. Gastric awareness is a feeling that draws the subject's attention to the gastric area, while discomfort is a more noticeable and uncomfortable feeling centered in the gastric area. Although one might think that epigastric awareness and epigastric discomfort would be difficult to distinguish, we find that many subjects readily distinguish between the two. Furthermore, we attribute special significance to gastric symptoms in the evolution of motion sickness. In our experience, gastric discomfort occurs late in the constellation of motion sickness symptoms and often immediately before frank nausea. As a result, we use gastric discomfort as hallmark symptom of the Malaise III (M-III) level motion sickness. The presence of significant levels of pallor, sweating, salivation, and drowsiness, along with gastric discomfort, usually completes our definition of M-III. In our experience, except for adaptation (see below), an individual tends to retain approximately the same order and severity of symptoms from test to test. Experienced laboratory personnel become skilled at ranking symptoms and often detect a characteristic pattern of motion sickness symptoms for an individual. A modified Graybiel Scale of Symptoms is perhaps the most accurate way to score motion sickness. With it, subjects can be brought to approximately the same endpoint of motion sickness on multiple occasions.

TABLE 1
Diagnostic Categorization of Different Levels of Severity of Acute Motion Sickness*

Category	Pathognomonic 16 points	Major 8 points	Minor 4 points	Minimal 2 points	AQS 1 point
Nausea syndrome	Vomiting or retching	Nausea II, III	Nausea I	Epigastric Discomfort	Epigastric Awareness
Skin color		Pallor III	Pallor II	Pallor I	Flushing
Cold sweating	III	II			
Increased salivation	III	II			
Drowsiness	III	II			
Pain					Headache
CNS					Dizziness

*Reproduced from Graybiel et. al., *Aerospace Med.*, 39, 453–455, 1968. With permission.

MOTIONS AND TEST CONDITIONS

This section reviews some of the more common test conditions and motion environments used for testing antimotion sickness drugs. Generally, all motion sickness studies have been conducted in one of two environments: the field or the laboratory. The following discusses the some of the problems associated with field tests and focuses on laboratory testing of antimotion sickness drugs.

FIELD TESTS

Although field tests of antimotion sickness drugs are still performed, there are fewer of this kind of test than in the past. Field testing of antimotion sickness drugs would at first seem ideal. The major advantage of a field test is that in most cases the drug is tested under the actual environment and conditions in which it will be used. However, there are significant practical and scientific problems associated with field testing, several of which are discussed below.

Field tests of antimotion sickness drugs have been conducted on boats, ships, planes and in various other environments. Field testing presents a practical problem for a university or industry based researcher. Ordinarily these workers do not have access to a boat, ship, plane or other specialized vehicle necessary to conduct field testing. Military workers, or researchers associated with a government or governmental agency, might have greater access to these test environments.

A major scientific objection to field testing is the lack of standardization and reproducible test conditions. The ability to reproduce the motion conditions in a boat off the coast of Florida is limited, to say the least. The exact sea conditions could never be reproduced. Results, therefore, cannot be compared from trial to trial, let alone between investigators. This inability to confirm data from test to test severely restricts the normal scientific process, which works through a alternating process of data corroboration and extension. Lack of control over the stimulus conditions also leads to unavoidable vomiting. Even when vomiting is used as an endpoint, the number of subjects vomiting is out of the direct control of the investigator. Brand and Perry[1] mentioned that the highly variable number of placebo or control responders in various studies presents a major difficulty in making comparisons. In most tests, the number of subjects responding in the control or placebo group gives some estimation of the motion severity or intensity involved in the test. Presumably, a more efficacious antimotion sickness drug will protect more subjects in a harsh motion environment than a less efficacious drug. How can we compare a drug that protects all subjects in a motion sickness trial that has a 20 percent placebo response rate, with one that protects all subjects in a trial with an 80 percent placebo response rate? Holling and his colleagues[37] propose the Index of Protection (IOP) to deal with these difficulties. The IOP is equal to the percentage of subjects responding with emesis after placebo, minus the percentage of subjects vomiting after drug, divided by the percentage of subjects responding with emesis after placebo. The result is then multiplied by 100. Although probably not a perfect solution to the differences in placebo response rate between trials, the IOP does allow some comparison between tests.

Some workers have attempted, where possible, to control the motion experience from one field test to another by establishing a standard motion protocol. In a plane, for example, the test could involve a series of standardized flight maneuvers. An example is NASA's KC-135 aircraft which has been used on a number of occasions for antimotion sickness drug testing (Figure 2). The aircraft flies a series parabolas which result in short period of hypo- and hypergravity conditions. Effective antimotion sickness drugs significantly increase the number of parabolic maneuvers tolerated.

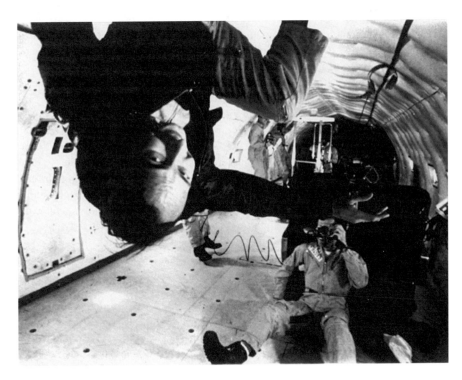

FIGURE 2   One of the authors (CDW) during the period of weightlessness aboard NASA's KC-135.

There are circumstances when field testing of antimotion sickness drugs is appropriate. For example, when the motion environment and test conditions are so unique, it may not be possible to stipulate the efficacy or side-effects of the drug in another test condition. Field testing for antimotion sickness drugs for use in the space program is a good example. Microgravity can be simulated only for 20 to 30 seconds in tests on earth. In addition, the physiological and biochemical changes that occur in space, called Space Adaptation Syndrome (SAS), are likely unique and not reproducible on earth.[38] SAS may result in altered bioavailability, especially for drugs given by the oral route. SAS may be sufficiently different from terrestrial motion sickness as to require drug tests in space.

LABORATORY TESTS

The laboratory conditions necessary to provoke motion sickness are stated in the Sensory Conflict Theory. The major perquisite is a conflict between present and anticipated sensory input. To be provocative the motion must be accelerative, because of the sensing capabilities of the receptors in the vestibular apparatus. The acceleration can be linear, angular or some combination thereof. The degree to which accelerative stimuli provoke motion sickness symptoms is directly proportional to the accelerative forces presented. However, motion need not be present. An optokinetic stimulus that generates a feeling of motion without corroborating input from the vestibular receptors, can also be provocative. Thus, there are three laboratory stimulus conditions to test antimotion sickness drugs: vestibular, optokinetic, or some combination of the two.

Vestibular stimulation can be produced by angular, linear or a complex accelerative force. Most devices used to provoke motion sickness by vestibular stimuli do so by rotating the subject around a vertical axis. This movement, combined with head movements out of the plane of rotation, produces a stimulus condition sometimes called Coriolis effect, or cross-coupled angular acceleration. Coriolis effect is accompanied by a tilt sensation about an axis orthogonal to the axis of rotation and a sense of increased rotation about the vertical axis. The accelerative forces generated, and hence the vestibular stress, is directly proportional to the horizontal rotational velocity and number of head movements performed.[36]

An optokinetic stimulus, such as a moving visual scene, can provoke motion sickness when the motion depicted by the visual scene is not corroborated by the vestibular system and non-vestibular proprioceptors. A stationary subject, presented with a moving visual scene, experiences an illusion of motion called vection. When delivered alone, visual stimuli are less effective at producing frank motion sickness than Coriolis stimulation. For example, although almost all individuals are susceptible to Coriolis stimulation, if applied at sufficient velocity and after a sufficient number of head movements, only approximately 60 percent of individuals experience nausea when viewing a rotating drum painted with alternating black and white stripes.[39] Higher frequency visual input is not necessarily more provocative. Symptoms of motion sickness increase in drum exposed subjects until the rotational velocity of the drum reaches 60 degrees per seconds. The incidence of frank sickness either plateaus or declines at higher drum velocities.[40]

Presented simultaneously, Coriolis and optokinetic stimuli combine in complex ways. The nauseogenic potential of the resulting stimulus depends upon whether the visual stimulus is discrepant, or in agreement with the sensations experienced by the vestibular apparatus. Figure 3 shows results of an experiment conducted in our laboratory which was designed to show the effects of combining a Coriolis and optokinetic stimulus on motion sickness development. The graph shows the number of head movements required to reach the Malaise III (M-III) level of motion sickness under various conditions. The test apparatus will be described in more detail later. Briefly, subjects performed head movements while seated on a rotating chair. Head movements were continued until the subject reached the M-III level of motion sickness on the Graybiel scale.[36] Surrounding the chair was a enclosure painted with white and black stripes. Both the chair and the visual surround (drum) were rotated clockwise either independently or simultaneously at velocities indicated in the figure. With the chair stationary and the visual surround rotated at 5 RPM, subjects tolerated 406 head movements before they reached the endpoint. When the subjects were blindfolded, allowing no visual stimulation, they tolerated fewer head movements when the chair was rotated at 7 RPM. However, when combined the resulting stimulus was greater than when either stimulus was presented alone. Notice the reduced number of head movements required to reach the endpoint when both the chair and the drum

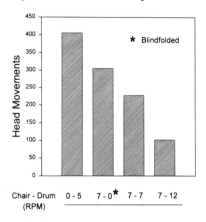

FIGURE 3   The number of head movements required to reach the M-III level of motion sickness after vestibular, optokinetic and combined vestibular and optokinetic stimuli. An optokinetic stimulus greatly increases the provocative nature of vestibular stimulation, especially when it provides discordant information.

were rotated at 7 RPM. This is explained by the added conflict involved in presenting vestibular stimulation without appropriate and corroborating visual input. Viewing the stripes rotating in the same direction and at the same speed as the chair, the subjects received the visual impression of standing still, but the vestibular apparatus and nonvestibular proprioceptors signaled rotation. The most provocative situation, however, is when the chair is rotated at 7 and the drum at 12 RPM. With the drum rotating faster than the chair, the painted stripes appear to move in the opposite direction. The conflict, therefore, is greater than when the chair and drum rotated at the same rate. The provocative nature of simultaneously applied vestibular and visual stimuli, therefore, is proportional to the algebraic sum of the conflict involved. The greater the conflict between vision and spatial receptor systems, the more provocative the combined stimulus.

The additive nature of vestibular and visual conflict might be use to extend or enhance the stressful nature of a motion sickness stimulus in drug testing protocols. There are two major instances where such a combined stimulus would find most use. One instance is where the protocol calls for the induction of motion sickness over a relatively short time. Combined stimuli, being more provocative, should cause subjects to reach an experimental endpoint more rapidly than when either stimulus is given alone. The other instance involves testing near maximally effective doses of an antimotion sickness drug, for example, in the course of constructing a dose response curve. Maximally effective doses of some drugs for example, will protect subjects so well that they never reach the experimental endpoint after receiving one provocative stimulus. In that case, adding a second stimulus that acts through another system, may allow for higher test doses, or bring certain especially resistant subjects to the experimental endpoint. Thus far, researchers have not taken advantage of combined stimuli in drug testing protocols. Studies should be conducted to test predicted utility of combined stimuli.

SLOW ROTATION ROOM

Motion around the vertical axis is perhaps the easiest motion to provide in the laboratory setting. The most famous, or infamous, apparatus of this type is the Slow Rotation Room (SRR) located in Pensacola, Florida. The SRR was used extensively by Graybiel and his colleagues throughout the '60s, '70s and early '80s. The SRR is a total living environment which rotates around the vertical axis at a controlled rotational velocity. The SRR has been used for both acute and chronic studies of motion sickness and antimotion sickness drugs. Ordinarily, both the experimental subjects and the investigators ride or live on the SRR. When the rotational velocity of the SRR is constant, the motion sickness stimulus is trivial, unless a person moves his head out of the plane of rotation. Investigators riding along to monitor symptoms or administer medications, can remain almost symptom free by immobilizing their head. On the other hand, experimental subjects can be exposed to standard motion sickness stimuli if they make standard head movements (Coriolis stimulation). To facilitate standard head movements, Graybiel and his colleagues developed the "Dial Test", where the subject was required to adjust the setting of 5 dials located at various points around the subject. The head movements associated with the dial setting served as a standard stimulus.[41] The SRR measures motion sickness susceptibility. Susceptibility is measured either by the duration of exposure, by the number of head movements performed, or the highest rotational velocity tolerated. Since subjects are usually not blindfolded in the SRR, the stimulus provided by the SRR is a combination of vestibular and optokinetic. Subjects receive vestibular stimulation from head movements, but the environment within the SRR appears stationary. The conflict produced is similar to that produced by the chair and drum both rotated at 7 RPM as described above.

ROTATING CHAIR

A more practical device for rotating subjects around the vertical axis is a rotating chair. Motorized chairs take a minimum of laboratory space and are inexpensive when compared with the expense of a rotating room. The chair shown in Figure 4 is manufactured by Contraves Goerz Corporation of Philadelphia, Pennsylvania. The chair is controlled by an external voltage in the minus to plus 5 volt range. This controlling voltage can be sent to the controller from a personal computer.

Many laboratories that use the rotating chair, either currently or in the past, use the Staircase Velocity Motion Test (SVMT) or some variant of it to induce motion sickness and test antimotion sickness drugs. In the SVMT, blindfolded subjects make standardized head movements while seated in the rotating chair. The head movements are made to headrests located on each side,

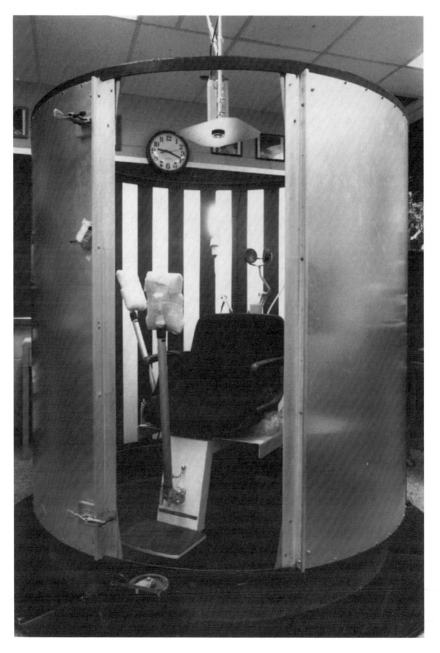

FIGURE 4   A rotating chair and visual surround. Notice the head rests located toward the front, back and sides of the chair.

front and back of the chair. The head rests are positioned so as to require a subject of average size to move from 20 to 45 degrees out of the vertical plane. Normally, the head movements are timed so that the subject makes 1 head movement every 3 seconds. The rotational velocity, and hence the Coriolis stimulus, is increased in steps. The initial velocity of the chair is set to 1 RPM. After 40 head movements, the rotational velocity of the chair is increased by 2 RPM. The test is continued until the subject reaches the desired endpoint or the rotational velocity reaches 35 RPM's. For most tests, we set our endpoint at the M-III level of motion sickness using the Graybiel Scale of Motion Sickness Symptoms. This is an advanced level of motion sickness short of actual vomiting.

Because of the standardized head movements and stepped rotational velocities involved, the number of head movements required to reach M-III, serves as a measure of relative motion sickness susceptibility. Without drug treatment, most naive subjects reach an advanced level of motion sickness after approximately 250 head movements. Effective antimotion sickness drugs increase the head movements required to reach M-III. For many subjects, for example, a maximal dose of scopolamine will allow the subject to tolerate the limit of the SVMT, which is a maximal of 35 RPM or 720 head movements. Since motion sickness susceptibility varies so much between subjects, we let each subject serve as his/her own control. For an experimental group, we often report the average difference in head movements between placebo and test treatment.

The SVMT requires too much time for some experimental situations. In these instances subjects can be brought to an advanced level of motion sickness faster by beginning rotation at an advanced rotational velocity. The rotational velocity used is sometimes selected for each subject based upon their relative susceptibility. For example, sometimes we use the highest rotational velocity tolerated by that individual in a training test administered prior to actual drug testing. In some subjects, head movements at chair rotational velocities in the range of 15 to 21 RPM produced an advanced level of motion sickness within minutes. Whatever protocol is chosen, it should not be varied in the course of testing. No one knows whether the response to drugs is similar when motion sickness is induced over a relatively short or long time. Another way to bring subjects to a motion sickness endpoint faster is to administered both Coriolis and optokinetic stimulation, as described above.

Another device used to rotate subjects around the vertical axis is the Stille-Werner Short-Arm Centrifuge. As the name implies, the centrifuge is meant for higher rotational velocities than a rotating chair. The motion sickness stimulus can be produced either by head movements within the centrifuge, or by a sudden stop procedure. Although sudden stop stimulus is used clinically to assess vestibular function, it is generally considered an ineffective stimulus for motion sickness. However, Graybiel and Lackner[42] found that a majority of individuals became motion sick if subjected to multiple accelerations and decelerations. In their protocol, blindfolded subjects were accelerated at 15 degrees per second per second, to a final velocity of 300 degrees per second. After 30 seconds of constant rotational speed, the centrifuge and subject were brought to a full stop in 1.5 seconds. Of course the accelerations and decelerations were sensed by the vestibular apparatus. The acceleration-deceleration procedure was repeated 20 times, or until the subject reached a mild nausea endpoint. If the stimulus procedure was not adequate to produce the desired sickness level, the 20 acceleration-deceleration procedures were repeated, only this time with the blindfold removed. With the blindfold removed, the subject was now able to view the six vertical stripes painted at 60-degree intervals around the inside drum surrounding the centrifuge. The additional visual stimuli enhanced the motion sickness stimuli as described previously. If the subject failed to reach the appropriate endpoint after the addition of optokinetic stimuli, then the procedure was repeated 20 times with the centrifuge rotated in the opposite direction. Reverse rotation would be highly emetogenic because some degree of adaptation is rapidly acquired during the test. Rotation in the opposite direction, after some adaptation to the initial rotational direction, would produce a greater discrepancy than if the procedure had been conducted in the same direction. The scoring system used reflected the increasing motion sickness stimuli in the three-staged test protocol: the score computed for each subject was equal to one-half the number of stops performed with eyes closed, plus the number of stops performed with eyes opened, plus two times the number of stops performed with the chair rotating in the reverse direction. The test procedure described is an excellent example of how motion sickness stimuli can be increased without actually increasing the rotational forces.

PROTOCOL AND TEST CONSIDERATIONS

The rules for good protocol design in studies of antimotion sickness drugs are no different than those for other types of clinical studies. However, there are several factors particular to clinical testing of antimotion sickness drugs. In the following, we assume that the drug testing will be conducted in the laboratory setting and that an appropriate dose has been selected for testing.

SUBJECT SELECTION

Subject recruiting and selection are issues which are specified by the human studies committee of the institution at which the studies will be conducted. Not all subjects willing to participate in experimental studies are willing to endure the unpleasant feelings experienced during antimotion sickness drug testing. Even if a subject expresses a willingness to participate, there are several disqualifying factors. Motion sickness is a physiological stress and only healthy individuals should be included in test protocols. A basic physical examination with a full complement of clinical laboratory measurements is important. No special tests of vestibular function are necessary since the subject's relative susceptibility to motion sickness is usually determined in a "training" session as described below. Recruiting from a relatively young subject population generally assures a healthy test group. However, even though we recruit predominately from college students, we have uncovered clinically significant abnormalities in several perspective test subjects. This is an often unstated benefit of human clinical research. Finally, there is the issue of illicit drug use. We routinely conduct urine screens for illicit drugs during the initial physical examination. Sometimes we ask each participant to donate a urine sample before each test. Of course the subjects are apprised of these possibilities before they agree to participate. Illicit drug use may be interfering factor in studies of antimotion sickness drugs. We have observed, although not documented, that subjects with positive screens for cannabinoids are especially refractory to the protective effects of antimotion sickness drugs.

TRAINING

If Coriolis stimulation is involved, then subjects must be trained to perform the head movements correctly. Timing sequences must be clearly understood. Furthermore, if the investigators decide to use a symptom scoring system that requires subject participation, such as the Graybiel Motion Sickness Symptom Scale described above, then the subject must be taught to identify and scale certain subjective motion sickness symptoms. This requires an understanding of the motion sickness symptoms, of what to expect, and an ability to articulate those subjective feelings experienced. The requirement that subjects be perceptive and articulate may influence recruiting efforts. Training should be conducted in one or more sessions before drug testing. When performed correctly, training sessions characterize the baseline motion sickness susceptibility of a subject.

BASIC DESIGN

A parallel-subject or cross-over design is often adequate for most tests of antimotion sickness drugs. A cross-over design study has the following advantages: 1) results for each treatment arm can be directly compared, 2) certain prognostic factors, like previous motion experience, need not be controlled, 3) between subject differences in motion sickness susceptibility can be accounted for and eliminated in the statistical analysis, 4) subjects can be asked for a subjective comparison of treatments, and 5) in general, fewer subjects are required to achieve the same power in a parallel-subject design than with other designs. One disadvantage of a parallel-subject design is the inability to detect interactions between treatment arms, for example, where the effects of a treatment influence the response to a subsequent treatment. We believe, however, that the advantages outweigh this potential disadvantage.

We also recommend double-blind and placebo control techniques. Blinding ensures that the outcome cannot be influenced by suggestion or expectation from either the subject or the investigator. Always include a placebo control, either a bogus capsule, tablet, liquid, or injection in the study. A properly placed placebo control also has another role in antimotion sickness drug testing. When combined with a training session, a strategically placed placebo trial can serve to warn the investigator of sudden changes in susceptibility. Changes in susceptibility may result from many sources including changes in the general health of the subject, dietary factors, lack of motivation and the development of protective adaptation as explained below.

ADAPTATION

If motion sickness stimuli are maintained long enough, symptoms of motion sickness diminish and eventually disappear. Protective adaptation, as this phenomenon is often called,[8] is an important consideration for designing drug testing protocols for antimotion sickness drugs. Adaptation occurs to both inertial and visual motion sickness stimuli. Most studies of adaptation use controlled Coriolis stimulation as the provocative stimulus. For example, if subjects are rotated around the vertical axis and make head movements after small changes (eg., 1 RPM) in rotational velocity until the sensations due to somatogyral or oculogyral effects are abolished, they typically reach otherwise intolerable angular velocities either symptom free or nearly so.[10,28] This suggests that acute tolerance or adaptation occurs under these conditions. Adaptation also can develop over longer periods. Nystagmus and oculogyral illusion, a consequence of repetitive semicircular canal stimulation, gradually decline over several days in the Slow Rotation Room.[43] Subjects rotated in a chair once daily for four days, require a gradually increasing number of head movements to reach a Malaise III endpoint of motion sickness.[44]

Adaptation also occurs to optokinetic stimuli. Stationary subjects viewing a rotating drum experience fewer symptoms of vection when exposed to the stimulus for two short periods immediately before testing.[45,46] Subjects show adaptation to vection when tested every 2, but not every 4 or 24 days.[47]

Adaptation is highly specific for the motion environment or stimulus that originally produced it. For example, subjects can make repetitive head movements to the right while rotating in the vertical axis and eventually, lose the nystagmic and illusory sensations associated with that movement. Movements to the left, however, will still produce sensations.[48] Other examples can be cited, but the point is that adaptation only occurs to the specific situation that originally produced it. Clearly, one way to avoid adaptation is to alter the motion stimulus. A more complete discussion of adaptation is available elsewhere.[8]

Adaptation can be problematic for investigators performing longitudinal studies of antimotion sickness drugs. The development of adaptation over days of testing is an additional experimental variable. Although randomization and appropriate statistical methods can account for adaptation, most investigators would be advised to avoid the issue by taking steps to avoid its development. One way to avoid the development of adaptation is to schedule consecutive tests far enough apart. Unfortunately, there are few data on the minimal inter-trial interval required to avoid adaptation. Our experience suggests that adaptation does not develop when subjects are brought to the M-III level of motion sickness in a rotating chair at weekly intervals. For example, the number of head movements to reach the M-III endpoint of motion sickness in 10 subjects tested on 4 occasions, once every 7 days was (group means $\pm$ SEM): 299 ($\pm$ 27), 342 ($\pm$ 46), 305.5 ($\pm$ 26) and 310 ($\pm$ 38) for tests 1 through 4, respectively. There was no statistical difference between tests. We advise, therefore, to keep all inter-trail intervals at least 1 week apart when scheduling multiple test sessions involving Coriolis stimulation. As a further precaution, if a rotational stimulus is involved, alternate the direction of rotation for each consecutive test session.

DIETARY STATUS

Another potentially important experimental variable, and one for which there is little information in the literature, is the influence of dietary status on susceptibility to motion sickness. This is quite surprising since the stomach plays such a central role in the expression of motion sickness symptoms. Recently, we conducted a study in which we compared the motion sickness susceptibility of subjects under fasted and fed conditions.[49] For the fed condition, we fed subjects yogurt immediately before the SVMT. We found subjects more susceptible after yogurt than after fasting, but the results may have been due to the rather large percentage of subjects in the study who found the taste of yogurt unappealing. The study should be repeated using a food acceptable to all participants. More recently, Stern's group reported that high levels of parasympathetic activity, such as that after feeding, was associated with lessened motion sickness symptoms produced by an optokinetic stimulus. They failed, however, to show unequivocal differences in motion sickness susceptibility between fed and fasted subjects.[50] Until the issue is clarified with acceptable data, motion sickness tests should be conducted using fasted subjects.

DATA NORMALIZATION

Although individuals maintain a consistent level of susceptibility from test to test, groups of subjects show very wide variations in susceptibility. Since all of our subjects are trained and treated similarly, we assume that this variation reflects an inherent difference in motion sickness susceptibility between individuals. This wide variation between subjects has important implications for subject design and data handling. We commonly normalize data, or find some way that allows each subject to serve has his own control. Calculating percent changes in susceptibility from control or placebo is one way to normalize data between individuals. In our rotating chair tests, we often use the difference in the number of head movements between placebo and drug tests as an indication of susceptibility and drug efficacy.

PHARMACODYNAMICS OF THE TEST DRUGS

The temporal characteristics of a drug should be carefully considered when designing drug protocols for testing antimotion sickness drugs. Antimotion sickness drugs show wide variations in time of peak effect and duration of action. Consequently, tests conducted at inappropriate times can severely underestimate the antimotion sickness efficacy of a drug. When tests involve comparisons of two or more drugs, the timing of the protocol might favor one or more drugs over another. The comparisons, therefore, might be grossly inaccurate. As an example, consider the case of parenteral scopolamine and promethazine shown in Figure 5. In the tests shown, scopolamine and promethazine were tested for antimotion sickness efficacy using the SVMT at various times after dosing. Notice that testing after 4 to 6 hours after IM drug administration would make promethazine appear much more efficacious than scopolamine.[51] Testing using a long duration motion would also favor promethazine. The temporal effects of a drug or series of drugs to be tested for antimotion sickness activity should be major consideration in test design.

ANIMAL MODELS

The list of practical animals for use in motion sickness research is somewhat limited since rodents and lagomorphs, two common laboratory animals, do not vomit.[52] Other animal species are susceptible to motion, including the dog, cat, and monkey, and exhibit vomiting when exposed to motion of sufficient intensity and duration. These have generally been the animals used for motion sickness research. To be valuable as an animal model for antimotion sickness drug screening, an animal should respond to the same stimuli, exhibit similar symptoms, have similar anatomy and physiology, and respond to drugs like man. Furthermore, acquisition and maintenance costs, along with practical consideration such as size, ease of handling and breeding characteristics are additional factors. Quantification of motion sickness in animal is another problem and until recently, was limited to the number and latency of emetic episodes. Some writers reject outright the notion of an animal model and feel that motion sickness and antimotion sickness drug testing is best performed using man.[8] Still, animal models are useful for procedures that cannot be performed in man. Animal studies confirmed the importance of the vestibular organs in the development of motion sickness.[53,54]

New methods and a new animal model may extend the usefulness of animals in antimotion sickness drug research. Investigators, carefully noting the sequence and changing intensity of certain overt behavioral signs of motion sickness, have developed symptom rating scales for cats and monkeys, similar to that proposed by Graybiel and his colleagues for use in humans. These symptom scales provide a means to quantify the degree of sickness present, the response to antimotion sickness drugs, and help in making comparisons between laboratories. Other workers have recognized certain non-emetic behaviors in rodents, which appear to correlate with motion sickness and which are quantitative. Their use in antimotion sickness drug research,

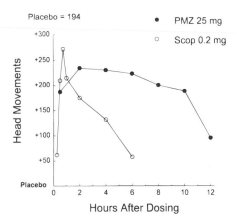

FIGURE 5 Number of head movements in excess of placebo required to reach the M-III endpoint of motion sickness at various times after 25 mg of promethazine (PMZ) and 0.2 mg of scopolamine (Scop) administered IM. Notice the vastly different pharmacodynamic profile for the drugs. (Reproduced from Wood, et. al., *J. Clin. Pharmacol.,* 32, 1008–1012, 1992. With permission.)

although currently limited, offers great potential. Finally, the development of the house musk shrew (Suncus) as an animal model for emetic and antiemetic drug research is one of the most exciting recent developments in the field. Developed by workers in Japan, the Suncus appears to respond to both emetic and antiemetic drugs like man. These new developments are described below.

DOGS

Dogs were used in a number of early studies of motion sickness and antimotion sickness drugs. Beginning in the early 1940s, Nobel conducted a series of studies that defined the motion response characteristics of dogs and the factors that determined their responsiveness to drugs.[55-57] Dogs were found to be particularly susceptible to linear horizontal motion. Nobel used a swing with a radius of 14.5 feet, a swing angle of 90 degrees and a frequency of 15 complete swings per minute. Although approximately 80 percent of animals vomited when subjected to the swing motion, there were large differences in the inherent susceptibility between animals. Animals could be divided into highly susceptible, moderately susceptible and nonsusceptible groups. Nobel found that the inherent susceptibility of an animal influenced its rate of adaptation to swing motion and responsiveness to drugs. Minimally susceptible animals adapted to the motion after weekly tests, while moderately and severely susceptible animals required either more frequent or prolonged exposures to show adaptation. Minimally susceptible animals responded to lower doses of an experimental antimotion sickness drug than moderately or highly susceptible animals.[55] Differences in adaptation and drug responsiveness were confounding factors in drug tests and led to Nobel's suggestion that drug testing be performed with dogs carefully selected for uniform susceptibility.

The dog lost favor as a model for antimotion sickness drug research when it was observed that dogs respond to drugs differently than man. Dogs were not protected from motion sickness stimuli by diphenhydramine, promethazine and scopolamine,[58] some of the most effective antimotion sickness drugs in man.

CATS

The cat *(Felis domesticus)* has been used for many studies of vestibular function, sensory neuroanatomy, physiology and biochemistry. The animal's low cost, availability, tractability, ease of care and handling all recommend it as an animal model. Suri and her colleagues[59] recently proposed the cat as an animal model for motion sickness and showed that the cat is susceptible to sinusoidal vertical linear accelerations. Cats were placed in a clear plastic box suspended from the ceiling by 3 springs. The box was propelled by hand to make sinusoid vertical movements with an amplitude of 0.7 meters and a frequency of 40 cycles per minute. After 20 minutes of stimulation, 22 percent of the animals became motion sick. Susceptible animals displayed varying degrees of salivation, panting, drowsiness, unusual postures, defecation and vomiting. These symptoms were formulated into a motion sickness symptom scale similar to that proposed by Graybiel and his colleagues for use in humans (see Table 2). According to the scale, salivation is scored in three levels: level 1, excessive licking and swallowing, level II, when drops form around the mouth area, and level III, when copious amounts of saliva are seen and the animal appears to be foaming. All other symptoms are divided into 5 levels and awarded points according to their severity. The points awarded are given in a geometric progression for each ascending level of sickness. The unique aspect of the rating scale is that symptom score is multiplied a weight factor for animals that responded

TABLE 2
Diagnostic Criteria For Grading The Severity of Acute Motion Sickness in the Cat*

Pathognomonic 16 points	Major 8 points	Minor 4 points	Minimal 2 points	QS* 1 point
Vomiting or Retching	Urination Defecation	Salivation III	Salivation II Panting	Salivation I Drowsiness Unusual Posture

*Reproduced from Suri et al., *Aviat. Space Environ. Med.,* 50, 614–618, 1979. With permission.

with emesis. Time (where time = T) to emesis is put in the formula, $1 + e^{-0.14T}$ and the result multiplied by the symptom score. If the animal did not vomit in the 20-minute session, then the weighing factor computes to 1. Using the symptom scores, the investigators successfully predicted responders and non-responders in a test of parabolic flight. In proposing the cat as an animal model for motion sickness and for the study of antimotion sickness drugs, the investigators recommend a 7- to 10-day inter-trial interval, and that each animal be used as its own control in a repeat measures design. They also recommended that only animals of extreme susceptibility be used. The response to test doses of scopolamine/dexedrine combination were not especially impressive. Additional drugs should be tested to further validate the predictive value of this animal model.

MONKEYS

Monkeys are in the same taxonomic order as man and are said to respond to the same motion sickness stimuli. Some species are more susceptible to motion sickness than others. Squirrel monkeys of the Bolivian, Peruvian and Guyanese phenotype will salivate, retch and vomit when rotated around the horizontal axis at 10 to 30 RPM.[60] The diurnal squirrel monkey (*Saimiri sciureus*) of the Bolivian phenotype is said to be most susceptible of all.[59] Bolivian squirrel monkeys are susceptible to Coriolis stimulation,[61] parabolic flight[62] and vestibular-visual conflict. Continuous rotation around the vertical axis (150 degs/sec) and rotation with intermittent sudden-stops produced vomiting in 0 of 10 rhesus, but vomiting in all of 10 squirrel monkeys tested. The relative resistance of the rhesus monkeys is apparently due to the animal holding its head motionless during rotation.[64] In this way the animal avoids Coriolis stress. Squirrel monkeys also are relatively resistant to rotation-induced motion sickness when they immobilize their head during the test.[65]

Although the monkey has been used for tests of antimotion sickness drugs in the past,[66] the first systematic study of drug responses was performed recently.[67] Cheung and his colleagues placed unrestrained squirrel monkeys of the Bolivian phenotype in a large lucite chamber and exposed them to horizonal angular rotation (25 RPM) and simultaneous sinusoidal vertical excursion (0.5 HZ). The animals were fed a standard meal of 20 grams of banana 20 to 30 minutes before testing. Each test lasted 60 minutes and animals were tested once every 10 days. Susceptible animals showed a progression of behavioral symptoms, beginning with licking the lips and progressing to salivation, chewing and finally vomiting. Several unusual postures were also noted. Some animals leaned their head against corner of the chamber, while others held their head down on the floor with their feet in the air. Other animals braced their lower limbs against the cage walls. From the behavioral signs observed, the investigators developed a rating scale similar to that proposed by Graybiel for use in humans (see Table 3). The scale, which

TABLE 3
Diagnostic Criteria For Acute Motion Sickness in the Squirrel Monkey*

Pathognomonic 16 points	Major 8 points	Minor 4 points	Minimal 2 points	Qualifying Symptoms* 1 point
Vomiting or retching	Frequent vigorous chewing	Salivation Occasional chewing	Reduced activity and alertness (drowsiness) Occasional licking of lips	Reduced activity and inquisitiveness Unusual posture

*Reproduced from Cheung et al., *J. Clin. Pharmacol.*, 32, 163–175, 1992. With permission.

is based on the progression of motion sickness symptoms observed, allows a maximum score of 31 points. Using the symptom scale they tested several antimotion sickness drugs and combinations of antimotion sickness drugs. Drugs tested included: scopolamine, dexamphetamine, a combination of scopolamine and dexedrine, promethazine, ephedrine sulfate, a combination of promethazine and ephedrine. The drugs were administered intravenously through the tail vein. The responses obtained were similar to those reported for man. Scopolamine was effective, as were combinations of promethazine and ephedrine, and scopolamine and dexedrine. Baseline scores for monkeys did not change when tested 5 times at 10-day intervals. It would appear, therefore, that 10 days is an appropriate inter-trial interval for the monkey.

One unique aspect of the work deserving of comment is the selection of dose for scopolamine. Rather than calculating from a human dose, or randomly selecting a test dose, the investigators based the dose tested (100 μg) on the ability of scopolamine to block the blood pressure depressor response to acetylcholine. They chose the 100 μg dose of scopolamine based on its ability to produce an approximately 10-fold dextral shift in the acetycholine dose response curve. This technique of selecting a dose for testing when no effective dose is known is highly appropriate. When possible, more studies should incorporate dose selecting criteria such as the one used in this study.

RATS

PICA

Although rats do not vomit, they exhibit several atypical behaviors when subjected to motion sickness stimuli.[68–70] Perhaps the most studied of these behaviors is pica, or the eating of a non-nutritive substance. Although there is some dispute as to the source of pica in rats exposed to motion, the weight of the evidence suggests that pica is an illness-response behavior related to the feelings of GI distress. Mitchell and his colleagues[71] demonstrated that rats rotated at 198 rpm for 1.5 hours preferentially consumed kaolin, a clay, rather than food. The preparation of kaolin was described in the original work. Briefly, the kaolin was of pharmaceutical grade and was prepared by mixing it with 1 percent acacia in distilled water. The resulting paste was extruded into molds and allowed to dry. The dried kaolin was made available to the animals as small pieces. The same group also demonstrated that the degree of kaolin consumption was directly proportional to the duration of motion stimuli and that kaolin consumption diminished when animals are subjected to the motion stimuli for 15 days, suggesting the presence of adaptation.[72] More recently, McCaffrey[73] performed several experiments that essentially confirmed these findings and suggested that kaolin consumption is an appropriate index of motion sickness and general GI malaise in the rat. Morita and his colleagues[74] also believe that pica is illness response behavior related to motion and they demonstrated that kaolin consumption was greater in animals exposed to double rotation with continually changing accelerative forces, than after rotation in a single plane with no accelerative component. Furthermore, they demonstrated that pica after motion is extinguished by bilateral labyrinthectomy[74] and diminishes after intraperitoneal diphenhydramine, methamphetamine, or transdermal scopolamine.[75] More drug studies are needed to confirm the usefulness of pica as a general screening technique for antimotion sickness drugs.

CONDITIONED TASTE AVERSION

One theory holds that vertebrates developed a defensive mechanism to protect the gastrointestinal tract from toxic substances. The defensive mechanism makes the animal associate the taste of a previously eaten substance with a delayed illness. After an initial experience, the animal avoids that taste or flavor in the future, a so-called conditioned taste aversion (CTA). Rats acquire a CTA when a novel taste is paired with GI distress. For example, when a novel taste, such as a vinegar/cider solution, is paired with immediate exposure to body rotation or other types of vestibular stimulation in rats, that animal will avoid that taste in the future.[76] This CTA after exposure to motion is taken as evidence for the presence of motion sickness. A similar behavior occurs in mice[77] guinea pigs,[78] quail[79] and in animals species capable of emesis, such as cats,[80] squirrel monkeys[81] and man.[82] Some maintain that the CTA response is mediated by the same neural mechanisms and pathways associated with the emetic reflex,[76] but some doubts have been raised. Grant[83] recently critically reviewed the claim that the CTA and emetic response are related and suggested that CTA may be associated with another component of the emetic reflex. Without exact knowledge of which component of the emetic reflex CTA measures, its value as an experimental endpoint is diminished. Wilpizeshi and Lowry[60] studied the development of CTA and motion sickness symptoms in squirrel monkeys exposed to rotation around the horizontal axis at 10 to 30 RPM. They demonstrated a close association between CTA and motion sickness. Bilateral labyrinthectomy for example, abolished both. They suggested that CTA is a subjective aversive state akin to nausea in man. Tests of CTA should be performed using antimotion sickness drugs of known efficacy. Inhibition of CTA by clinically effective antimotion sickness drugs might help establish the rat as an animal model for motion sickness.

Designing protocols to study antimotion sickness drugs using either pica or CTA as the measured response might at first seem simple. However, antimotion sickness drugs often have effects on the central nervous system and the gastrointestinal tract. In most cases, we know little about drug effects on such complex behaviors as feeding. As a result, it might be wise to administer drug and placebo treatments to animals both exposed and not exposed to the test motion. Testing in both motion-exposed and stationary animals would control for confounding drug effects on feeding behavior or taste discrimination.

SUNCUS

Suncus murinus, commonly known as the house musk shrew, was recently proposed as an experimental model for motion sickness by Ueno and his colleagues.[84] The Suncus, which belongs to the family *Soricidae* in the order *Insectivore,* is found widely distributed in tropical and subtropical areas of the world. The animal has recently become commercially available in Japan.[85]

The physical and reproductive characteristics of the Suncus make it an attractive laboratory animal. Adult males weight from 50 to 80 grams, while adult females range from 30 to 50 grams. The animals eat a high protein and high lipid diet and their gestation period is 30 days. Females typically have from 3 to 4 young and their life span appears to be greater than 2 years.[85]

The Suncus also is an attractive animal model because unlike rodents and lagomorphs, it responds with the oral expulsion of GI contents (emesis) after the same emetic stimuli that produce vomiting in man. For example, the Suncus vomits in response to copper sulfate, emetine, lobeline, nicotine, pilocarpine, veratrine, bleomycin, cisplatin, (IV and IP), cyclophosphamide, 5-FU, methotrexate, mitomycin, bromocriptine, and serotonin. Interestingly, the animal does not respond to apomorphine, L-dopa or digitalis. It does respond to bromocriptine however, indicating the presence of dopamine D2 receptors.[85]

The Suncus also responds with retching and vomiting when exposed to intense motion of certain kinds. The animal is most susceptible to movement in the horizontal plane; back and forth, right and left, and rotation around the horizontal axis induces motion sickness and emesis to an equal extent. Vertical motion is far less effective.[86] Mild reciprocal shaking at amplitudes of 10 to 40 mm and frequencies of 1 to 3 Hz produced vomiting in 60 to 100 percent of the animals within 5 minutes, an amazingly high incidence and short latency to vomiting. The lack of visual development of the Suncus may actually be an advantage for motion sickness research since the stimuli would is more purely vestibular. Scopolamine (100 mg/kg), chlorpromazine(8 mg/kg), promethazine (50 mg/kg), diphenhydramine (20 mg/kg), chlorphenylamine (20 mg/kg) and methamphetamine (2mg/kg) given subcutaneously decrease the incidence of motion sickness in Suncus. Pyrilamine(20 mg/kg), meclizine (20 mg/kg) and dimenhydrinate (32 mg/kg) are much less effective. A typical index of protection may be used to quantify drug responses [(% of vomiting in control—% vomiting in treated)/(% vomiting in control) $\times$ 100] in the Suncus.[84]

Adaptation is an important experimental consideration with the Suncus. When the Suncus is repeatedly exposed to a motion stimulus every 2 to 3 days, there is a decreased percentage of animals responding with emesis, a reduced number of vomiting episodes in those responding, and an extended latency to emesis.[84] Even ineffective motions may produce adaptation. Animals exposed to a motion which does not produce motion sickness in itself, will after 14 consecutive days, reduce the susceptibility of the animals to a previously effective motion.[86] The adaptation developed may be long lasting. The number of animals responding to a provocative motion was reduced for as long as 40 days after adaptation.[84] There are no studies which more carefully characterize the temporal development of adaptation in the Suncus.

SUMMARY AND CONCLUSIONS

Testing methods for antimotion sickness drugs are available for both man and animals. Human tests generally involve exposing individuals to a provocative motion under drug and placebo conditions. The motion used must be accelerative to produce a stimulation of the vestibular receptors required to induce motion sickness. Perhaps the most practical motion device for most investigators contemplating antimotion sickness drug testing is a rotating chair. When subjects make head movements out of the plane of rotation while seated in a rotating chair an accelerative force is applied to their vestibular receptors which is proportional to the rotational velocity of the chair. A common test protocol using a rotating chair is the Staircase Velocity Motion Test. In the SVMT subjects make standardized and time head movements while seated in a rotating chair. Initially, subjects perform head movements at a low rotational velocity (e.g. 1 RPM). The rotational velocity of the chair is increased after every so many head movements. Nearly every subject is susceptible to the SVMT and most respond with an advanced level of motion sickness before the maximal rotational rate of 35 RPM and 720 head movements.

The experimental endpoint is a major consideration in drug testing protocols. Although advocated by some, vomiting is not an acceptable experiment endpoint in human tests. Instead, some reproducible level of motion sickness short of vomiting should be employed. The level of motion sickness present can best be assessed using a combination of subjective symptoms experienced by the subject and objective observations scored by trained laboratory personnel. The motion sickness symptom scale devised by Graybiel and his colleagues uses both subjective and objective symptoms to produce an overall motion sickness score. Motion sickness scores of from 12 to 16 points are an advanced level of motion sickness and are reproducible from test to test within the same individual.

One common test protocol for testing antimotion sickness drugs uses the SVMT and the Graybiel's motion sickness rating scale. After drug or placebo administration the SVMT is conducted and the test is continued until the subject reaches a certain symptom score on the rating scale. The number of head movements required to reach the predefined symptom level scores the degree of motion sickness susceptibility for that test. Individuals trained to recognize the endpoint in one or more training sessions reach similar symptom levels by making a similar number of head movements when tested on more than one occasion. Training tests also allow laboratory personnel to assess the sometimes unique order, intensity and duration of motion sickness symptoms in an experimental subject. Ideally the subjects selected for participation in tests of antimotion sickness drugs should be healthy, articulate and motivated. In general, a parallel subject or cross-over design has several advantages over other study designs and is appropriate for antimotion sickness drug testing. One potentially important variable is adaptation, or the development of decreased susceptibility after repeated testing. Adaptation can be minimized by spacing trials at 7- to 10-day intervals. Dietary status has an unknown effect on motion sickness susceptibility. As a consequence, subjects should be tested in the fasted state. Drug dose and pharmacodynamics are also important considerations.

Antimotion sickness drug testing in animals has been hampered in the past by lack of a practical animal species. Some of the more common laboratory animals either do not respond to motion or do not respond to drugs like man. The cat and monkey are acceptable animal models for testing antimotion sickness drugs. A symptom rating scale, similar to one proposed for man, has been developed for each animal. Both animals exhibit a wide range of susceptibility to motion. In the case of the cat, the differences are likely inherent differences in motion sickness susceptibility between animals. Phenotypic differences in motion sickness susceptibility in monkeys likely reflect the animals response to a motion environment. The rhesus monkey immobilizes its head in a motion environment which effectively reduces the motion sickness stimulus. The Bolivian Squirrel monkey appears most susceptible to motion sickness and responds to antimotion sickness drugs like man.

In addition to cats and monkey, rats are candidates for antimotion sickness drug testing. Although previously disqualified because they do not vomit, rats exhibit unusual behaviors after intense motion. Pica, or the eating of a non-nutritive substance, and conditioned taste aversion, are two behaviors that appear to be specifically associated with motion in the rat. Furthermore, the degree to which both are manifested appears to be directly proportional to the degree of sickness or GI malaise present. Therefore, both of these behaviors may be useful for quantification of motion sickness.

The house musk shrew *(Suncus murinus)* is the most exciting new animal model for antiemetic and antimotion sickness drug research. In addition to its practical size, ease of handling and desirable breeding characteristics, the animal responds to motion with sickness that culminates in the oral expulsion of GI contents. Vomiting is used as an experimental endpoint in tests with the Suncus. Furthermore, the animal appears to respond to a wide range of antimotion sickness drugs in approximately the same order as man.

REFERENCES

1. **Brand, J. J., Perry, W. L. M.,** Drugs used in motion sickness: A critical review of the methods available for the study of drugs of potential value in its treatment and of the information which has been derived by these methods, *Pharmacol. Revs.* 18, 895–924, 1966.

2. **Tyler, D. B., Bard, P.,** Motion sickness, *Physiol. Rev.* 29, 311–370, 1949.

3. **Chinn, H. I., Smith, P. K.,** Motion sickness, *Pharmacol. Rev.,* 7, 33–83, 1953.

4. **Money, K. E.,** Motion sickness, *Physiol. Revs.* 50, 1–39, 1970.

5. **Irwin, J. A.,** The pathology of seasickness, *Lancet,* 907–909, 1881.

6. **Marti-Ibanez, F.,** Philosophical perspectives of motion sickness, *Intern. Record Med.,* 167, 621–626, 1954.

7. **James, W.,** The sense of diziness in deaf mutes, *Am. J. Otol.,* 4, 239–250, 1882

8. **Reason, J. T., Brand, J. J.,** *Motion Sickness,* Academic Press, New York, 1975.

9. **Oman, C. M.,** Motion sickness: A synthesis and evaluation of the sensory conflict theory. *Can. J. Physiol. Pharmacol.,* 68, 294–303, 1990.

10. **Reason, J. T.,** Motion sickness adaptation: A neural mismatch model., *J. R. Soc. Med.,* 71, 819–829, 1978.

11. **von Holst, E.,** Relations between the central nervous system and the peripheral organs, *Br. J. Anim. Behav.,* 2, 89–94, 1954.

12. **Held, R.,** Exposure history as a factor in maintaining stability of perception and coordination, *J. Nerv. Ment. Dis.,* 132, 26–32, 1961.

13. **Ruckenstein, M. J., Harrison, R. V.,** Motion sickness: Helping patients tolerate the ups and downs, *Postgrad. Med.,* 89, 139–144, 1991.

14. **Gay, L. N., Carliner, P. E.,** The prevention and treatment of motion sickness, I. Seasickness, *Science,* 109, 359, 1949.

15. **Homick, J. L., Reschke, M. F., Vanderploeg, J. M.,** Space adaptation syndrome, Incidence and operational implication for the space transportation system program. Advisory group for Aerospace Research & Development, NATO sponsored conference on Motion sickness: Mechanisms, prediction, prevention and treatment.

16. **Bagian, J.,** First intramuscular administration in the U. S. Space Program., *J. Clin. Pharmacol.,* 31, 920, 1991.

17. **Graybiel, A., Johnson, W. H.,** A comparison of the symptomatology experienced by healthy persons and subjects with loss of labyrinthine function when exposed to unusual patterns of centripetal force in a counter-rotating room, *Ann. Otol. Rhin. Laryngol.,* 72, 357–373, 1963.

18. **Guyton, Arthur C.,** *Textbook of Medical Physiology,* 8th ed., Saunders, Philadelphia, 1990, pp. 610–615.

19. **Berne, R. M., Levy, M. N.,** The vestibular system, in *Physiology,* C. V. Mosby, St. Louis, Mo. 1988, pp. 179–187.

20. **Wang, S. C., Chinn, H. I.,** Experimental motion sickness in dogs. Importance of labyrinth and vestibular cerebellum, *Amer. J. Physiol.,* 185, 617–623, 1956.

21. **Brizzee, K. R., Ordy, J. M., Mehler, W. R.,** Effect of ablation of area postrema in frequency and latency of motion sickness-induced emesis in squirrel monkey. *Physiol. Behav.,* 24, 849–853, 1980.

22. **Borison, H. L.,** A misconception of motion sickness leads to false therapeutic expectations, *Aviat. Space Environ. Med.,* 56, 66–68, 1985.

23. **Schwab, R. S.,** The nonlabyrinthine causes of motion sickness. *Intern. Record Med.,* 167, 631–637, 1954.

24. **Stewart, J. J., Wood, M. J., Wood, C. D.,** Electrogastrograms after rotation-induced motion sickness in fasted and fed subjects, *Aviat. Space Environ. Med.,* 60, 214–217, 1989.

25. **McClure, J. A., Fregly, A. R., Molina, E., Graybiel, A.,** Response from arousal and thermal sweat areas during motion sickness, Naval Aerospace Medical Research Laboratory Report, NAMRL-1142, Pensacola, Fla.

26. **Gordon, C. R., Ben-Aryeh, H., Szargel, R., Attias, J., Rolnick, A. Laufer, D.,** Salivary changes associated with experimental motion sickness condition in man. *J. Auton. Nerv. Syst.,* 22, 91–96, 1988.

27. **Graybiel, A., Knepton, J.,** Sopite sydrome: A sometimes sole manifestation of motion sickness, *Aviat. Space and Environ. Med.,* 47, 873–882, 1976.

28. **Reason, J. T., Graybiel, A.,** Changes in subjective estimates of well-being during the onset and remission of motion sickness symptomatology in the slow rotation room. *Aerospace Med.,* 41, 166–171, 1970.

29. **Barber, H. O., Basser, W., Johnson, W. H., Takahashi, P.,** The laboratory assessment of anti-motion sickness and anti-vertigo drugs, *Can. Med. Assoc. J.,* 97, 1460–1465, 1967.

30. **Sunahara, F. A., Farewell, J., Mintoz, L., Johnson, W. H.,** Pharmacological interventions for motion sickness: cardiovascular effects, *Aviat. Space Environ. Med.,* 58, A270–276, 1987.

31. **Cowings, P. S., Naifeh, K. H., Toscano, W. B.,** The stability of individual patterns of autonomic responses to motion sickness stimulation, *Aviat. Space Environ Med. 61,* 399–405, 1990.

32. **Daimond, S. G., Markham, C. H., Money, K. E.,** Instability of ocular torsion in zero gravity: Possible implications for space motion sickness, *Aviat. Space Environ Med.,* 61, 899–905, 1990.

33. **Warwick-Evans, L. A., Church, R. E., Hancock, C., Jochim, E., Morris, P. H., Ward, F.,** Electrodermal activity as an index of motion sickness, *Aviat Space Environ. Med.,* 58, 417–423, 1987.

34. **Dichgans, J., Brandt, Th.,** Optokinetic motion sickness and pseudo-coriolis effects induced by moving visual stimuli, *Acta Otolaryng.,* 76, 339–348, 1973.

35. **Wood, C. D., Graybiel, A., McDonough, R. C.,** Human centrifuge studies on the relative effectiveness of some antimotion sickness drugs, *Aerospace Med.,* 37, 187, 1966.

36. **Graybiel, A., Wood., C. D., Miller, E. F., Cramer, D. B.,** Diagnostic criteria for grading the severity of acute motion sickness, *Aerospace Med.,* 39, 453–455, 1968.

37. **Holling, H. E., McArdle, B., Trotter, W. R.,** Prevention of seasickness by drugs, *Lancet,* 1, 127–129, 1944.

38. **Lathers, C. M., Charles, J. B., Bungo, M. W.,** Pharmacology in space. Part 1. Influence of adaptive changes on pharmacokinetics, *Trends Pharmacol. Sci.,* 10(5), 193–200, 1989.

39. **Stern, R. M., Hu, S., Anderson, R. B., Leibowitz, H. W., Koch, K. L.,** The effects of fixation and restricted visual field on vection-induced motion sickness, *Aviat. Space Environ. Med.,* 61, 712–715, 1990.

40. **Hu, S. Stern, R. M., Vasey, M. W., Koch, K. L.,** Motion sickness and gastric myoelectric activity as a function of speed of rotation of a circular vection drum, *Aviat. Space Environ. Med.,* 60(5), 411–414, 1989.

41. **Graybiel, A., Wood, C. D., Knepton, J., Hocke, J. P., Perkins, G. F.,** Human assay of antimotion sickness drugs. *Aviat. Space Environ. Med.,* 46, 1107–1118, 1975.

42. **Graybiel, A., Lackner, J. R.,** A sudden-stop vestibulovisual test for rapid assessment of motion sickness manifestations, *Aviat. Space Environ. Med.,* 51, 21–23, 1980.

43. **Guedry, F. E., Jr., Graybiel, A.,** Compensatory nystagmus conditioned during adaptation to living in a rotating room, *J. Appl. Physiol.,* 17, 398–404, 1962

44. **Wood, C. D., Manno, J. E., Manno, B. R., Odenheimer, R. C., Bairnsfather, L. E.,** The effect of antimotion sickness drugs on habituation to motion, *Aviat. Space Environ. Med.,* 57, 539–542, 1986.

45. **Hu, S. Q., Stern, R. M., Koch, K. L.,** Effects of pre-exposures to a rotating optokinetic drum on adaptation to motion sickness. *Aviat. Space Environ. Med.* 62, 53–56, 1991.

46. **Hu, S., Grant, W. F., Stern, R. M., Koch, K. L.,** Motion sickness severity and physiological correlates during repeated exposures to a rotating optokinetic drum. *Aviat. Space Environ. Med.,* 62, 308–314, 1991.

47. **Stern R. M., Hu, S. Q., Vasey, M. W., Koch, K. L.,** Adaptation to vection-induced symptoms of motion sickness. *Aviat. Space Environ. Med.,* 60, 566–572, 1989.

48. **Guedry, F. E., Graybiel, A., Collins, W. E.,** Reduction of nystagmus and disorientation in human subjects. *Aerospace Med.,* 33, 1356–1360, 1962

49. **Stewart, J. J., Wood, M. J., Wood, C. D.,** Electrogastrograms after rotation-induced motion sickness in fasted and fed subjects, *Aviat. Space Environ. Med.,* 60, 214–217, 1989.

50. **Uijtdehaage, S. H., Stern, R. M., Koch, K. L.,** Effects of eating on vection-induced motion sickness, cardiac vagal tone, and gastric myoelectric activity. *Psychophysiol.,* 29(2), 193–201, 1992.

51. **Wood, C. D., Stewart, J. J., Wood, M. J., Mims, M. E.,** Effectiveness and duration of intramuscular antimotion sickness medications, *J. Clin. Pharmacol.* 32, 1008–1012, 1992.

52. **Hatcher, R. A.,** The mechanism of vomiting. *Physiol. Rev.,* 4, 479–504, 1924.

53. **Money, K. E., Friedberg, J.,** The role of the semi-circular canals in causation of motion sickness and nystagmus in the dog, *Can. J. Physiol. Pharmacol.,* 42, 793–801, 1964.

54. **Igarashi, M., McLeod, M. E., Graybiel, A.,** Clinical pathological correlations in squirrel monkey after suppression of semicircular canal function by streptomycin sulfate, NSAM-940, US Naval Sch. Aviat. Med., 1–33, 1965.

55. **Noble, R. L.,** Methods of assaying motion sickness preventives on dogs, *Can. J. Res.,* 23E, 226–234, 1945.

56. **Noble, R. L.,** Observations on various types of motion causing vomiting in animals. *Can. J. Res.,* 23E, 212–225, 1945.

57. **Noble, R. L.,** Adaptation to experimental motion sickness in dogs, *Am. J. Physiol.,* 154, 433–450, 1948.

58. **Chinn, H. I., Plotnikoff, N. P.,** Evaluation of various techniques for screening antimotion sickness drugs, *J. Appl. Physiol.,* 5, 392–394, 1953.

59. **Suri, K. B., Crampton, G. H., Daunton, N. G.,** Motion sickness in cats: A symptom rating scale used in laboratory and flight tests, *Aviat. Space Environ. Med.,* 50, 614–618, 1979.

60. **Wilpizeski, C. R., Lowry, L. D.,** A two-factor model of rotation-induced motion sickness syndrome in squirrel monkeys. *Am. J. Otolaryngol.,* 8, 7–12, 1987.

61. **Ordy, J. M., Brizzee, K. R.,** Motion sickness in the squirrel monkey, *Aviat. Space Environ. Med.,* 51, 215–223, 1980.

62. **Meek, J. C., Graybiel, A., Beischer, D. E., Riopelle, A. J.,** Observations of canal sickness and adaptation in chimpanzees and squirrel monkeys in a "slow rotation room," *Aerospace Med.,* 33, 571–578, 1962.

63. **Daunton, N. G.,** Animal model for motion sickness research. Symposium Proceedings, Space Motion Sickness, Lyndon B. Johnson Space Center, Nov. 15–17, 64–65, 1978.

64. **Corcoran, M. L., Fox, R. A., Daunton, N. G.,** The susceptibility of rhesus monkeys to motion sickness, *Aviat. Space Environ. Med.,* 61, 807–809, 1990.

65. **Fox, R. A., Daunton, N. G., Coleman, J.,** Susceptibility of the squirrel monkey to several different motion conditions, *Neurosci. Abst.,* 8, 698, 1982.

66. **Johnson, W. H., Ireland, P. E.,** Suppression of motion sickness by thiethylperazine (Torecan), *Aerospace Med.,* 37, 181–183, 1966.

67. **Cheung, B. S. K., Money, K. E., Kohl, R. L., Kinter, L. B.,** Investigation of anti-motion sickness drugs in the squirrel monkey, *J. Clin. Pharmacol.,* 32, 163–175, 1992.

68. **Griffith, C. R.,** The effect upon the white rat of continued bodily rotation. *Am. Natural.,* 54, 524–534, 1920.

69. **Riccio, D. C., Thach, J. S.,** Response suppression produced by vestibular stimulation in the rat, *J. Exp. Analysis Behav.,* 11, 479–488, 1968.

70. **Eskin, A., Riccio, D. C.,** The effects of vestibular stimulation on spontaneous activity in the rat, *Psychol. Rec.,* 16, 523–527, 1966.

71. **Mitchell, D., Laycock, J. D., Stephens, W. F.,** Motion sickness-induced pica in the rat, *Am. J. Clin. Nutr.,* 30, 147–150, 1977.

72. **Mitchell, D., Krusemark, M. L., Hafner, E.** Pica: a species relevant behavioral assay of motion sickness in the rat, *Physiol. Behav.,* 18, 125–130, 1977.

73. **McCaffrey, R. J.,** Appropriateness of kaolin consumption as an index of motion sickness in the rat, *Physiol. Behav.,* 35,151–156, 1985.

74. **Morita, M., Takeda, N., Kibo, T., Matsunaga, T.,** Pica as an index of motion sickness in rats, *J. Otorohinolaryngol. Relat. Spec.,* 50, 188–192, 1988.

75. **Morita, M., Takeda, N., Kubo, T., Yamatodani, A., Wada, H., Matsunaga, T.,** Effects of anti-motion sickness drugs on motion sickness in rats. *J. Otorhinolaryngol. Relat. Spec.,* 50, 330–333, 1988.

76. **Garcia, J., Lasiter, P. S., Bermudez-Rattoni, F., Deems, D. A.,** A general theory of aversion learning, *Ann. NY Acad. Sci.,* 443, 8–21, 1985.

77. **Fox, R. A., Lauber, A. H., Daunton, N. G., Phillips, M., Diaz, L.,** Off-vertical rotation produces conditioned taste aversion and suppressed drinking in mice, *Aviat. Space Environ. Med.,* 55, 632–635, 1984

78. **Ossenkopp, K.-P., Ossenkopp, M. D.,** Motion sickness in guinea pigs (Cavia porcellus) indexed by body rotation-induced conditioned taste aversions, *Physiol. Behav.,* 47, 467–470, 1990.

79. **Ossenkopp, K.-P., Tu, G. S.,** Motion sickness in quail: Body-rotation-induced conditioned fluid avesions in *C. coturnix japonica, J. Comp. Psychol.,* 98, 189–193, 1984

80. **Corcoran, M., Fox, R., Brizzee, K., Crampton, G., Daunton, N.,** Area postrema ablations in cats: Evidence for separate neural routes for motion- and xylazine-induced CTA and emesis, *Physiologist,* 28, 330, 1985

81. **Roy, A., Brizzee, K. R.,** Motion sickness-induced food aversions in the squirrel monkey, *Physiol. Behav.,* 23, 39–41,1979.
82. **Mellor, C. S., White, H. P.,** Taste aversions to alcoholic beverages conditioned by motion sickness, *Am. J. Psychiat.,* 135, 125–126, 1978.
83. **Grant, V. L.,** Do conditioned taste aversions result from activation of emetic mechanism? *Psychopharmacol.,* 93, 405–415, 1987.
84. **Ueno, S., Matsuki, N. and Saito, H.,** Suncus murinus as a new experimental model for motion sickness, *Life Sci.,* 43, 413–420, 1988
85. **Matsuki, N., Torii, Y., Ueno, S., Saito, H.,** Suncus murinus as an experimental animal model for emesis and motion sickness, in *Mechanisms and Control of Emesis,* A. L. Bianchi, L. Grelot, A. D. Miller, G. I. King, Eds., Colloque, INSERM/John Libbey Eurotext Ltd, 1992, 223, 323–329.
86. **Kaji, T., Saito, H., Ueno, S., Matsuki, N.,** Comparison of various motion stimuli on motion sickness and acquisition in Suncus Murinus, *Jikken Dobutsu,* 39, 75–79, 1990.

15 Evaluation of Visceral Pain

Gerald F. Gebhart and Jyotirindra N. Sengupta

INTRODUCTION

Current understanding of pain mechanisms has been derived primarily through the use of models of cutaneous pain. In general, such models have been well-characterized in animals and have proven to be of value in the evaluation of new drugs for pain control. For example, the effects of opioids in the standard tail flick flexor withdrawal reflex, evoked by noxious thermal stimulation of the skin of the tail of a rat, reliably reproduces the rank order of analgesic potency of opioids in man.[1,2]

It has been appreciated for some time, however, that pain arising from the viscera significantly differs in many important ways from pain that arises from cutaneous structures (see[3,4,5] for reviews). Knowledge about deep pain mechanisms is not nearly as extensive as is our knowledge of cutaneous pain mechanisms. Deep pain, particularly that arising from the viscera, differs significantly from cutaneous pain. Cutaneous pain is well localized and typically produces rapid, reflex motor responses to appropriate stimuli. In contrast, visceral pain is poorly localized and diffuse in character. Visceral pain is typically referred to superficial structures and often produces cutaneous hyperalgesia.[6] In addition, visceral pain is often associated with exaggerated motor and autonomic reflexes.

Because cutaneous structures are easily accessible and adequate, noxious stimuli are well documented, the development and study of cutaneous pain models progressed rapidly. One reason for the relative lack of knowledge about visceral pain mechanisms is that reliable models of visceral pain have been more difficult to develop. Notwithstanding that pain is the predominant sensation arising from the viscera, models of visceral pain have not been widely developed because adequate, noxious visceral stimuli are not well understood. Before describing the models we have developed for the study of visceral pain mechanisms, it is instructive to consider briefly (1) criteria important in the development of models of pain in non-human animals and (2) stimuli that are "adequate" for the viscera.

CRITERIA FOR DEVELOPMENT OF MODELS OF PAIN

Among criteria that are important to consider in developing models of pain in non-human animals, the following are perhaps most important:

- the stimulus should reproduce as much as possible a natural stimulus for the tissue or organ;
- application of the stimulus should be as non-invasive as possible;
- the stimulus should be reproducible and subject to control (onset, intensity and duration) by the experimenter;

- the responses produced should be quantifiable; and
- the model should be able to be used in unanesthetized animals.

These criteria apply equally well to models of cutaneous or deep pain, although the nature of the stimulus becomes more problematic when dealing with tissues other than the skin. The most important requirement in the development of new models of pain in non-human animals is to establish that the stimulus produces a behavior(s) in the animal consistent with it being noxious, hence the criterion that the stimulus should be able to be used in unanesthetized animals. Associated with this essential requirement are a number of ethical considerations:

- the intensity of the stimulus should be the minimum required to evoke the measured behavior;
- the duration of the stimulus should be limited to that necessary to evoke the measured behavior;
- the interval between stimuli should be long enough to prevent tissue damage;
- the animal, by its behavior, should be able to terminate or escape the stimulus; and
- the duration of the experiment should be as short as possible.

In the models of visceral pain described below, we have used balloon distension of the gastrointestinal tract because distension of hollow organs reproduces a natural visceral stimulus. Balloons can often be inserted into a viscus via a natural body orifice and models using balloon distension need not be particularly invasive. Balloon distension of the gastrointestinal tract is a mechanical stimulus that can be reproducibly and reliably administered and which produces responses (e.g., autonomic responses or motor responses) that can be readily quantified.

ADEQUATE STIMULI FOR THE VISCERA

A noxious stimulus is commonly defined as one which produces tissue damage or threatens to damage tissue. This definition was developed by Sherrington[7] and has served well in the study of pain arising from cutaneous structures; as discussed below, this definition of "noxious" is not applicable to the viscera. The specialized neurons in the skin that respond to mechanical or thermal stimuli that are tissue damaging or threatening are called nociceptors. These specialized sensory receptors respond to a specific quality of the stimulus, called the *adequate stimulus* for the receptor. Unfortunately, sensory receptors in the viscera are not as well understood as are sensory receptors in the skin. For example, it is not certain that nociceptors exist in the viscera.[8] Consequently, adequate, noxious stimuli for the viscera are not generally known, but it is clear that stimuli which do produce visceral pain in humans are not the same as those which are noxious when applied to the skin. For example, when tissue-damaging stimuli are applied to hollow viscera, neither sensation (i.e., pain) nor autonomic or motor responses are produced. Indeed, it was argued at the turn of the 20th century that the viscera were *in*sensate because stimuli which clearly produced pain when applied to the skin (e.g., cutting, crushing or burning) were ineffective when applied to the viscera.[9] Accordingly, the relationship between frank tissue damage (a noxious *cutaneous* stimulus) and the production of pain does not apply when the viscera are involved. We now know that some solid viscera, like the liver or the kidneys, are insensitive to all stimuli and no sensation is associated with their manipulation unless and until the capsule which contains them becomes distended or inflamed. Although the term "noxious" is not, strictly speaking, applicable to the viscera, it will be used here for convenience to refer to visceral stimuli that have been associated with the sensation of pain in humans—understanding that tissue damage is not necessarily a component of the adequacy of a visceral stimulus.

Given the foregoing, what constitutes an adequate, noxious stimulus for the gastrointestinal tract? Hurst[10] was the first to suggest, based on studies in humans, that tension on gastrointestinal muscles was an adequate visceral stimulus associated with the sensation of pain. He determined that distension of the stomach resulted in sensations that ranged from fullness to pain depending upon the rate and magnitude of distension. He concluded that abnormal tension on the muscle was probably the adequate stimulus for the production of pain in the stomach and, as has been documented since, all along the gastrointestinal tract. The results of numerous studies in humans have subsequently established that balloon distension of the esophagus, stomach, jejunum, gall bladder, or colon can produce pain.[11–16, see 5 for review]

Balloon distension of hollow organs can be applied as either a constant volume stimulus or as a constant pressure stimulus. Which is most appropriate? Lipkin and Sliesenger,[12] using controlled, constant pressure distension of the esophagus, established that the relation between pressure and sensation was reliable and documented that constant pressure stimulation is 1) reproducible and 2) produces the same sensations when tested in the same individuals over time. Accordingly, the appropriate distending stimulus for hollow viscera is one which is applied and maintained at a constant pressure.

In addition to distending stimuli, other adequate stimuli for many of the hollow viscera include irritation or inflammation of the tissue or organ and spasm or strong contraction of muscles, typically accompanied by ischemia. In an experimental context, ischemia or irritation/inflammation are more difficult to control in terms of onset, intensity, duration and reproducibility. Further, in unanesthetized animals, such stimuli may raise ethical concerns. For example, a commonly used "visceral" pain model in rodents is intraperitoneal administration of irritant chemicals or hypertonic saline. There is little doubt that this stimulus produces a behavior (writhing) suggestive that the stimulus is noxious. However, the intensity of the stimulus is unknown and its site(s) of action is similarly unknown. More importantly, because the animal can neither terminate nor escape from the stimulus, ethical concerns are associated with the use of irritant chemicals given intraperitoneally to unanesthetized animals. From a scientific point of view, the stimulus lacks reproducibility and reliability, is questionably related to human pathology and, further, non-analgesic drugs are also effective in attenuating the writhing behavior[17] (i.e., the model falsely identifies non-analgesic drugs as efficacious).

In consideration of the above, the models we have developed to investigate visceral pain include balloon distension of the descending colon/rectum, stomach and esophagus, all in the rat.

METHODS

COLORECTAL DISTENSION (CRD)

Colorectal distension was the first model we undertook to develop. As a stimulus, balloon distension of the colon of the rat nicely satisfies the criteria previously suggested as important for development of a model of visceral pain in non-human animals:

- CRD reproduces a natural visceral stimulus;
- CRD is non-invasive (a balloon is inserted via the anus);
- the onset, magnitude and duration of CRD can be easily controlled;
- CRD produces easily quantifiable pseudaffective reflexes (e.g., changes in mean arterial pressure, changes in heart rate and a visceromotor response recorded from the peritoneal musculature); and
- CRD can be used in unanesthetized, behaving animals to assess its nociceptive character.

BEHAVIORAL ASSESSMENT OF CRD

We first established that CRD affected behavior in a manner consistent with it being aversive or noxious to the rat. Because CRD in the unanesthetized, unrestrained rat typically produces a cessation of movement, it was difficult to use an operant behavioral paradigm. We adapted instead a passive avoidance behavioral paradigm modified after Jarvic and Essman.[18] Rats, when placed on a platform about 10 cm above the floor of an open field, normally step down from the platform to explore the environment. The latency to step down can be easily measured and was defined as the time from placing the rat on the raised platform until it placed both forepaws on the floor. After insertion of the balloon into the colon, rats were placed on the raised platform and, when they stepped down to explore the environment, the colon was distended for 20 seconds. Typically, 10–15 trials are given at an intertrial interval of 5–10 minutes. A more detailed description of this procedure is given elsewhere.[19,20] Figure 1 illustrates the intensity-dependent effects of CRD on acquisition of this passive avoidance behavior. At distending pressures of 40 or 80 mmHg (when rats stepped off the platform), rats learned after several trials to passively avoid CRD by remaining on the platform. The behavior of rats when distending pressures of 20 or 30 mmHg were given when stepping down from the platform was not different from rats which received no CRD in association with their behavior. Accordingly, we interpreted these results to suggest that CRD at pressures greater than 30 mmHg (20 sec) could be considered noxious in the rat.

Balloons

The colonic balloons we have used are 7–8 cm long and made of latex. Previously, we used children's party balloons. Currently, we use condoms or cut the fingers from latex surgical gloves (large size) and fabricate balloons by inserting a length of tygon flexible plastic tubing (3/16 inch outer diameter, 1/8 inch inner diameter) into the condom or finger from the surgical glove and tying the open end tightly around the tygon tubing with silk suture. The length of tygon flexible plastic tubing that is inserted into the condom or finger from the surgical glove is approximately 6 cm; this portion of the tubing is repeatedly perforated (about 20 holes) with a hole punch tool (hole punch #35, available from Cook Inc., P. O. Box 489, Bloomington, IN 47402). Examples of perforated tygon flexible plastic tubing before and after insertion into a

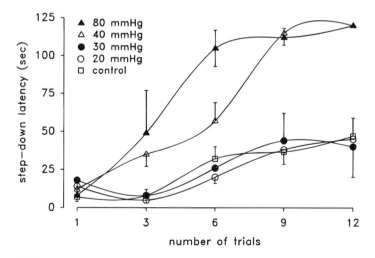

FIGURE 1 Acquisition of a passive avoidance behavior produced by colorectal distension (CRD). Rats were placed on a raised platform and the latency to step-down from the platform was measured (in sec, vertical axis). Different groups of rats ($n = 10$/group) received different intensities of CRD (20, 30, 40 or 80 mmHg, 20 sec) when both forepaws were placed on the floor. The behavior of rats receiving 20 or 30 mmHg CRD did not differ from rats which received no CRD (control). The behavior of rats receiving 40 or 80 mmHg CRD significantly differs from all other groups.

latex condom and fabrication into a balloon are shown in Figure 2. Because the latex from which the balloons are fabricated offers inherent resistance to inflation, it is necessary before use to inflate the balloons and maintain them fully inflated for a period of at least several hours; we typically leave them inflated overnight. This is necessary to insure that the balloon does not leak and has a diameter greater than the distended colon and thus itself offers no resistance to inflation when the colon is distended. In this regard, the latex condoms from which colonic balloons are made have a greater non-distended diameter than do the fingers cut from latex surgical gloves. The surgical gloves, on the other hand, are less expensive; we have noted no differences in any response measures related to the starting material from which the balloons are made. Depending on the means of distension (see below), this also insures that the intraluminal pressure which is monitored is an accurate representation of the distending pressure. An example of a pre-distended balloon ready for experimental use is also illustrated in Figure 2.

For insertion into the colon via the anus, the surface of the balloon is lubricated either with a water soluble surgical lubricant or with saline and can be inserted in unanesthetized animals. In initial work, we briefly sedated rats by exposure to either ether or halothane for insertion of the balloon into the colon. We have learned that it is unnecessary to sedate rats for insertion of the balloons and no longer do so. We also find it useful to fast the rats the night before an experiment to reduce the amount of feces in the colon. After insertion into the colon, the balloon assembly is kept in position by taping the tygon flexible plastic tubing to the base of the rat's tail; the balloon is inserted such that the end of the balloon is about 1 cm from the anus (the tygon tubing is pre-marked; see Figure 2). Figure 3 shown an intracolonic balloon *in situ* distended to approximately 100 mmHg.

BALLOON INFLATION

Inflation of the balloon with air can be achieved by a variety of methods. The simplest way to inflate the colonic balloon is to connect the end of the tygon tubing to larger diameter tubing that is connected to a syringe (e.g., 25 ml syringe) with a side arm manometer. This method is straightforward and easy, but lacks precision and reproducibility.

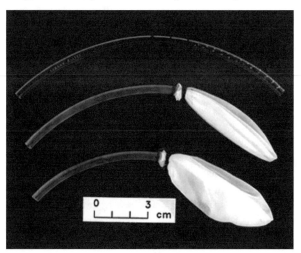

FIGURE 2   Examples, from top to bottom, of the perforated tygon flexible plastic tubing, the distending balloon constructed from a latex condom before and (bottom) after it has been inflated to overcome its inherent resistance to distension. The flaccid balloon shown at the bottom is then lubricated and inserted *via* the anus into the colon; the tygon flexible plastic tubing is taped to the base of the rat's tail to retain the balloon in the colon.

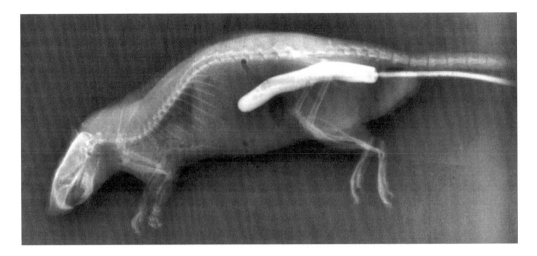

FIGURE 3   Radiograph of an intracolonic balloon distended with a radiopaque medium to approximately 100 mmHg in an anesthetized rat.

For our experimental work, we designed and constructed a distension control device.[21] The distension control device is a stand-alone unit with solenoid valves and timing circuits associated with a large air reservoir maintained at a constant pressure by a tank of compressed air. We chose to use air as the distending medium because it is compressible and has a low resistance to flow (low viscosity). These characteristics are responsible for the stability of the constant pressure in the air reservoir in the presence of reflex contractions of the colon. Fluids have also been used as distending media, but fluids have low compressibility and greater viscosities than air and thus reflex contractions of hollow organs filled with fluid can cause relatively large, undesirable transient increases in intraluminal pressure. With this pressure control device, the time to establish a constant pressure within the distending balloon in the colon is a function of the volume of air that must be moved and the diameter of the tubing connecting the distension control device to the balloon in the colon. Generally, the connecting tubing should be as short in length as is practical and its inner diameter should not be less than 3/16 inch (which snugly fits around the end of the tygon flexible plastic tubing that is used in fabrication of the distending balloon). Due to air's low resistance to flow, a near instantaneous on/off constant pressure stimulus can be provided by opening of the solenoid valve connecting the distending balloon with the large volume constant pressure reservoir. The reservoir provides air to the balloon and pressure is relatively unaffected because the volume of air that flows into the distending balloon can be made insignificant relative to the volume of the air reservoir. According to Boyle's Law (pressure $\times$ volume = a constant), the pressure in the air reservoir will vary less than 1% if the volume of the distending balloon is less than 1/100th of the volume of the reservoir. Additional details about this distension control device, including electronic schematics, have been published.[21]

More recently, we have simplified the means by which the colon is distended. The constant pressure air reservoir that we now use is a tank of compressed nitrogen fitted with a two–stage pressure regulator (0–3 psi output for nitrogen, Matheson Gas Products, PO Box 23029, Newark, NJ 07189; model 8-2-580; 0.1 psi $\approx$ 5 mmHg) which is used to set the distending pressure. Inflation of the balloon is effected by opening a solenoid valve placed between the cylinder of compressed nitrogen (which acts as a large constant pressure reservoir) and the intracolonic balloon. The intensity of CRD is set with the regulator and the onset and duration of CRD is controlled by a computer. The distending stimulus is terminated by closing the first solenoid valve and simultaneously opening a second solenoid valve that gates the nitrogen in the inflated balloon to room air. The solenoid valves we use for CRD in the rat (or gastric distension, see below) are available from General Valve Co. (202 Fairfield Road, Fairfield, NJ 07006; part # series I 12 volt DC-GVCP-NI-17-900). An interface (B482C Valve Interface, Bioengineering, The University of Iowa, 54 MRF, Iowa City, IA 52242) completes the distension device. It provides an interface between the computer and the solenoid valves and also includes a manual on/off switch. This device for CRD is less expensive to build than the distension control device described above and can be easily constructed. Both devices have the requirement that the distending pressure must be set before each distension (if the distending pressures from one trial to the next are different).

RESPONSES TO CRD

In awake rats, CRD produces an increase in arterial blood pressure, an increase in heart rate and a visceromotor response, each of which can be readily quantified. An indwelling arterial catheter (e.g., femoral artery) can be surgically placed for subsequent access in unanesthetized, unrestrained rats. Arterial pressure and heart rate can be monitored continuously by conventional techniques and CRD-produced changes in either measurement can be readily quantified. The visceromotor response to CRD is a contraction of the peritoneal (skeletal) musculature in response to distension of the colon. We quantify this response electromyographically after surgically implanting electromyographic (EMG) electrodes in the external oblique musculature just above the inguinal ligament. We typically implant both EMG electrodes and intra-arterial catheters during the same surgery; both the arterial catheter and the bipolar EMG electrode leads are externalized at the back of the head of the rat for easy access. For the EMG electrodes, we use multi-stranded, teflon-insulated, 40–gauge stainless-steel wires (Cooner Wire Co., Chatsworth, CA 91311). The EMG signal is amplified ($\times$ 10,000, 300–1,000 Hz), filtered (200 Hz high pass), digitized at 1,000 Hz and integrated. Typical responses to phasic CRD in unanesthetized, unrestrained rats are illustrated in Figure 4. We typically distend the colon to between 5 and 80 or 100 mmHg; in initial work, we determined that the mean minimum distending pressure that ruptured the colon/rectum was 141 $\pm$ 3 mmHg (range 120–155 mmHg).[19] Accordingly, we do not distend the colon to intensities greater than 100 mmHg.

Colorectal distension can be given either as a phasic stimulus or as a ramped, incrementing stimulus. In most of our work, we have used phasic CRD at intensities between 5–100 mmHg, quantifying changes in blood pressure, heart rate, and the visceromotor response, typically in the same rat. In unanesthetized rats, both cardiovascular and visceromotor responses to CRD are reproducible, graded, and normally distributed.[19] Colorectal distension when used as a ramped, incrementing stimulus provides the opportunity to determine a threshold for response, particularly the visceromotor response. The visceromotor response is observed as a sudden "hunching" of the rat at some intensity of CRD and threshold can be determined either by observing this behavior or by monitoring EMG activity recorded from the external oblique musculature. An example of the EMG record from a rat in which the threshold for the visceromotor response was defined as an increase in the EMG to 350% above the resting EMG is given in Figure 5. The utility of applying CRD as a phasic stimulus in some experiments and incrementing stimulus in other experiments is that modulation of responses by pharmacological treatments can give information about attenuation of response magnitude and change in response threshold. Of course, the stimulus-response function to phasic CRD can also be used to extrapolate by linear regression a response threshold for any measure. The extrapolated thresholds to which CRD first produces a measurable increase in blood pressure, heart rate or the EMG are typically between 17–25 mmHg.[19,22] We have, in a number of reports, examined the pharmacological modulation of responses to CRD, but these will not be discussed further here.[19,22,23]

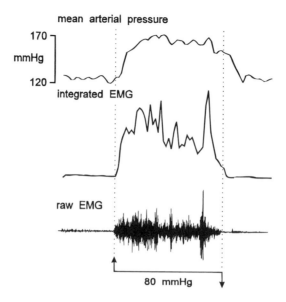

FIGURE 4 Examples of cardiovascular and visceromotor responses to phasic colorectal distension (CRD). In unanesthetized rats, phasic CRD produces a pressor effect (top) and tachycardia (not illustrated) which is sustained and related temporally to the period of distension. The electromyogram (EMG), recorded from the external oblique musculature, is shown as the original (raw) EMG recording as well as after rectification and integration (examples from Burton and Gebhart, unpublished). The cardiovascular and visceromotor responses to phasic CRD in the unanesthetized rat are graded with increasing intensities of CRD.[19]

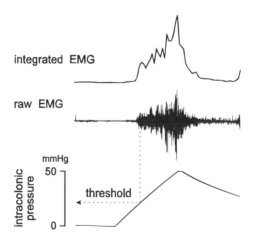

FIGURE 5 Example of the electromyogram (EMG) recorded from the external oblique musculature in an unanesthetized rat during ramped, incrementing colorectal distension (CRD). It is possible, using this method, to determine the threshold at which the visceromotor response occurs in response to CRD. Both the original (raw) EMG recording and the integrated EMG are shown as is the threshold for response, defined as a change in the EMG 350% greater than baseline before distension; (examples from Burton and Gebhart, unpublished).

It is important to appreciate that anesthetic agents affect all of the pseudaffective responses to CRD. In pentobarbital- or α-chloralose-anesthetized rats, the pressor and tachycardic responses produced by CRD in unanesthetized rats become depressor and bradycardic effects. Figure 6 illustrates the effects of preparation and anesthetics on the cardiovascular responses to CRD (80 mmHg, 20 sec). Two points merit emphasis with respect to these data. First, both the cardiovascular and visceromotor (data not shown) responses to CRD are unaffected in decere-brated rats, but are significantly attenuated in spinal-transected rats. Thus, pseudoaffective responses to CRD are representative of spinobulbar-spinal reflexes and clearly require supraspinal integration. That is, the pressor response to CRD is not the result of a distension-produced reduction in blood flow to the colon (i.e., ischemia) and consequent redistribution of blood volume and increase in blood pressure. The second point to emphasize is that although CRD produces depressor and bradycardic effects in pentobarbital- and α-chloralose-anesthetized rats, response magnitude can be readily quantified and the use of anesthetic agents does not necessarily mitigate against the utility of hollow organ distension as a visceral stimulus. However, depth of anesthesia is important and both cardiovascular and visceromotor responses in deeply anesthe-tized rats are significantly attenuated.[24,25]

ESOPHAGEAL DISTENSION (ED)

Because of its easy accessibility, balloon distension of the esophagus has been widely used to evaluate sensations arising from the human esophagus.[12–14] We undertook development and characterization of a model of ED in the rat using controlled, constant volume distension. We were unable to develop a means of constant pressure ED in the rat because of the unavailability of appropriately sized, low-compliance balloons and the relative inelasticity (nondistensibility) of the esophagus because of its striated muscle composition. We therefore used constant volume as the distending stimulus and were able to establish that both neuronal and behavioral responses to ED were graded with increasing volume of ED.

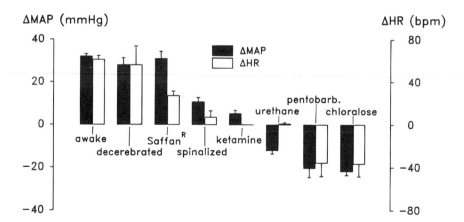

FIGURE 6   Effect of preparation (intact, decerebrated or spinal transected) and anesthetics on the cardio-vascular responses to noxious colorectal distension (CRD; 80 mmHg, 20 sec). Data are presented as change in mean arterial pressure (△MAP) in mmHg and change in heart rate (△HR) in beats per minute (bpm). Pressor (filled bars, left vertical axis) and tachycardic (unfilled bars, right vertical axis) responses to CRD are vigorous in both the awake and decerebrated conditions, but significantly attenuated or absent in spinal-transected rats. In the presence of anesthesia, the pressor and tachycardic responses normally produced by CRD become depressor and bradycardic responses, which also can be quantified.

TABLE 1
Relationship Between Volume of Esophageal Distension and Diameter of the Balloon *Ex Corpo* and External Diameter of the Esophagus *In Corpo*

Inflation Volume, ml	Esophageal Diameter *In Corpo,* cm	Length of Distended Esophagus, cm	Balloon Diameter *Ex Corpo,* cm
0.50	0.43 ± 0.04	0.8 ± 0.1	0.40
0.75	0.50 ± 0.01	1.5 ± 0.1	0.70
1.00	0.53 ± 0.02	1.7 ± 0.2	1.00
1.25	0.57 ± 0.03	1.9 ± 0.1	1.10
1.50	0.62 ± 0.02	2.1 ± 0.1	1.25

Values in Esophageal Diameter *in Corpo* and Length of Distended Esophagus are means ± SE. Length of the non-distended balloon, 0.8 cm.

BALLOONS

Esophageal distension is produced by air inflation of a Swan-Ganz catheter (Baxter Health-care, Santa Anna, CA; size 7F) inserted orally into the mid-thoracic esophagus. The mid-thoracic esophagus is reached by inserting the catheter about 9 cm from the rat's incisors, depending on age and weight. Table 1 presents information about the relation between the volume of balloon inflation, balloon diameter and esophageal diameter during distension. Because constant volume stimulation was used, it was achieved by connecting a 2 ml syringe to the end of the size 7 F Swan-Ganz catheter; volumes of distension ranged from 0.5–1.5 ml. Accordingly, ED in rats requires no special equipment and is straightforward and simple. Figure 7 shows an esophageal balloon *in situ* inflated to 1.25 ml. Esophageal distension similarly meets criteria for developing a visceral pain model in that ED reproduces a natural stimulus, is non-invasive, and is easily controlled by the investigator. Most of our work has been done in rats sedated with pentobarbital or halothane in which the esophageal balloon can be easily inserted via the mouth. In such experiments, ED produces intensity-dependent increases in mean arterial blood

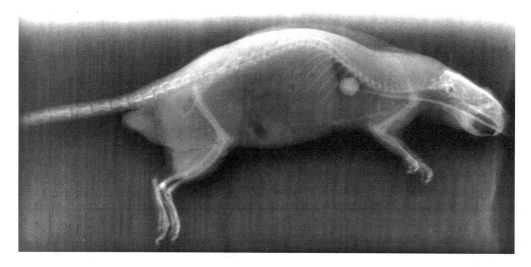

FIGURE 7   Radiograph of an esophageal balloon distended with radiopaque medium to 1.25 ml in an anesthetized rat.

pressure and visceromotor responses. Esophageal distension, however, can be used in unanesthe-tized, unrestrained rats, but such experiments require surgical preparation of the rats.

For experiments in unanesthetized, unrestrained rats, the same Swan-Ganz catheter is surgi-cally implanted into the mid-thoracic esophagus via the stomach through the lower esophageal sphincter in deeply anesthetized rats. The end of the catheter is exteriorized at the back of the head for later connection with a syringe for air distension of the esophagus. These experiments are typically performed within 12 hours after surgical placement of the Swan-Ganz catheter into the esophagus; subcutaneous injections of dextrose in saline are given to avoid dehydration and provide some nutrition. Using the same passive avoidance step-down paradigm described previously, inflation of the esophageal balloon with 1.25 ml air, but not 0.75 ml air, leads to rapid acquisition of the avoidance behavior. We estimate on the basis of these data that 1.0 ml ED or greater is noxious in rats.

RESPONSES TO ED

As described for CRD above, ED also produces two robust, quantifiable pseudaffective responses: a visceromotor response that can be measured by EMG recordings in the pectoral or massetter muscles and cardiovascular pressor and tachycardic responses. These pseudaffective responses are produced in unanesthetized rats or rats which are very lightly anesthetized (sedated) with either pentobarbital or halothane. The increase in blood pressure, increase in heart rate and visceromotor response to phasic ED are reliable and intensity dependent.[26]

GASTRIC DISTENSION (GD)

The stomach is also easily accessible and balloon distension of the stomach in humans has been documented to be painful.[10,11] The most recent model we have developed is gastric distension (GD) in the rat using controlled, constant pressure balloon inflation. Like CRD and ED, GD reproduces a natural stimulus which is experimentally reproducible and reliable and produces easily quantified responses. Unlike CRD or most experiments with ED, however, GD in the rat is only achieved after surgical placement of the balloon.

BALLOONS AND SURGICAL PREPARATION

The fabrication of balloons for GD is very similar to the method described earlier for colonic balloons. The GD balloons are 2.0–2.5 cm long and are made from latex condoms. The end of a condom is fabricated into a balloon for GD by inserting a length of polyethylene tubing (PE 240; Intramedic Polyethylene Tubing, Clay Adams division of Becton Dickenson and Co., Parsippany, NJ 07054) and tying the open end of the condom tightly around the polyethylene tubing with silk suture. The length of polyethylene tubing that is inserted into the condom is approximately 2 cm; this portion of the tubing is repeatedly perforated with a hole punch (hole punch #25, available from Cook Inc., P. O. Box 489, Bloomington, IN 47402). Examples of the materials used to fabricate these gastric balloons are shown in Figure 8. Because the latex from which the balloons are made has some inherent resistance to inflation, it is necessary to fully inflate them for a period of several hours before use experimentally (see figure 8).

Under deep surgical anesthesia, a gastric balloon is placed in the stomach through the fundus; the balloon occupies approximately two-thirds of the proximal stomach. When placed properly and not inflated, the pylorus is not obstructed and there is no blockage of gastric emptying. The polyethylene tubing for air inflation of the gastric balloon is exteriorized at the back of the neck. Experiments in unanesthetized, unrestrained rats with permanently placed

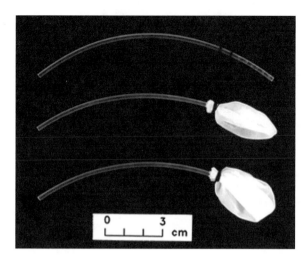

FIGURE 8 Examples, from top to bottom, of the perforated polyethylene tubing, the gastric distending balloon constructed from a latex condom before and (bottom) after it has been inflated to overcome its inherent resistance to distension.

gastric balloons have been carried out 72 hours after surgery. In acute electrophysiological experiments, the gastric balloons are placed in the stomach in the same manner as described above and the recording of afferent fiber activity or second order neurons in the spinal cord or brainstem follows. Figure 9 shows the intragastric balloon *in situ* inflated to approximately 30 mmHg.

BALLOON INFLATION AND RESPONSES TO GD

The same methods of balloon inflation described above for CRD can be used for GD. Currently, we use the most recent computer-controlled distension device for GD (2-stage regulator, compressed nitrogen gas, solenoid valves and valve interface). Our use of GD experimentally has primarily focused on electrophysiological studies of gastric afferent fibers and thus has

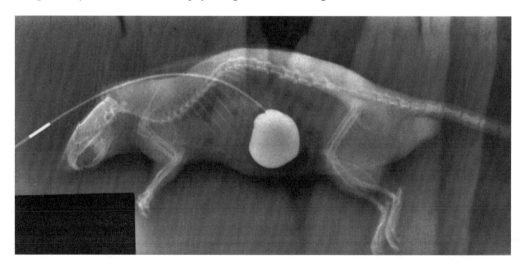

FIGURE 9 Radiograph of an intragastric balloon distended with radiopaque medium to approximately 30 mmHg in an anesthetized rat.

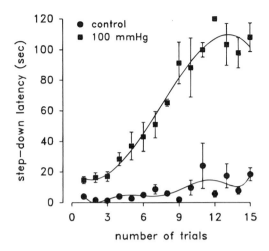

FIGURE 10 Acquisition of a passive avoidance behavior produced by gastric distension (GD). Rats were placed on a raised platform and the latency to step-down from the platform was measured (in sec, vertical axis). Different groups of rats, both with surgically implanted gastric balloons, received either no distension (control group) or 100 mmHg gastric distension when both forepaws were placed on the floor. The behavior of rats receiving GD significantly differed from rats receiving no GD.

been carried out principally in anesthetized rats after surgical placement of the distending balloon. However, because we needed to first establish that GD was an adequate, noxious stimulus in the rat, we examined the behavioral effects of GD as well as the cardiovascular pseudaffective responses to GD in unanesthetized, unrestrained rats.

Using the passive avoidance paradigm described earlier for CRD, unanesthetized, unrestrained rats which, 72 hours previously, had gastric balloons surgically implanted were placed on a raised platform above an open field and the latency to step down from the platform measured in seconds. When rats in the control group stepped down from the platform, the previously placed gastric balloons were not inflated. When rats in the GD group stepped down from the platform, the previously placed gastric balloons were inflated to 100 mmHg for 20 seconds. The results are illustrated in Figure 10; it is clear that rats receiving GD when stepping down from the raised platform learn after three trials to passively avoid the stimulus. Accordingly, 100 mmHg GD produces behavior in rats consistent with an interpretation that the stimulus is noxious. We did not examine the effects of GD in an intensity-dependent manner and thus cannot report the intensity at which GD significantly changes this passive avoidance behavior. In other rats in which gastric balloons were placed, GD produced intensity-dependent pressor and tachycardic pseudaffective responses; the threshold for producing a measurable increase in mean arterial pressure was about 20 mmHg GD. Gastric distension in rats, because surgical placement of the distending balloons is required, is more invasive as a noxious visceral stimulus and there is thus greater concern for animal well-being in these experiments.

SUMMARY AND CONCLUSIONS

Three models of visceral pain have been developed, all of which rely on balloon distension of hollow organs. Balloon distension of the gastrointestinal tract in humans has consistently demonstrated that the pain produced experimentally is similar, if not identical, in intensity, quality and localization to pain associated with pathologies of the gastrointestinal tract (see[5] for review and references). Thus, balloon distension of hollow organs experimentally reproduces a natural stimulus and, in addition, satisfies other criteria for development of models of pain in non-human animals. The model that has been best studied is CRD, which in our hands is a reliable and reproducible visceral stimulus that produces easily quantifiable responses. Colorectal distension as a noxious visceral stimulus is regularly used in unanesthetized, unrestrained rats as well as in electrophysiological experiments in deeply anesthetized rats. In unanesthetized rats, the ethical concerns associated with this model are diminished compared with chemical irritation of the peritoneal cavity because the distending stimulus is of short duration and is non-invasive. We have also examined the nociceptive quality of ED and GD in unanesthetized, unrestrained rats and distension of either the esophagus or stomach also leads to rapid acquisition of a passive avoidance behavior, supporting the nociceptive character of ED and GD. Both ED and GD, however, are relatively more invasive to the rat than is insertion of a balloon into the colon via the anus for CRD. Most of our work with ED or GD thus has been done in sedated or anesthetized rats where both stimuli, because of behavioral evidence, can be considered adequate, noxious visceral stimuli.

Ischemia and inflammation are also natural events which can lead to visceral pain. In an experimental context, however, neither stimulus is reliably reproducible nor produces easily quantifiable responses. We consider inflammation to be an experimentally useful "conditioning" stimulus, for which there is clinical support. For example, Wolf's patient Tom reported that mechanical stimulation of the gastric mucosa was not perceived until the gastric mucosa had been irritated experimentally by mustard powder, whereupon the same stimuli now produced pain.[16] Experimentally, inflammation of the colon with chemicals (e.g., turpentine, acetic acid, etc.) shifts the stimulus-response function of CRD to the left (see[26,27] for illustrations and discussion), similar to the altered sensations to balloon distension reported in patients with functional bowel disorders (e.g., irritable bowel syndrome).[15] We consider that experimental use of well-characterized, controllable visceral stimuli will aid in our understanding of visceral pain mechanisms and present opportunities for investigation of mechanisms of altered sensation from the viscera that heretofore have not kept pace with advances in cutaneous pain mechanisms.[28]

REFERENCES

1. **Hammond, D. L.,** Inference of pain and its modulation from simple behaviors, in *Issues in Pain Measurement,* Loeser, J. and Chapman, C. R., Eds., Raven Press, New York, 1989, 69.
2. **Taber, R. I.,** Predictive value of analgesic assays in mice and rats, in *Narcotic Antagonists,* Braude, M. C., Harris, L. S., May, E. L., Smith, J. P. and Villarreal, J. E., Eds., Advances in Biochemical Psychopharmacology, volume 8, Raven Press, New York, 1973, 191.
3. **Cervero, F.** Visceral pain, in *Proceedings of the Vth World Congress on Pain,* Dubner, R., Gebhart, G. F. and Bond, Eds., Elsevier, Amsterdam, 1988, 216.
4. **Gebhart, G. F. and Ness T. J.,** Mechanisms of visceral pain, in *Proceedings of the VIth World Congress on Pain,* Bond, M. R., Charlton, J. E. and Woolf, C. J., Eds., Elsevier, Amsterdam, 1991, 351.
5. **Ness, T. J. and Gebhart, G. F.,** Visceral pain: a review of experimental studies, *Pain,* 41, 167, 1990.
6. **Hardy, J. D., Wolff, H. G. and Goodell, H.,** Experimental evidence on the nature of cutaneous hyperalgesia, *J. Clin. Invest.,* 29, 115, 1950.
7. **Sherrington, C. S.,** *The Integrative Action of the Nervous System,* Yale University Press, New Haven, 1906.
8. **Sengupta, J. N. and Gebhart, G. F.,** Gastrointestinal afferent fibers and sensation, in *Physiology of the Gastrointestinal Tract,* Third Edition, Johnson, L. R., Ed., Raven Press, New York, 1994, 483.
9. **Lennander, K. G.,** Uber die Sensibilität der Bauchhöhle und über lokale und allgemeine Anästhesie bei Bruch und Bauchoperationen, *Zentralbl. Chir.,* 28, 200, 1901.

10. **Hurst, A. F.,** The sensibility of the alimentary canal in health and diseases, *Lancet* (1), 1051, 1911.

11. **Bloomfield, A. L. and Polland, W. S.,** Experimental referred pain from the gastrointestinal tract. I. Stomach, duodenum and colon, *J. Clin. Invest.,* 10, 453, 1931.

12. **Lipkin, M. and Sliesenger, M. H.,** Studies of visceral pain: measurements of stimulus intensity and duration associated with the onset of pain in esophagus, ileum, and colon, *J. Clin. Invest.,* 37, 28, 1958.

13. **Payne, W. W. and Poulton, E. P.,** Experiments on visceral sensation. I. The relation of pain to activity in the human esophagus, *J. Physiol. Lond.,* 65, 157, 1929.

14. **Polland, W. S. and Bloomfield, A. L.,** Experimental referred pain from the gastrointestinal tract. I. The esophagus. *J. Clin. Invest.,* 10, 435, 1931.

15. **Ritchie, J.,** Pain from distension of the pelvic colon by inflating a balloon in the irritable colon syndrome, *Gut,* 14, 125, 1973.

16. **Wolf, S.,** *The Stomach,* Oxford, New York, 1965.

17. **Hendershot, L. C. and Forsaith, J.,** Antagonism of the frequency of phenylquinone-induced writhing in the mouse by weak analgesics and nonanalgesics, *J. Pharmacol. Exp. Ther.,* 125, 237, 1959.

18. **Jarvic, M. E. and Essman, W. B.,** A simple 1-trial learning situation for mice, *Psychol. Rep.,* 6, 290, 1960.

19. **Ness, T. J. and Gebhart, G. F.,** Colorectal distension as a noxious visceral stimulus: physiologic and pharmacologic characterization of pseudaffective reflexes in the rat, *Brain Res.,* 450, 153, 1988.

20. **Ness, T. J., Randich, A. and Gebhart, G. F.,** Further behavioral evidence that colorectal distension is a noxious visceral stimulus in rats, *Neurosci. Lett.,* 131, 113, 1991.

21. **Anderson, G. H., Ness, T. J. and Gebhart, G. F.,** A distension control device useful for quantitative studies of hollow organ sensation, *Physiol. Behav.* 41, 635, 1987.

22. **Danzebrink, R. M. and Gebhart, G. F.,** Antinociceptive effects of intrathecal adrenoceptor agonists in a rat model of visceral nociception, *J. Pharmacol. Exp. Ther.,* 253, 698, 1990.

23. **Maves, T. J. and Gebhart, G. F.,** Antinociceptive synergy between intrathecal morphine and lidocaine during visceral and somatic nociception in the rat, *Anesthesiol.,* 76, 91, 1992.

24. **Clark, S. J. and Smith, T. W.,** Opiate-induced inhibition of the visceral distension reflex by peripheral and central mechanisms, *Naunyn-Schmiedeberg's Arch. Pharmacol.,* 330, 179, 1985.

25. **Lembeck, F. and Skofitsch, G.,** Visceral pain reflex after pretreatment with capsaicin and morphine, *Naunyn-Schmiedeberg's Arch. Pharmacol.,* 321, 116, 1982.

26. **Gebhart, G. F., Meller, S. T., Euchner-Wamser, I. and Sengupta, J. N.,** Modeling visceral pain, in *New Trends in Referred Pain and Hyperalgesia,* Vecchiet, L., Albe-Fessard, D., Lindblom, U. and Giamberardino, Eds., Elsevier, Amsterdam, 1993, 129.

27. **Gebhart, G. F.,** Visceral pain mechanisms, in *Current and Emerging Issues in Cancer Pain,* Chapman, C. R. and Foley, K. M., Eds., Raven Press, New York, 1993, 99.

28. **Mayer, E. A. and Gebhart, G. F.,** Basic and clinical aspects of visceral hyperalgesia, *Gastroenterol.,* 107, 271, 1994.

16 The Gut as a Model of Opioid Dependence

Thomas F. Burks

INTRODUCTION

Because the enteric nervous system shares many features in common with the brain, preparations of gastrointestinal tissues have often been used to examine actions of opioids that can be extrapolated to the central nervous systems (CNS). The preparation most widely employed in this regard has been the isolated ileum of the guinea pig. The intact guinea pig ileum, or, most often, the guinea pig ileum longitudinal muscle-myenteric plexus preparation, has in fact become the standard assay for opioids to determine their biological actions at mu and kappa receptors and to assess opioid tolerance and dependence. Few model systems have achieved the status of the guinea pig ileum as standards in pharmacological testing of drugs and in studies of neural mechanisms of opioid tolerance and dependence.

In vivo models are also employed in opioid studies, including the gastrointestinal effects of opioids, but are complicated by multiple sites of opioid action that affect gastrointestinal function, by the pharmacokinetic considerations that must apply, and by loss of precision in comparison with *in vitro* systems. However, *in vivo* models are indispensable for some types of studies, such as those that are designed to investigate brain-gut interactions or to study opioid effects on certain functions of the gastrointestinal tract that occur only *in vivo*.

One preparation that has been used to study functional aspects of opioid intestinal effects is the dog isolated *(ex vivo)* intestine. While this preparation does not lend itself to routine bioassays, it provides a useful spectrum of opioid actions at multiple receptors and allows measurement of circular muscle activity. Unlike the guinea pig ileum preparation, mu and delta opioids are primarily stimulatory in dog intestine.

GUINEA PIG ILEUM

HISTORY

Opioid Actions

The isolated ileum of the guinea pig has been used for study of opioid actions for nearly four decades. Schaumann reported in 1955 that morphine inhibited contractions induced by transmural electrical stimulation of longitudinally suspended ileum in an isolated muscle chamber.[1] The morphine inhibition of contractions was concentration-dependent and reversible upon washout. It was subsequently discovered that the inhibitory effect of morphine is related to ability of the opiate to depress release of acetylcholine from the terminals of intramural cholinergic motor neurons.[2,3] It has since been established that the magnitude of the opioid effect is dependent on

0-8493-8304-8/96/$0.00+$.50

375

the electrical stimulation parameters which are used.[4] Acetylcholine released by high frequency electrical stimulation is much less sensitive to inhibition by morphine than is low frequency-induced release. The advantage of the guinea pig ileum preparation is that it provides a stable baseline rarely interrupted by spontaneous contractions of the longitudinal muscle, thus allowing reproducible twitch responses to transmural electrical stimulation (Table 1). However, the electrical stimulation and many drugs can also produce contraction of the circular muscle which can interfere with measurement of the contraction amplitudes of the longitudinal muscle. For this reason, isolated strips of longitudinal muscle with adherent myenteric plexus have more often been used in recent times for studies of opioid actions.

The assay preparation most used today is the guinea isolated ileum longitudinal muscle-myenteric plexus preparation, a modification of the method originally introduced by Rang.[5,6] Excised ilea are generally placed in Krebs-bicarbonate solution (bubbled with 95% O_2-5% CO_2). The segment of ileum within 10 cm of the cecum is discarded because terminal ileum is less sensitive to opioids than non-terminal ileum. Several 3 cm segments of ileum can be prepared. Each segment is threaded over a glass rod and thin strips of longitudinal muscle are gently dissected, generally with the use of an iris forceps and a buffer-saturated cotton swab. The strips (1–3 cm in length) with adherent myenteric plexus are attached to gold jeweler's chains (to avoid metal interactions with the highly oxygenated buffer) with surgical suture and are suspended in chambers (50–60 ml) where they are bathed in oxygenated Krebs-bicarbonate solution at 37°C. One chain is attached to an isometric recording transducer for measurement of twitch height. Platinum plate or ring electrodes connected to a stimulator are placed on each side of the longitudinal muscle strip for stimulation with supramaximal voltage at 0.1 Hz, 0.5–2.0 ms pulse duration. Tension on the strips is adjusted to produce a twitch height of convenient amplitude (usually about 1 g of tension). Once the preparations have stabilized, they maintain consistent pharmacological responses for periods of several hours. Many longitudinal muscle strips can be prepared from the ileum of one guinea pig.

Activation of either mu or kappa opioids receptors produces concentration-dependent inhibition of twitch height, due to acetylcholine antirelease effects on cholinergic motor neurons.[4] Cholinergic motor neurons in guinea pig longitudinal muscle do not possess functional delta opioid receptors. Because of the sensitivity and reproducibility of responses to opioid agonists, the guinea pig ileum longitudinal muscle-myenteric preparation has been widely employed for bioassay of opioid agonists and antagonist drugs.[7] As agonist activity at the cholinergic nerve

TABLE 1
Characteristics of Guinea Pig Isolated Ileum Preparation for Studies of Opioids

Advantages	Disadvantages
Simple, economical	Provides no functional insights
Highly quantitative	Diminished utility for mixed agonists-antagonists
Consistent between preparations	Does not respond to δ opioids
Measures neural effects of opioids	Sensitive to muscarinic antagonists
Responds to μ and κ opioids	Sensitive to AChE inhibitors
Can assess both tolerance and dependence	
Tolerance and dependence can be induced *in vivo* or *in vitro*	
Little cross-tolerance develops	
Can assess both affinity and efficacy	
Can assess both full and partial agonists	
Useful for opioid antagonists	

AChE = acetylcholinesterase.

terminal in the longitudinal muscle preparation is caused mainly by actions at mu opioid receptors, there is a close correlation between opioid in vitro actions in longitudinal muscle myenteric plexus and as analgesic drugs in humans.

Opioid Receptors

The first direct demonstration of ligand binding to opioid receptors occurred with preparations of brain and myenteric plexus.[8] Subsequent studies showed a relationship between the in vitro pharmacological activity of opioids and their ability to bind to intestinal neural receptors.[9] Multiple types of opioid receptors were identified in studies of guinea pig ileum longitudinal muscle-myenteric plexus and mouse vas deferens preparations.[10] Electrically-induced contractions of guinea pig ileum longitudinal muscle were found to be inhibited primarily by agonists acting at mu receptors, whereas electrically-induced contractions of mouse *vas deferens* were inhibited primarily by agonists acting at delta opioid receptors. Differential activity of agonist ligands in the guinea pig ileum bioassay in comparison with the mouse *vas deferens* bioassay has been used extensively to determine the relative selectivity of opioid ligands for mu and delta receptors.[11–14] Both the guinea pig ileum longitudinal muscle myenteric plexus and the mouse *vas deferens* preparations possess kappa opioid receptors.[15,16] The mu, kappa and delta opioid receptors in guinea pig ileum and mouse *vas deferens* are similar to those found in brain.[17]

TOLERANCE TO OPIOIDS

Tolerance to the inhibitory effect of opioids on electrically-induced contractions of the guinea pig ileum longitudinal muscle-myenteric plexus preparation can be induced in two ways, *in vivo* by treatment of the donor guinea pig with the opiate (generally morphine) or *in vitro* by incubation of tissue with opiate. In practice, guinea pigs commonly receive 4 morphine pellets each containing 75 mg free base implanted s.c. for 96 hours before use.[18] Such treatment generally produces a 5 to 10-fold increase in the IC_{50} values for a mu agonist in the guinea pig ileum longitudinal muscle-myenteric plexus taken from morphine-treated donor animals in comparison with placebo-treated donor animals (Figure 1). Alternatively, strips of guinea pig longitudinal muscle can be incubated in various concentrations of morphine for 2–6 hours to induce tolerance.[19] In both chronic and acute tolerance models, responses to exogenously applied acetylcholine are not altered, indicating that the site of tolerance is at the opioid receptor mechanism at the terminals of cholinergic motor neurons.[18–20] However, responses to exogenously administered 5-hydroxytryptamine (5-HT) are enhanced in morphine tolerant longitudinal muscle strips of guinea pig ileum, leading to the suggestion that alterations in neurotransmitter receptor sensitivity may be involved in opioid tolerance.[21] However, morphine was not found to alter release of 5-HT from guinea pig ileum myenteric plexus.[22] It is more likely that supersensitivity in morphine-tolerant ileial strips to 5-HT, electrical stimulation, and potassium is caused by an increase in neuronal excitability, possibly brought about by membrane depolarization, rather than changes in receptors for particular neurotransmitters.[23]

Acute tolerance can be produced *in vitro* by incubation of guinea pig ileum or longitudinal muscle preparations with morphine or other opioid agonists.[19,24,25] Typically, strips of longitudinal muscle-myenteric plexus are incubated for 4–8 hours in concentrations of morphine or other opioid ranging from 0.5–2 times IC50 of the opioid in non-tolerant preparations. The development of tolerance is generally maximum at 4–6 hours and can range from about 10-fold to more than 100-fold.[23]

OPIOID DEPENDENCE

Guinea pig ileum longitudinal muscle myenteric preparations can display opioid withdrawal responses *in vitro*, characterized by contracture of the longitudinal muscle smooth (Figure 1).

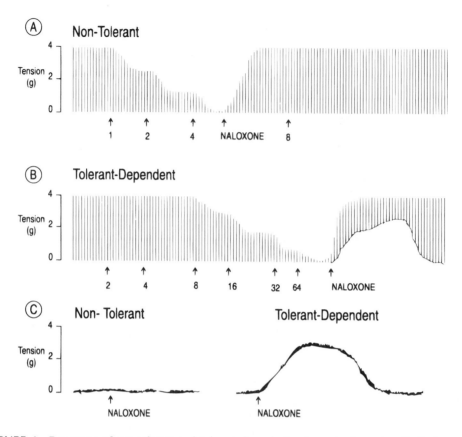

FIGURE 1 Responses of non-tolerant and tolerant-dependent guinea pig ileum longitudinal muscle-myenteric plexus preparations to a mu opioid. Panel A: non-tolerant preparations show concentration-dependent inhibition of twitch height in response to cumulative doses of mu opioids, such as morphine or normorphine. Addition of naloxone blocks mu receptors and restores twitch height to original level. In the presence of naloxone, even high doses of mu agonist are antagonized. Panel B: Responses of morphine tolerant-dependent preparations. The tissue is resistant to inhibitory effects of mu agonists, thereby requiring large doses to inhibit twitch height. Addition of naloxone induces a characteristic withdrawal contracture measured as a sustained increase in baseline tension. Panel C: naloxone given alone has no effect in nonstimulated, non-tolerant preparations but produces a characteristic withdrawal contracture in morphine tolerant-dependent preparations. Even in the absence of electrical stimulation, the addition of naloxone results in a sustained increased in baseline tension. (The numerical values represent arbitrary concentrations of mu opioid agonists. This composite figure was redrawn from records from the author's laboratory.)

Dependence characterized by an abstinence response can be produced in strips taken from opioid-treated guinea pigs or in strips incubated with appropriate opioid agonists *in vitro*.[26,27] The abstinence contraction can be produced either by withdrawal of opioid from the bathing solution or by administration of an opioid antagonist, such as naloxone. Dependence can be demonstrated only in strips in which opioid tolerance has been produced. Thus, opioid dependence is linked to tolerance in this isolated tissue. However, it has been postulated that tolerance can occur without concomitant dependence.[28] There is a rapid loss of tolerance after opioid withdrawal.[23,29,30]

The electrophysiological basis for the abstinence contracture in guinea pig ileum longitudinal muscle may be activation of S-type neurons, some of which are motor neurons to the longitudinal muscle.[31] Depolarization in S neurons evoked by naloxone in tolerant-dependent tissue may result in release of excitatory neurotransmitters from nerve terminals innervating longitudinal muscle.

CROSS-TOLERANCE AND DEPENDENCE

Opioids may induce either specific or nonspecific tolerance and dependence in guinea pig ileum longitudinal muscle-myenteric plexus. Tolerance and dependence that develops in longitudinal muscle-myenteric plexus after treatment of the donor guinea pigs with opioids or after incubation of muscle strips with opioids *in vitro* can be highly specific for the type of opioid receptor, and stereospecific.[25,32–35] There is little cross-tolerance or cross-dependence between agents selective for mu receptors with those selective for kappa receptors. However, there is cross-tolerance and cross-dependence among opioid agonists that act at mu opioid receptors. Lack of cross-tolerance and cross-dependence has been utilized to differentiate opioids with primary actions at mu receptors from those acting primarily at kappa receptors.

The tolerance observed before a withdrawal response is relatively specific for the type of agonist responsible for induction of tolerance, whereas residual tolerance observed after withdrawal *in vitro* may be nonspecific.[18,30] The nonspecific tolerance may extend to agents such as epinephrine, norepinephrine, clonidine, and 2-chloroadenosine.[36] It has been postulated that the tolerance observed after prolonged pre-treatment of guinea pigs with morphine consists of at least two components.[23] One component, present prior to morphine withdrawal, is of high degree, decays within minutes or hours after removal of the opioid from the receptor, and is specific for the class of opioid agonist used to induce it. The other component of tolerance is more modest in degree, decays slowly and is nonspecific. The nonspecific tolerance may be related to alterations in membrane excitability of motor neurons in the myenteric plexus.[31]

MECHANISMS OF TOLERANCE AND DEPENDENCE

Opioid tolerance and dependence in guinea pig ileum longitudinal muscle-myenteric plexus has not been shown, despite many efforts, to be related to alterations in affinity of neural opioid receptors.[37,38] Likewise, the tolerance and dependence appear not to result from changes in sensitivity of the smooth muscle to intrinsic neurotransmitters.[23] While the withdrawal contracture induced by naloxone in opioid tolerant-dependent tissue evidently results from release of acetylcholine and substance P, the motor effect is probably secondary to changes in neuronal excitability rather than changes in neurotransmitter receptors.[27,31,39] Both cholera toxin and pertussis toxin were found to attenuate naloxone precipitated withdrawal contracture in opioid tolerant-dependent longitudinal muscle-myenteric plexus.[40] These results indicate that expression of the withdrawal sign in longitudinal muscle-myenteric plexus requires excitatory input of neurons by way of guanosine triphosphate-binding proteins.[28]

Whereas changes in opioid receptor sensitivity have not been observed in tolerant-dependent longitudinal muscle-myenteric plexus, opioid tolerance appears to be associated with decreased reserves of spare opioid receptors in myenteric neurons.[41,42] Greater concentrations of the irreversible opioid antagonist, beta-chlornaltrexamine, were required in naive than tolerate preparations to induce nonsurmountable antagonism of responses to normorphine. Calculations of dissociation constants and the fraction of receptors remaining unblocked allowed the conclusion that the number of spare receptors for normorphine was reduced. Further, the dissociation constant and sensitivity to naloxone is decreased in morphine-tolerant longitudinal muscle-myenteric plexus.[30,38,43]

In contrast to isolated longitudinal muscle-myenteric plexus preparations, the intact guinea pig ileum may show enhanced sensitivity to acetylcholine during tolerance and dependence.[44,45]

In the intact ileum *in vitro,* sensitivity of the peristaltic reflex to acetylcholine was increased during morphine tolerance and the number of peristaltic waves per minute was increased during morphine withdrawal. Again, these phenomena may be related to neuronal hyperexcitability during tolerance and withdrawal.

The observation that very gradual increases in the concentration of naloxone in the organ bath containing tolerant-dependent guinea pig ileum *in vitro* can block opioid receptors without inducing withdrawal contractions has led to the formulation of extremely interesting theories of rate coupled phenomena in drug-effector systems.[46,47] The novel theory predicts that drug-receptor-effector complexes become inactivated at a rate that is independent of the rate of chemical association. Thus, depending on rate of administration, a system may become refractory to either agonist or antagonist drugs. This theory could explain the decrease in receptor reserve associated with morphine tolerance.

IN VIVO MODELS

In vivo models allow assessment of opioid actions on many physiological variables that cannot be effectively studied *in vitro* (Table 2). For example, opioid effects in mammals on gastric emptying, gastrointestinal motility, gastrointestinal propulsion and gastric secretion can be examined more readily *in vivo* than *in vitro*. At the same time, *in vivo* studies are limited by pharmacokinetic characteristics of agonists and antagonist drugs as well as multiple sites of opioid action that regulate gastrointestinal function. Opioid agonists are known to act in the brain and spinal cord, as well as locally in the enteric nervous system, to affect gastrointestinal

TABLE 2
Characteristics of *In Vivo* Models for Studies of Gastrointestinal Effects of Opioids

Advantages	Disadvantages
Rat	
Opioids effects on gastric emptying, small intestinal propulsion, colonic propulsion, fecal output and gastric secretion can be measured	Most measures require prior surgical preparation Opioids *in vivo* act at multiple sites
Withdrawal diarrhea and weight loss are characteristic	
Motility can be measured	
Both tolerance and dependence occur	
Mouse	
Economical	Opioids *in vivo* act at multiple sites
Opioid effects on gastric emptying and gastrointestinal propulsion can be measured	Difficult to separate effects on gastric emptying from those on intestinal propulsion
Withdrawal diarrhea and weight loss are characteristic	Colonic propulsion difficult to assess
Both tolerance and dependence occur	
Dog	
Opioid effects on motility and MMC activity can be measured	Opioids *in vivo* act at multiple sites
Model of opioid stimulant actions	Most measures require prior surgical preparation
Tolerance occurs	Expensive
	Propulsion difficult to assess
	Dependence difficult to assess

functions.[48–50] Most *in vivo* experiments cannot rule out opioid actions at remote sites that affect gastrointestinal activity.

RAT

Development of tolerance to the intestinal antipropulsive effects of morphine *in vivo* was first demonstrated in rats.[51] In these experiments, the intestinal distribution of a nonabsorbable marker ($Na_2^{51}CrO_4$) was determined after intraduodenal instillation in unanesthetized rats. Access to the duodenum was provided by an indwelling catheter previously implanted under surgical anesthesia. In naive animals, acute administration of morphine (20 mg/kg) produced marked inhibition of propulsion of ^{51}Cr. Animals that had been administered morphine (60 mg/kg per day in 3 divided doses) for 7 days were essentially refractory to the antipropulsive effects of morphine.

The gastrointestinal tract is also involved in morphine dependence. Loss of body weight produced in tolerant-dependent rats by administration of naloxone is one of the most consistent, reliable, quantitative measures of the degree of opioid dependence.[52] The rapid loss of body weight associated with precipitated opioid withdrawal results primarily from increased fecal excretion which may progress to diarrhea. The rate of development of gastrointestinal tolerance-dependence with chronic administration of morphine is slower than the rate of tolerance-dependence induction to many other withdrawal signs.[53]

MOUSE

Opioid tolerance-dependence can also be produced by chronic opioid treatment of mice.[54] Typically, mice are treated with subcutaneously implanted pellets containing 75 mg of morphine base per pellet. Peak tolerance-dependence occurs at 72 hours after implantation of pellets. Among other withdrawal signs, such as jumping behavior, precipitated withdrawal elicited by naloxone is associated with the appearance of diarrhea and acute loss of body weight. It is clear from studies in mice that the central nervous system plays an important role in opioid withdrawal *in vivo*. Systemically administered naloxone acts at opioid receptors in the central nervous system and the periphery. However, peptidic opioid antagonists with high selectivity for mu opioid receptors do not readily cross the blood-brain barrier.[55,56] When administered intracerebro-ventricularly (i.c.v.) in morphine tolerant-dependent mice, a peptidic mu antagonist caused dose-related increases in defecation and weight loss which were equal to or greater in magnitude than those caused by i.c.v. naloxone.[57] When administered intrathecally in morphine tolerant-dependent mice, the peptidic mu opioid antagonist elicited behavioral signs of withdrawal but not loss of body weight or diarrhea.[58] It would appear that supraspinal mu opioid receptors are largely responsible for the increased fecal output and loss of body weight associated with antagonist-precipitated morphine withdrawal responses in mice.

DOG

In dogs, mu and delta agonist opioids increase the amplitude and frequency of small intestinal circular muscle contractions.[59,60] The dog thus serves as a useful model of the stimulatory effects of opioids on intestinal motility. Tolerance to the stimulatory effect of morphine in dogs has been demonstrated.[61] Dogs were treated with morphine for 8 or 9 days in incrementing doses until a daily dosage of 30 mg/kg was reached. Small intestinal intraluminal pressure was measured in anesthetized animals. Responses to morphine in the morphine-treated dogs were markedly reduced in comparison with saline-treated animals. Stimulatory effects of morphine were diminished in morphine-treated dogs in both the duodenum and the ileum. In contrast, intestinal stimulatory responses to 5-hydroxytryptamine were not altered by chronic morphine treatment. Thus, the diminished intestinal responses to morphine appeared to reflect development of specific morphine tolerance. These experiments, however, were potentially complicated by the presence of anesthesia.

Morphine tolerance was also demonstrated in unanesthetized dogs.[62,63] Myoelectric activity was recorded from serosal electrodes surgically implanted on the small intestine of anesthetized dogs. After full recovery from surgery, dose-response data were obtained for myoelectric changes induced by intravenous boluses of morphine in doses of 30–300 μg/kg during a specific part of the migrating motor complex of the small intestine. Morphine produced characteristic dose-dependent increases in myoelectric spiking activity indicative of circular muscle contractions. Dogs were subsequently given morphine in doses up to 40 mg/kg/day by continuous intravenous infusion. During continuous administration of morphine, the intestinal stimulatory effects of the boluses doses were lost. Further, the changes in motility associated with initial infusions of morphine disappeared after 2–4 days of continuous infusion and motility patterns returned to normal. Thus, tolerance to the effects of morphine was demonstrated in two ways. First, the normal patterns of interdigestive myoelectric activity turned toward normal when a particular dose level of morphine administered by continuous infusion was maintained for several days. Second, effects of acute bolus doses of morphine diminished during morphine tolerance. Development of tolerance to bolus administration of morphine was more prominent during infusion of higher dose levels of morphine. After discontinuation of morphine infusion, withdrawal signs, including diarrhea, occurred. Motility patterns were disrupted for up to one week following discontinuation of morphine, indicating that physical dependence had developed and that a withdrawal sign was elicited by abstinent withdrawal.[63]

It is difficult to assess effects of precipitated withdrawal in unanesthetized dogs. In animals that are highly tolerant to morphine, administration of naloxone results in behavioral agitation and motor activity so pronounced as to make myoelectric recording nearly impossible.

DOG ISOLATED INTESTINE

Dog intestine provides a model for the intestinal stimulatory effects of mu and delta opioid agonists.[64] While only a few studies of morphine tolerance have been carried out with isolated dog intestine, the technique has great potential utility (Table 3).

TABLE 3
Characteristics of Canine Small Intestine *Ex Vivo* for Studies of Opioids

Advantages	Disadvantages
Adequately quantitative	Complex
Mainly neural effects of opioids	Expensive
Responds to μ and δ opioids	Variability between preparations
Tolerance occurs	Poorly responsive to κ opioids
Both affinity and efficacy can be assessed	Incompletely characterized
Can assess both full and partial agonists	Sensitive to muscarinic agonists
Useful for opioid antagonists	Sensitive to AChE inhibitors
Functionally relevant	
Model of stimulatory opioid effects	

AChE = acetylcholinesterase.

PREPARATION

Isolated segments of small intestine are prepared from anesthetized dogs by cannulation of juxtaintestinal mesenteric arteries supplying small (8–10 cm) sections of jejunum or proximal ileum.[65] The arterial supply is perfused with Krebs-bicarbonate solution warmed to 37°C and bubbled with 95% O_2-5%CO_2. The intestinal segment is ligated on both sides of the perfused mesenteric arcade and is surgically divided and removed from the animal. Intraluminal pressure is measured by a pressure transducer from a small balloon tied into the lumen of the intestine. Perfusion pressure is monitored from a T connection between the pump and the perfused artery.

Drugs for continuous perfusion are dissolved in the reservoir of Krebs-bicarbonate solution. Bolus doses of drugs are administered directly in the arterial cannula. Contractions of the isolated intestinal segments are measured as the maximum increases in intraluminal pressure in response to stimulatory agents.

OPIOID TOLERANCE

Tolerance to morphine stimulatory actions in isolated vascularly perfused intestinal segments has been observed in tissues taken from morphine-treated dogs and in segments perfused *ex vivo* with morphine.[61,66] For induction of morphine tolerance in donor dogs, the animals were treated for 9 days with daily doses of morphine incrementing from 5 mg/kg to 30 mg/kg. Each morphine-treated dog was, thereafter, maintained at a dose level of 30 mg/kg for either 7 or 8 additional days. The last dose of morphine was administered 24 hours before experiments were performed.[61] Control segments were removed from dogs treated identically with injections of saline rather than morphine. Intestinal segments removed from morphine-treated dogs showed diminished responses to morphine. Morphine dose-response curves were shifted approximately 400-fold to the right in preparations from morphine-treated dogs in comparison with preparations from saline-treated dogs. Dose-response curves to bethanechol and 5-hyroxytryptamine (5-HT) were not altered by morphine treatment of donor animals. These experiments indicated that tolerance to the intestinal stimulatory effects of morphine develops in chronically morphine-treated dogs. The lack of effect of prior morphine treatment on responses to bethanechol and 5-HT indicates that the tolerance to morphine was specific, not nonspecific.

Tolerance to morphine and levorphanol was also induced by vascular perfusion with buffer solution containing morphine (2 μg/ml) or levorphanol (0.2 μg/ml).[66] Perfusion with morphine induced acute tolerance to morphine shown by virtual obliteration of stimulatory responses to bolus doses of morphine. Response to bethanechol, dimethylphenylpiperazinium (DMPP), and 5-HT were not diminished by morphine tolerance. Again, these data indicate that the tolerance to morphine was selective, and did not extend to stimulatory agonists acting either directly on smooth muscle or on enteric motor neurons. Perfusion with levorphanol likewise diminished stimulatory responses to morphine selectively without reducing responses to bethanechol, DMPP, or 5-HT.

The patterns of intestinal responsiveness observed with acute morphine or levorphanol tolerance were strikingly similar to responses of intestinal segments removed from dogs treated chronically for 16 days with morphine.[61] In both cases, responsiveness to morphine was reduced, whereas responses to cholinergic agonists and 5-HT were essentially unchanged. These data suggest that tolerance to morphine in the dog reflects events at the opioid receptor or opioid receptor-coupled mechanisms, not events at neurotransmitter receptors or smooth muscle.

SUMMARY AND CONCLUSIONS

The gastrointestinal preparation most used for opioid bioassay and studies of opioid tolerance and dependence is the longitudinal muscle myenteric plexus *in vitro* preparation of guinea pig ileum. Transmural electrical stimulation of the ileum excites cholinergic motor neurons and induces twitch responses of the smooth muscle. Mu and kappa opioid agonists act prejunctionally at cholinergic motor neurons to decreased release of acetylcholine, thereby reducing twitch amplitude in a concentration-dependent manner. Treatment of donor guinea pigs with opioids produces tolerance in excised strips of ileal longitudinal muscle preparations. Opioid tolerance can also be induced by *in vitro* incubation of muscle strips with opioid agonists. Administration of naloxone to tolerant-dependent longitudinal muscle-myenteric plexus preparations results in withdrawal contracture, a quantitative measure of physical dependence.

In vivo models of gastrointestinal opioid tolerance and dependence are also useful, especially for functional studies. Opioid tolerance can be demonstrated after chronic opioid treatment by diminished responsiveness to acute doses of opioid on parameters such as small intestinal propulsion. Dependence can be demonstrated by naloxone-precipitated withdrawal signs including diarrhea and weight loss. Rats and mice have been employed for these purposes. Tolerance to morphine intestinal stimulatory effects has also been demonstrated *in vivo* in anesthetized and unanesthetized dogs.

Dog isolated vascularly perfused small intestinal segments exhibit stimulatory responses to morphine characterized by contractions of circular smooth muscle. Chronic treatment of donor dogs or perfusion with opioids *ex vivo* have been shown to induce selective morphine tolerance in intestinal segments. This preparation is particularly useful in studies of the stimulatory effects of opioids.

ACKNOWLEDGMENTS

The author is grateful to Ms. Christine Goodwin for preparation of this manuscript. Supported by a U.S. Public Health Service Grant number DA02163 from the National Institute on Drug Abuse.

REFERENCES

1. **Schaumann, W.,** The paralysing action of morphine on the guinea-pig ileum, *Br. J. Pharmacol.,* 10, 456, 1955.
2. **Schaumann, W.,** Inhibition by morphine of the release of acetylcholine from the intestine of the guinea-pig, *Br. J. Pharmacol.,* 12, 115, 1957.
3. **Paton, W. D. M.,** The action of morphine and related substances on contraction and on acetylcholine output of coaxially stimulated guinea-pig ileum, *Br. J. Pharmacol.,* 12, 119, 1957.
4. **Leslie, F. M.,** Methods used for the study of opioid receptors, *Pharmacol. Rev.,* 39, 197, 1987.
5. **Rang, H. P.,** Stimulant actions of volatile anaesthetics on smooth muscle, *Br. J. Pharmacol.,* 22, 356, 1964.
6. **Kosterlitz, H. W., Lydon, R. J., and Watt, A. J.,** The effects of adrenaline, noradrenaline, and isoprenaline on inhibitory α- and β-adrenoceptors in the longitudinal muscle of the guinea-pig ileum, *Br. J. Pharmacol.,* 39, 398, 1970.
7. **Gyang, E. A., and Kosterlitz, H. W.,** Agonist and antagonist actions of morphine-like drugs on the guinea-pig ileum, *Br. J. Pharmacol.,* 27, 514, 1966.
8. **Pert, C. B., and Snyder, S. H.,** Opiate receptor: demonstration in nervous tissue, *Science (Washington),* 179, 1011, 1973.
9. **Creese, I., and Snyder, S. H.,** Receptor binding and pharmacological activity of opiates in the guinea-pig intestine. *J. Pharmacol. Exp. Ther.,* 194, 205, 1975.
10. **Lord, J. A. H., Waterfield, A. A., Hughes, J., and Kosterlitz, H. W.,** Endogenous opioid peptides: multiple agonists and receptors. *Nature (London),* 267, 495, 1977.

11. **Handa, B. K., Lane, A. C., Lord, J. A. H., Morgan, B. A., Rance, M. J., and Smith, C. F. C.,** Analogues of β-LPH$_{61-64}$ possessing selective agonist activity at μ-opiate receptors, *Eur. J. Pharmacol.,* 70, 531, 1981.

12. **Mosberg, H. I., Hurst, R., Hruby, V. J., Gee, K., Yamamura, H. I., Galligan, J. J., and Burks, T. F.,** Bis-penicillamine enkephalins possess highly improved specificity towards δ opioid receptors, *Proc. Natl. Acad. Sci. U. S. A.,* 80, 5871, 1983.

13. **Chang, K. J., Wei, E. T., Killian, A., Chang, J. K.,** Potent morphiceptin analogs: structure activity relationships and morphine-like properties. *J. Pharmacol. Exp. Ther.,* 227, 403, 1983.

14. **Davis, T. P., Gillespie, T. J., Shook, J., Kramer, T. H., Hoyer, G., Hawkins, K., Davis, P., Yamamura, H. I., and Burks, T. F.,** Changes in opioid receptor selectivity following processing of peptide E: effect on gut motility, *Gastroenterology,* 100, 1603, 1991.

15. **Chavkin, C., James, I. F., and Goldstein, A.,** Dynorphin is a specific endogenous ligand of the κ opioid receptor, *Science (Washington),* 215, 413, 1982.

16. **Cox, B. M., and Chavkin, C.,** Comparison of dynorphin-selective kappa-receptors in mouse vas deferens and guinea-pig ileum, *Molecular Pharmacology,* 23, 36, 1983.

17. **Leslie, F. M., Chavkin, C., and Cox, B. M.,** Opioid binding properties of brain and peripheral tissues: evidence for heterogenity in opioid ligand binding sites. *J. Pharmacol. Exp. Ther.,* 214, 395, 1980.

18. **Goldstein, A. and Schulz, R.,** Morphine-tolerant longitudinal muscle strip from guinea- pig ileum, *Br. J. Pharmacol.,* 48, 655, 1973.

19. **Kosterlitz, H. W. and Waterfield, A. A.,** An analysis of the phenomenon of acute tolerance to morphine in the guinea-pig isolated ileum, *Br. J. Pharmacol.,* 53, 131, 1975.

20. **Cox, B. M.,** Characteristics of the increased response to electrical stimulation of ileum preparations from morphine-treated guinea pigs, *Life Sciences,* 24, 1503, 1979.

21. **Schulz, R. and Goldstein, A.,** Morphine tolerance and supersensitivity to 5-hydroxytryptamine in the myenteric plexus of the guinea-pig, *Nature (London),* 244, 168, 1973.

22. **Schulz, R. and Cartwright, C.,** Effect of morphine on serotonin release from myenteric plexus of the guinea pig, *J. Pharmacol. Exp. Ther.,* 190, 420, 1974.

23. **Johnson, S. M. and Fleming, W. W.,** Mechanisms of cellular adaptive sensitivity changes: applications to opioid tolerance and dependence, *Pharmacol. Rev.,* 41, 435, 1989.

24. **Schulz, R. and Herz, A.,** Aspects of opiate dependence in the myenteric plexus of the guinea-pig, *Life Sci.,* 19, 1117, 1976.

25. **Rezvani, A., Huidobro-Toro, J. P., Hu, J., and Way. E. L.,** A rapid and simple method for the quantitative determination of tolerance development to opiates in the guinea-pig ileum in vitro, *J. Pharmacol. Exp. Ther.,* 225, 251, 1983.

26. **Lujan, M. and Rodriguez, R.,** Pharmacological characterization of opiate physical dependence in the isolated ileum of the guinea-pig, *Br. J. Pharmacol.,* 73, 859, 1981.

27. **Chahl, L. A.,** Contracture of guinea-pig ileum on withdrawal of methionine[5]-enkephalin is mediated by substance P, *Br. J. Pharmacol.,* 80, 741, 1983.

28. **Schulz, R.,** Opioid tolerance/dependence in isolated organs, in *Handbook of experimental Pharmacology,* Vol. 104/II, Herz, A. (ed.), Spring-Verlag, Berlin, p. 597, 1993.

29. **Gillan, M. G. C., Kosterlitz, H. W., Robson, L. E., and Waterfield, A. A.,** The inhibitory effects of presynaptic α-adrenoceptor agonists on contractions of guinea-pig ileum and mouse vas deferens in the morphine-dependent and withdrawn states produced in vitro, *Br. J. Pharmacol.,* 66, 601, 1979.

30. **Ward, A. and Takemori, A. E.,** Studies on the narcotic receptor in the guinea-pig ileum, *J. Pharmacol. Exp. Ther.,* 199, 117, 1976.

31. **Johnson, S. M., Williams, J. T., Costa, M. and Furness, J. B.,** Naloxone-induced depolarization and synaptic activation of myenteric neurons in morphine-dependent guinea-pig ileum, *Neuroscience,* 21, 595, 1987.

32. **Schulz, R., Wü, M., Rubini, P., and Herz, A.,** Functional opiate receptors in the guinea-pig ileum: their differentiation by means of selective tolerance development, *J. Pharmacol. Exp. Ther.,* 219, 547, 1981.

33. **Schulz, R., Seidl, E., Wüster, M., and Herz, A.,** Opioid dependence and cross-dependence in the isolated guinea-pig ileum, *Eur. J. Pharmacol.,* 84, 33, 1982.

34. **Schulz, R. and Herz, A.,** Opioid tolerance and dependence in light of the multiplicity of opioid receptors, *Natl. Inst. Drug Abuse Res. Monograph Series,* 54, 70, 1984.

35. **Schulz, R.,** Dependence and cross-dependence in the guinea-pig myenteric plexus, *Naunyn-Schmeideberg's Arch. Pharmacol.,* 337, 644, 1988.

36. **Taylor, D. A., Leedham, J. A., Doak, N., and Fleming, W. W.,** Morphine tolerance and nonspecific subsensitivity of the longitudinal muscle myenteric plexus preparation of the guinea-pig to inhibitory agonists, *Naunyn-Schmiedeberg's Arch. Pharmacol.,* 338, 553, 1988.

37. **Höllt, V., Dum, J., Blasig, J., Schubert, P., and Herz, A.,** Comparison of in vivo and in vitro parameters of opiate receptor binding in naive and tolerant/dependent rodents, *Life Sci.,* 16, 1823, 1975.

38. **Cox, B. M. and Padhya, R.,** Opiate binding and effect in ileum preparations from normal and morphine pretreated guinea-pigs, *Br. J. Pharmacol.,* 61, 271, 1977.

39. **Gintzler, A. R. and Scalisi, J. A.,** Effects of opioids on noncholinergic responses of the guinea pig isolated ileum: inhibition of release of substance P, *Br. J. Pharmacol.,* 75, 199, 1982.

40. **Lux, B. and Schulz, R.,** Effect of cholera toxin and pertussis toxin on opioid tolerance and dependence in the guinea-pig myenteric plexus, *J. Pharmacol. Exp. Ther.,* 237, 995, 1986.

41. **Porreca, F. and Burks, T. F.,** Affinity of normorphine for its pharmacologic receptor in the naive and morphine-tolerant guinea-pig isolated ileum. *J. Pharmacol. Exp. Ther.,* 225, 688, 1984.

42. **Chavkin, C. and Goldstein, A.,** Opioid receptor reserve in normal and morphine-tolerant guinea pig ileum myenteric plexus, *Proc. Natl. Acad. Sci. U. S. A.,* 81, 7253, 1984.

43. **Tallarida, R. J., Robinson, M. J., Porreca, F., and Cowan, A.,** Estimation of the dissociation constant of naloxone in the naive and morphine-tolerant guinea-pig isolated ileum: analysis by the constrained Schild plot, *Life Sci.,* 31, 1691, 1982.

44. **Kromer, W. and Woinoff, R.,** Peristalsis in the isolated guinea-pig ileum during opiate withdrawal. Naunyn-Schmiedeberg's *Arch. Pharmacol.,* 314, 191, 1980.

45. **Kromer, W. and Steigemann, N.,** Opiate tolerance/dependence in the isolated guinea pig ileum is associated with an increased sensitivity to acetylcholine, *Pharmacology,* 25, 294, 1982.

46. **Villarreal, J. E., Cruz, S. L., Herrera, J. E., and Salazar, L. A.,** Pharmacologic intrinsic activity in rate coupled receptor systems, *Proc. West. Pharmacol. Soc.,* 30, 373, 1987.

47. **Villarreal, J. E., Cruz, S. L., and Salazar, L. A.,** Theory for stationary state responses of drug-receptor-effector systems in the rate occupation continuum, *Proc. West. Pharmacol. Soc.,* 31, 241, 1988.

48. **Burks, T. F.,** Central sites of action of gastrointestinal drugs, *Gastroenterology,* 74, 322, 1978.

49. **Galligan, J. J. and Burks, T. F.,** Opioid peptides inhibit intestinal transit in the rat by a central mechanism, *Eur. J. Pharmacol.,* 85, 61, 1962.

50. **Porreca, F. and Burks, T. F.,** The spinal cord as a site of opioid effects on gastrointestinal transit in the mouse, *J. Pharmacol. Exp. Ther.,* 227, 22, 1983.

51. **Weisbrodt, N. W., Badial-Aceves, F., Dudrick, S. J., Burks, T. F., and Castro, G. A.,** Tolerance to the effect of morphine on intestinal transit, *Proc. Soc. Exp. Biol. Med.,* 154, 587, 1977.

52. **Way, E. L.,** Opioid tolerance and physical dependence and their relationship, in *Handbook of Experimental Pharmacology,* vol. 104/II, A. Herz (ed.), Springer-Verlag, Berlin, p. 573, 1993.

53. **Bläsig, J., Herz, A., Reinhold, K., and Zieglgänsberger, W.,** Development of physical dependence on morphine in respect to time and dosage and quantification of the precipitated withdrawal syndrome in rats, *Psychopharmacologia,* 33, 19, 1972.

54. **Way, E. L., Loh, H. H., and Shen, F. H.,** Simultaneous quantitative assessment of morphine tolerance and physical dependence, *J. Pharmacol. Exp. Ther.,* 167, 1, 1969.

55. **Shook, J. E., Pelton, J. T., Wire, W. S., Hirning, L. D., Hruby, V. J. and Burks, T. F.,** Pharmacological evaluation of a cyclic somatostatin analog with antagonist activity at mu opioid receptors in vitro, *J. Pharmacol. Exp. Ther.,* 240, 772, 1987.

56. **Shook, J. E., Pelton, J. T., Lemcke, P. K., Porreca, F., Hruby, V. J., and Burks, T. F.,** Mu opioid antagonist properties of a cyclic somatostatin octapeptide in vivo: identification of mu receptor related functions, *J. Pharmacol. Exp. Ther.,* 242, 1, 1987.

57. **Shook, J. E., Pelton, J. T., Kazmierski, W., Lemcke, P. K., Villar, R. G., Hruby, V. J., and Burks, T. F.,** A cyclic somatostatin analog that precipitates withdrawal in morphine-dependent mice, *National Institute on Drug Abuse Research Monograph,* 76, 295, 1986.

58. **Shook, J., Kazmierski, W., Hruby, V., and Burks, T. F.,** Precipitation of spinally mediated withdrawal signs by intrathecal administration of naloxone and the mu-receptor antagonist CTP in morphine-dependent mice, *National Institute on Drug Abuse Research Monograph,* 81, 143, 1988.

59. **Burks, T. F., Galligan, J. J., Hirning, L. D., and Porreca, F.,** Brain, spinal cord and peripheral sites of action of enkephalins and other endogenous opioids on gastrointestinal motility, *Gastroenterol. Clin. Biol.,* 11, 44B, 1987.

60. **Kromer, W.,** Endogenous and exogenous opioids in the control of gastrointestinal motility and secretion, *Pharmacol. Rev.,* 40, 121, 1988.

61. **Burks, T. F., Jaquette, D. L., and Grubb, M. N.,** Development of tolerance to the stimulatory effect of morphine in dog intestine, *Eur. J. Pharmacol.,* 25, 302, 1974.

62. **Burks, T. F., Castro, G. A., and Weisbrodt, N. W.,** Tolerance to intestinal stimulatory actions of morphine, in *Opiates and Endogenous Opioid Peptides,* Kosterlitz, H. W. (ed.), North-Holland, Amsterdam, p. 369, 1976.

63. **Weisbrodt, N. W., Thor, P. J. Copeland, E. M. and Burks, T. F.,** Tolerance to the effects of morphine on intestinal motility of unanesthetized dogs, *J. Pharmacol. Exp. Ther.,* 215, 515, 1980.

64. **Hirning, L. D., Porreca, F., and Burks, T. F.,** Mu, but not kappa, opioid agonists induce contractions of the canine intestine, ex vivo, *Eur. J. Pharmacol.,* 109, 49, 1985.

65. **Burks, T. F. and Long, J. P.,** Responses of isolated dog small intestine to analgesic agents, *J. Pharmacol. Exp. Ther.,* 158, 264, 1967.

66. **Burks, T. F. and Grubb, M. N.,** Sites of acute morphine tolerance in intestine, *J. Pharmacol. Exp. Ther.,* 191, 518, 1974.

17 Methods for Studying Splanchnic Blood Flow

Karen D. Crissinger and D. Neil Granger

INTRODUCTION

Milestones in development of techniques to measure intestinal blood flow in the modern era began in 1868 when Carl Ludwig invented the stromuhr, or "stream clock".[1] This device was first used in the splanchnic circulation by Burton-Opitz[2] in 1908. By the early 1940s, the intestinal circulatory relationships to absorption and secretion had been described. The next significant advance in techniques came from Grim and Lindseth[3] in 1958 when the microsphere technique made possible the measurement of the distribution of intestinal blood flow among the various layers of the bowel wall. Development of the arteriovenous oxygen content difference analyzer by Shepherd[4] in 1977 provided a means to continuously monitor the interactions between intestinal blood flow and oxygenation. In 1982, Shepherd[5] introduced the laser-Doppler flowmeter for continuous measurement of mucosal and muscularis blood flow.

This chapter will discuss many of the techniques currently available for measurement of gastrointestinal perfusion. Although none of the currently employed techniques fulfills the criteria outlined by Jacobson[6] for the ideal method, i.e., safe, noninvasive, continuous, quantitative, accurate, reproducible, measures intramural distribution, and does not alter blood flow, all of these methods do appear to provide a useful measure of tissue perfusion in the splanchnic circulation. For ease of comparison, these techniques have been divided into those used to measure total organ blood flow versus those employed for determination of blood flow distribution among layers of the bowel wall.

TECHNIQUES MEASURING TOTAL ORGAN BLOOD FLOW

VENOUS OUTFLOW

This technique measures blood flow by timed collections of venous blood draining the intestine. It is the gold-standard against which other techniques for measuring blood flow are validated. Continuous measurements may also be performed by using a drop counter. A disadvantage is that this technique cannot be used in the clinical setting or in chronic animal studies. It also provides no information on flow distribution to different layers or regions in an organ; and the organ or segment under study must be drained by a single vein.[7]

ELECTROMAGNETIC FLOW

Blood flow measurement using electromagnetic flow probes is based on the principle of electromagnetic induction by flowing blood. It requires cannulation of a vessel or placement of a perivascular sensor to measure volume flow. This technique allows continuous, instantaneous, and quantitative measurement of flow. The use of perivascular sensors allows for the vessel to remain intact, doesn't interfere with flow, permits flow measurement in situ, and can be used in acute or chronic animal studies. The major disadvantages of this technique are its invasiveness and the need to occlude the vessel to obtain zero flow calibration. Flow must also be temporarily interrupted to insert a cannulating flow probe; or the perivascular cuff may disturb the nervous supply surrounding the vessel during its placement.[8]

PULSED DOPPLER

The pulsed Doppler technique for measuring blood flow involves placement of a single piezoelectric crystal that emits a 20 mHz ultrasonic signal. The same crystal receives the reflected signal from passing red blood cells in the interval between ultrasonic pulses. The major advantages include continuous measurements, chronic implantation of multiple flow probes in small animals, minimal interference of vessels during placement of the crystals, and the capability of determining zero flow electronically. The disadvantages of this technique are the necessity for surgical implantation and the inability to measure volume flow quantitatively (although percentage change in flow can be calculated accurately).[9–10]

DOPPLER FLOWMETRY

The technique of Doppler flowmetry involves measurement of the average velocity of moving red blood cells using an ultrasonic duplex scanner to combine pulsed Doppler with real-time imaging. The velocity obtained is multiplied by the cross-sectional area of the vessel to obtain volume flow. The advantages are that it is a non-invasive method that does not use ionizing radiation. The disadvantages are multiple. A major source of error in determining *absolute* blood flow involves estimation of the average velocity which varies across the vessel diameter and is affected by vessel size, geometry, and wall composition as well as the cardiac and respiratory cycles. The angle of insonation also affects estimation of average velocity. The cosine of the angle of Doppler shift frequency is used in the calculation and the error thus increases with the angle. Another source of error is determination of the vessel cross-sectional area, particularly in veins which are not perfectly circular and whose diameter can change with respiration and alterations in intravascular pressure. Small errors in measurement of diameter lead to large errors in cross-sectional area. Thus, due to the magnitude of potential errors in flow estimation, the use of Doppler ultrasound to make absolute measurements of flow is considered unreliable. Nonetheless, this technique may be useful to measure *changes* in flow in the same vessel over time. Repeated measurements in the individual subject do, however, exhibit a large variability in baseline flow. Group data may be more reliable because changes in baseline flow are minimized.[11–13]

TECHNIQUES MEASURING FRACTIONATED BLOOD FLOW

RADIOACTIVE MICROSPHERES

Measurement of blood flow with radioactive microspheres is based on the assumption that the number of microspheres trapped in an organ is proportional to blood flow. In the intestinal circulation, the microsphere technique has long been used to measure intramural distribution of blood flow. Although this method has no clinical applicability, it has been widely used in animals to study blood flow to organs without manipulation of the vessels supplying those organs. Disadvantages of the technique, however, are that only single measurements of flow in time can be made, flow may be underestimated due to arteriovenous shunting of spheres or movement of spheres after injection due to vasodilation, and microspheres may be impeded from reaching some tissues in series-coupled vascular beds if the size of the spheres exceeds 12 μm.[14–17]

Aminopyrine Clearance

The aminopyrine clearance method capitalizes on the fact that aminopyrine is a weak base which is freely permeable in tissues at pH 7 and above. At a pH less than 3, however, it dissociates and is no longer permeable. In the stomach, it is cleared from gastric mucosal blood, diffuses into the gastric lumen, and becomes "trapped" via dissociation at a pH of 3 in the

TABLE 1
Summary of Techniques Used to Measure Total Organ Blood Flow

Technique	Clinical Applicability	Major Advantages	Major Disadvantages
Venous outflow	No	1. Easy/accurate 2. Repeated measurements possible	1. No application to clinical or chronic animal studies 2. Organ or segment must be drained by single vein
Electromagnetic flowmeter	No	1. Continuous instantaneous, and quantitative 2. Perivascular sensors leave the vessel intact, do not interfere with flow, and permit flow measurement *in situ* 3. Can be used in chronic animal studies	1. Invasive 2. Must occlude vessel to obtain zero flow calibration 3. Must interrupt flow to insert cannulating flow probe 4. Disturbs perivascular nervous supply when placing non-cannulating cuff on vessel 5. Requires intimate vessel-probe contact
Pulsed Doppler flowmeter	No	1. Continuous measurement 2. Chronic, long-term implantation of crystals 3. Minimal interference with vessel during placement of crystal 4. Can determine zero flow electronically	1. Necessity for surgical implantation 2. Inability to measure volume flow quantitatively 3. Affected by vessel diameter 4. Susceptible to local radiofrequency transmissions (e.g. taxis, television stations)
Duplex Doppler flowmetry	Yes	1. Noninvasive 2. Useful to measure *changes* in flow 3. Problems with individual variations in baseline flow minimized by using group data	1. Unreliable *absolute* flow measurements (see text) 2. Repeated measurements in individual subjects show large variability in baseline flow

Reprinted with permission from Crissinger, K. D. and Granger, D. N., in *Splanchnic Ischemia and Multiple Organ Failure,* Maraton, A., Bulldey, G. B., Fiddian-Green, R. G., and Haglund, U. H., Edward Arnold, London, 1989, 42.

gastric lumen. Gastric mucosal clearance of aminopyrine should provide an accurate estimate of gastric mucosal blood flow if: 1) aminopyrine is completely cleared by the gastric mucosa from the circulation in a single passage, 2) aminopyrine is not actively transported into the gastric lumen, and 3) clearance of aminopyrine is blood flow limited. The major advantages of this technique are that it measures gastric mucosal (rather than total) blood flow, it provides a continuous measurement of blood flow, it can be used in unanesthetized animals and humans, and it provides simultaneous acid secretory data. It has been used extensively for studying the relationship of mucosal blood flow to gastric acid secretion during the administration of various agents. Major disadvantages of this technique include significant metabolism of ^{14}C-aminopyrine within the body, dependence of the clearance calculation on the volume of acid secretion, and significant overestimation of blood flow at high rates of blood flow, suggesting that aminopyrine clearance measures a combination of blood flow and parietal cell activity.[18-20]

USE OF INERT GAS

Inert gases rapidly diffuse into tissues due to their high lipid solubility. The rate of elimination of an inert gas from a tissue is flow-limited and therefore flow rates in whole organs or parts of organs can be estimated from the rate of washout of radioactive isotopes of inert gases ([133]xenon and [85]krypton). An inert gas may be introduced into a tissue via the intravascular route or by injecting it directly into the tissue. In the intestine the gas may be placed into the intestinal lumen or into the peritoneal space. The major advantages of this technique are that no sampling of blood or tissue is necessary and clinical applications are possible. Disadvantages include the fact that it is a discontinuous measurement of blood flow, flow must be constant during the entire measurement period (15 min), trauma to the microvasculature may occur from injection into the tissue, and countercurrent exchange may significantly affect mucosal blood flow estimates in the small intestine.[21-22]

IODOANTIPYRINE CLEARANCE

The technique of iodoantipyrine clearance is based on the assumption that this highly diffusible tracer distributes in tissue as a function of the rate of blood flow to the tissue. The major advantages of this method are that the spatial resolution is so well-defined that blood flow can be measured even in single villi, it is minimally affected by the countercurrent exchange mechanism, regional flow and microscopic anatomy can be closely correlated, and there is no need for anesthesia or surgery before measuring blood flow. Major disadvantages include the need for biopsy specimens, blood flow measurement is discontinuous, fluid in the lumen leads to underestimation of blood flow due to diffusion of iodoantipyrine into this compartment, and radioactive material must be used.[23-25]

HYDROGEN CLEARANCE

The hydrogen gas clearance technique is based on the principle that the disappearance of hydrogen, a highly diffusible, biologically inert gas, from a perfused tissue is determined by the rate of venous outflow from that tissue. A 3% hydrogen-20% oxygen mixture is inhaled and a platinum electrode (which can be affixed to an endoscope) that is in contact with the tissue surface generates a current that is proportional to the hydrogen concentration in the tissue. The advantages of this technique are its clinical applicability to the stomach and colon without the need for anesthesia or laparotomy and the capability of using a nontoxic, nonradioactive marker. Also, no tissue destruction or vessel cannulation is required. The disadvantages are that

TABLE 2
Summary of Techniques Used to Measure Fractionated Blood Flow

Technique	Clinical Applicability	Major Advantages	Major Disadvantages
Microspheres	No	1. Can determine distribution of flow within an organ 2. No vessel manipulation 3. Five or six measurements can be made without disturbing tissue	1. Discontinuous measurement 2. Possible underestimation of flow due to shunting or movement of spheres after injection 3. Impedence of spheres from reaching some tissue layers due to sphere size ($> 12 \ \mu m$)
Aminopyrine clearance	Yes	1. Measures gastric mucosal blood flow 2. Can be measured continuously 3. Can be used in chronic studies 4. Provides simultaneous acid secretory data	1. Metabolism of ^{14}C-aminopyrine within the body leads to overestimation of flow 2. Clearance calculation is dependent on volume of acid secretion 3. Overestimation of blood flow at high flow rates
Inert gas washout	Yes	1. Sampling of blood/tissue unnecessary 2. Clinical application possible 3. May instill intraluminal gas to measure small intestinal blood flow 4. May instill IP gas to evaluate ischemic intestine	1. Discontinuous measurement 2. Countercurrent exchange may affect results in small intestine 3. Tissue injection causes microvascular injury 4. Equipment costly and interpretation of washout curves complex
Iodoantipyrine clearance	Yes (Endoscopy)	1. Minimally affected by counter-current exchange 2. Can measure flow in very small dimensions including simple villi 3. No need for anesthesia or surgery 4. Can closely correlate regional flow and microscopic anatomy	1. Needs biopsy specimens 2. Discontinuous measurement 3. Luminal fluid leads to underestimation of blood flow 4. Requires radioactive tracer
Hydrogen gas clearance	Yes (Endoscopy)	1. Non-toxic and non-radioactive tracer 2. Clinically applicable 3. No tissue destruction 4. No vessel manipulation 5. No anesthesia or surgery	1. Discontinuous, focal measurement 2. Constant flow for 15–30 minutes required 3. May alter blood flow due to tissue compression or mechanical stimulation by platinum electrode 4. Affected by countercurrent exchange in small intestine
Laser Doppler velocimetry	Yes (Endoscopy)	1. Continuous measurement 2. Unaffected by countercurrent exchange 3. Potential clinical applications	1. Depth of resolution not clarified 2. No absolute units of blood flow 3. May alter blood flow due to tissue compression or mechanical stimulation 4. Difficulty in maintaining constant optical coupling due to tissue motion 5. Decreased correlation with total blood flow as flow Increases

TABLE 2
(*continued*)

Technique	Clinical Applicability	Major Advantages	Major Disadvantages
In vivo microscopy	No	1. Correlation of intestinal vascular responses to specific types, sizes, and tissue locations of microvessels 2. Determination of flow to discrete layers or regions in an organ	1. No clinical application 2. Cannot use in chronic animal studies 3. Requires surgical manipulation to exteriorize tissue 4. Optical resolution of system may limit the accurate determination of vessel diameter and RBC velocity

Reprinted with permission from Crissinger, K. D. and Granger, D. N., in *Splanchnic Ischemia and Multiple Organ Failure,* Maraton, A., Bulkley, G. B., Fiddian-Green, R. G., and Haglund, U. H., Edward Arnold, London, 1989, 44.

it provides discontinuous measurement of flow, and blood flow must be constant during the 15–30 minute measurement period. The platinum electrode may alter blood flow due to tissue compression or mechanical stimulation. Countercurrent exchange limits its application in the small intestine of some species. Finally, the spatial (depth) resolution of the technique remains uncertain.[24,26–30]

LASER DOPPLER VELOCIMETRY

This technique works on the principle that light scattered by moving red cells undergoes a shift in frequency such that the mean Doppler frequency provides an estimate of blood flow. Fiber optic guides, which conduct laser light to the tissue and return scattered light back to a photodetector, are placed directly on the tissue of interest. The advantages of the technique are that it provides a continuous measurement and it is unaffected by countercurrent exchange in the small intestine. It also can be used clinically via endoscopy without the need for anesthesia or surgery. There are, however, major difficulties associated with this method. The depth resolution has not been clarified, with some investigators finding a resolution of 0.5–1.0 mm while others give a value > 3 mm, which roughly corresponds to total intestinal thickness. Another problem with this method is that it does not provide a measure of blood flow in absolute units. There is also difficulty in maintaining constant optical coupling between the probe and tissue, due to peristalsis. Finally, blood flow may be altered due to tissue compression or mechanical stimulation by the flow probe.[24,27,31–35]

IN VIVO MICROSCOPY

Using direct visualization of microvessels and photometric measurement of red blood cell velocity, blood flow is calculated from measurements of vessel cross-sectional area and red blood cell velocity. The upper limit of vessel diameter for accurate measurement of velocities is about 70 μm. Advantages of the technique are 1) the capability of correlating intestinal vascular responses to specific types, sizes, and tissue locations of microvessels and 2) the capability of determining flow to discrete layers or regions in an organ. Disadvantages of the technique include the need for anesthesia, the necessity of surgical manipulation and exterioriza-

TABLE 3
Resting Blood Flow Values and Transmural Distribution (ml min^{-1} 100 g^{-1})

		Stomach	Small Intestine	Large Intestine	References
Human	Total wall		8–77	8–44	38–40
	Mucosa-submucosa[b,d]	38–77	7–103	9–55	29,38–40
	Muscle-serosa[d]		5–38	10–34	40–41
Dog	Total wall	20–45	30–80	30–74	41–50
	Mucosa-submucosa[a,b]	23–110	58–87	91–112	26–27,30,50
	Muscle-serosa	13–24	27–49	12–48	41,50
Cat	Total wall	26–32	20–78	11–39	35,39,40,51–54
	Mucosa-submucosa[a]	35–42	42–119	13–58	39–40,53,55
	Muscle-serosa		7.5–18	1.1–17	39–40,53
Rat	Total wall	32–118	68–346	29–87	56–60
	Mucosa-submucosa[a,b,c]	23–136	75–140	30–41	25,28–29,60
	Muscle-serosa	2	2.5–7.5	1–5	60
Piglet					
1 day	Total wall		40–128	22–53	61–63
	Mucosa-submucosa[a]		50–78		63
	Muscle-serosa		20–38		63
3 day	Total wall	75–140	55–188	33–118	61–62,64–66,=
	Mucosa-submucosa[a]		95–237		65–66,=
	Muscle-serosa		15–95		65–66,=
2 week	Total wall		49–96	35–52	67–68,=
	Mucosa-submucosa[a]		57–102		=
	Muscle-serosa		43–49		=
1 mo	Total wall		27–57	19–49	61,63–64,=
	Mucosa-submucosa[a]		30–60		63
	Muscle-serosa		10–20		63

[a]Radioactive microspheres, [b]H$_2$ gas clearance, [c]iodo(^{14}C)antipyrine, [d]Inert gas washout. = from unpublished data for expts. from Crissinger K. D., Granger D. N.[63]

Reprinted with permission from Crissinger, K. D. and Granger, D. N., in *Textbook of Gastroenterology,* Yamada, T., Alpers, D. H., Owyang C., Powell, D. W., and Silverstein, F. E., J. B. Lippincott Company, Philadelphia, 1995.

tion of the tissue, and optical resolution which can limit the accurate determination of vessel diameter and red cell velocity.[36–37]

Recently hydrogen gas clearance has become available as a noninvasive means to measure gastric and colonic blood flow endoscopically in humans. Laser Doppler flowmetry is also amenable to measurement of changes in gastric and colonic blood flow, although absolute units and spatial resolution remain to be clarified. Experimental animals are used extensively to study gastrointestinal blood flow, with possible applications to human disease states. Tables 1 and 2 compare and contrast the various techniques used to measure intestinal blood flow and indicate whether they may be applied for clinical use. Table 3 summarizes basal values of total and fractionated blood flow obtained in several commonly used experimental animals. One must be cognizant that widely variable values have been obtained within a given experimental preparation or model.

It is important to point out that measurements of indices of oxygenation are crucial in evaluating the relationship of changes in blood flow to gastrointestinal function and pathology. Tissue oxygen uptake can be estimated from the product of blood flow and arteriovenous oxygen

TABLE 4

Resting Values for Arteriovenous Oxygen Content Difference (ml O_2/100ml), Oxygen Uptake (ml min^{-1} $\cdot$ 100 g^{-1}) and Tissue pO_2 (mm Hg)

		Stomach	Small Intestine	Large Intestine	References
Dog	A-V O_2 difference	3.0–3.7	3.5–4.5	3.0–4.4	34,43–44,47–49
	Oxygen uptake	1.0–1.5	1.5–2.2	1.56–1.68	34,42–44,46–49,69
Cat	A-V O_2 difference		4.6		52
	Oxygen uptake		1.4		52
Rat	A-V O_2 difference		4.5		56
	Oxygen uptake		4.8		56
	Villous pO_2		14–17		37,71
	Muscle pO_2		21–26		37,71
Piglet					
1 day	A-V O_2 difference		3.4–3.8		61–62
	Oxygen uptake		2.9–4.3		61–62
3 day	A-V O_2 difference		3.1–4.2		61–62,64,66
	Oxygen uptake		2.0–2.9		61–62,64–66
2 week	A-V O_2 difference		3.3–4.8		61–62
	Oxygen uptake		2.4–3.0		61–62
1 month	A-V O_2 difference		4.3–4.5		61,64,69
	Oxygen uptake		1.8–2.4		61,64,69

Reprinted with permission from Crissinger, K. D. and Granger, D. N., in *Textbook of Gastroenterology,* Yamada, T., Alpers, D. H., Owyang C., Powell, D. W., and Silverstein, F. E., J. B. Lippincott Company, Philadelphia, 1995.

difference. In addition, there are a limited number of studies that have utilized measurements of tissue oxygen tension as an index of tissue oxygenation.

Table 4 lists representative values for resting arteriovenous oxygen difference, oxygen uptake and tissue pO_2 (where available).

SUMMARY AND CONCLUSIONS

Several techniques are available for the measurement of total and fractionated blood flow in the splanchnic circulation. None of the methods in current use fulfills the criteria outlined by Jacobson as being ideal, i.e., safe, noninvasive, continuous, quantitative, accurate, reproducible, measures intramural distribution, and does not alter blood flow, particularly as relates to clinical application. Nonetheless, each of these methods provides a useful measure of tissue perfusion which, when combined with measurements of tissue oxygenation, may facilitate our understanding of the relationships among ischemia, tissue hypoxia, and subsequent mucosal injury.

REFERENCES

1. **Granger, D. N. and Shepherd, A. P.,** The intestinal circulation: a historical perspective, in *Physiology of the Intestinal Circulation,* Shepherd, A. P. and Granger, D. N., Eds., Raven Press, New York, 1984, 4.

2. **Burton-Opitz, R.,** Ueber die stroemung des blutes in dem frebiete der pfortader, *Arch f ges Physiol,* 124, 469, 1908.

3. **Grim, E. and Lindseth, E. O.,** Distribution of blood flow to the tissues of the small intestine of the dog, *Univ Minn Med Bull,* 30, 138, 1958.

4. **Shepherd, A. P. and Burgar, C. G.,** A solid state arteriovenous oxygen difference analyzer for flowing whole blood, *Am J Physiol,* 232, H437, 1977.

5. **Shepherd, A. P. and Riedel, G. L.,** Continuous measurement of intestinal mucosal blood flow by laser-Doppler flowmetry, *Am J Physiol,* 242, G668, 1982.

6. **Jacobson, E. D.,** Criteria for an ideal method of measuring blood flow to a splanchnic organ, in *Measurement of Blood Flow: Applications to the Splanchnic Circulation,* Granger, D. N. and Bulkley, G. B., Eds., Williams & Wilkins, Baltimore, 1981, 5.

7. **Larsen, K. R. and Moody, F. G.,** Selection of appropriate methodology for the measurement of blood flow in the gut, in *Measurement of Blood Flow: Applications to the Splanchnic Circulation,* Granger, D. N. and Bulkley, G. B., Eds., Williams & Wilkins, Baltimore, 1981, 514.

8. **Charbon, G. A. and Van Der Mark, F.,** Use of electromagnetic flowmeters for the study of splanchnic blood flow, in *Measurement of Blood Flow: Applications to the Splanchnic Circulation,* Granger, D. N. and Bulkley, G. B., Eds., Williams & Wilkins, Baltimore, 1981, 125.

9. **Haywood, J. R., Shaffer, R. A., Fastenow, C., et al.** Regional blood flow measurement with pulsed Doppler flowmeter in conscious rat, *Am J Physiol,* 241, H273, 1981.

10. **Van Orden, D. E., Farley, D. B., Fastenow, C., and Brody, M. J.,** A technique for monitoring blood flow changes with miniaturized Doppler flow probes, *Am J Physiol,* 247, H1005, 1984.

11. **Burns, P. N. and Jaffe, C. C.,** Quantitative flow measurements with Doppler ultrasound: techniques, accuracy and limitations, *Radiol Clin North Am,* 23, 641, 1985.

12. **Gill, R. W.,** Measurement of blood flow by ultrasound: accuracy and sources or error, *Ultrasound Med Biol,* 11, 625, 1985.

13. **Gibson, R. N., Gibson, P. R., Donlan, J. D., and Padmanabhan, R.,** Modified Doppler flowmetry in the splanchnic circulation, *Gastroenterology,* 105, 1029, 1993.

14. **Dregelid, E., Haukaas, S., Amundsen, S., et al,** Microsphere method in measurement of blood flow to wall layers of small intestine, *Am J Physiol,* 250, G670, 1986.

15. **Maxwell, L. C., Shepherd, A. P., and McMahan, C. A.,** Microsphere passage through intestinal circulation: via shunts or capillaries?, *Am J Physiol,* 248, H217, 1985.

16. **Maxwell, L. C., Shepherd, A. P., and Riedel, G. L.,** Vasodilation or altered perfusion pressure moves 15-um spheres trapped in the gut wall, *Am J Physiol,* 243, H123, 1982.

17. **Maxwell, L. C., Shepherd, A. P., Riedel, G. L., and Morris, M. D.,** Effect of microsphere size on apparent intramural distribution of intestinal blood flow, *Am J Physiol,* 241, H408, 1981.

18. **Kauffman, G. L. and Grossman, M. I.,** Use of aminopyrine clearance as a measure of gastric mucosal blood flow, in *Measurement of Blood Flow: Applications to the Splanchnic Circulation,* Granger, D. N. and Bulkley, G. B., Eds., Williams & Wilkins, Baltimore, 1981, 203.

19. **Holm-Rutili, L. and Berglindh, T.,** Pentagastrin and gastric mucosal blood flow, *Am J Physiol,* 250, G575, 1986.

20. **Sack, J. and Spenney, J. G.,** Aminopyrine accumulation by mammalian gastric glands: an analysis of the technique, *Am J Physiol,* 243, G313, 1982.

21. **Lundgren, O.,** Use of inert gas washout for studying blood flow and flow distribution in the intestine, in *Measurement of Blood Flow: Applications to the Splanchnic Circulation,* Granger, D. N. and Bulkley, G. B., Eds., Williams & Wilkins, Baltimore, 1981, 227.

22. **Gharagozloo, F., Bulkley, G. B., Zuidema, G. D., et al,** The use of intraperitoneal xenon for early diagnosis of acute mesenteric ischemia, *Surgery,* 95, 404, 1985.

23. **Dugas, M. C. and Wechsler, R. L.,** Validity of iodoantipyrine clearance for measuring gastrointestinal tissue blood flow, *Am J Physiol,* 243, G155, 1982.

24. **Granger, D. N. and Kvietys, P. R.,** Recent advances in measurement of gastrointestinal blood flow, *Gastroenterology,* 88, 1073, 1985.

25. **Hudson, D., Scremin, O. U., and Guth, P. H.,** Measurement of regional gastroduodenal blood flow with Iodo (^{14}C) antipyrine autoradiography, *Am J Physiol,* 248, G539, 1985.

26. **Ashley, S. W. and Cheung, L. Y.,** Measurements of gastric mucosal blood flow by hydrogen gas clearance, *Am J Physiol,* 247, G339, 1984.

27. **Gana, T. J., Huhlewych, R., and Koo, J.,** Focal gastric mucosal blood flow by laser-Doppler and hydrogen gas clearance: a comparative study, *J Surg Research,* 43, 337, 1987.

28. **Leung, F. W., Guth, P. H., Scremin, O. U., et al.,** Regional gastric mucosal blood flow measurements by hydrogen gas clearance in the anesthetized rat and rabbit, *Gastroenterology,* 87, 28, 1984.

29. **Murakami, M., Moriga, M., Miyake, T., and Uchino, H.,** Contact electrode method in hydrogen gas clearance technique: a new method for determination of regional gastric mucosal blood flow in animals and humans, *Gastroenterology,* 82, 457, 1982.

30. **Soybel, D. I., Wan, Y. L., Ashley, S. W., et al,** Endoscopic measurements of canine colonic mucosal blood flow using hydrogen gas clearance, *Gastroenterology,* 92, 1045, 1987.

31. **Ahn, H., Lindhagen, J., Nilsson, G. E., et al,** Assessment of blood flow in the small intestine with laser Doppler flowmetry, *Scand J Gastroenterology,* 21, 863, 1986.

32. **Ahn, H., Lindhagen, J., and Lundgren, O.,** Measurement of colonic blood flow with laser Doppler flowmetry, *Scand J Gastroenterology,* 21, 871, 1986.

33. **DiResta, G. R., Kiel, J. W., Riedel, G. L., et al,** Hybrid blood flow probe for simultaneous H_2 clearance and laser-Doppler velocimetry, *Am J Physiol,* 253, G573, 1987.

34. **Kiel, J. W., Riedel, G. L., and Shepherd, A. P.,** Local control of canine gastric mucosal blood flow, *Gastroenterology,* 93, 1041, 1987.

35. **Kvietys, P. R., Shepherd, A. P., and Granger, D. N.,** Laser-Doppler, H_2 clearance, and microsphere estimates of mucosal blood flow, *Am J Physiol,* 249, G221, 1985.

36. **Bohlen, H. G.,** *In vivo* microscopy of the intestinal microcirculation, in *Measurement of Blood Flow: Applications to the Splanchnic Circulation,* Granger, D. N. and Bulkley, G. B., Eds., Williams & Wilkins, Baltimore, 1981, 89.

37. **Bohlen, H. G.,** Intestinal tissue pO_2 and microvascular responses during glucose exposure, *Am J Physiol,* 238, H164, 1980.

38. **Forrester, D. W., Spence, V. A., and Walker, W. F.,** The measurement of colonic mucosal-submucosal blood flow in man, *J Physiol (London),* 299, 1, 1980.

39. **Hulten, L., Jodal, M., Lindhagen, J., and Lundgren, O.,** Colonic blood flow in the cat and man as analyzed by an inert gas washout technique, *Gastroenterology,* 70, 36, 1976.

40. **Hulten, L., Lindhagen, J., and Lundgren, O.,** Sympathetic nervous control of intramural blood flow in the feline and human intestines, *Gastroenterology,* 72, 41, 1977.

41. **Kvietys, P. R. and Granger, D. N.,** Regulation of colonic blood flow, *Fed Proc,* 41, 2106, 1982.

42. **Kvietys, P. R., Miller, T., and Granger, D. N.,** Intrinsic control of colonic blood flow and oxygenation, *Am J Physiol,* 128, G478, 1980.

43. **Granger, H. J. and Norris, C. P.,** Intrinsic regulation of intestinal oxygenation in the anesthetized dog, *Am J Physiol,* 238, H836, 1980.

44. **Shepherd, A. P. and Riedel, G. L.,** Optimal hematoctrit for oxygenation of canine intestine, *Circ Res,* 51, 233, 1982.

45. **Kiel, J. W. and Shepherd, A. P.,** Optimal hematocrit for canine gastric oxygenation, *Am J Physiol,* 256, H472, 1989.

46. **Kiel, J. W., Riedel, G. L., and Shepherd, A. P.,** Effects of hemodilution on gastric and intestinal oxygenation, *Am J Physiol,* 256, H171, 1989.

47. **Bulkley, G. B., Kvietys, P. R., Perry, M. A., and Granger, D. N.,** Effects of cardiac tamponade on colonic hemodynamics and oxygen uptake, *Am J Physiol,* 244, G604, 1983.

48. **Kvietys, P. R. and Granger, D. N.,** Relation between intestinal blood flow and oxygen uptake, *Am J Physiol,* 242, G202, 1982.

49. **Perry, M. A., Bulkley, G. B., Kvietys, P. R., and Granger, D. N.,** Regulation of oxygen uptake in resting and pentagastrin-stimulated canine stomach, *Am J Physiol,* 242, G565, 1982.

50. **Chou, C. C. and Grassmick, B.,** Motility and blood flow distribution within the wall of the gastrointestinal tract, *Am J Physiol,* 235, H34, 1978.

51. **Granger, D. N., Richardson, P. D. I., and Taylor, A. E.,** Volumetric assessment of the capillary filtration coefficient in the cat small intestine, *Pfluegers Arch,* 381, 25, 1979.

52. **Granger, D. N., Kvietys, P. R., and Perry, M. A.,** Role of exchange vessels in the regulation of intestinal oxygenation, *Am J Physiol,* 242, G570, 1982.

53. **Premen, A. J., Banchs, V., Womack, W. A., et al.** Importance of collateral circulation in the vascularly occluded feline intestine, *Gastroenterology,* 92, 1215, 1987.

54. **Kvietys, P. R., Smith, M. S., Grisham, M. B., and Manci, E. A.,** 5-Aminosalicylic acid protects against ischemia/reperfusion-induced gastric bleeding in the rat, *Gastroenterology* 94, 733, 1988.

55. **Groenbech, J. E., Matre, K., Stangeland, L., Svanes, K., and Varhaug, J. E.,** Gastric mucosal repair in the cat: role of the hyperemic response to mucosal damage, *Gastroenterology,* 95, 311, 1988.

56. **Anzueto, L., Benoit, J. N., and Granger, D. N.,** A rat model for studying the intestinal circulation, *Am J Physiol,* 246, G56, 1984.

57. **Hernandez, L. A., Kvietys, P. R., and Granger, D. N.,** Postprandial hemodynamics in the conscious rat, *Am J Physiol,* 251, G117, 1986.

58. **Ulrich-Baker, M. G., Hollwarth, M. E., Kvietys, P. R., and Granger, D. N.,** Blood flow responses to small bowel resection, *Am J Physiol,* 251, G815, 1986.

59. **Tuma, R. F., Vasthare, U. S., Irion, G. L., and Wiedeman, M. P.,** Considerations in use of microspheres for flow measurements in anesthetized rat, *Am J Physiol,* 250, H137, 1986.

60. **Benoit, J. N., Womack, W. A., Korthuis, R. J., Wilborn, W. H., and Granger, D. N.,** Chronic portal hypertension: effects on gastrointestinal blood flow distribution, *Am J Physiol,* 250, G535, 1986.

61. **Crissinger, K. D., Kvietys, P. R., and Granger, D. N.,** Developmental intestinal vascular responses to venous pressure elevation, *Am J Physiol,* 254, G658, 1988.

62. **Crissinger, K. D. and Granger, D. N.,** Intestinal blood flow and oxygen consumption: responses to hemorrhage in the developing piglet, *Pediatr Res,* 26, 102, 1989.

63. **Crissinger, K. D. and Granger, D. N.,** Characterization of intestinal collateral blood flow in the developing piglet, *Pediatr Res,* 24, 473, 1988.

64. **Nowicki, P. T. and Miller, C. E.,** Autoregulation in the developing postnatal intestinal circulation, *Am J Physiol,* 254, G189, 1988.

65. **Szabo, J. S., Mayfield, S. R., Oh, W., and Stonestreet, B. S.,** Postprandial gastrointestinal blood flow and oxygen consumption: effects of hypoxemia in neonatal piglets, *Pediatr Res,* 21, 93, 1987.

66. **Nowicki, P. T., Stonestreet, B. S., Hansen, N. B., Yao, A. C., and Oh, W.,** Gastrointestinal blood flow and oxygen consumption in awake newborn piglets: effect of feeding, *Am J Physiol,* 245, G697, 1983.

67. **Mortillaro, N. A. and Taylor, A. E.,** Interaction of capillary and tissue forces in the cat small intestine, *Circ Res,* 39, 348, 1976.

68. **Grogaard, B., Parks, D. A., Granger, D. N. et al.,** Effects of ischemia and oxygen radicals on mucosal albumin clearance in intestine, *Am J Physiol,* 242, G448, 1982.

69. **Crissinger, K. D., Kvietys, P. R., and Granger, D. N.,** Autoregulatory escape from norepinephrine infusion: roles of adenosine and histamine, *Am J Physiol,* 254, G560, 1988.

70. **Bulkley, G. B., Kvietys, P. R., Parks, D. A., et al,** Relationship of blood flow and oxygen consumption to ischemic injury in the canine small intestine, *Gastroenterology,* 89, 852, 1985.

71. **Bohlen, H. G.,** Intestinal mucosal oxygenation influences absorptive hyperemia, *Am J Physiol,* 239, H489, 1980.

18 Isolation and Characterization of Rat Intestinal Mucosal Mast Cells

Elyse Y. Bissonnette, Beth Chin, and A. Dean Befus

INTRODUCTION

Mast cells (MC) are found throughout the body, often closely associated with the nervous system or the vasculature.[1–3] Their presence in the gastrointestinal tract has been known for several decades, although until the mid 1960s, there was significant controversy about their abundance.[4,5] This was because formalin-based fixatives, normally used in histology, inhibit dye binding to this MC type. In 1966, Enerbáck rigorously defined appropriate fixation and staining procedures so that that gastrointestinal mucosa could be characterized as a tissue with an abundance of MC.[6]

Gastrointestinal MC can be found in the lamina propria, the submucosa, the epithelium, the muscularis mucosa and the muscle.[6–8] MC hyperplasia is characteristic of several inflammatory bowel diseases such as celiac disease, ulcerative colitis, and Crohn's disease, as well as reflux gastritis and chronic gastritis.[9–12] Although MC appear to be important in these diseases, there are few studies on the pharmacological characteristics of human intestinal mucosal MC because it is difficult to acquire the tissues, and isolate and purify these cells. In addition, the impressive heterogeneity among MC populations makes their study challenging.

MAST CELL HETEROGENEITY

The heterogeneity of MC within rodent tissues is well documented.[13–17] There are at least two distinct populations of MC: connective tissue MC (CTMC) usually isolated from the rat peritoneum and the mucosal MC (MMC) from the intestine (IMMC). Both populations are found in the rodent intestine, with CTMC in the submucosal and muscle layers and IMMC predominating in the lamina propria.[13,19] These two cell populations differ in several aspects (Figure 1) including obvious morphologic differences such as size and granule structure. There are both qualitative and quantitative differences in their mediator content (eg., histamine, proteases, proteoglycan, eicosanoids, and cytokines) and in their IgE receptors.[14,19–23]

In addition to their physical distinctions, these MC populations differ functionally. Although both CTMC and IMMC produce and secrete histamine in response to several stimuli, a number of secretagogues, including many neuropeptides, induce secretion by CTMC but are without effect on IMMC.[22] These MC populations also differ markedly in their responsiveness to some anti-allergic drugs such as cromoglycate and theophylline.[21,23,24] The majority of these studies used histamine release as the measure of MC function. However, studies using serotonin or eicosanoids release showed that MC can differentially release mediators upon activation.[25,26]

CTMC   IMMC

	CTMC	IMMC
Histamine	15-20 pg/cell	1-2 pg/cell
Proteoglycans	Heparin	Cs di B and E
Proteases	Chymase 1, 5 Tryptase Carboxypeptidase	Chymase 2 ?
Eicosanoids	PGD_2	PGD_2, LTB_4, LTC_4
Cytokines	IL-1,3,4,5,6,8,10,LIF,IFNγ	?
TNFα	0.89 pg/cell	0.17 pg/cell

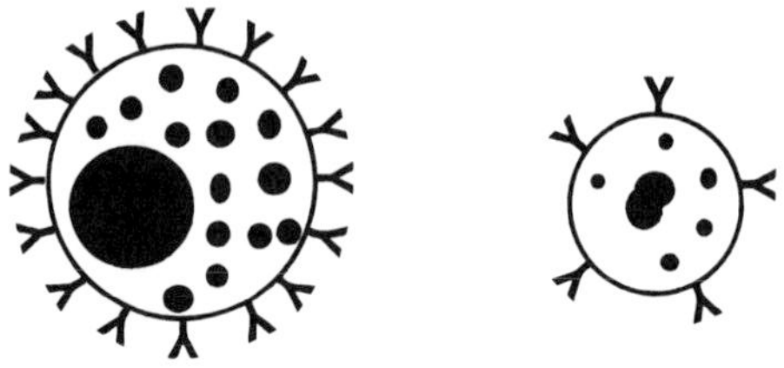

FIGURE 1 Heterogeneity of rat connective tissue and intestinal mucosal mast cells. RMCPI: rat mast cell protease I; RMCPII: rat mast cell protease II; CS: chondroitin sulfates; PG: prostaglandin; Lt: leukotriene; IFN: interferon; TNFα: tumor necrosis factor α; Y: IgE receptor.

Thus, the modulation of the release of different MC mediators may differ. For example, MC have been shown to be an important source of a potent inflammatory mediator, tumor necrosis factor α (TNFα).[27] Interestingly, the release of histamine and TNFα by MC can be modulated differently by interferon within and between MC types.[28] Whereas interferon treatment inhibits histamine and TNFα release from CTMC, the same treatment inhibits only TNFα release from IMMC without affecting histamine release. These studies show how critically important it is to investigate modulatory effects of MC functions with the appropriate MC population and mediator.

Heterogeneity is also evident in human MC. As in rodents, the best discriminating markers in human MC are their neutral proteases. One MC population most abundant at mucosal surfaces such as the intestine contains only tryptase, whereas the other population, which is abundant in certain connective tissue sites such as the skin, contains both tryptase and chymase.[29] Because of their physical similarities and overlapping distribution, human MC subpopulations are difficult to separate and characterize.[14] However, dispersed mixtures of intestinal cells containing up to 30% MC have been obtained.[30] Within these dispersed cells from human intestine, MC histochemically analogous to both CTMC and IMMC of rats have been identified. Whether these human MC populations are functionally distinct as in the rat remains to be confirmed.

The main problem in studying functional heterogeneity in MC is to obtain a pure suspension of MC belonging to each subpopulation. In efforts to provide such pure populations, *in vitro* culture systems have been established. Large numbers of bone marrow-derived cultured MC (BMCMC) can be generated with growth factors derived from activated T cells or fibroblasts.[31–33] The first MC growth factor identified was interleukin-3 (IL-3).[34] Further investigations showed that IL-4 and IL-10 potentiate IL-3-dependent growth and that stem cell factor (SCF) can induce proliferation and maturation of MC.[35–37]

Mouse BMCMC that are IL-3-dependent were originally classified as "mucosal type" because of their staining properties, proteoglycan content, low levels of histamine and functional responsiveness.[38] This identification was based on comparisons with *in vivo*-derived IMMC from rats rather than mice because the *in vivo*-derived mouse IMMC had not been isolated or functionally characterized. Indeed, this has proved to be extremely difficult and there are no published reports of the isolation or characterization of *in vivo*-derived mouse IMMC. Repeated attempts were made to isolate mouse IMMC, but were unsuccessful (personal observation), despite our considerable experience with the isolation of rat IMMC. One of the problems that makes the isolation of mouse IMMC more difficult than rat IMMC may be the short half life of mouse IMMC compared to rat IMMC.[39]

The presence of IL-3 in rat bone marrow cultures also generates MC with some IMMC characteristics.[40] However, it is now widely accepted that BMCMC are not IMMC, but rather immature MC which can acquire characteristics of either CTMC-like or IMMC-like MC under appropriate circumstances *in vitro*.[33,37]

In addition to cultured MC, mastocytomas or leukemic cells have been used to isolate MC lines which express some characteristics of MMC, but also have some characteristics that distinguish them from *in vivo*-derived MMC.[41] Immortalization of MC by use of viruses such as Kirstein murine sarcoma virus gave a spectrum of MC lines frozen in different phases in the ontogeny of MC, some with CTMC characteristics and some with MMC characteristics.[42–44] These studies of cultured MC and MC lines have shed important light on different aspects of MC ontogeny and phenotype, but caution must be expressed about the relationship of these cultured cells to *in vivo* populations of MC or to their development. Thus, it is critically important to study *in vivo*-derived MC to define their characteristics, responsiveness to anti-allergic drugs, and functions.

CELL SEPARATION

The intestine is composed of a variety of different cell types. To understand the function of these cells and their pharmacologic properties, it is important to work with dispersed cell populations that are as pure as possible. In mixed cell populations, the effects of drugs on other cell types can modify the effect on the cell population targeted. Thus, the purification of a cell population is an initial and critical step for these types of studies.

Different techniques based on cell size or density have been developed to purify cell types.[45] The most widely used parameter to purify MC is their high density. Isolated rat peritoneal MC can be enriched to near 100% purity by centrifugation on density gradients of Percoll.[46] This technique is designed to select for dense cells such as MC or small lymphocytes. Fortunately, given the small number of lymphocytes in peritoneal lavage, high purity of peritoneal MC is easily obtained.

In contrast to peritoneal lavage, the intestine contains a large number of lymphocytes which makes it more difficult to purify MC from dispersed populations of intestinal cells. To add to the difficulty of their purification, MMC have fewer granules than CTMC and are thus less dense than CTMC.[19] Given these characteristics of intestinal cell populations, IMMC have been enriched to ~65% purity using density gradients of Percoll.[47] Another characteristic of the cell population, namely its size distribution was then used to further enrich IMMC. Velocity sedimentation at unit gravity, a procedure which separates cells largely on the basis of their size, increased IMMC purity up to 95%.[48]

Although IMMC have been isolated from sheep, at the present time the rat is the main source of *in vivo*-derived MMC, so that they may be directly compared with CTMC (represented by peritoneal MC).[49–52] The technique described here is not widely used because it requires care and rigor, is time consuming (requires about 8 h to 65% and 12 h to > 90% purity), and the yield of IMMC per rat is small (approximately 2×10^6). However, this is the only technique available that gives access to highly enriched MMC. Thus, we will describe in detail the technique developed to purify rat IMMC using density gradients of Percoll and velocity sedimentation at unit gravity.

HELMINTH INFECTION

Although MC are present in the intestine of a normal rat (approximately 3–4 MC/villus crypt unit), to improve the yield of IMMC, we induced intestinal mastocytosis by infection with the nematode, *Nippostrongylus brasiliensis*.[53] This infection induces high levels of IgE and a reproducible intestinal mastocytosis with >50 IMMC/villus crypt unit between days 19–26 of infection (Figure 2).[53–56] In addition of provoking mastocytosis and infiltration of eosinophils into the lamina propria, helminth infection also induced alterations in epithelial secretion, goblet cell hyperplasia, mucus secretion, and smooth muscle reactivity.[57] Peak levels of IgE in serum of infected Sprague Dawley rats were observed on day 11 post infection.[58] The increment of other classes of Ig was small compared to the elevation of IgE level in serum. During infection, MC become sensitized to worm allergens and subsequent exposure to allergens causes systemic anaphylaxis.[59] However, IMMC from infected rats are similar to MMC from normal rats in their average size and histamine and protease content.[47]

N. brasiliensis uses its rodent host for reproductive purposes.[60,61] Eggs are secreted in feces of infected animals. Stage one larvae hatch from the eggs and feed upon fecal bacteria. They moult to larva stages two and three; third stage larvae are infective to rats. Rats are infected with 3000 L_3 injected subcutaneously in the scruff of the neck.[53] The larvae migrate to the lungs and approximately 3 days later moult to the fourth stage.[62] Lung larva migrate up the trachea, are swallowed and reach the small intestine where they molt to adult worms. Eggs begin to be passed in the feces by the 6th day.[59] Thus, to maintain *N. brasiliensis* in the laboratory, feces containing eggs are collected from animals infected 6 to 10 days previously and blended with water, charcoal and vermiculite to obtain a mixture with a consistency similar to that of garden soil. L_3 appear at day 5 or 6 in these cultures and are infectious for up to 3 weeks.

The number of IMMC decreased in the early stages following infection between days 10–14 in infected Lewis rats, but increased dramatically between day 15 and 19 to levels about 20 times normal.[53] The timing of these responses varies among strains.[53–56,61] Although the worms are localized in the proximal jejunum, MC hyperplasia is observed throughout the intestine.[63] The maximum sensitivity to systemic anaphylaxis in the small intestine of infected rats is reached between days 20 and 35 following infection.[59] During the course of infection and especially near the time of worm expulsion, there is a dramatic inflammation of the intestinal mucosa including goblet cell hyperplasia and excess mucus production and secretion.[64] We found that it was difficult to isolate large numbers of viable leukocytes from the intestinal lamina propria when this acute inflammation was present (Table 1). However, after the goblet cell hyperplasia and acute inflammation have subsided (> day 20), the average yields were 120×10^6 leukocytes (Table 1). Thus, for isolation of IMMC we use rats infected for 35 to 40 days. Experiment should be initiated 5 to 6 weeks before cell isolation.

SPECIFIC METHODOLOGY

To isolate IMMC from three rats and to enrich the IMMC to approximately 65% purity using a density gradient of Percoll takes about 8 hours. Some time can be saved by preparing materials and supplies for the experiment the day before.

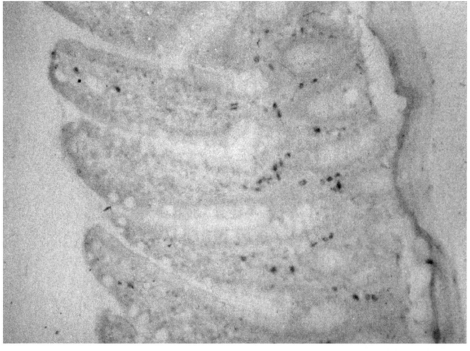

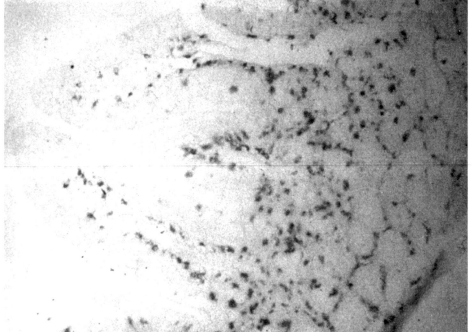

FIGURE 2 (Left) Intestine from uninfected rat. A small number of mast cells is present. (Right) Intestine from *N. brasiliensis* infected rat 35 days after infection. The number of mast cells in the mucosa is increased. Photographs were provided by Dr. J. L. Wallace, University of Calgary.

TABLE 1
Effects of *N. Brasiliensis* Infection of Total Cell Yields From Rat Intestine

Days	Yield/rat
0	43.9×10^6 (n = 10)
11–17	17.0×10^6 (n = 4)
>20	120×10^6 (n = 35)

ADVANCE PREPARATION

Rats are fasted the day before to minimize intestinal contents and to facilitate cleaning the bowel of contents (see below). Nylon wool columns (14 columns) used to remove debris from the cell suspensions can be prepared before the day of the experiment. The nylon wool (Du Pont Canada Inc., Mississauga, Ontario, Canada) is weighed (300 mg/column) and the fibers are teased apart and aligned in parallel to minimize problems of clogging the columns. The nylon wool fibers are placed in 10 ml syringe and packed so in total they are at the level of 10 ml. Parafilm is used to plug the bottom of the syringes that will be filled with Hanks' balanced salt solution (HBSS; Gibco, Grand Island, NY) the day of the experiment.

Some solutions can also be prepared the day before an experiment, whereas others are made the day of the experiment. Table 2 outlines the list of the solutions required. Given the number of IMMC recovered per rat ($2.1 \pm 0.28 \times 10^6$, n=33), the bowels of three rats are normally used for each experiment.

The protein supplement for basal tissue culture media (CLEX; Dextran Products Ltd., Scarborough, Ontario, Canada) must be heat inactivated (45 min at 56°C) before use. The phosphate buffered saline (PBS) with calcium and magnesium and the calcium and magnesium free HBSS containing HEPES (United States Biochemical Corp., Cleveland, Ohio) buffer (20 mM) can be prepared the day before (Table 3). The solutions should be at pH 7.2 and the osmolarity at 283 ± 10 mosmoles/kg H_2O to be isotonic with the serum of rats. These sterile solutions can be kept over night at 4°C.

The glassware used for velocity sedimentation, the STA-PUT (see below), must be siliconized to avoid MC adherence to the glass. This procedure should be done in a fume hood. The reservoir and the small loading chamber (Figure 3) of the STA-PUT are siliconized using 10%

TABLE 2
Solutions for IMMC Isolation From Three Rats

	(ml)
PBS (with Ca^{++} and Mg^{++})	2250
HBSS (Ca^{++} and Mg^{++} free) + HEPES (20 mM)	3000
CLEX	200
EDTA (1.3 mM) in HBSS + HEPES	900
complete HBSS (Ca^{++} and Mg^{++} free) (+HEPES + 20% CLEX)	800
Collagenase (~25 U/ml) in complete HBSS	600

PBS: phosphate buffered saline; HBSS: Hanks' balanced salt solution; HEPES: N-(2-hydroxyethyl) piperazine-N'-(2-ethanesulfonic acid); CLEX: supplement for basal tissue culture media; EDTA: disodium ethylenediamine tetraacetate.
* All solutions should be at pH 7.2 and osmolarity at 283 ± 10 mosmoles/kg H_2O.

TABLE 3
Recipe for Solutions Used for IMMC Isolation

	HBSS (+HEPES)	EDTA (+HBSS +HEPES)
HEPES	14.304g	5.364 g
HBSS 10x	300 ml	85 ml
ddH2O	2700 ml	815 ml
EDTA	—	0.45 g
Total	3000 ml	900 ml

* All solutions should be at pH 7.2 and osmolarity at 283 ±10 mosmoles/kg H_2O.

silane (SIGMA, St. Louis, MO) in chloroform. This procedure involves completely coating the inner surfaces and can be accomplished by "swirling" the silane solution around in the glassware, thereby prolonging the time of contact. This procedure should be repeated 2 to 3 times. The glassware is subsequently washed twice with distilled water and rinsed three times with PBS before air drying. The glassware should be sealed to keep free of dust and contamination.

It is also recommended to set up the working area the day before. Diapers (this procedure is very messy), surgical instruments (3 small scissors and 3 forceps), 2 funnels (~8 cm diameter), Erlenmeyer flasks (4 × 250 ml for EDTA and collagenase treatment and 2 × 500 ml for discarding waste), 6 petri dishes (~14 cm diameter), gauze, plastic kitchen sieve with ~2 mm pore size, filter paper (Whatman, 14 cm diameter, quality 1), 4 × 50 ml and 400 ml plastic beakers, and paper towels. A desk lamp is very useful to illuminate the working area for cutting the intestine (see below).

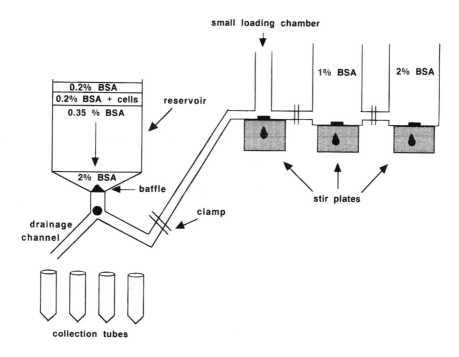

FIGURE 3 STA-PUT. This diagram shows the STA-PUT set up.

PREPARATION ON THE EXPERIMENTAL DAY

EDTA (1.3 mM)

EDTA (Sigma, St. Louis, MO) solution (Table 3) can be prepared the morning of the experiment and put in a water bath at 37°C (warming the HBSS solution to 37°C helps dissolve the EDTA). HBSS (Ca^{++} and Mg^{++} free) solution should be divided into two containers where 1 liter stays at 4°C and 2 liters are at 37°C (for washes). Cold HBSS will be used in the first part when the intestine is isolated, cleaned and cut into small strips.

Gradients of Percoll

Before starting the experiment, gradients of Percoll should be prepared to minimize the time that cells wait on the bench. The number of gradients required depends upon the number of dispersed cells obtained after collagenase digestion and mechanical disruption of the tissues (see below). However, about 10 gradients should be set up. If the number of cells is greater than expected, a few more gradients can be prepared at the last minute. Table 4 shows the solutions used to prepare the 30% and 80% Percoll (Pharmacia Ltd., Uppsala, Sweden). Fifteen ml of 80% Percoll are put in the bottom of 50 ml clear polystyrene tubes (Corning) and 20 ml of 30% Percoll are slowly layered on top to maintain a sharp 30%–80% interface. The gradients are kept at 4°C until needed.

STA-PUT Solutions

The sterile solutions for the STA-PUT (see below) including four concentrations of bovine serum albumin (BSA; Sigma, St. Louis, MO) in PBS (250 ml of 2%; 250 ml of 1%; 25 ml of 0.35%; 50 ml of 0.2%) should be prepared the same day. However, these solutions and the set-up of the STA-PUT can be prepared during incubation times in the cell isolation procedure.

PROCEDURES

TISSUE COLLECTION

Prior to the sacrifice of the rats, the accessories needed to flush the intestines of their contents should be prepared. These include three syringes of 20 ml of cold PBS in a 250 ml beaker containing about 100 ml PBS and 2 × 250 ml beakers containing about 30 ml of PBS on ice.

Rats are put down by light anaesthesia with few drops of metofane in a jar and killed by cervical dislocation. Animals are then exsanguinated by severing the jugular vein. The intestine

---

TABLE 4
Percoll Gradients

Final concentration of percoll	RPMI (ml)	Isotonic stock percoll* (ml)
30%	154	66
80%	32	128

For gradients use 20 ml of 30% and 15 ml of 80%.

*Isotonic stock Percoll: 200 ml Sterile Percoll, 18 ml HBSS (10X), 2 ml 1 M HEPES, adjust pH at 7.2 with 1 N HCl.

is cut free of the stomach below the pylorus and at the ileocaecal junction. It can be removed by gently pulling from the pyloric end and carefully cutting the mesentery as necessary. Care must be taken to avoid cutting or tearing the intestine as holes make the procedure for removing luminal contents difficult. The intestine is put directly into the beaker containing ~30 ml of ice cold PBS. Flush the contents from the intestine as quickly as possible using the 20 ml syringes of cold PBS inserted in the pyloric end. Make sure that the end of the intestine is placed directly and firmly around the syringe opening to ensure a tight seal. If everything goes well, only 2 syringes are needed, but one more syringe should be ready in case needed. The flushed intestine is put in a clean beaker containing 30 ml ice cold PBS. The same procedure is repeated for each rat (3) as quickly as possible. It should take about 10 min per rat.

TISSUE PROCESSING

Removal of Peyer's Patches

Each intestine is placed in a glass petri dish (14 cm) containing cold HBSS. The tissue is then placed on paper towel and, with good lighting, look meticulously for Peyer's patches. The Peyer's patches contain a large number of lymphocytes and few MC and are thus removed with scissors. The remaining intestinal tissue is put into another petri dish with cold HBSS. When all Peyer's patches have been removed, each piece of intestine is laid on paper towel with the mesentery facing up. The tissue is flattened and the mesentery is removed because it contains large numbers of CTMC. The mesentery is discarded and the intestine is cut longitudinally and opened. At this point, missed Peyer's patches can be detected and removed. The tissue is put in a petri dish with fresh HBSS. The cold HBSS is left on the bench so that it warms up slowly which will gradually bring the tissues to room temperature. When the mesentery has been removed from all the tissues, they are washed by stirring with forceps.

Strips

The next step is to cut the tissue into small pieces to facilitate enzymatic digestion. Fragments of tissue are spread, one at a time, mucosal side down on Whatman paper to remove mucus. Each fragment is cut into thin strips (1–2 mm). Strips are collected and put into fresh HBSS. Up to this point, the work should be done as quickly as possible to keep the tissues and cells healthy. It is recommended that three people work together, each doing the equivalent of one intestine. After cutting the tissues into small strips, one person can conduct the rest of the experiment, although we recommend that two persons work together to complete the cell isolation as quickly as possible. A sketch of the procedure is shown in Figure 4.

EDTA

Strips of tissues are washed and collected by filtering through two layers of gauze placed in a funnel. To collect the strips, it is easier if the gauze is tightly stretched on the funnel. Then, forceps or a small fork can be used to collect the strips and put them into 2×250 ml Erlenmeyer flasks containing 150 ml of the warm (37°C) EDTA solution with a stirring bar. The flasks are incubated at 37°C on a stirring plate for 10 minutes. The tissue should be moving slowly without accumulation in the bottom. If the stirring is too fast, MC will be damaged making it difficult to isolate them because of alterations in their density and size characteristics which are used to purify them.

The first EDTA incubation can be prolonged to 15 minutes if there is a lot of mucus. The tissue can be stirred a little faster to help eliminate the mucus. After incubation with EDTA, the strips are allowed to settle and the supernatants are decanted slowly into a petri dish. The

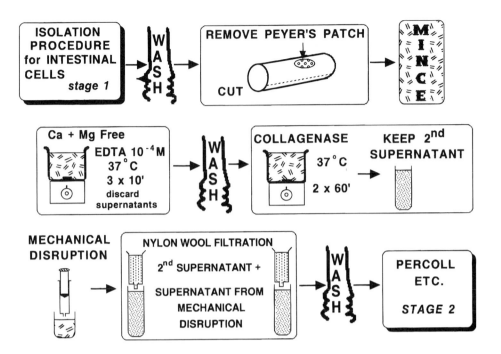

FIGURE 4   IMMC isolation stage 1. Sketch of IMMC isolation procedure.

strips are washed twice with a small volume of warm HBSS, swirling and decanting. Then, strips are collected by filtration through gauze as described earlier (help to clean the mucus) and put back into two Erlenmeyer flasks containing 150 ml of fresh warm (37°C) EDTA solution. This process removes mucus and epithelial cells. This EDTA incubation is carried out three times. The supernatants are discarded after each incubation and strips are washed.

Collagenase

At the end of the third incubation with EDTA, strips are thoroughly washed with HBSS three to four times to remove EDTA since its presence can inhibit the cation-dependent collagenase activity. After the washes, the tissue strips are put into clean Erlenmeyer flasks containing 150 ml of ~25 U/ml (approximately 200 U/mg) of collagenase (E.C. number: 3.4.2.4.3, Gibco, Grand Island, NY) in HBSS containing 20% CLEX and incubated at 37°C on a stirring plate (slow speed) for 60 minutes. The exact concentration of the collagenase to be used should be determined for every batch purchased because the efficiency of the collagenase for IMMC isolation differs from batch to batch. It is believed that the collagenase is not the only active component in the purchased enzyme in the digestion of the intestine, but that contaminants such as neutral proteases are important and the concentration of these contaminants varies from batch to batch. Thus, we recommend buying a large quantity of collagenase and testing three different concentrations of the preparation on intestinal digestion to optimize the recovery of viable MC. The optimal concentrations to be used should be re-evaluated as the enzyme approaches its expiry date.

After the first collagenase incubation, the strips are washed as mentioned previously and the supernatant discarded. Although this supernatant was kept in earlier experiments, IMMC purity is greater when this supernatant is discarded because it contains a large number of eosinophils which are important contaminating cells in IMMC preparations. Thus, the tissues are put into fresh collagenase and incubated for an additional 60 minutes on a stirring plate (slow speed). The second collagenase treatment is filtered through gauze into 50 ml tubes.

These supernatants contain some MC which are recovered by centrifugation at $150 \times g$ at room temperature for 10 minutes. The remaining tissues are collected from the gauze and put into a 40 ml plastic beaker containing 20–25 ml HBSS supplemented with 10% CLEX (complete HBSS) at room temperature. With a new 10 ml syringe, the tissues are mechanically disrupted by firmly syringing the tissue in solution up and down 10 times. The supernatant is decanted into a sieve over a 400 ml plastic beaker (MC can adhere to glass) and 10 ml of complete HBSS is poured on the tissue to wash it. Then, using forceps, strips are collected and added to fresh complete HBSS and the syringing process is repeated. This procedure should be done until the supernatant is clear (approximately 5 times).

Nylon Wool Column

During cell centrifugation, the previously prepared nylon wool columns can be submerged with complete HBSS. Make certain that there are no air pockets in the columns. The cells pelleted from the second collagenase digestion should be resuspended in approximately 15 ml complete HBSS and combined with the supernatants from the syringing. When cells and supernatants are pooled, the volume is adjusted to $\sim$300 ml with complete HBSS. At this point, the parafilm on the nylon wool columns is removed, thereby draining the syringes. Two beakers of 40 ml, one containing 20 ml complete HBSS and the other one 20 ml of the cell suspension, are prepared. The columns are filled with $\sim$8 ml of complete HBSS immediately followed by well-mixed cell suspension and the continuous rapid and smooth out-flow is collected. The rest of the complete HBSS is added (without stopping the flow) to wash the column and collect the effluent. These nylon wool columns minimize debris in the cell suspensions. The columns can be kept and put in a test tube rack on top of 50 ml tubes that are in a rack holder and seven columns are done sequentially.

After the cell suspension has gone through the nylon wool columns, cells are pelleted by centrifugation at $150 \times g$ for 10 minutes at room temperature. The cells are resuspended in 50 ml RPMI supplemented with 5% FBS and containing 15 µg/ml DNase (2000 units/mg, Boehringer Mannheim). The DNase minimizes clumping due to DNA from dead cells and thus, increases cell yields. The total cells are counted ($120 \pm 9 \times 10^6$ cells/rat, n = 35) and the viability ($48 \pm 2\%$, n = 35) using trypan blue noted. Large numbers of nonviable epithelial cells are present in the suspension.

Percoll

A maximum of 40×10^6 cells in 5 ml of RPMI can be loaded on top of one Percoll gradient (20 ml 30%, 15 ml 80%). Cells are spun at $600\ g$ for 20 minutes at 10°C (Figure 5). Average yields are $2.1 \pm 0.3 \times 10^6$ MC (n = 35) are obtained per rat with a purity of $65.7 \pm 1.6\%$ and a total cell viability of $72.2 \pm 2.5\%$. The contaminating cells are predominantly small lymphocytes, but some epithelial cells and eosinophils are also seen. IMMC recovery from the Percoll gradients represents approximately 20% of loaded IMMC. Many IMMC are trapped in the thick interface bands, presumably because of their lower density or because of contaminating cells. Recovered IMMC show no obvious morphological signs of damage due to the enrichment procedure as assayed by light microscopy. The effects of this isolation procedure have been tested on peritoneal MC and effects on histamine and TNFα release are minimal. These controls have been conducted repeatedly in several studies and the results are consistent.[19–22,28,47,64] Most functional studies we have conducted use IMMC enriched to this extent (72%). However, IMMC can be purified further using the STA-PUT (Figure 5).

STA-PUT

This phase of the procedure is run at 4 °C and should be performed in an area of little or no traffic or activity to avoid disrupting the shallow and fragile BSA gradient used. Centrifuges

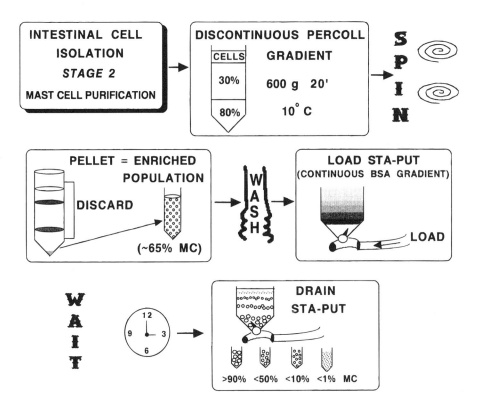

FIGURE 5   IMMC isolation stage 2. Sketch showing the Percoll and STA-PUT enrichment procedures for IMMC.

or even the door of the cold room can disrupt the gradient. Before assembly, the reservoir base and stopcock should be greased. When all the glassware and tubing are assembled (Figure 3), all tubing is clamped and reservoir placed in its holder. The metal baffle in the bottom of the funnel must be centered.

The sterile 2% and 1% BSA solutions are added into the appropriate vessels (see Figure 3), making sure that the stir bars can move freely. Solutions are allowed to flow into the tubing connecting these vessels, but mixing should be avoided. The idea is to remove all trapped air. After re-clamping, the tubing is gently massaged between fingers to dislodge any air bubbles remaining in/attached to the tubing.

The small loading chamber is filled with 25 ml of 0.2% BSA. The clamp is released and the flow rate (~2 min) is adjusted. The loading chamber should not be drained completely before re-clamping. There should not be any air in any of the pieces of tubing. The STA-PUT (Johns Scientific Co.) is now ready to be loaded with the IMMC suspension.

Percoll purified IMMC ($>5 \times 10^6$ cells) are resuspended in 0.2% BSA to a final volume of 15 ml and put into the small loading chamber. The clamp is removed and the cells are allowed to flow into the reservoir, but the tubing should be re-clamped before air enters. Then, the small loading chamber is rinsed twice with PBS while the clamps are still in place.

The loading chamber is then loaded with 25 ml of 0.35% BSA. The clamp is released to allow slow flow into the reservoir. Immediately after, the clamp between the 2% and 1% BSA chambers is loosened followed by the loosening of the clamp between the 1% BSA and small loading chamber. The stir plates are turned on to a slow speed to avoid bubble formation. It should take approximately 15 to 25 minutes for the BSA chambers to empty. Then, the stir plates can be turned off.

The loaded STA-PUT should be left in place for 3 hours. Extreme care should be taken to avoid disturbing the gradient. This includes care with the cold room door. At the end of this incubation, the reservoir is drained from the bottom via the port that is not connected to the BSA chambers (Figure 5). The flow should be continuous and the cells are collected into 50 ml fractions, each fraction taking approximately 30 minutes to complete. The flow can be adjusted using the stopcock, but precaution has to be taken not to disturb the gradient.

All fractions are centrifuged at $200 \times g$ for 12 min at 4°C. The supernatants should be removed carefully because IMMC are easily resuspended. Each fraction is resuspended in RPMI or PBS and counted. Fraction I contains ~95% pure IMMC which represent 84% of the total MC loaded. Fraction II contains 14% IMMC, whereas fractions III and IV contain very few IMMC (<2%).

TIMING

This procedure is time consuming. The day has to be well prepared to do this experiment within 12 hours. As mentioned above, some solutions as well as the nylon wool columns can be prepared the day before.

Two people can prepare 10 Percoll gradients (30 min) while one person kills the rats and collects the intestines (30 min). From the collection of the intestine to EDTA incubation, it takes about 1 hour per person per intestine. The strips from three intestines are separated into two equal parts into 250 ml Erlenmeyer flasks and it takes 5 to 6 hours for two people to process the tissue from the EDTA incubation to Percoll purified IMMC. During incubation times (3×10 min and 2×60 min), different solutions such as collagenase, complete HBSS, and BSA concentrations can be prepared, and the nylon wool columns can be submerged with complete HBSS. Further purification using velocity sedimentation at unit gravity (STA-PUT) takes around 4 hours after the apparatus is siliconized and set up.

TROUBLE SHOOTING

To obtain a good yield of viable IMMC some steps are critical. The time between tissue collection and EDTA incubation should be as short as possible. The passage from EDTA to collagenase is also critical. The strips should be extensively washed after EDTA treatment, because EDTA inhibits collagenase activity. In addition, the activity of collagenase decreases with time. If the collagenase is old, increased concentrations should be used once properly identified.

The mechanical disruption using a 10 ml syringe is also an important step. This process destroys the tissue and liberates the cells. Thus, it should not be too strong which will degranulate MC, but it should be strong enough to liberate the cells.

The last purification step, STA-PUT, is a tricky procedure. It takes experience and patience to achieve good results reproducibly.

FUTURE DIRECTIONS

Given the time consuming nature of the isolation procedure for IMMC, attempts were made to develop other techniques. Flow cytometry is a powerful technique to purify cells using parameters such as size, shape, cytoplasmic granularity, surface antigens, lectin binding, total protein, basic protein, DNA and RNA content.[66,67] The specificity of the marker is an important determinant in the purification of cell population. The high affinity receptor for IgE (FcεRI) which is specific for MC, basophils and epidermal Langerhans cells, has been used to analyze human basophils by flow cytometry, but no purification of the basophils was attempted.[68–71] Preliminary experiments using FcεRI to purify IMMC by flow cytometry were disappointing (personal observation) because of interference of the low affinity receptor for IgE present on a variety of cell types. The presence of cell debris in the preparation also created problems for the analysis. A preenrichment of the cell population with elimination of debris before the flow cytometric analysis may help to improve the efficacy of this technique. However, to purify MC by fluorescence activated cell sorting will be a long process because the cell sorting rate is low.

Many other strategies such as density gradients, affinity chromatography, negative selection and rosetting using IgE, have been described in attempts to purify basophils from whole blood.[72–77] Unfortunately, most of these techniques cannot be extrapolated for the isolation of MMC for different reasons such as cost, availability of products, the mixture of cells, and the presence of debris. However, recently a new technique using magnetic beads has been used to isolate human lung MC. Bradding et al. purified human lung MC using 65% continuous Percoll gradient followed by 30 minutes incubation with an antibody to c-kit receptor (receptor for SCF).[78] Cells were then washed and incubated for 60 minutes with a suspension of magnetic beads coated with goat anti-mouse IgG antibody. Purified MC attached to magnetic beads were removed from the suspension with a magnet. This process seems to be applicable for the purification of IMMC, as all MC that have been studied express SCF receptors. However, dead cells and some unwanted cell types should be eliminated by using a gradient of Percoll before treatment with antibody. Furthermore, care has to be taken not to activate the MC because SCF has been previously shown to potentiate mediator release by MC.[79] Thus, it will be critical to employ a concentration of the antibody to c-kit that will allow for their isolation but not for their activation. This technique has the potential to be easier and faster than using the STA-PUT.

The ability to obtain highly enriched populations of MMC is critical for pharmacological studies. However, pure MMC are not easily accessible and, as discussed above, cultured MC are not necessarily representative of *in vivo* MMC. The rat lamina propria MC represents an unusual, *in vivo*-derived MC population that will continue to provide important information about MMC functions. Although the isolation procedure is difficult and time consuming, new techniques or new specific surface markers for MC will allow the development of easier ways to study these cells.

REFERENCES

1. **Wilhelm, D. L., Yong, L. C. J., and Watkins, S. G.,** The mast cell: distribution and maturation in the rat, *Agents & Actions,* 8, 146, 1978.
2. **Stead, R. H., Tomioka, M., Quinonez, G., Simon, G. T., Felten, S. Y., and Bienenstock, J.,** Intestinal mucosal mast cells in normal and nematode-infected rat intestines are in intimate contact with peptidergic nerves, *Proc. Natl. Acad. Sci. USA,* 84, 2975, 1987.
3. **Bienenstock, J., Perdue, M., Blennerhassett, M., Stead, R., Kakuta, N., Sestini, P., Vancheri, C., and Marshall, J.,** Inflammatory cells and the epithelium. Mast cell/nerve interactions in the lung *in vitro* and *in vivo, Am. Rev. Respir. Dis.,* 138, S31, 1988.
4. **Lindholm, S.,** Mast cells in the wall of the alimentary canal, *Acta Pathol. Microbiol. Scand.* (Suppl), 46, 10, 1959.
5. **Kraft, S. C. and Kirsner, J. B.,** Mast cells and the gastrointestinal tract, *Gastroenterology,* 39, 764, 1960.
6. **Enerbäck, L.,** Mast cells in rat gastrointestinal mucosa. 1. Dye-binding and metachromatic properties, *Acta Path. Microbiol. Scandinav.,* 66, 303, 1966.
7. **Norris, H. T., Zamcheck, N., and Gottlieb, L. S.,** The presence and distribution of mast cells in the human gastrointestinal tract at autopsy, *Gastroenterology,* 44, 448, 1963.
8. **Dobbins, W. O., Tomasini, J. T., and Rollins, E. L.,** Electron and light microscopic identification of the mast cell of the gastrointestinal tract, *Gastroenterology,* 56, 268, 1969.

9. **Strobel, S., Busuttil, A., and Ferguson, A.,** Human intestinal mucosal mast cells: expanded population in untreated coeliac disease, *Gut,* 24, 222, 1983.

10. **Balazs, M., Illyes, G., and Vadasz, G.,** Mast cells in ulcerative colitis. Quantitative and ultrastructural studies, *Virchows Arch. Cell. Pathol.,* 57, 353, 1989.

11. **Dvorak, A. M., Monoham, R. A., Osage, J. E., and Dickersin, G. R.,** Crohn's disease: transmission electron microscopic studies. Immunologic inflammatory response. Alteration of mast cells, basophils, eosinophils, and microvasculature, *Hum. Pathol.,* 11, 606, 1980.

12. **Mangham, D. C. and Newbold, K. M.,** Mucosal mast cells in reflux gastritis and chronic (type B) gastritis, *Histopathology,* 15, 531, 1989.

13. **Lee, T. D. G., Swieter, M., Bienenstock, J., and Befus, A. D.,** Heterogeneity in mast cell populations, *Clin. Immunol. Rev.,* 4, 143, 1985.

14. **Benyon, R. C., Lowman, M. A., Rees, P. H., Holgate, S. T., and Church, M. K.,** Mast cell heterogeneity, in *Asthma Reviews* Vol. 2, Morley, J., Ed., Academic Press, London, 1989, 151.

15. **Kitamura, Y.,** Heterogeneity of mast cells and phenotypic change between subpopulations, *Annu. Rev. Immunol.,* 7, 59, 1989.

16. **Befus, A. D.,** Mast cells are that polymorphic!, *Reg. Immunol.,* 2, 176, 1989.

17. **Galli, S. J.,** New insights into "The riddle of the mast cells": microenvironmental regulation of mast cell development and phenotypic heterogeneity, *Lab. Invest.,* 62, 5, 1990.

18. **Enerbäck, L.,** The gut mucosal mast cell, *Monogr. Allergy,* 17, 222, 1981.

19. **Befus, A. D., Pearce, F. L., Gauldie, J., Horsewood, P., and Bienenstock, J.,** Mucosal mast cells I. Isolation and functional characteristics of rat intestinal mast cells, *J. Immunol.,* 128, 2475, 1982.

20. **Swieter, M., Chan, B. M. C., Rimmer, C., McNeill, K., Froese, A., Befus, D.,** Isolation and characterization of IgE receptors from rat intestinal mucosal mast cells, *Eur. J. Immunol.,* 19, 1879, 1989.

21. **Pearce, F. L., Befus, A. D., Gauldie, J., and Bienenstock, J.,** Mucosal mast cells II. Effects of anti-allergic compounds on histamine secretion by isolated intestinal mast cells, *J. Immunol.,* 128, 2481, 1982.

22. **Shanahan, F., Denburg, J. A., Fox, J., Bienenstock, J., and Befus, D.,** Mast cell heterogeneity: effects of neuroenteric peptides on histamine release, *J. Immunol.,* 135, 1331, 1985.

23. **Shanahan, F., Lee, T. D. G., Bienenstock, J., and Befus, A. D.,** Mast cell heterogeneity: effect of anti-allergic compounds on neuropeptide-induced histamine release, *Int. Archs. Allergy Appl. Immun.,* 80, 424, 1986.

24. **Church, M. K.,** Modulation of mast cell mediator secretion by drugs used in the treatment of allergic diseases, in *Mast Cells, Mediators and Disease,* Holgate, S. T., Ed., Boston: Kluwer Academic Press, 1988, 259.

25. **Theoharides, T. C., Kops, S. K., Bondy, P. K., and Askenase, P. W.,** Differential release of serotonin without comparable histamine under diverse conditions in the rat mast cell, *Biochem. Pharmacol.,* 34, 1389, 1985.

26. **Heavey, D. J., Ernst, P. B., Stevens, R. L., Befus, A. D., Bienenstock, J., and Austen, K. F.,** Generation of leukotriene C_4, leukotriene B_4, and prostaglandin D_2 by immunologically activated rat intestinal mucosa mast cells, *J. Immunol.,* 140, 1953, 1988.

27. **Gordon, J. R. and Galli, S. J.,** Mast cells as a source of both preformed and immunologically inducible TNFα-/cachectin, *Nature,* 346, 274, 1990.

28. **Bissonnette, E. Y., Chin, B., and Befus, A. D.,** Heterogeneity of mast cells and the regulation of their mediator release by interferons, CSI Spring Meeting, Alberta, March 1993.

29. **Schwartz, L. B.,** Preformed mediators of human mast cells and basophils, in *Mast Cells, Mediators and Disease,* Holgate, S. T., Ed., Boston: Kluwer Academic Press, 1988, 129.

30. **Befus, A. D., Dyck, N., Goodacre, R., and Bienenstock, J.,** Mast cells from the human intestinal lamina propria. Isolation, histochemical subtypes, and functional characterization, *J. Immunol.,* 138, 2604, 1987.

31. **Ginsburg, H., Olson, E. C., Huff, T. F., Okudaira, H., Ishizaka, T.,** Enhancement of mast cell differentiation *in vitro* by T cell factor(s), *Int. Arch. Allergy Appl. Immunol.,* 66, 447, 1981.

32. **Yung, Y.-P. and Moore, M. A. S.,** Long-term *in vitro* culture of murine mast cells. III. Discrimination of mast cell growth-factor and granulocyte CSF, *J. Immunol.,* 129, 1256, 1982.

33. **Ginsburg, H., Ben-Shahar, D., and Ben-David, E.,** Mast cell growth on fibroblast monolayers. Two cell entities, *Immunology*, 45, 371, 1982.

34. **Ihle, J. N., Keller, J., Oroszlan, S., Henderson, L. E., Copeland, T. D., Fitch, F., Prystowsky, M. B., Goldwasser, E., Schrader, J. W., Paraszynski, E., Dy, M., and Lebel, B.,** Biologic properties of homogeneous interleukin-3. I. Demonstration of WEHI-3 growth-factor activity, mast cell growth-factor activity, P cell-stimulating factor activity and histamine-producing cell-stimulating factor activity, *J. Immunol.*, 131, 282, 1983.

35. **Hamaguchi, Y., Kanakura, Y., Fujita, J., Takeda, S.-I., Nakano, T., Tarui, S., Honjo, T., and Kitamura, Y.,** Interleukin 4 as an essential factor for *in vitro* clonal growth of murine connective tissue-type mast cells, *J. Exp. Med.*, 165, 268, 1987.

36. **Thompson-Snipes, L., Dhar, V., Bond, M. V., Mosmann, T. R., Moore, K. W., and Rennick, D. M.,** Interleukin 10: a novel stimulatory factor for mast cells and their progenitors, *J. Exp. Med.*, 173, 507, 1991.

37. **Tsai, M., Takeishi, T., Thompson, H., Langley, K. E., Zsebo, K. M., Metcalfe, D. D., Geissler, E. N., and Galli, S. J.,** Induction of mast cell proliferation, maturation, and heparin synthesis by the rat c-*kit* ligand, stem cell factor, *Proc. Natl. Acad. Sci. USA*, 88, 6382, 1991.

38. **Sredni, B., Friedman, M. M., Bland, C. E., and Metcalfe, D. D.,** Ultrastructural, biochemical, and functional characteristics of histamine-containing cells cloned from mouse bone marrow: tentative identification as mucosal mast cells, *J. Immunol.*, 131, 915, 1983.

39. **Alizadeh, H., and Wakelin, D.,** Comparison of rapid expulsion of *Trichinella spiralis* in mice and rats, *Int. J. Parasitol.*, 12, 65, 1982.

40. **Shanahan, F., Lee, T. D. G., Denburg, J. A., Bienenstock, J., and Befus, A. D.,** Functional characterization of mast cells generated *in vitro* from the mesenteric lymph node of rats infected with *Nippostrongylus brasiliensis, Immunology*, 57, 455, 1986.

41. **Seldin, D. C., Adelman, S., Austen, K. F., Stevens, R., Hein, A., Caulfield, P. P., and Woodbury, R. G.,** Homology of the rat basophilic leukemia cell and the rat mucosal mast cell, *Proc. Natl. Acad. Sci. USA*, 82, 3871, 1985.

42. **Pierce, J. H., Di Fiore, P. P., Aaronson, S. A., Potter, M., Pumphrey, J., Scott, A., and Ihle, J. N.,** Neoplastic transformation of mast cells by Abelson-MuLV: abrogation of IL-3 dependence by a nonautocrine mechanism, *Cell*, 41, 685, 1985.

43. **Rein, A., Keller, J., Schultz, A. M., Holmes, K. L., Medicus, R., and Ihle, J. N.,** Infection of immune mast cells by Harvey Sarcoma Virus: immortalization without loss of requirement for interleukin-3, *Mol. Cell Biol.*, 5, 2257, 1985.

44. **Reynolds, D. S., Serafin, W. E., Faller, D. V., Wall, D. A., Abbas, A. K., Dvorak, A. M., Austen, K. F., and Stevens, R. L.,** Immortalization of murine connective tissue-type mast cells at multiple stages of their differentiation by coculture of splenocytes with fibroblasts that produce Kirsten Sarcoma virus, *J. Biol. Chem.*, 263, 12783, 1988.

45. **Pretlow, T. G. and Pretlow, T. P. Eds.** *Cell separation, methods and selected applications,* Vol. 1, New York, 1982, 330.

46. **Enerback, L. and Svensson, I.,** Isolation of rat peritoneal mast cells by centrifugation on density gradients of Percoll, *J. Immunol. Methods*, 39, 135, 1980.

47. **Lee, T. D. G., Shanahan, F., Miller, H. R. P., Bienenstock, J., and Befus, A. D.,** Intestinal mucosal mast cells: isolation from rat lamina propria and purification using unit gravity velocity sedimentation, *Immunology*, 55, 721, 1985.

48. **Miller, R. G.,** Separation of cells by velocity sedimentation, in *New techniques in biophysics and cell biology,* Vol. 1, Pain, R. H. and Smith, B. J. Eds, J. Wiley & Son, New York, 1973, 87.

49. **Huntley, J. F., Wallace, G. R., and Miller, H. R. P.,** Quantitative recovery of isolated mucosal mast cells and globule leucocytes from parasitised sheep, *Res. Vet. Sci.*, 33, 58, 1982.

50. **Befus, A. D., Bienenstock, J., and Denburg, J. A., Eds.,** *Mast cell differentiation and heterogeneity,* New York, Raven Press, 1986, 426.

51. **Galli, S. J. and Austen, K. F., Eds.,** *Mast cell and basophil differentiation and function in health and disease,* New York, Raven Press, 1989, 425.

52. **Abe, T., Swieter, M., Imai, T., Den Hollander, N., and Befus, A. D.,** Mast cell heterogeneity: two-dimensional gel electrophoretic analyses of rat peritoneal and intestinal mucosal mast cells, *Eur. J. Immunol.*, 20, 1941, 1990.

53. **Befus, A. D., Johnston, N., and Bienenstock, J.,** *Nippostrongylus brasiliensis:* mast cells and histamine levels in tissues of infected and normal rats, *Exp. Parasit.,* 48, 1, 1979.

54. **Wells, P. D.,** Mast cell, eosinophil and histamine levels in *Nippostrongylus brasiliensis* infected rats, *Exp. Parasit.,* 12, 82, 1962.

55. **Keller, R.,** *Nippostrongylus brasiliensis* in the rat: failure to relate intestinal histamine and mast cell levels with worm expulsion, *Parasitology,* 63, 473, 1971.

56. **Kelly, J. D. and Ogilvie, B. M.,** Intestinal mast cell and eosinophil numbers during worm expulsion in nulliparous and lactating rats infected with *Nippostrongylus brasiliensis, Int. Archs. Allergy,* 43, 497, 1972.

57. **Moqbel, R.,** Helminth-induced intestinal inflammation, *Trans. Roy. Soc. Trop. Med. Hyg.,* 80, 719, 1986.

58. **Ramaswamy, K. and Befus, D.,** IgE antibody responses in bronchoalveolar spaces of rats infected with *Nippostrongylus brasiliensis, Exp. Parasitol.,* 76, 23, 1993.

59. **Keller, R.,** Immune reactions to *Nippostrongylus brasiliensis* in the rat, I. Characteristics of primary and secondary immune response *in vivo, Int. Arch. Allergy,* 37, 197, 1970.

60. **Rothwell, T. L. W.,** Immune expulsion of parasitic nematodes from the alimentary tract, *Int. J. Parasitol.,* 19, 139, 1989.

61. **Miller, H. R. P. and Jarrett, W. F. H.,** Immune reaction in mucous membranes, I. Intestinal mast cell response during helminth expulsion in the rat, *Immunology,* 20, 277, 1971.

62. **Kassi, T.,** *Handbook of Nippostrongylus brasiliensis (nematode),* Akadémiai Kiadó, Budapest, 1982, 15.

63. **MacDonald, T. T., Murray, M., and Ferguson, A.,** *Nippostrongylus brasiliensis:* mast cell kinetics at various small intestinal sites in infected rats, *Exp. Parasitol.,* 49, 9, 1980.

64. **Koninkx, J. F. J. G., Mirck, M. H., Hendriks, H. G. C. J. M., Mouwen, J. M. V. M., and van Dijk, J. E.,** *Nippostrongylus brasiliensis:* histochemical changes in the composition of mucins in goblet cells during infection in rats, *Exp. Parasitol.,* 65, 84, 1988.

65. **Befus, A. D., Spencer, J. A., McDermott, M. R., McLaughlin, B., and Bienenstock, J.,** Isolation and characteristics of small intestinal lamina propria cells from normal and nematode (*Nippostrongylus brasiliensis*)-infected rats, *Int. Archs Allergy Appl. Immun.,* 75, 345, 1984.

66. **Loken, M. R. and Stall, A. M.,** Flow cytometry as an analytical and preparative tool in immunology, *J. Immunol. Methods,* 50, R85, 1982.

67. **Shapiro, H. M.,** Multistation multiparameter flow cytometry: a critical review and rationale, *Cytometry,* 3, 227, 1983.

68. **Froese, A.,** Receptors for IgE on mast cells and basophils, *Prog. Allergy,* 34, 142, 1984.

69. **Wang, B., Rieger, A., Kilgus, O., Ochiai, K., Maurer, D., Födinger, D., Kinet, J. P., and Stingl, G.,** Epidermal Langerhans cells from normal human skin bind monomeric IgE via Fc epsilon RI, J. *Exp. Med.* 175, 1353, 1992.

70. **Bochner, B. S., McKelvey, A. A., Schleimer, R. P., Hildreth, J. E. K., and MacGlashan, D. W.,** Flow cytometric methods for the analysis of human basophil surface antigens and viability, *J. Immunol. Methods,* 125, 265, 1989.

71. **Gane, P., Pecquet, C., Lambin, P., Abuaf, N., Leynadier, F., and Rouger, P.,** Flow cytometric evaluation of human basophils, *Cytometry,* 14, 344, 1993.

72. **Leonard, E. J., Roberts, R. L., and Skeel, A.,** Purification of human blood basophils by a single step isopycnic banding on Percoll, *J. Leukoc. Biol.,* 35, 169, 1984.

73. **Miroli, A. D., Bridget, M. B., James, M. B., and Spitz, M.,** Single step enrichment of human peripheral blood basophils by Ficoll-Paque centrifugation, *J. Immunol. Methods,* 88, 91, 1986.

74. **MacGlashan, D. W. and Lichtenstein, L. M.,** The purification of human basophils, *J. Immunol.,* 124, 2519, 1980.

75. **Landry, F. J. and Findlay, S. R.,** Purification of human basophils by negative selection, *J. Immunol. Methods,* 63, 329, 1983.

76. **Bjerke, T., Nielsen, S., Helgestad, I., Nielsen, B. W., and Schiøtz, P. O.,** Purification of human blood basophils by negative selection using immunomagnetic beads, *J. Immunol. Methods,* 157, 49, 1993.

77. **Schroeder, J. T. and Hanrahan, L. R.,** Purification of human basophils using mouse monoclonal IgE, *J. Immunol. Methods,* 133, 269, 1990.

78. **Bradding, P., Feather, I. H., Howarth, P. H., Mueller, R., Roberts, J. A., Britten, K., Bews, J. P. A., Hunt, T. C., Okayama, Y., Heusser, C. H., Bullock, G. R., Church, M. K., and Holgate, S. T.,** Interleukin 4 is localized to and released by human mast cells, *J. Exp. Med.* 176, 1381, 1992.

79. **Bischoff, S. C. and Dahinden, C. A.,** C-kit ligand: a unique potentiator of mediator release by human lung mast cells, *J. Exp. Med.,* 175, 237, 1992.

19 Molecular Biology Methods in Gastrointestinal Pharmacology

Charles D. Ulrich, II and Laurence J. Miller

INTRODUCTION

Since the discovery of porcine secretin by Bayliss and Starling in 1902,[1] an increasing number of gastrointestinal peptide hormones have been isolated and characterized. A variety of whole animal, isolated perfused organ, and cellular models have been utilized to study the pharmacology of these polypeptides and their binding proteins. However, the sparse number of receptors in native cellular membranes, in conjunction with the inability to purify these binding proteins, significantly limited attempts to understand the molecular interactions between these hormones and their binding proteins. Such knowledge may greatly facilitate the efficient and timely design of pharmacologically useful agonists and antagonists.

The advent of molecular biology ushered in a new era in gastrointestinal pharmacology. The ability to clone cDNA's encoding hormones and receptors, express these proteins in high copy numbers in a variety of systems, and characterize them functionally, has provided us with the tools necessary to overcome many of the traditional limitations in this field.

In this chapter, we will review the basic concepts of molecular biology; the techniques available to generate probes, clone full length cDNA's, and express the encoded proteins; and the methods and models that have been designed to utilize these tools in the detailed study of the molecular interactions between ligands and their receptors.

ENDOGENOUS LIGANDS AND RECEPTORS: CLASSIFICATION AND DIVERSITY

Appropriately, the first hormone identified in 1902, secretin, is a gastrointestinal peptide having the pancreas as its primary target.[1] Since then, a large number of gastrointestinal hormones have been isolated and characterized.[2] A partial list of these peptides and their functions is illustrated in Table 1. Interesting features of these peptides include not only their ability to regulate a variety of gastrointestinal events, but their important roles in extraintestinal physiology. Among the most extensively characterized peptides and receptors in this field, the cholecystokinin (CCK)/gastrin family exemplifies these features.

The CCK/gastrin hormone family contributed the first gastrointestinal hormone to be isolated in sufficient purity to allow determination of its peptide sequence by classical chemical means.[3] Delineation of the amino acid sequence for these peptides confirmed significant homology, with identity of the five amino acids at the carboxyl terminus.[4] Cholecystokinin regulates gallbladder

TABLE 1
Gastrointestinal Peptides and Their Major Biological Actions

Cholecystokinin (CCK)	Stimulates gallbladder contraction, pancreatic enzyme secretion and growth, muscarinic pathways, and substance P release; inhibits contraction of sphincter of Oddi and gastric emptying; induces satiety
Gastrin	Stimulates gastric acid secretion and fundic mucosal growth
Gastrin releasing peptide	Mediates release of antral gastrin
Secretin	Stimulates pancreatic bicarbonate and enzyme secretion, biliary secretion; inhibits gastric emptying
Vasoactive intestinal peptide (VIP)	Relaxation of the lower esophageal sphincter (LES), sphincter of Oddi, and anal sphincter; reflex vasodilation of the small intestine; descending relaxation of the peristaltic reflex; stimulation of intestinal chloride secretion
Gastric inhibitory peptide (GIP)	Enhances insulin release in the presence of hyperglycemia
Glucagon	Inhibits LES tone, intestinal motility, pancreatic secretion
Enteroglucagon	Stimulates intestinal growth; inhibits gastric acid secretion and gastric emptying
Motilin	Initiates interdigestive migrating motor complex
Somatostatin	Inhibits CCK, gastrin, secretin, PP, GIP, motilin, insulin, and glucagon release; directly inhibits salivary, gastric acid, small intestinal chloride, biliary, and pancreatic secretion
Pancreatic polypeptide (PP)	Inhibits pancreatic secretion, hepatic glucose production
Peptide YY (PYY)	Inhibits pancreatic secretion, gastric emptying, intestinal transit
Neuropeptide Y	Vasoconstrictor, stimulates food intake, inhibits colonic motility, alters circadian rhythms
Endogenous opioids	Inhibits intestinal motility and pain; enhances intestinal fluid and electrolyte absorption
Neurotensin	Inhibits peristalsis, gastric acid secretion, gastric emptying, intestinal blood flow, intestinal secretion; stimulates pancreatic secretion
Substance P	Stimulates intestinal smooth muscle contraction, pain perception
Calcitonin gene-related peptide	Sensory transmission of gut reflexes
Galanin	Inhibits VIP release from enteric nerves

contraction, pancreatic enzyme secretion and growth, and gastric emptying, while gastrin regulates gastric acid secretion and promotes fundic mucosal growth.[4] These peptides have also been implicated in the control of satiety, schizophrenia, and panic disorder, and in the regulation of peripheral neural (muscarinic) pathways.[4]

The receptors for these peptides have been defined based on their relative affinities for naturally-occurring hormones and hormone fragments and analogues. For example, the pharmacophoric domain of CCK for recognition by the CCK-A receptor represents the carboxyl-terminal heptapeptide-amide including a sulfated tyrosine, with smaller fragments possessing little activity.[5] While structure-activity studies utilizing a variety of amino acid substituted analogues and peptide fragments have allowed limited characterization of ligand-receptor interactions, the molecular basis for agonist binding has essentially remained a mystery.

Recently, the ability to clone cDNA's encoding receptors has broadened our perspective of receptor subtypes. While ion channel, guanylyl cyclase, cytokine, tyrosine kinase and serine-threonine kinase receptors have now been characterized, G protein-coupled receptors appear to be most important quantitatively and physiologically for the control of secretory and motor events along the gastrointestinal tract. These seven transmembrane proteins are typically glycosylated, contain extracellular cysteine residues for potential disulfide bond formation, and are thought to be arranged in a cylindrical configuration with residues critical for ligand binding potentially residing in both extracellular and transmembrane domains. Following agonist binding, the receptor couples to a guanine nucleotide-binding protein (G protein), which leads to the activation of cascades that may result in intracellular lipid hydrolysis, Ca^{2+} release, cAMP generation, and tyrosine kinase activation. These events are known to regulate such cellular events as vesicular transport and secretion, transcription, and growth. Desensitization, reduced cellular response to agonist stimulation, is generally felt to be regulated through receptor phosphorylation events.[6]

Although structure-activity studies utilizing a variety of amino acid substituted analogues and peptide fragments allowed limited characterization of ligand-receptor interactions, the detailed knowledge of G protein-coupled receptor structure and function has been obtainable only through the techniques of molecular biology. Indeed, a basic understanding of molecular biology is now almost necessary to study the pharmacology of gastrointestinal hormone receptors, and to read relevant literature.

FROM GENE TO PROTEIN: DNA, RNA, AND AMINO ACIDS

Any discussion of techniques in molecular biology presumes a basic knowledge of protein biochemistry. Since the description of the structure of DNA by Watson and Crick in 1953,[7] our understanding of the steps involved in protein synthesis has expanded exponentially. The nucleic acids, enzymes, and pathways leading from genomic DNA to mature protein have formed the basis for many techniques in molecular biology. Prior to discussing molecular methods in gastrointestinal pharmacology, a review of the intracellular events involved in protein biosynthesis is therefore in order.

Genomic DNA, made up of two strands of deoxyribonucleic acids linked by a sugar-phosphate backbone, forms the blueprint for life. The ability of purines, adenine and guanine, to form hydrogen bonds with pyrimidines, thymine and cytosine, results in the noncovalent bonding of complementary strands with the formation of a double helix. These double stranded pieces of DNA form chromosomes, each encoding hundreds (or even thousands) of proteins. While certain regions of this blueprint contain sequences that encode proteins (exons), other regions do not (introns).[8] DNA also contains sequences which have a regulatory role in transcription.[9]

Once transcription is activated, RNA polymerases catalyze the synthesis of a strand of RNA complementary to regions in genomic DNA encoding a protein.[10] This RNA strand consists of the ribonucleic acids adenine, guanine, uracil, and cytosine, and is termed messenger RNA (mRNA). This mRNA is processed by splicing out the introns and it is transported out of the nucleus, where it can interact with rough endoplasmic reticulum or free ribosomes (dependent on whether it encodes a membrane protein, protein for export, or a soluble protein).

There, as the mRNA strand is fed through the ribosomes, triplets of transfer RNA (tRNA), or anti-codons, linked to specific amino acids are matched sequentially to complementary triplets, codons, in the mRNA strand.[11] These amino acids are linked sequentially by amide bonds to form a protein molecule. Following post-translational events such as acylation, glycosylation, and folding, the tertiary molecule is either utilized within the cell or transported in vesicles to the cell surface, where it may become part of the plasmalemma or may be secreted.

Based on this background, a number of innovative investigators have developed techniques allowing the sequencing, replication, and manipulation of DNA fragments. The remainder of this chapter will explore these molecular methods and their implications for gastrointestinal pharmacology.

MOLECULAR CLONING: FIRST THINGS FIRST

BASIC CONCEPTS AND TERMINOLOGY, AN HISTORICAL PERSPECTIVE

While the earliest work in molecular biology focused on the identification of factors regulating transcription, the inability to reproducibly replicate and manipulate DNA fragments provided a barrier to subsequent work. Finally, in the mid-1960s, Robert Holley and his associates at Cornell University sequenced the yeast alanine tRNA molecule utilizing enzymes that cut the tRNA chains reproducibly into smaller and smaller fragments.[12] In 1976, Walter Fier's laboratory reported the complete sequence of the RNA chromosome of the RNA phage MS2, describing the exact codons specifying amino acids as well as the translation terminators in these genes.[13] Subsequently, numerous enzymes that reproducibly cleave at specific sites in nucleotide sequences, termed restriction endonucleases, were utilized to digest fragments of DNA creating smaller fragments of specific sizes.[14] Following electrophoresis, a process utilizing an electrical field to move DNA molecules through porous agarose gels, ethidium bromide staining, and illumination with ultraviolet (UV) light, a specific pattern or restriction map of these smaller fragments could be visualized.

These DNA fragments were sequenced directly with a variety of techniques, the most commonly used method described by Sanger in 1977.[15] This utilized DNA polymerase, radiolabeled deoxynucleoside triphosphates (dNTP's) and chain termination by $2',3'-$dideoxynucleoside triphosphates (ddNTP's), followed by electrophoresis on a denaturing polyacrylamide gel, and autoradiography. The chemical synthesis of oligonucleotides followed soon afterwards.

Following cleavage of DNA with certain restriction endonucleases, it was recognized that smaller double-stranded DNA fragments with single stranded overhangs, or "sticky" ends, that could be annealed with a DNA ligase were generated.[16] The concurrent identification of plasmids, circular fragments of DNA containing a large number of unusual restriction sites as well as promoter sequences, allowed the insertion of these DNA fragments into these "vectors" and the production of large amounts of the sequence of interest.

Since the first experiments describing this technique by Herbert Boyer and Stanley Cohen in 1973 utilizing the *E. coli* plasmid pSC101,[17] a number of prokaryotic and eukaryotic plasmids and phages, essentially protein coated plasmids, have been described. Through disruption of the cell membrane (plasmids), or binding of their protein coat to the cell membrane (phages), these vectors containing DNA inserts could be introduced into their host cell (transformation), with the resulting replication (cloning) of plasmids and/or phages, and recombinant protein expression. An essential feature of these molecules is their organization into transcriptional regulation domains, a polylinker domain containing multiple unique restriction endonuclease sites in order to facilitate ligation of digested DNA fragments, and domains conferring antibiotic resistance and color selectivity allowing the selection for and identification of bacteria or eukaryotic cells containing these vectors. These are the concepts and techniques that facilitated the transformation of molecular biology into a commonplace tool.

Later, in the mid-1980s, Kary Mullis further revolutionized molecular genetics through the description of the polymerase chain reaction technique (PCR).[18] This method utilizes oligonucleotide primers which are complementary to known sequences in combination with DNA and the DNA polymerase of Thermus aquaticus (Taq DNA polymerase—a thermostable enzyme) which are used through repeated cycles of annealing, extension, and heating to separate strands of DNA to generate millions of copies of a specific DNA fragment.

The first step is mixture of a predetermined cocktail containing either isolated RNA, with subsequent generation of a complementary strand of DNA (cDNA) using Reverse transcriptase, or double-stranded DNA as a template; oligonucleotides (primers) complementary to both the coding (sense) and anti-coding (anti-sense) strands of the double-stranded molecule; Taq DNA polymerase; magnesium as a cofactor; equal amounts of dATP, dTTP, dGTP, and dCTP; and a buffer to maintain pH. This is followed by denaturation of the double-stranded template into single strands by heating to 94°C, cooling to allow annealing of the oligonucleotide primers to their complementary segments, and heating to 72°C allowing chain extension. The specificity (stringency) of the match between primer and template is determined by both the annealing temperature and the magnesium concentration. This thermal cycle is repeated with a theoretical doubling of the template pool at each stage. The products of this reaction are then separated by agarose gel electrophoresis.

This powerful technique allows the amplification of millions of copies of specific DNA fragments from a mixed pool of RNA or DNA. While this provides a method of generating bulk quantities of DNA fragments, a certain amount of caution must be taken given the infidelity, or misincorporation rate, of Taq DNA polymerase, at approximately one per ten thousand nucleotides. More recently, thermostable DNA polymerases with lower rates of misincorporation have become available.

METHODS OF CLONING PEPTIDE HORMONE AND RECEPTOR cDNA'S

Obviously, the cloning of high fidelity cDNA's encoding hormones and receptors became an important hurdle preceding the expression, characterization, and manipulation of these recombinant proteins. Features key to the cloning of these cDNA's included probe generation and isolation, obtaining a source of high fidelity DNA, and the development of techniques to screen this source for the DNA fragment(s) of interest and isolate them to sufficient purity to facilitate specific protein expression.

Probe Generation

The first step is to generate probes with adequate specificity to allow successful screening of DNA sources. These may be either oligonucleotides, PCR products, or ligands such as antibodies or peptides, depending on the information available and techniques used.

First, if accurate nucleotide sequence is available for the DNA fragment of interest, specific oligonucleotides may be synthesized and radiolabeled either during synthesis, or afterwards using phosphorylation or primer extension methods.[19] In addition, specific primers, in combination with RNA or DNA from a particular source, may be used in PCR[20] with labeling of the product of interest either during PCR utilizing limiting amounts of labeled dNTP,[21] or after PCR through nicking, phosphorylation, or primer extension. It is important at this point to note that even under optimal conditions, amplification of undesired products in the expected size range may occur. The identity of any PCR products should be confirmed with either nested PCR, or direct nucleotide sequencing.

In a second scenario, limited peptide sequence may be available for the protein of interest.[22] This provides sufficient information to synthesize a mixture of primers all of which could encode the peptide sequence of interest (remember that multiple codons may encode the same amino acid, the redundancy of the genetic code). These degenerate primers may then be used in mixed oligonucleotide primed amplification of cDNA (MOPAC).[22] In this case, degenerate primers are used with a cDNA source in PCR under varying conditions, the products in the expected size range ligated into vectors, transformed into cells, isolated, and sequenced. Once a sequence of interest is identified, probes can either be removed by restriction cleavage and labeled, or amplified by PCR and labeled. Of note, if a PCR product of adequate purity is obtained from these methods, PCR sequencing may be used to confirm the amplified sequence,[23] obviating the need for subcloning the product into a vector.

In a third scenario, only the peptide or nucleotide sequence for a related family member(s) is known.[22] Two tacts may be taken in this case. First, a nucleotide probe identical to a family member is generated, labeled, and utilized in low stringency screening. Secondly, degenerate primers based on conserved regions of peptide or nucleotide sequence within a hormone or receptor family may be used in a number of low stringency PCR techniques. Identification and labeling of the resulting sequences of interest would be identical here to that following MOPAC PCR.

Finally, if no peptide or nucleotide sequence is available for either the protein of interest or related family members, expression cloning can be utilized with an antibody or other ligand.[24] Expression cloning techniques have rapidly evolved into extremely powerful tools (discussed below).

Library Screening

Once a probe has been generated and labeled in sufficient quantity, it is used to screen an appropriate high-fidelity DNA source. The traditional source of high-fidelity DNA is a library. While both cDNA and genomic DNA libraries are available, the purpose of this chapter is to discuss recombinant protein expression and not gene regulation. While a number of the techniques discussed will be appropriate to both sources, we will restrict our discussion to cDNA libraries.

A library is a collection of cDNA's from a particular tissue or cell type which are ligated into a vector. Think of each different cDNA as a book on a library shelf, the total collection of books makes up the library. The challenge is making a good library that contains the whole book, or a full-length cDNA encoding the protein of interest.

When making a cDNA library,[25,26] one first identifies the tissue or cell type of interest. Total RNA may then be isolated from the selected source utilizing cellular disruption in a guanidinium isothiocyanate or guanidinium HCl solution followed by either serial phenol extractions and precipitations, single-step extraction and precipitation, CsCl gradient ultracentrifugation, or serial low ethanol precipitations.[27,28] In any case, mRNA is subsequently isolated from total cellular RNA based on its polyadenylation utilizing oligo-dT. Either oligo-dT or random primers are then used along with reverse transcriptase to generate a complementary strand of cDNA. This product must then be converted to double-stranded DNA with one method utilizing nicking of the RNA with RNase H followed by a fill-in reaction with DNA polymerase. The resulting blunted fragments of double-stranded DNA are then ligated on both ends to short fragments of DNA containing specific restriction sites, with subsequent restriction cleavage in order to generate sticky ends, and size-selection by gel electrophoresis in order to remove degraded fragments. These fragments are then ligated into a plasmid or phage precut with the appropriate restriction enzymes, the resulting library transformed into appropriate bacteria, grown-up in selective media, and stored in aliquots.

So we have a probe and a cDNA library, how do we find the cDNA or book of interest. The method depends on both the type of probe and library vector. If the probe is a labeled oligonucleotide or segment of labeled double-stranded DNA, plaque (phage) or colony (plasmid) screening are the methods of choice.[19,29] In these methods, aliquots of library transformed into bacteria are either plated out using a top-agar method with the production of phage plaques on the surface, or by spreading the bacteria over selective media with the formation of colonies. In either case, the density of plaques or colonies must be optimized to allow screening of a maximal number of library members while avoiding complete coalescence. The plaques or colonies of interest are then "lifted" onto nitrocellulose filters, the bacteriasplysed and proteins denatured in an alkaline solution, and the remaining DNA covalently bound to the nitrocellulose through baking in a vacuum desiccator or ultraviolet cross-linking. The resulting filters are then washed, pre-hybridized to salmon sperm DNA or its equivalent in order to reduce non-specific background signals, hybridized to denatured labeled probe, and washed at varying stringencies based on both the wash temperature and the sodium concentration of a sodium chloride/sodium citrate/0.1% SDS solution. The higher the temperature and the lower the sodium concentration, the higher the stringency or specificity of the screen.[20] When looking for exact nucleotide complementation, high stringency screening will eliminate false positives. When using a probe to identify related family members, screening at a lower stringency is necessary but also increases the number of false positives.

Putative positive plaques or colonies are identified by the relative intensity of the label signal compared to background, cored from the plate, replated at a lower density, and screened again in a similar fashion. Isolated positive colonies are then selected, and the vector containing the DNA insert of interest isolated and sequenced in order to confirm its identity. While these represent traditional methods of library screening that have been used to isolate a number of gastrointestinal hormone receptors, a number of innovative alternatives are also available and merit further discussion.

PCR Methods

Again, while some authors have advocated the use of primer specific and degenerate primer PCR in the amplification of full-length cDNA's from mRNA or from cDNA libraries, the low fidelity of Taq DNA polymerase makes this less definitive than higher fidelity techniques.[30] This limitation can be avoided by performing cycle sequencing of the PCR product,[23] rather than subcloning it and sequencing that. One variant of this technique utilizes oligonucleotide primers preceded by promoters for RNA transcription. The resulting radiolabeled RNA fragments are separated by gel electrophoresis, the sequence representing the average of the PCR product pool and not one specific clone. While this minimizes any contribution of misincorporation, errors occurring in early cycles may still dominate the pool, and the PCR product needs to be of sufficient purity to allow clean sequencing.

One PCR method that has proven useful in extending incomplete cDNA fragments to full-length clones was termed rapid amplification of cDNA ends (RACE) by Frohman and associates in 1988.[31] In this method, either end of a partial cDNA clone may be extended utilizing a combination of primers based on the known cDNA sequence and polyadenylation. The resulting products should then be sequenced by the cycle (PCR) method in order to minimize misincorporation error. Following restriction cleavage of both the original cDNA fragment and the PCR product, the resulting full-length cDNA clone should be sequenced to confirm the accuracy of the added sequence.

As discussed above, in the circumstance where no peptide or nucleotide sequence is available for either the protein of interest or related family members, alternate strategies for isolation of cDNA's from libraries must be used. The most commonly used methods in this setting are based on expression cloning. In this strategy, aliquots or pools of a library are transfected into prokaryotic or eukaryotic cells, the resulting protein expressed in high copy numbers, and the cells screened in order to identify putative positives within each pool. Once a potential positive is identified within a pool, the DNA is isolated from that pool by subselection through splitting into smaller pools, and rescreened. This process continues until a single clone containing the cDNA insert of interest is isolated for sequencing.

Commonly used screening techniques in expression cloning include radiolabeled peptide binding, ligand coupling to a solid support, fluorescent-activated cell sorting (FACS), and antibody recognition. The former was the method used to isolate the cDNA's encoding the gastrin[32] and secretin receptors.[33] In an analogous approach, RNA can be synthesized from an aliquot of a unidirectional cDNA library, injected into the oocytes of the African clawed toad Xenopus laevis, and the cells expressing the receptor of interest detected electro-physiologically or with luminescence.[34] This was the method used to isolate the bombesin receptor.[35] While these powerful techniques continue to be used in attempts to identify novel GI peptide hormone receptors, new techniques that overcome traditional limitations seem to be described on almost a monthly basis.

EXPRESSION OF RECOMBINANT PROTEINS

Once a cDNA with a full length open reading frame is isolated, the next step is to express the encoded protein for identity verification and further characterization. A variety of expression systems are available.[36] Expression can be facilitated in both prokaryotic (i.e. yeast and *E. coli*), and eukaryotic (i.e. monkey kidney (COS) and chinese hamster ovary (CHO)) cells.[37] Initial requirements for protein expression include a full length cDNA encoding the protein of interest, its orientation in the proper direction downstream from a promoter recognized by the cell line, and a plasmid containing regions conferring resistance to antibiotics or other agents allowing selection of transfected cells from the pool. In addition, the cell line selected should not contain the protein of interest prior to transfection. Once these criteria are met, the plasmids of interest are "transfected" into the chosen cell line, there may be selection based on plasmid-conferred resistance, and the cells are allowed to express protein for a fixed period of time. In some cases, such as in COS cells, expression of recombinant protein overwhelms the cellular machinery resulting in cell death within a matter of days (transient transfection). In others, such as in CHO cells, cell lines stably expressing recombinant protein may be enriched by subcloning or by techniques such as fluorescence-activated cell sorting (FACS). Viral systems, such as Vaccinia or Baculovirus, may be used when a particularly high-level of protein expression is required.[38] When expression is optimal, the recombinant protein may be characterized biochemically in intact cells or following isolation from cytosol or within membranes.

There are a number of possible problems with expression systems. First, there is no guarantee that the cell's ribosomal machinery will recognize the appropriate initiator codon in the chosen construct. Remember that initiation sites for translation are preferred based on the surrounding nucleotide sequence.[39] If the selected cell line prefers an initiation site other than that encoding the protein, a misread may occur impairing protein translation. Once this obstacle is overcome, one has to deal with differences in post-translational processing, which may alter the functional characteristics of the protein, or preclude expression in the plasmalemma altogether. Even if the protein is appropriately expressed, overexpression of protein may overwhelm limited numbers of important components such as G proteins.[40] The host cell may also have inadequate numbers of other signal-transduction components leading to an impaired ability to measure traditionally-activated signal cascades, or the detection of spurious activation of cascades not normally activated by the protein. The level of recombinant protein expressed in stable cell lines may diminish with time, especially if its presence leads to counter-selection. Finally, effects observed in the selected cell line may not extrapolate to the level of the tissue or whole organism.

While these represent potentially serious limitations of expression systems, in almost all cases they can be overcome. Changes in the nucleotide sequence at the 5' end of the cDNA can create a more favorable milieu for the initiator codon. Characterization of the glycosylation and acylation state of the expressed protein will confirm similarities and differences with native protein. Cell lines with inadequate numbers of G proteins may be transfected with appropriate cDNA's and selected prior to transfection with receptor cDNA.[41,42] Similar techniques may be used to overcome deficiencies in other components of signal cascades. Stable cell lines must be rechecked periodically in order to ensure adequate expression of recombinant protein. As always, any effects seen in cultured cells must be extended to isolated native cell or whole organ models in order to confirm their validity. This may present a difficult task in and of itself. Obviously, the ability to overcome these limitations is critical for the successful expression of structurally-intact, functional recombinant proteins.

EXPLORING LIGAND-RECEPTOR BINDING AND FUNCTION

MOLECULAR METHODS OF STUDYING LIGAND-RECEPTOR BINDING

The ability to clone and successfully express structurally and functionally intact receptors has been pivotal in extending our understanding of the molecular basis of ligand-receptor interactions. Once a recombinant receptor is expressed, its structural and functional integrity are generally assessed with competition-binding studies and measurement of second messenger responses to agonist binding. This is straightforward when the identity of the receptor is known. What if a cDNA is isolated with open reading frame and subsequent hydrophobicity analysis predicting a seven transmembrane protein of unclear identity? This is not an uncommon problem and the encoded proteins are initially termed "orphan" receptors. The identity of an orphan receptor can be difficult to ascertain.[43] Comparison of the predicted amino acid sequence to other members of the G protein-coupled receptor branch of the phylogenetic tree may provide clues as to the family to which the receptor belongs. Following successful expression of the recombinant receptor, a variety of ligands can be used in competition-binding studies or functional assays. Techniques such as Northern blotting, RNase protection assays, and *in situ* hybridization may provide clues based on the cellular distribution of the mRNA encoding the predicted receptor. This later technique is probably the least helpful as our identification of the number of differing receptors in certain cells continues to grow. In many cases, the identity of the receptor becomes clear, in others, it remains a mystery.

Once the receptor's identity is confirmed, formal characterization of its binding domain may take place. Prior to the advent of molecular biology, traditional methods of characterizing receptor-binding domains included structure-activity studies using substituted or truncated peptide hormone analogues, as well as intrinsic or extrinsic "affinity" labeling with similar analogues, followed by protease digestion, separation of the resulting fragments by 2–dimensional electrophoresis or HPLC, and subsequent immunoblotting or sequencing of the separated labeled-peptide fragments. While these studies gave us clues about some residues or regions of receptors critical to ligand binding, molecular biology has allowed us to study these interactions in substantially greater detail at a molecular level.

One method that has proven extremely useful in binding domain characterization is the generation of chimeras and site-directed mutagenesis.[44] A chimera is, as the name implies, a hybrid of two receptor sequences. In essence, fragments of one receptor cDNA are substituted into analogous segments of another, the open reading frame remaining intact. Chimeras are most useful when cDNA's encoding two closely related receptors with differing binding affinities are available. The areas selected for substitution are generally based on important differences between the two predicted amino acid sequences in extracellular and transmembrane domains, as well as any clues provided by prior traditional biochemical studies. Generally, a number of chimeras are generated, expressed, and characterized through competition-binding studies. Based on these results, regions of interest are identified for point mutations. In this method, termed "site-directed mutagenesis," a single codon is altered resulting in a single amino acid change. A variety of techniques are currently available to facilitate site-directed mutagenesis.[45] These utilize a primer containing the desired point mutation to replicate the entire insert-containing double-stranded plasmid. Again, a number of constructs are generated containing varying numbers of point mutations, expressed, and characterized through competition-binding studies. This allows the identification of specific residues that are critical to high affinity binding. An important adjunct to these techniques is the use of peptide hormone analogues with modifications of key residues. This allows the confirmation of specific interactions between hormone and receptor binding domain residues. Applications to gastrointestinal pharmacology have already included the identification of the residue critical to receptor specific recognition of CCK antagonists,[46] as well as the residues important in binding of ligands to the histamine H_2 receptor.[47]

Computer simulations are potentially complementary to mutagenesis methods in specifically characterizing ligand-receptor interactions on a molecular level. Molecular dynamics simulations such as CHARMM utilize specific structural data on a protein in a computer model that calculates the energy forces acting on each atom within the molecule at any point in time. Sequential calculations predict the movement of atoms within the molecule until an energy-minimized or preferred configuration is attained. This allows us to speculate about the proximity of residues to one another within the molecule, and identify regions that would act as suitable binding domains. Once such domains have been identified, ligands can be introduced into the system and predictions of specific sites of ligand-receptor interactions can be made. Despite the potential of computer modeling in gastrointestinal pharmacology, its current effectiveness is quite limited.

Prior to successful computer modeling, detailed data on the structure of the receptor molecule in the lipid bilayer must be obtained. This has proven exceptionally difficult utilizing x-ray crystallographic methods. Attempts to obtain such data with nuclear magnetic resonance spectroscopy are also underway. In addition, developing a reliable theoretical model of a lipid bilayer containing the receptor for simulations has been difficult. These obstacles are being overcome by a small but growing number of investigators, the most successful currently characterizing rhodopsin.[48] Studies applying these methods to a number of gastrointestinal receptors and ligands are currently underway.

MOLECULAR METHODS OF STUDYING LIGAND-RECEPTOR FUNCTION

While a detailed understanding of molecular interactions between ligand and receptor is critical to streamlining the development of new pharmacologic agents, one must also define the receptor's physiologic role. A number of important molecular techniques have been developed specifically to address this issue.

Transgenic "knock-outs" were initially hailed as the ultimate method of determining the functional role of any protein.[49] In one method, a plasmid containing an altered sequence homologous to the endogenous gene fragment of interest is introduced into embryonic stem cells, the cells incorporating the plasmid DNA selected based on their plasmid-conferred resistance, with subsequent injection into blastocysts, and the eventual production of mice failing to express the protein of interest in various tissues. Other methods are available as well. Unfortunately, a true phenotype is not always obtained, and even when it is, the specific role the deleted receptor plays in the animals altered physiology is not always clear.[50] Indeed, examples of animals with altered phenotypes compensating for the deficiencies through other mechanisms have been described.[51] In addition, the genetic deletion may affect other proteins and pathways, further clouding the issue.

Selective inhibition of receptor translation through the use of antisense RNA strands is another method to assess receptor physiology on a cellular level.[52,53] In this method, the cDNA encoding the receptor of interest is ligated into a plasmid in an antisense direction with respect to the promotor region. One option is to incorporate this plasmid into a phage, with subsequent introduction of the plasmid into receptor-expressing cells, and binding of resultant antisense RNA to the mRNA of interest, preventing translation. Alterations in the cellular responses to ligand in the absence of receptor are then observed. Limitations of this technique include limited stability of the antisense RNA *in vivo,* difficult delivery, and non-specific effects.

A number of mutations of native receptors have been identified and may provide insights into their function.[54] This has led to the development of pharmaceutical agents specifically recognizing these mutants, and not unaltered native receptor (wild-type), potentially allowing for selective inhibition of mutant receptors.

Finally, as we eluded to earlier, cellular localization of mRNA encoding the receptor of interest may infer novel physiologic roles. Standard methods available include Northern blot hybridization, RNase protection assays, and *in situ* hybridization.[55] Each method is based on the hybridization of RNA or DNA probes to mRNA encoding the protein of interest. Northern blotting utilizes either total or messenger RNA separated by formaldehyde/agarose gel electrophoresis, with subsequent transfer to a nylon or nitrocellulose membrane, hybridization to the probe of interest, washing at high stringency, and autoradiography. While this is sufficient for mRNA localization on a tissue level, true cellular localization may require cell isolation to near purity. In RNase protection assays, antisense RNA probes are hybridized to the mRNA of interest, with subsequent RNase digestion of unhybridized single-stranded RNA, separation on a denaturing acrylamide gel, and autoradiography. It has the same limitations as Northern blotting but with a much higher sensitivity. *In situ* hybridization is an elegant method for demonstrating message within cells. In this method, tissue sections are fixed on slides, prehybridized with yeast RNA or its equivalent, hybridized to the antisense RNA probe of interest, washed at predetermined stringencies, and the signal detected either radiographically or colorimetrically. Following development of the signal, the slides are then counterstained, allowing visualization of signal over specific cells. While this technique works well in systems where large amounts of message are expressed, success rates in native receptor-bearing cells are variable. Obviously, the localization of mRNA does not confirm protein expression. In addition, detailed studies need to be performed on isolated cells in order to delineate the receptor's role in normal cellular physiology. Even so, identification of receptor mRNA in novel sources has allowed us to extend our knowledge of their roles in extraintestinal systems.

APPLICATIONS TO CLINICAL PHARMACOLOGY

AGONIST AND ANTAGONIST DESIGN

The utility of molecular cloning and expression in characterizing ligand-receptor interactions rests in our ability to apply the resultant tools and knowledge to improved drug design and screening methods. Techniques such as combinatorial library screening in combination with improved systems for the detection of ligand binding or receptor activation have substantially streamlined analogue development. In addition, a number of novel therapeutic approaches have been taken in attempts to utilize analogues, recombinant receptors, and their cDNA's.

In combinatorial library screening, one utilizes large collections of synthetic molecules in rapid bioassays attempting to identify the agent of choice from within that library.[56] Initially, a peptide library is generated containing all possible combinations of amino acids in a chain of specified length. Bioassays assessing ligand binding are performed on 20 subsets (pools) of this library, each pool containing peptides beginning with a different amino acid. Once a pool is identified as promising, 20 more pools all starting with that same amino acid but with different amino acids in position 2 are synthesized. Similar bioassays are performed and promising pools are extended to 20 more pools based on differing amino acids at position 3. This process is continued until specific peptides are identified with a high affinity for the receptor of interest. This process allows the screening of an enormous number of analogues in a short period of time. For example, in order to identify a heptapeptide, seven cycles screening 20 pools per cycle should be adequate.

Combinatorial peptide libraries may be used coupled to a solid support or free in solution.[56,57] Peptides may also be spatially arranged on chips using a photolithographic process with subsequent fluorescent detection of receptor binding; displayed on the surface of a phage with alternation of binding steps and growing up of the selected phage population; or specifically labeled with nucleotides, allowing identification of small amounts of bound peptide utilizing PCR methods. This technique may be applied not only to peptides, but oligonucleotides and other polymers as well. Indeed, it has been shown repeatedly that specific oligonucleotides (aptamers) may bind selectively and with high affinity to certain receptors.[58]

Obviously, most screening methods, including combinatorial methods, are dependant on the type of bioassays available and the speed with which they can be performed. The speed of performing selected bioassays has improved dramatically with the development of scintillation-proximity assays, novel β-counters, and automated filtration systems to enhance detection of radioligand binding. Recently, nonradioactive detection methods have grown in popularity. Stimulation of cultured cells expressing high numbers of recombinant receptor may result in quantitative changes in acidification rates as measured by microphysiometry.[59] Small changes in mass resulting from ligand binding to immobilized recombinant receptor, or visa versa, may be measured by surface plasmon resonance. Coupling of regulatory DNA elements to reporter genes allows the detection of transcriptional regulation in response to ligand binding to recombinant binding-protein.[60] These biochemical techniques, among others, are growing in popularity, substantially enhancing analogue screening.

Computer modeling strategies could potentially complement biochemical approaches to analogue development. Based on predicted interactions between known agonists and specific residues in receptor binding domains, analogue design may be streamlined by screening only those peptides or oligonucleotides potentially fulfilling those requirements. Once a promising ligand is identified, it could be included in a molecular dynamics simulation predicting its configuration and specific interactions within the binding domain. While the previously discussed limitations of molecular modeling approaches apply to these applications as well, this remains an exciting possible adjunct to traditional biochemical approaches.

THERAPEUTIC APPROACHES

Once an analogue with promising agonistic or antagonistic characteristics has been identified, appropriate animal and, if warranted, human trials testing its safety and efficacy must be undertaken. The phrase "many are called but few are chosen" certainly applies to this process. The leap from novel design and more efficient screening of analogues to clinical applications is a large one. While the cDNA's encoding a number of important gastrointestinal receptors have been, or are in the process of being cloned, attempts to study ligand-receptor interactions on a molecular level utilizing recombinant receptors are in their infancy. Although a number of traditionally designed agonists and antagonists to G protein-coupled receptors have either already impacted on clinically important gastrointestinal processes (e.g. H_2 antagonists, octreotide, cisapride), or are still in the process of being studied (e.g. CCK and gastrin receptor antagonists), eventual applications of novel agonists and antagonists resulting from more molecular approaches remain years in the offing.

Innovative methods of applying the tools of molecular biology to clinical therapy have expanded beyond the simple concept of receptor agonists and antagonists. Indeed, purified recombinant receptor, or fragments thereof, have been utilized in "receptor therapy" strategies where receptors can potentially act as scavengers for toxins, viruses, or excess signalling molecules, attenuating their physiologic impact. Gene therapy, a potentially powerful method of correcting genetic mutations (e.g. cystic fibrosis[61]), has been hailed as the wave of the future. In one method, the cDNA of interest is ligated into a retroviral vector;[62] introduced into the cell line of interest; the viral DNA containing domains conferring antibiotic resistance, transcriptional promotion, and the cDNA of interest incorporated into host genomic DNA; and transfected cells selected based on antibiotic resistance. The predominant cell types used have included fertilized eggs, hematopoietic cells, skin fibroblasts, and hepatocytes. Cells expressing wild-type receptor may then be introduced into the animal of interest, hopefully correcting the genetic "mistake". Alternate strategies more relevent to gene therapy in whole animals include the use of adenoviral vectors and liposomes.

While gene therapy provides hope for thousands of patients inflicted with genetic defects, enormous hurdles must be overcome before it becomes a reality at the bedside. Although transfection of isolated cells in culture is generally straightforward, introduction of adequate numbers of these cells into the host while insuring their viability and continued expression of wild-type protein in adequate numbers, has proven difficult. In some cases, prohibitive numbers of cells are required to correct defects in larger animals. In others, cellular viability is compromised, or the host suppresses expression of the desired protein. When transfection of whole animals is attempted, the effects of protein expression in cells not normally expressing that protein mast be assessed. If cell selectivity is achieved through the use of monoclonal antibodies or other cell specific markers, adequate protein expression must occur, and viral replication must be kept in-check while minimizing the immune response. In short, gene therapy holds exciting promise with enormous but not insurmountable obstacles.

FUTURE DIRECTIONS

In this chapter, we have reviewed the concepts of molecular biology, the methods available to generate probes and clone cDNA's, and the hurdles to be overcome in successful protein expression. We have also discussed the techniques available to study ligand-receptor interactions on a molecular level, and possible applications of the resultant knowledge and tools to the pharmacotherapy of certain gastrointestinal disease states.

It is safe to say that while molecular cloning, mutagenic, cellular localization, and computer modeling strategies have and/or will provide important insights into ligand and receptor structure and function, application of this knowledge at the bedside is still in the distance. Novel agonists and antagonists will require extensive study in animal models prior to their application to humans. Receptor therapy, while intriguing, has a limited number of potential applications, and has been used sparingly. Gene therapy offers the greatest potential benefit in disease states due to genetic mutations, but substantial hurdles must be overcome, and broad clinical applications are still years down the road. The delay from cloning to pharmacotherapy is an expected one, and in no way should deter one from pursuing molecular approaches to solving clinical problems. Indeed, the future of gastrointestinal pharmacology depends on present and future molecular methods.

REFERENCES

1. **Bayliss, W. M., Starling, E. H.,** On the causation of the so-called "peripheral reflex secretion" of the pancreas, *Proc. R. Soc. Lond. [Biol],* 69, 352, 1902.
2. **Miller, L. J.,** A historical perspective of gastrointestinal endocrinology—The new age of molecular receptorology, *Gastroenterology,* 102, 2168, 1992.
3. **Gregory, H., Hardy, P. M., Jones, D. S., Kenner, G. W., Sheppard, R. C.,** The antral hormone gastrin. Structure of gastrin, *Nature,* 204, 931, 1964.
4. **Mutt, V.,** Cholecystokinin: isolation, structure, and functions, *Gastrointestinal hormones,* Glass, G. B. J., Ed., Raven Press, New York, 1980, p169.
5. **Ondetti, M. A., Rubin, B., Engel, S. L., Pluscec, J., Sheehan, J. T.,** Cholecystokinin-pancreozymin. Recent developments, *Am. J. Dig. Dis.,* 15, 149, 1970.

6. **Lefkowitz, R. J., Cotecchia, S., Kjelsberg, M. A., Pitcher, J., Koch, W. J., Inglese, J., Caron, M. G.,** Adrenergic receptors: recent insights into their mechanism of activation and desensitization, *Adv. Second Messenger Phosphoprotein Res.,* 28, 1, 1993.

7. **Watson, J. D., Crick, F. H. C.,** Molecular structure of nucleic acids: a structure for deoxyribose nucleic acid, *Nature,* 171, 737, 1953.

8. **Chambon, P.,** Split genes, *Sci. Am.,* 244, 60, 1981.

9. **Jacob, F., Monod, J.,** Genetic regulatory mechanisms in the synthesis of proteins, *J. Mol. Biol.,* 3, 318, 1961.

10. **Hurwitz, J., Bresler, A., Diringer, R.,** The enzymatic incorporation of ribonucleotides into polyribonucleotides and the effect of DNA, *Biochem. Biophys. Res. Commun.,* 3, 15, 1960.

11. **Crick, F. H. C.,** On protein synthesis. Biological replication of macromolecules, *Symp. Soc. Exp. Biol.,* 12, 138, 1958.

12. **Holley, R. W.,** The nucleotide sequence of a nucleic acid, *Sci. Am.,* 214, 30, 1966.

13. **Fiers, W., Contreras, R., Duerinck, F., Haegeman, G., Iserentant, D., Merregaert, J., MinJou, W., Molemans, F., Raeymaekers, A., Berghe, V., Volckaert, G., Ysebaert, M.,** Complete nucleotide sequence of bacteriophage MS2 RNA: primary and secondary structure of replicase gene, *Nature,* 260, 500, 1976.

14. **Roberts, R. J.,** Restriction and modification enzymes and their recognition sequences, *Nucleic Acids Res.,* 11, r135, 1983.

15. **Sanger, F., Nicklen, S., Coulson, A. R.,** DNA sequencing with chain-terminating inhibitors, *Proc. Natl. Acad. Sci. USA,* 74, 5463, 1977.

16. **Mertz, J. E., Davis, R. W.,** Cleavage of DNA by RI restriction endonuclease generates cohesive ends, *Proc. Natl. Acad. Sci., USA,* 69, 3370, 1972.

17. **Cohen, S., Chang, A., Boyer, H., Helling, R.,** Construction of biologically functional bacterial plasmids *in vitro, Proc. Natl. Acad. Sci., USA,* 70, 3240, 1973.

18. **Mullis, K. B.,** The unusual origin of the polymerase chain reaction, *Sci. Am.,* 262, 56, 1990.

19. **Grunstein, M., Hogness, D. S.,** Colony hybridization: a method for the isolation of cloned DNAs that contain a specific gene, *Proc. Natl. Acad. Sci., USA,* 72, 3961, 1975.

20. **Lathe, J.,** Synthetic oligonucleotide probes deduced from amino acid sequence data: theoretical and practical considerations, *J. Mol. Biol.,* 183, 1, 1985.

21. **Schowalter, D. B., Sommer, S. S.,** The generation of radiolabeled DNA and RNA probes with polymerase chain reaction, *Anal. Biochem.,* 177, 90, 1989.

22. **Hanks, S.,** Homology probing: identification of cDNA clones encoding members of the protein-serine kinase family, *Proc. Natl. Acad. Sci. USA,* 84, 388, 1987.

23. **Scharf, S. J., Horn, G. T., Erlich, H. A.,** Direct cloning and sequence analysis of enzymatically amplified genomic sequences, *Science,* 233, 1076, 1988.

24. **D'Andrea, A. D., Lodish, H. F., Wong, G. C.,** Expression cloning of the murine erythropoietin receptor, *Cell,* 57, 277, 1989.

25. **Okayama, H., Berg, P.,** High-efficiency cloning of full length cDNA, *Mol. Cell Biol.,* 2, 161, 1982.

26. **Gubler, U., Hoffman, B. J.,** A simple and very effective method for generating cDNA libraries, *Gene,* 25, 263, 1983.

27. **Chomczynski, P., Sacchi, N.,** Single-step method of RNA isolation by acid guanidinium thiocyanate-phenol-chloroform extraction, *Anal. Biochem.,* 162, 156, 1987.

28. **Han, J. H., Stratowa, C., Rutter, W. J.,** Isolation of full-length putative rat lysophospholipase cDNA using methods for mRNA isolation and cDNA cloning, *Biochemistry,* 26, 1617, 1987.

29. **Benton, W. D., Davis, R. W.,** Screening lambda-gt recombinant clones by hybridization to single plaques *in situ, Science,* 196, 180, 1977.

30. **Keohavong, P., Thilly, W. G.,** Fidelity of DNA polymerases in DNA amplification, *Proc. Natl. Acad. Sci. USA,* 86, 9253, 1989.

31. **Frohman, M. A., Dush, M. K., Martin, G. R.,** Rapid production of full-length cDNAs from rare transcripts: amplification using a single gene-specific oligonucleotide primer, *Proc. Natl. Acad. Sci. USA,* 85, 8998, 1988.

32. **Kopin, A. S., Lee, Y. M., McBride, E. W., Miller, L. J., Lu, M., Lin, H. Y., Kolakowski, L. F., Beinborn, M.,** Expression cloning and characterization of the canine parietal cell gastrin receptor, *Proc. Natl. Acad. Sci. U. S. A.,* 89, 3605, 1992.

33. **Ishihara, T., Nakamura, S., Kaziro, Y., Takahashi, T., Takahashi, K., Nagata, S.,** Molecular cloning and expression of a cDNA encoding the secretin receptor, *EMBO J.,* 10, 1635, 1991.

34. **Giladi, E., Spindel, E. R.,** Simple luminometric assay to detect phosphoinositol-linked receptor expression in Xenopus oocytes, *BioTech.,* 10, 744, 1991.

35. **Spindel, E. R., Giladi, E., Brehm, P., Goodman, R. H., Segerson, T. P.,** Cloning and functional characterization of a complementary DNA encoding the murine fibroblast bombesin/gastrin-releasing peptide receptor, *Mol. Endocrinol.,* 4, 1956, 1990.

36. **Moss, B., Elroy-Stein, O., Mizukami, T., Alexander, W. A., Fuerst, T. R.,** New mammalian expression vectors, *Nature,* 348, 91, 1990.

37. **Payette, P., Gossard, F., Whiteway, M., Dennis, M.,** Expression and pharmacological characterization of the human M1 muscarinic receptor in Saccharomyces cerevisiae, *FEBS Lett.,* 266, 21, 1990.

38. **Miller, L. K.,** Insect baculoviruses: powerful gene expression vectors, *BioEssays,* 11, 91, 1989.

39. **Shine, J., Dalgarno, L.,** The 3′–terminal sequence of Escherichia coli 16S ribosomal RNA: complementarity to nonsense triplets and ribosome binding sites, *Proc. Natl. Acad. Sci. USA,* 71, 1342, 1974.

40. **King, K., Dohlman, H. G., Thorner, J., Caron, M. G., Lefkowitz, R. J.,** Control of yeast mating signal transduction by a mammalian beta 2–adrenergic receptor and Gs alpha subunit, *Science,* 250, 121, 1990.

41. **Felgner, P. L., Gadek, T. R., Holm, M., Roman, R., Chan, H. M., Wenz, M., Northrop, J. P., Ringold, G. M., Danielson, M.,** Lipofection: a highly efficient, lipid-mediated DNA-transfection procedure, *Proc. Natl. Acad. Sci. USA,* 84, 7413, 1987.

42. **Shigekawa, K., Dower, W. J.,** Electroporation of eukaryotes and prokaryotes: a general approach to the introduction of macromolecules into cells, *BioTech.,* 6, 742, 1988.

43. **Libert, F., Schiffmann, S. N., Lefort, A., Parmentier, M., Gerard, C., Dumont, J. E., Vanderhaeghen, J. J., Vassart, G.,** The orphan receptor cDNA RDC7 encodes an A1 adenosine receptor, *EMBO J.,* 10, 1677, 1991.

44. **Zoller, M. J.,** New molecular biological methods for protein engineering, *Curr. Opin. Struct. Biol.,* 1, 605, 1991.

45. **Deng, W. P., Nickoloff, J. A.,** Site-directed mutagenesis of virtually any plasmid by eliminating a unique site, *Anal. Biochem.,* 200, 81, 1992.

46. **Beinborn, M., Lee, Y. -M., McBride, E. W., Quinn, S. M., Kopin, A. S.,** A single amino acid of the cholecystokinin-B/gastrin receptor determines specificity for non-peptide antagonists, *Nature,* 362, 348, 1993.

47. **Gantz, I., Delvalle, J., Wang, L., Tashiro, T., Munzert, G., Guo, Y. J., Konda, Y., Yamada, T.,** Molecular basis for the interaction of histamine with the histamine H2 receptor, *J. Biol. Chem.,* 267, 20840, 1992.

48. **Khorana, H. G.,** Rhodopsin, photoreceptor of the rod cell. An emerging pattern for structure and function, *J. Biol. Chem.,* 267, 1, 1992.

49. **Jaenisch, R.,** Transgenic animals, *Science,* 240, 1468, 1989.

50. **Li, E., Sucov, H. M., Lee, K. F., Evans, R. M., Jaenisch, R.,** Normal development and growth of mice carrying a targeted disruption of the alpha1 retinoic acid receptor gene, *Proc. Natl. Acad. Sci. USA,* 90, 1590, 1993.

51. **Erickson, H. P.,** Gene knockouts of c-src, transforming growth factor beta1, and tenascin suggest superfluous, nonfunctional expression of proteins, *J. Cell Biol.,* 120, 1079, 1993.

52. **Wahlestedt, C., Pich, E. M., Koob, G. F., Yee, F., Heilig, M.,** Modulation of anxiety and neuropeptide Y–Y1 receptors by antisense oligodeoxynucleotides, *Science,* 259, 528, 1993.

53. **Weintraub, H. M.,** Antisense RNA and DNA, *Sci. Am.,* 262, 40, 1990.

54. **Strader, C. D., Gaffney, T., Sugg, E. E., Candelore, M. R., Keys, R., Patchett, A. A., Dixon, R. A. F.,** Allele-specific activation of genetically engineered receptors, *J. Biol. Chem.,* 266, 5, 1991.

55. **Alwine, J. C., Kemp, D. J., Stark, G. R.,** Method for the detection of specific RNAs in agarose gels by transfer to diazobenzyloxymethyl-paper and by hybridization with DNA probes, *Proc. Natl. Acad. Sci. USA,* 74, 5350, 1977.

56. **Houghten, R. A.,** Peptide libraries: criteria and trends, *Trends Genet.,* 9, 235, 1993.

57. **Houghten, R. A., Pinilla, C., Blondelle, S. E., Appel, J. R., Dooley, C. T., Cuervo, J. H.,** Generation and use of synthetic peptide combinatorial libraries for basic research and drug discovery, *Nature,* 354, 84, 1991.

58. **Bock, L. C., Griffin, L. C., Latham, J. A., Vermaas, E. H., Toole, J. J.,** Selection of single-stranded DNA molecules that bind and inhibit human thrombin, *Nature,* 355, 564, 1992.

59. **Owicki, J. C., Parce, J. W., Kersco, K. M., Sigal, G. B., Muir, V. C., Venter, J. C., Fraser, C. M., McConnell, H. M.,** Continuous monitoring of receptor-mediated changes in the metabolic rates of living cells, *Proc. Natl. Acad. Sci. USA,* 87, 4007, 1990.

60. **Peterson, M. G., Baichwal, V. R.,** Transcription factor based therapeutics: drugs of the future?, *Trends Biotechnol.,* 11, 11, 1993.

61. **Rich, D. P., Anderson, M. P., Gregory, R. J., Cheng, S. H., Paul, S., Jefferson, D. M., McCann, J. D., Klinger, K. W., Smith, A. E., Welsh, M. J.,** Expression of cystic fibrosis transmembrane conductance regulator corrects defective chloride channel regulation in cystic fibrosis airway epithelial cells, *Nature,* 347, 358, 1990.

62. **Eglitis, M. A., Anderson, W. F.,** Retroviral vectors for introduction of genes into mammalian cells, *BioTech.,* 6, 608, 1988.

INDEX

Mannitol, 95
Manometry, 273–275, 292
  Dent Sleeve, 277–278
  perfused catheters, 277–281
Marker-dilution technique, 9–10
Mast cell hyperplasia, 401, 404
Mast cells, 401
  cell separation, 403
  heterogeneity, 401–403
  histamine, 402
  human intestinal mucosal, 401
  tumor necrosis factor alpha, 402
Mastocytosis, 404
MC
  See Mast cells
McN-A-343, 290
M-current, 242
Meal, 40
Mean transit time, 169
Mebumal, 44
Mechanical activity, 175–176
Meissner's plexus, 85
Membrane depolarization, 192
Membrane potential, 117, 237, 287
Membrane resistance, 254–255
Mercury strain gages, 177–178
Mesenteric vascular bed, 127
Messenger RNA, 421
  reverse transcription, 153
Metabolic inhibitors, 107
Metabolism
  within the lumen, 88
Methacrylate, 173
[Methionin]enkephalin, 233
Methoxyflurane, 74
Methylene blue, 131
4-methylhistamine, 22
Microdialysis, 307
Microelectrode recordings, 251
Microelectrodes, 29
  distension-evoked synaptic potentials, 260
  drup application, 260–262
  electrical stimulation, 260
  intracellular, 251
  membrane potential recordings, 259
  single electrode voltage clamp, 259–260
  types, 251
Microinjection, 52
  into the nuclei, 303–304
    microintophoretic technique, 303
    volumes, 308
Microintophoretic technique, 308
Microminiature force transducer, 182–183
Microsurgical techniques, 252
Microtransducers, 278
Migrating motor complexes, 285–286, 298
  effect of yohimbine, 324
Migrating myoelectric complexes
  See Migrating motor complexes
Miniature intraluminal transducer, 183
Miniature pigs, 91

Mixed oligonucleotide primed amplification of cDNA, 427
MMC
  See Migrating motor complexes
M3-muscarinic cholinergic receptor, 156
Molecular cloning, 426
  electrophoresis, 427
  vectors, 426
Morphine, 92
  and acetylcholine, 375–376
  antitransit effect, 308
  inhibition of contractions, 375
  intracerebroventricular administration
    rats, 201
  tolerance, 377
Morphine tolerance
  and bethanechol, 383
  and dimethylphenylpiperazinium, 383
  dogs, 382
    effect of naloxone, 382
    myoelectric activity, 382
  and 5-hydroxytryptamine, 383
  rats, 381
Morphometric analysis
  smooth muscle cells, 284–285
Motilin, 232
Motilin receptors, 232
Motility
  choice of techniques, 163–164
  definition, 164
  gastrointestinal transit, 166
  general approach, 163–164
  historical perspective, 164–165
  parameters, 165
    intraluminal pressure, 165
    muscle contraction, 165
    transit, 165
    wall motion, 165
Motion sickness, 331
  adaptation, 345–346
  animal models, 347–351
    cats, 348–349
    dogs, 348
    monkeys, 349–350
    rats, 350–351
    suncus murinus, 351
  and central nervous system, 334
  conditioned taste aversion, 355
  Coriolis stimulation, 344–346
  drugs, 348
    promethazine, 348
    scopolamine, 348
  Graybiel Motion Sickness Symptom Scale, 344
  optokinetic stimulus, 340–342, 344, 345
  Slow Rotation Room, 345
  subject selection, 344–345
  symptoms, 334, 344
    dizziness, 334–335
    emetic reflex, 334
    headache, 334–335
    nystagmus, 334–335